Staying
· WELL ·
Your Complete Guide
to Disease Prevention

Also by Harvey B. Simon, M.D.

The Athlete Within:
A Personal Guide to Total Fitness
(with Steven R. Levisohn, M.D.)

Tennis Medic
(with Steven R. Levisohn, M.D.)

Staying
·WELL·
Your Complete Guide
to Disease Prevention

HARVEY B. SIMON, M.D.
Harvard Medical School

Illustrated by
Casserine Toussaint

HOUGHTON MIFFLIN COMPANY

Boston · New York · London
1992

For information about permission to reproduce selections from this
book, write to Permissions, Houghton Mifflin Company, 215 Park
Avenue South, New York, New York 10003.

Library of Congress Cataloging-in-Publication Data

Simon, Harvey B. (Harvey Bruce), date.
    Staying well : your complete guide to disease prevention / Har-
vey B. Simon ; illustrated by Casserine Toussaint.
      p.   cm.
    Includes bibliographical references and index.
    ISBN 0-395-53762-2
    1. Medicine, Popular. 2. Medicine, Preventive.   I. Title.
RC82.S565   1992
613 — dc20   92-6429
                                                    CIP

Printed in the United States of America

AGM 10 9 8 7 6 5 4 3 2 1

None of the information presented here is intended to substitute
for personal medical care and advice. Before you start the regimens presented in this book, consult your own physician to make
sure that they are suitable for you. If you have problems or questions related to your own health and fitness, you should direct
them to your physician.

for Rita

All things to one person

Every man desires to live long,
but no man would be old.
— Jonathan Swift

We have met the enemy, and he is us.
— Pogo (Walt Kelly)

Acknowledgments

S*taying Well* could never have been written without the help of many people. I have only myself to blame for the book's shortcomings, but there are many to thank for its merits. At the cost of omitting many sources of inspiration and assistance, I would like to express my particular gratitude:

To my patients, both for the privilege of caring for them during the past 25 years and for the questions and concerns that motivated me to write this book. In a real sense, this book speaks to them.

To my students, whose questions teach me so much and whose enthusiasm reinforces the excitement of learning new answers.

To the medical scientists, clinical investigators, and writers whose work has provided the information and insights on which this book is based.

To the physicians who have taught me with such patience, and to the many who teach me daily. Among them I am particularly grateful to my late father, Dr. Kona Simon, for his unmatched example of humanism, caring, and love; to Dr. Sheldon M. Wolff for showing me the elegance of laboratory science and clinical investigation; to Dr. Alexander Leaf for his many insights into nutrition and prevention; and to Dr. Morton M. Swartz, whose brilliance and humility have informed and inspired me through my professional life.

To the doctors, nurses, and secretaries who took such wonderful care of my patients each time I traded stethoscope for pencil. A special thanks to Dr. Richard Pingree; it's a wonder my patients have returned from his office to mine.

To Ruth Hapgood and her colleagues at Houghton Mifflin who have been so supportive, instructive, and helpful at each stage in my work.

To Robert Becker, who can decipher my hieroglyphics as well as any pharmacist, turning them on his word processor into a real manuscript.

Above all, to my family. To my daughter Ellie, a constant source of energy and joy. To my daughter Stephanie, a skilled journalist whose careful reading and warm support have contributed so much to my poor prose. And to my wife, Rita, who has done more for me than I can convey.

Contents

Preface   xiii

Part One: Health and Prevention

1   Prevention Is the Best Medicine   3

Part Two: Preventable Illnesses—and How to Prevent Them

2   Heart Disease   25
3   High Blood Pressure and Blood Vessel Diseases   54
4   Stroke and Other Neurological Disorders   74
5   Lung and Respiratory Tract Diseases   92
6   Diseases of the Stomach and Intestinal Tract   112
7   Diseases of the Liver and Gallbladder   133
8   Musculoskeletal Disorders   143
9   Disorders of the Breast and Reproductive Systems   158
10   Disorders of the Kidneys and Urinary Tract   182
11   Diseases of the Blood and Immune System   193
12   Metabolic Disorders: Diabetes and Obesity   204
13   Disorders of the Eyes and Ears   233
14   Disorders of the Teeth, Mouth, and Throat   246
15   Skin Disorders   261
16   Infectious Diseases   273
17   Accidents and Occupational Disorders   298
18   Substance Abuse: Tobacco, Alcohol, and Drugs   315

Part Three: A Comprehensive Program for Health Enhancement

19 Psychological Health   337
20 Nutritional Health   357
21 Exercise, Fitness, and Health   415
22 The Environment and Your Health   448
23 Preventive Medical Care   483
24 Keeping Up with New Developments in Prevention   503

    Index   515

Preface

In my 25 years of medical practice, I have seen hundreds — perhaps thousands — of people die needlessly. And I cannot begin to count the thousands of patients I have seen suffering through illnesses that could have been prevented. As much as I love the practice of medicine, I must confess that I'm growing a bit weary of patching up problems that never should have happened in the first place.

Nine of the ten leading causes of death in the United States are preventable. Chapter 1 lists our ten leading killers. Only one of ten, diabetes, is an inherited disease; all the others are affected much more by what we do than by who we are. And since diabetes itself can often be controlled by diet, weight loss, and exercise, it is fair to say that changes in the American lifestyle could help control all of the ten leading American "death styles."

Of course, no amount of prevention can eliminate disease, much less death. But preventive measures *can* prolong your life. And, at the same time, prevention *can* keep you more active, productive, and happy; there is more to health than just the absence of illness.

Prevention is simple. On virtually every day of my professional life patients have asked me for blood tests or x rays to detect diseases or for pills or shots to prevent illness. They are missing the point. In most cases disease prevention depends much more on the patient than on the doctor. Preventive *medicine* is only a small part of the solution. Prudent *living* is the best way to stay healthy.

In fact, disease prevention depends on a partnership between patients and doctors. Sad to say, up until now neither has been doing their part. Patients subject their bodies to an amazing array of abuses — and then ask for help. But doctors are guilty as well. American medicine, the best in the world, has focused chiefly on diagnoses and treatment. We have made wonderful progress indeed. But sophisticated — and expensive — technological advances would be much less necessary if doctors spent more time working with patients to prevent disease.

Heart disease is a good example. With the stroke of a pen I can arrange any number of fancy tests to detect heart trouble. With a simple prescription I can obtain powerful medications to reduce the symptoms of cardiac disease. And with a phone call I can schedule angiograms or arrange heart surgery for my patients. I am proud to be able to offer so much help. But I am also ashamed to need these tools. The major causes of heart disease should be known to every doctor and every patient: high cholesterol, high blood pressure, lack of exercise, smoking, stress, obesity, diabetes, and heredity. You cannot trade in your grandparents, but you can correct all the other causes of heart disease. Although I am delighted to prescribe medications that help my heart patients feel better, I ask myself with every prescription where they — and I — went wrong.

Prevention is not a fantasy. Heart attacks were almost unknown before the industrial revolution. Even today they are a rarity in agricultural societies. But I am not asking you to go back to the farm to protect your heart. Even in an industrial giant like Japan, the risk of heart disease is very much lower than in the United States.

We are making progress with heart disease in America; during the past 30 years the incidence of heart disease has declined by 44 percent. But heart disease is still our leading killer. Medical science must go on developing new ways to treat sick hearts. And even more important, we must all do much more to eliminate the bodily abuse and disuse that cause atherosclerosis.

An old joke tells of the patient who gave up eggs and steak to prevent a heart attack. It worked — but he died of cancer. It's not a very funny joke, but it's often used by people as an excuse for continued self-neglect. But, like so many jokes, it does have a grain of truth. To be truly effective, prevention cannot focus on just one problem, but must deal with the whole person and his or her whole life.

That's why I wrote *Staying Well*. The book is a comprehensive approach to preventing disease. Even so, the program is simple — and achievable. You can understand your body — how it works, what threatens its good function, and how to fight back. You can deal with your doctor; you should know what tests and treatments really will help keep you well. And, above all, you can change. You can get control of your health. And you will enjoy the longer, healthier life that you have earned.

Harvey B. Simon, M.D.
Stockbridge, Massachusetts

■ O N E ■

Health and
Prevention

▪ 1 ▪

Prevention Is
the Best Medicine

American medicine is the best in the world, but American health is not. Throughout the twentieth century America has been the clear leader in biomedical research and technology. Our scientists have made great discoveries in every area of medicine, ranging from basic research in molecular biology to applied science in biomedical engineering. Our medical schools are the world's best. American medical textbooks and journals are the most prestigious and widely read in every country where modern medicine is practiced. People come from all over the world to have puzzling illnesses diagnosed and to have difficult illnesses treated. The United States is the best place to have a cardiac bypass operation or a kidney transplant. Surely we can be proud of American medicine.

American society is willing to pay for superior medical research and technology. In 1991 we spent $756 billion on health care, over 12 percent of the gross national product. Government economists place the 1992 figure even higher, at $817 billion, more than 14 percent of the GNP. This means that we are paying more than $2,400 for the health care of each man, woman, and child in the United States each year — more than twice the average for other industrialized countries. Surely this is an impressive allocation of America's resources.

America is the world's leader in medical science and education — yet we rank only sixteenth among the nations in life expectancy. The United States spends more for health care than any other country — yet we rank twenty-fourth in infant mortality. We should be proud of American medicine and American wealth but ashamed of American health.

The reasons for this paradox are many and complex. The causes and remedies of the gap between our potential and our performance is beyond the scope of this book. But I would suggest that one explanation of this gap is our neglect of preventive medicine. And prevention, indeed, is our topic.

Dr. Woods Hutchinson wrote in the *Journal of the American Medical Association* that "our system's philosophy might be condensed in the motto 'millions for health care and not a penny for prevention.'" Dr. Hutchinson wrote these words in 1896! Things have changed in the century that followed: we have spent hundreds of billions for health care — but we still devote less than three cents of each health care dollar to prevention and education.

Why is preventive health care so woefully neglected? The responsibility is widely shared. Ultimately it lies with each individual: if you don't look after your health, who will? It's a sad fact that most people don't think about health until it's lost. But even though common sense can go a long way toward preserving health, few people can develop the expertise needed to make major decisions about health and medicine. I hope that you will have such expertise by the time you finish this book. But if we had proper leadership and education in prevention, this book would not have been necessary in the first place.

My profession certainly deserves its share of the blame for our neglect of prevention. Medical research is devoted principally to discovering the causes and treatment of disease — and so it should be. Once we understand causes, however, our mission should be to reverse those causes, to prevent damage before treatment is even necessary. Unfortunately, there is little profit in prevention; funding for research and compensation for clinical care make illness our major priority rather than health. Not surprisingly, the prestige and glamour in medicine are reserved for the molecular biologist and cardiac surgeon rather than the nutritionist or the epidemiologist. Nor are things likely to change in the near future. Among the 6,938 medical training programs in the United States, only 36 offer residencies in preventive medicine; this means that in 1991 we trained 82,902 physicians in specialties ranging from anesthesia to urology but only 202 in preventive medicine.

Medical research and training neglect health and prevention. Despite this neglect, we have learned a lot about prevention. But most doctors don't incorporate this knowledge into their practices. A majority of practitioners do not follow the guidelines for screening tests and preventive medicine that have been developed and published by their own professional organizations. Fewer than 20 percent of office visits deal with prevention and health education. And fewer than 10 percent of all physicians describe themselves as being very successful in promoting healthful behavior in their patients.

I acknowledge the prevention failings of my profession, but the blame does not rest solely with us. Unfortunately, there is plenty to go around. For one thing, even when we want to order a preventive test or treatment, we are often thwarted by financial restraints. Whether you know it or not, your insurance premiums, often staggeringly high, are buying you not health insurance but illness insurance. All insurance carriers will pay for diagnosis and treatment of illness, but most reject claims for procedures aimed at maintaining health. For example, until 1991 Medicare did not pay for the screening mammograms recommended by the American Cancer Society, nor did private insurance companies in 13 states; even now, Medicare will pay for mammograms only every two years instead of the annual exams that are recommended. Until 1991 Medicare did not even pay for the very inexpensive Pap smears that have helped reduce the mortality rate from cervical cancer by 75 percent since 1950. Similarly, neither Medicare nor private insurance will pay for cholesterol screening, routine blood pressure checks, tetanus or influenza shots, or health maintenance counseling. In a sense, the health insurance industry promotes risk rather than safety. Can you imagine an auto insurance company giving you a discount for a bad driving record? This terribly shortsighted policy is actually *costing* health carriers money because prevention is cheaper than treatment. Worse, it is costing you your health.

In the final analysis the reasons for our neglect of prevention extend far beyond the medical trinity of patient, physician, and payer to our society as a whole. Corporate America concentrates on the bottom line rather than the lifeline. Sadly, there seems to be more profit in fast convertibles than in air bags, in alcohol than in fruit juice, in tobacco than in clean air, in fast food than in whole grain. We may spend $817 billion annually for health care, but we also spend $65.6 billion for alcohol and $41.7 billion for tobacco.

Madison Avenue also contributes to America's passion for dangerous living. Have you ever seen an ad glamorizing eight hours of sleep or routine dental care? And the media do little to counter the barrage of subliminal urgings to overeating, overdrinking, promiscuity, and sloth. Corporate advertising revenues keep broadcasters on the air and newspapers in print. The tobacco industry alone spends $7 million *a day* on advertising! All too often journalistic principles vanish in the face of economic pressures, both overt and implied. In particular, information about the enormous health risks of tobacco, alcohol, and fast automobiles is suppressed or at least understated. Surely we can find a way to preserve our valued First Amendment guarantees of free speech while still providing the facts the public needs to choose a life-style that will protect health.

With all these problems, it's a wonder that prevention has any chance at all. But it does. To stay well, depend not on preventive *medicine* but on preventive *health*. The key is prudent living rather than medical technology. You can make the personal changes necessary to prevent illness and enhance the quality of life. And if enough of us act together, we can promote the social changes needed to make this world of ours a lot healthier for all of us.

How to proceed? In the next few pages let's explore the origins of disease and then the principles of prevention. In the chapters that follow, you'll be able to learn the practical details that will enable you to prevent illness so that you will live longer *and* live better.

■ What Determines Health?

Almost all of us are lucky enough to be born healthy, yet most of us will at some time fall ill. Society accepts disease as an inevitable part of the human condition; indeed, it is unrealistic to expect that we can avoid all ailments. But the diseases that cause *the majority* of disability and death in the United States today are far from inevitable; in fact they result from the self-inflicted problems of bodily abuse or disuse, or from exposure to environmental hazards. And they can be prevented.

What causes illness? Human health is limited by four factors:

1. genetics and human biology
2. personal behavior
3. environmental influences
4. health care

Of these, only the first is beyond our control. Our genes set limits for our physical and mental abilities, and in some cases our genes dictate disabilities. We can't trade in our grandparents, but in many cases (such as sickle cell anemia in blacks and Tay-Sachs disease in Jews) genetic testing and counseling can prevent our children from inheriting inborn diseases.

Exciting research in genetics will expand the list of inherited diseases that can be prevented by testing or treated by gene engineering. But even with these advances, human biology will ultimately limit longevity. It is up to each of us, however, to control our personal behavior, minimize exposure to environmental harm, and obtain optimal health care. With these interventions we can realize the full potential of human biology. The limits of that potential are unknown. Sir Richard Doll, the eminent epidemiologist at Radcliffe Infirmary at Oxford, doubts that prolongation of life to 100 years is achievable, but he predicts that an average life span of 90 years *is* attainable. Preventive health measures can make those 90 years vigorous and enjoyable. Prevention means more than eliminating disease; it means enhancing health and function.

Genetics and human biology set our limits, but it's up to each of us to push those limits and to prevent illness. For most of us health will depend not on who we are but on how we live. The body you have at 20 depends on your genes, but the body you have at 40, 60, or 80 is the body you deserve, the body that reflects your behavior.

Even the most optimistic of us must concede that the prevention of illness is complex. The *personal behaviors* necessary for remaining healthy include diet, exercise, automotive and industrial safety, safe sex, and stress control and avoiding abuse of tobacco, alcohol, and drugs. The *environmental hazards* that must be minimized include biological agents that cause infection, chemical exposures, radiation, and physical and climatic trauma. And *medical care* involves immunizations to prevent infection, screening tests to detect latent or early disease, and sometimes even preventive medications.

Is it realistic to think that we can prevent disease? Let's take a closer look at the origins of illness. Perhaps by reviewing the causes of disease we can rediscover the basic behavioral and environmental factors that are suited to our genetic material and will keep us healthy.

■ The Origins of Illness: Historical Perspectives

The human species, *Homo sapiens,* appeared on earth about 40,000 years ago. Even though it seems like a very long time ago, in evolutionary terms it's little more than a tick of the clock: it took about 1 billion years for evolution to produce humans. In view of this time scale, it's not surprising to learn that humanity's genetic material has changed very little in the past 40,000 years. In terms of our DNA we are still in the Stone Age. But if our genes have not changed, the world around us has changed enormously: the simple life of the hunter-gatherer has been altered immeasurably and would surely be unrecognizable to our Paleolithic progenitors.

This mismatch between our genes and our life-style is responsible for many of the diseases that afflict us today. We can't change our genes, but we can change our ways. Let's look at the origins of disease over the past 40,000 years to learn how we can live in the modern world without modern diseases.

How much do we know about the patterns of health and disease in human prehistory? Clearly there are enormous gaps in our knowledge. But we do have enough information to offer intelligent speculation about health and disease over the millennia. This information comes from three sources. First, paleontologists can study both fossils and mummies to discover information about nutrition, exercise, and trauma and to find traces of certain diseases. Second, anthropologists can study primitive population groups living in isolated areas of the world today. Finally, physicians and biologists can extrapolate from what we know about human biology and behavior. It may sound rather obscure, but many scientists have made enormous contributions to this field, including anthropologists and physicians such as Thomas McKeown, Mark Nathan Cohen, Melvin Konner, and S. Boyd Eaton.

The historical patterns of human health and disease can be divided into four basic eras, two of which are in the past, one in the present, and the fourth, I fear, in the future.

The Primitive Era: Diseases of Deprivation

Human life changed but little in the first 30,000 years of our species. Beginning about 40,000 years ago in the late Paleolithic era, people lived in small bands that roamed over modest areas. Human population was sparse: scant resources and low fertility limited people to a density of one per square mile. Social organization was simple, with most members of the group doing the same tasks. First and foremost among these tasks was the quest for food. There were no domesticated animals, and farming was unknown, so life depended entirely on wild resources. Stone Age people hunted and trapped game and fish and gathered wild fruits, tubers, nuts, and seeds. Because there was no way to store food, it was consumed as soon as it was available, resulting in periods of plenty and periods of scarcity.

The Stone Age diet was high in protein but very low in fat. Even though meat was a major source of protein and calories, wild game was lean. Dairy products were unknown, and carbohydrate intake was highly variable, but the primitive diet was very high in fiber and had plenty of vitamins, iron, and minerals — except for salt, which was scarce. Needless to say, primitive

humans got lots of exercise. Tobacco and alcohol were, of course, unknown, and motor vehicles were beyond the realm of fantasy.

Life span was short in the Paleolithic era and is short even in primitive
tribes leading a Stone Age existence today. The major causes of death were
trauma and exposure. Starvation was probably quite uncommon, and heart
disease, strokes, and many types of cancer were practically unknown. Measurements of people leading primitive lives today show spectacularly good
levels of blood pressure and cholesterol. Obesity and diabetes are rare,
and aerobic capacities and physical fitness are excellent. Contemporary
hunter-gatherers are also remarkably free from many of the "minor" ailments that afflict modern man, including hemorrhoids, hernias, appendicitis, varicose veins, gallstones, kidney stones, hearing loss, and dental
cavities.

The Agricultural Era: Diseases of Contagion

About 10,000 years ago life began to change. The main agent of change was
the development of agriculture. The introduction of farming and the domestication of animals seem simple enough, but the changes that resulted
were so profound that anthropologists describe them as a broad-spectrum
or Neolithic revolution.

With the introduction of farming, people became linked to cultivated
land and ceased to wander. Population centers began to appear and progressively increased in size, leading ultimately to the development of cities.
Until the rise of irrigated farming, about 6,000 years ago, the largest human
settlements were villages of perhaps 300 people; within just a few generations improved farming techniques led to the establishment of cities, some
with populations of 100,000.

As life grew complex, it became increasingly difficult for the individual
to be self-sufficient. No longer able to perform all the tasks needed for survival, people began to specialize and to become interdependent. With specialized tasks came social classes and hierarchies. It's not far-fetched, I
think, to speculate that psychological stress had its origins in these first
attempts at social organization that ultimately led to civilization as we
know it today, with all its blessings and blemishes.

Although it seems intuitively obvious that farming and domestication
of animals would lead to improved nutrition, this is probably not the case.
Cereals and tubers became the main vegetable foods, replacing wild fruits
and nuts. One of the earliest by-products of cultivated grain was beer, first
brewed from barley 10,000 years ago; the process of fermenting fruits into
wine began 5,000 years ago. Foods derived from animals changed just as
dramatically as domesticated animals and dairy products replaced wild
game. The result: a diet higher in fat and calories and lower in fiber. Because it became dependent on a few crops, the agricultural diet was also
less diversified than the hunter-gatherer diet; hence, nutritional deficiency
diseases began to appear.

Agricultural people learned to store food, helping to moderate the plenty-scarcity cycles of more primitive life. But with farming came dependence on climate, rainfall, and crop yields. Crops were also vulnerable to agricultural blights and pests. Coupled with a growing population, these problems produced new threats to health: malnutrition and starvation.

Man learned to use tools in the agricultural period, but physical labor was still the way of life, so exercise remained necessary for survival. Despite exercise, the increased intake of fat and calories resulted in increased body fat, which helps to explain the earlier onset of menstruation and the increased fertility rates of agricultural-era women. Human population grew steadily throughout the agricultural period, but growth depended on increased birth rates rather than declining death rates. In fact, the life expectancy of agricultural people did not improve over the longevity of the hunter-gatherer, remaining at about 30 years.

Agricultural-era people were able to overcome partially the major threats to life in the Stone Age — trauma and exposure. But life span did not increase in agricultural society because new diseases were acquired. Many factors conspired to produce the rise of infectious diseases. As human population density increased, people passed bacteria, viruses, and parasites to one another. The close proximity of domesticated animals allowed microbes from animals to infect people. Food storage led to food spoilage. The rise of population centers amplified the effects of poor hygiene and sanitation. The net result was the spread of infection. And as people began to explore, travel, and trade, they took infections with them. Terrible epidemics resulted when new germs reached populations that had no previous exposure and immunity. For example, the Mongols introduced plague to Europe, and the Europeans brought measles, mumps, and smallpox to the New World while carrying syphilis back with them on their return. But the chronic diseases that are the major killers in twentieth-century Western society remained as rare in the agricultural era as they were in the age of the hunter-gatherer.

The Industrial Era: Diseases of Abuse and Disuse

A dominant characteristic of human history is that the rate of change has accelerated progressively and dramatically. Hunter-gatherers appeared on earth about 40,000 years ago, and their way of life prevailed for about 30,000 years. Agricultural life began 10,000 years ago, and remained the human norm until the nineteenth century. Despite all the historical events and cultural developments that occurred during this era, life expectancy did not increase.

The industrial revolution produced spectacular changes in life — changes that continue even today. In the past 200 years we have created machines, harnessed the energy of nature, and have even succeeded in creating energy. The many changes that have followed from these spectacular achievements have altered immutably the basic patterns of human life. In the nineteenth century about 30 percent of all the energy used for industry and agriculture in the United States was derived from human physical labor; with industrialization this rapidly declined to less than 1 percent. No longer dependent on the work of their bodies for daily survival, people became dependent instead on their minds.

From the point of view of health, the triumph of human intellect has been a mixed blessing. The population bomb exploded, resulting in previously unthinkable densities of human population. Crowded cities with terrible sanitation and poor nutrition intensified the infectious diseases that were the main killers of the agricultural era. In fact, life expectancy did not improve at all until the late nineteenth century.

But early in the twentieth century health began to change. Improvements in sanitation and hygiene began to limit the spread of infection. Immunizations have become extremely effective means of preventing many infections, and antibiotics have dramatically improved survival from bacterial infections. With the control of infection and infant mortality, life expectancy has finally increased, more than doubling in the last 100 years. Only after millennia of human progress has life expectancy finally exceeded the biblical ideal of three score and ten years.

But even as the great contagions of the agricultural era have yielded to sanitation and medical science, a new class of diseases has appeared. Freed from starvation and exposure, from diseases of deficiency, we find our new wealth has made us vulnerable to diseases of excess. The major chronic diseases that account for 75 percent of deaths in the United States today are diseases of this century. They are often called diseases of civilization, but I dislike this term because it implies two things that are untrue: that our society is more "civilized" than earlier cultures, and that we would have to turn back our social system to prevent these diseases. These are often called diseases of affluence, but I dislike this term, too, for two reasons: it overlooks the fact that the poorest members of our society are the most vulnerable to many of these diseases, and it implies erroneously that we must abandon affluence to control disease. In my view the diseases of the modern industrial era can be captured best in another term: diseases of abuse and disuse.

Let us reflect briefly on why we are so vulnerable to heart disease, stroke, cancer, chronic lung disease, diabetes, and hypertension — diseases that were all but unknown in the primitive and agricultural eras. What has happened is this: humankind's Stone Age genetics have survived, but its life-style has not. We're now living in the fast lane, but our genes haven't kept up with our pace. Like the hunter-gatherers', our metabolism is designed to cope with the risk of starvation but not with today's hazardous overnutrition. We have not evolved the means to cope with high-fat, high-calorie, high-salt, low-fiber diets. We have no way of dealing adaptively with tobacco, alcohol, and drugs. There are neither substitutes for lost exercise nor antidotes to newfound stress. In a very literal sense, we are killing ourselves with progress.

We cannot speed up genetic adaptations to modern life, nor should we even aspire to adapt ourselves to unnecessary toxins. But we *can* remove the health hazards of the industrial era without undoing the magnificent benefits of the twentieth century's many triumphs. We can go back to the basics for our bodies while continuing onward with the progress of our minds.

This book will explain how we can prevent disease in the modern world while also leading a happier and more productive life. We have the means to achieve these goals here and now. But to preserve these benefits, we must also look ahead at the diseases that may threaten us in the next era.

The Technological Era: Diseases of Environmental Contamination

As we enter the twenty-first century, we confront increasing dangers from a new class of illness — environmental diseases. The health hazards of the primitive era — trauma and exposure — resulted in large part from Paleolithic peoples' inability to control the environment. In the agricultural era some measure of control was achieved, but poverty led to the rise of infectious diseases. The industrial era saw humans dominate their environment, but diseases of abuse and disuse have resulted from the consumption of our newfound wealth. And with the rise of technology in the twentieth century, we are faced with diseases caused by environmental hazards resulting from the production of wealth.

Environmental diseases are as old as the industrial revolution. But over the years industrial pollutants have progressively accumulated. Nuclear wastes and accidents increase the stakes by orders of magnitude. The pesticides that have increased food production more than thirtyfold have introduced new chemical hazards into the food chain. The incredible population explosion, which has increased human numbers from less than 1 billion to more than 5 billion in only ten generations, has produced enormous demands for energy and has generated enormous quantities of wastes. Collectively these influences are actually changing the environment itself, depleting the ozone layer and warming the globe.

It is no surprise that the external environment can affect our internal environment, that exposure to radiation, chemicals, and contaminants can cause disease. But when it comes to controlling the diseases of environmental origin, a new element is present: the need for collective action. To a great extent all of us can protect ourselves from the diseases of abuse and disuse through simple life-style changes. And it is true that we can reduce our exposure to some environmental hazards by exercising care at work and at home, by monitoring our water, food, and air whenever possible, and by manipulating our microenvironment to minimize risk. Yet many environmental hazards now occur with a subtlety that subverts personal surveillance and on a scale that precludes individual remedies. We will need to work together to prevent the new environmental diseases of the technological era that lies ahead. We will need the best efforts of physicists, chemists, and engineers to make the means of production safe. We will need the work of biologists to detect environmental hazards and of physicians to detect environmental diseases. We will need the help of educators and economists to turn the prospects of change into realities. Above all, we will need the political will to insist on the primacy of health as a long-term goal, even at the cost of short-term economic sacrifice.

The stakes are enormous. The diseases of earlier eras have caused suffering and premature death without reducing fertility or overall longevity. But the environmental diseases of the future have the potential to do both, ultimately threatening our species itself.

■ American Health: A Contemporary Crisis

Although I find these historical perspectives fascinating, I live not in the Paleolithic era but in the twentieth century, and I don't practice anthropology, I practice medicine. I believe, however, that we can learn from our past, and that these insights can serve us well both today and tomorrow. In fact, diseases from all four health eras — primitive, agricultural, industrial, and technological — are present in America today.

American Health during the Twentieth Century

Let's look at the changes in disease patterns that have occurred in our country during the present century. In 1900 the leading causes of death were pneumonia, influenza, and tuberculosis — infectious diseases promoted by crowded living conditions, poor sanitation, and undernutrition. During the twentieth century socioeconomic advances have improved living conditions, and medical science has developed antibiotics and vaccines that have helped control infections. Tuberculosis has become an uncommon cause of death, and pneumonia and influenza have dropped from first place to sixth, an improvement that is simultaneously an indictment of our health care system, since we have vaccines that could further control these infections if they were administered as recommended.

But as we have controlled diseases of poverty and contagion in mainstream America, we have simultaneously created a new epidemic. Diseases of disuse and abuse are now the leading cause of death, with heart disease, cancer, and stroke the top three. Life expectancy *has* improved during the twentieth century: a male born in 1900 had a life expectancy of 47 years, whereas a male born in 1990 has a life expectancy of 74 years. This gain of 27 years is dramatic, but it's actually less impressive than it seems. Most of the improvement is due to progress in reducing infant mortality caused by childhood illnesses and infections. An American who made it past these hazards to reach adulthood in 1900 lived almost as long as an adult in 1990; contemporary American adults have gained only four additional years of life over their ancestors of 100 years ago.

We've come to accept heart disease, cancer, stroke, and other contemporary killers as facts of life. The medical textbooks categorize these as "degenerative diseases," implying that people who live long enough will inevitably succumb to one of them. But history teaches us that these dis-

eases are *not* inevitable. Far from being an intrinsic part of the human condition, they are the products of civilization as we have created it, caused by
overnutrition, underexercise, overdrinking, voluntary and involuntary exposure to tobacco smoke and other toxins, and excessive stress. All of these
hazards can be avoided — and so can the "degenerative" diseases they
have given us. All in all, about 75 percent of deaths in America today are
premature, caused by self-administered bodily abuse and disuse, and fully
60 percent of these deaths could be significantly postponed, preventing
500,000 people from dying prematurely each year.

A close look at heart disease, the number one cause of death, should
prove the point. Heart attacks are so common that they have been accepted
by physicians and patients alike as an intrinsic part of human biology. But
the first heart attack in the United States was not reported in the American
medical literature until 1912. And our current epidemic of heart disease did
not really get started until the 1930s. Can it be a coincidence that the first
commercially rolled cigarettes were marketed a decade earlier?

The International Health Gap

Could it be that American genes, rather than the American habits, are responsible for the health gap? Not likely in a country as genetically diverse
as ours. But we can prove that life-style is the major factor by comparing
heart disease in Japan and America.

In Japan the risk of dying from a heart attack is only about one sixth as
high as the risk in the United States. You might argue that there is less heart
disease in Japan because there are more early deaths from other disease,
but in fact the current overall life expectancy in Japan (79 years) is four
years longer than in the United States (75 years). But as Japanese migrate
from their homeland to Hawaii, their diet and activity patterns change,
their blood cholesterol levels rise — and their heart attack risk increases.
And Japanese who live on the American mainland and have acquired the
American life-style have exactly the same heart attack risk as Americans
from other ethnic backgrounds. Nor is the disparity confined to heart disease; Japanese men have eleven times more prostate cancer and Japanese
women six times more breast cancer in Hawaii than in Japan. How sad that
America has a health deficit as well as a trade deficit!

The Burden of Preventable Illnesses

Preventable diseases place a staggering burden on American society.

We can measure this burden in terms of mortality. More than 60 percent
of all American deaths are premature. Of the 2 million deaths in the United
States each year, more than half are due to just nine diseases: heart disease,
stroke, diabetes, emphysema, lung cancer, breast cancer, cervical cancer,
colon and rectal cancer, and cirrhosis of the liver. These are all chronic
diseases; they have identifiable precursors that can be detected and treated
in early stages. More important, we understand causes of these diseases
and could actually *prevent* many of them if we made personal and social

changes early enough. In all, premature death costs American society 12 million person-years of productive life annually.

We can measure this burden in terms of morbidity, the sum of disability and suffering caused by disease. Again using cardiovascular disease as an example, we can see the enormous impact of preventable diseases: in 1980 alone cardiovascular disease accounted for 50 million days of hospitalization and 900 million days of disability (to say nothing of nearly 1 million deaths). During the same year tobacco abuse and overnutrition each led to more than 16 million days of hospitalization, high blood pressure to nearly 10 million, and alcohol to more than 3 million. In total, one third of all hospital stays could be eliminated by simple life-style changes. And prevention could have a similar impact on diseases that do not require hospitalization. All in all, we could — and should — be preventing more than one third of the acute disabilities and more than two thirds of the chronic disabilities that afflict Americans today.

We can measure the burden in economic terms as well. Medical care in America will consume more than $817 billion in 1992, and the cost is growing at a terrifying rate of more than 10 percent each year. We spend more than $1 billion on coronary angioplasties — billions that could be saved since we *can* prevent coronary artery disease. Even more staggering is the cost of smoking: $52 billion in direct health expenses and lost productivity, well over $200 for each American every year.

American industry pays about 25 percent of all medical costs. At $3,605 per worker, corporate America is now spending more on employee health care each year than it distributes in corporate profits. Ultimately, of course, those costs are passed on to the consumer; when you buy an American car, about $500 of the price goes to pay workers' medical bills. As a result, American industry is placed at a tremendous competitive disadvantage. Industry blames high medical charges, but costs could be cut dramatically by simple life-style changes. For example, a study conducted by the Control Data Corporation found that a 40-year-old employee who smokes, is overweight, does not exercise, and does not wear a seat belt costs his employer an average of $1,282 in medical bills annually — more than twice the $631 of another 40-year-old worker who simply avoids these four health hazards. Nor are these hazards unique to Control Data employees; throughout the country at least 25 percent of the population smokes, 30 percent are overweight, 40 percent do not use seat belts, and 60 percent are sedentary. How much money could we save if we invested in prevention, spending on health care instead of disease care, on preserving and enhancing wellness instead of patching up unnecessary illnesses?

Disparities in Health and Illness

These enormous burdens of illness, the burdens of mortality, morbidity, and money, are not distributed uniformly in our society.

Death and disability rates depend on geography: in Michigan, for example, the annual death rate from the nine major chronic diseases cited earlier is 58 percent higher than in Hawaii.

The burdens of illness are dependent on gender: the life expectancy for women is 79 years, for men only 74.

The toll of ill health varies, too, with race: white males live six years longer than nonwhite males, and white females four years longer than nonwhite females. Because the life expectancy of black Americans has *decreased* each year since 1988 while that of white Americans has increased, the gap is widening. Add poverty and inner-city life, and the disparities are shocking: a black man in Harlem, in New York City, is less likely to reach age 65 than a man in Matlab, Bangladesh.

There are, of course, many reasons for these disparities. Health habits such as smoking, diet, exercise, and drinking vary greatly. Exposure to pollutants and toxins is also a major variable. Differences in education, economics, and access to medical care play a role: 34 million Americans lack health insurance, including many of the people who need it most. Other social factors are also important, including stress, violence, sexual behavior, adolescent pregnancies, and drug abuse. From a nationwide perspective, all these factors must be addressed if we are to bring prevention within the reach of our entire population.

Hawaii is a useful example for our other 49 states. Since 1974 Hawaii has had a program of universal health insurance; at present 98 percent of Hawaiians are insured, while only 86 percent of other Americans are covered. Despite its much higher than average cost of living, health care costs in Hawaii are much lower than average; yet Hawaiians have the lowest risk of major chronic diseases and the highest life expectancy in the country. It may be a result of the diet or even the climate, but Hawaii's success story may also be due to its insurance plan's strong emphasis on preventive services.

If the burden of disease is distributed unevenly in our country, global inequities are even more glaring. As we struggle with diseases of excess and affluence, much of the world struggles with diseases of poverty. The World Health Organization estimates that more than 20 percent of all humankind suffers from severe health problems. Some, of course, are common to both industrialized and underdeveloped countries: worldwide, 12 million people die each year from cardiovascular disease, 5 million from cancer, 3 million from chronic lung disease, and at least .25 million from AIDS. But other causes of death are linked strongly to poverty, including 5 million from diarrhea, 5 million from pneumonia, 3 million from tuberculosis, and more than 1 million each from measles, malaria, and hepatitis. The obstacles that stand in the way of controlling diseases of poverty are enormous. In many cases the necessary medical technology is available, but limitations imposed by economics, health care delivery, education, cultural and religious practices, nutrition, sanitation, and politics prevent its use. The situation is grim but not hopeless. Remember that a brilliant worldwide campaign eliminated smallpox from the face of the earth, banishing forever this historic scourge of humanity.

Even with such a success story to inspire, we must admit that preventing disease around the globe and equalizing health care in the United

States are complex, multifaceted problems, well beyond the scope of this book. But this bad news serves to emphasize some good news: most readers of this book are very fortunate indeed, and should find it much easier to make the personal, and even the communal, changes needed to prevent disease.

Let's get started.

■ Can Prevention Work?

With the appalling burden of illness in our country, to say nothing of the world, it's hard to muster much optimism that the simple strategies of prevention can make a difference. Cheer up — they can.

What Keeps Us Well?

In 1972 Drs. Nedra Belloc and Lester Breslow examined the impact of basic health habits on the health of Californians. The seven habits they studied were startlingly simple: eating breakfast, eating regular meals, eating moderately, abstaining from alcohol or using it in moderation, not smoking, exercising regularly, and sleeping seven to eight hours a night. They found that even these very simple habits had a major impact on health: a middle-aged adult with three or fewer of these habits had a life expectancy of only 67 years, whereas an individual with four or five had a life expectancy of 73 years, and a person with six or seven could expect to live for 78 years. I think you'll agree that this is an impressive demonstration of the power of prevention, and it works for both sexes, all ages, and all economic strata. Remember that all the medical progress in the United States between 1900 and 1990 increased the life span of the average adult by only four years, and you'll be even more impressed by the 11-year gain that can be achieved with simple life-style changes.

My list of crucial health practices for the 1990s is only slightly longer than Belloc and Breslow's, and it's nearly as simple:

1. Don't use tobacco or drugs — at all.
2. Don't consume more than two ounces of alcohol per day.
3. Eat a diet low in fat, cholesterol, and salt but high in fiber, fruits, vegetables, and fish.
4. Exercise regularly: one hour each week is helpful, three hours is ideal.
5. Stay lean.
6. Use air bags or wear seat belts, drive prudently, and never drink before you drive.
7. Avoid excessive stress.
8. Minimize your exposure to radiation, ultraviolet rays, chemical pollutants, and other environmental hazards.
9. Protect yourself from sexually transmitted diseases.
10. Obtain regular medical care, including immunizations and screening tests.

The impact of these Ten Commandments of Prevention should be even greater than the seven habits studied in 1972. Only one item, the tenth, requires help from the medical establishment. You can do the rest yourself — and this book explains exactly how to do it.

Why Prevention Works

Why should ten simple interventions have such a powerful impact on preventing disease? The answer is obvious when you look at the ten leading causes of death along with the controllable factors that cause or contribute to each:

1. Heart disease	Tobacco abuse
	High blood pressure
	High cholesterol
	Lack of exercise
	Excessive stress
	Diabetes
	Obesity
2. Cancer	Tobacco abuse
	Radiation
	Environmental exposures
	Improper diet
	Alcohol abuse
3. Stroke	Tobacco abuse
	High blood pressure
	High cholesterol
4. Accidents	Alcohol and drug abuse
	Tobacco abuse
	Not using seat belts
	Fatigue, stress, and recklessness
5. Chronic lung disease	Tobacco abuse
	Environmental exposures
6. Pneumonia and influenza	Chronic lung disease
	Environmental exposures
	Tobacco abuse
	Alcohol abuse
	Lack of immunizations
7. Diabetes	Obesity
	Improper diet
	Lack of exercise
8. Suicide	Excessive stress
	Alcohol and drugs
9. Liver disease	Alcohol
	Exposure to toxins
	Lack of immunization

10. Atherosclerosis   Tobacco abuse
                             High cholesterol
                             Lack of exercise
                             High blood pressure

In addition to these controllable causes there are, of course, risk factors that we can't control, such as the genetic influences that contribute to many cases of diabetes and some cases of heart disease, the bacteria and viruses that cause infections, and the complex, still obscure factors that lead to some cancers and mental disorders.

But even if prevention is not perfect, the potential benefits of simple life-style changes is little short of astounding. Note that the correctable causes of the ten leading killers overlap considerably. This means that if we could eliminate tobacco, we could save 350,000 American lives each year. Controlling hypertension could save 300,000 lives, as would preventing overnutrition. If we could eliminate alcohol abuse, we would be able to save another 100,000 lives each year. All in all, we could prevent nearly 25 percent of all cancer deaths and almost 50 percent of all deaths from heart disease and stroke. And even an inherited disease like diabetes can be controlled, since more than 50 percent of the lethal complications can be prevented. The net result could be the prevention of two thirds of the premature deaths in the United States. Prevention is not yet perfect — but it's potent indeed!

Implementing Prevention: Tasks and Rewards

To save hundreds of thousands of lives (and billions of dollars), we need to make major changes in the fabric of society. We should all help advance these changes. The task is complex, involving education and public information, continued medical research, environmental cleanup, new standards for nutrition, balanced controls on advertising, industrial safety, improved health care delivery, socioeconomic changes to fight poverty and deprivation, and a realignment of many of our national values and priorities.

Prevention is a huge task, but it offers huge benefits. We've barely begun to implement it, but progress can be measured even now; for example, although cardiovascular disease remains the leading cause of death in the United States, the mortality rate from heart disease has declined by 44 percent in the past three decades; credit for this improvement is shared equally between the medical community (improved diagnosis and treatment) and the public (life-style changes). Similarly, the mortality from stroke has declined by 50 percent since 1950, largely owing to improved treatment of high blood pressure. And while we are congratulating ourselves, let's remember that dreadful infections such as paralytic polio and congenital rubella have been nearly eliminated in the United States.

Even as we nudge our leaders and our neighbors into doing what's good for all of us, we can implement preventive life-style changes for each of us. What can you gain on your own? If you don't smoke, you'll live 6.1 years longer than a smoker if you are a man, and at least 2.1 years longer if you are a woman. If you maintain your ideal body weight, you'll live 3.6 years longer than someone who is 30 percent overweight. Preventing radiation exposure is worth nearly a year. And if you exercise regularly, you'll out-live a couch potato by more than a year on average.

We all agree that life expectancy is very important. But there is more to prevention. If you follow the Ten Commandments of Prevention, you'll also get more from life. By obeying these simple rules, you'll actually enhance your health; you'll feel better, look better, and function better every day of your life. I don't think it's at all unrealistic for us to aim for vigor, produc-tivity, and enjoyment well into old age.

The life-style changes that form the basis for preventive health are con-ceptually simple, even obvious. But implementing these changes is harder than merely understanding them; many will take hard work, some will take time, and a few may require professional help. Still, if you understand *why* each change is important, *what* your goals should be, and exactly *how* to achieve these goals, you can succeed in preventing disease.

I have seen many patients, colleagues, and friends succeed. And I've experienced both the difficulties and rewards of change myself. My educa-tion at Yale and Harvard notwithstanding, when I graduated from medical school I was an overnourished, overstressed, sedentary smoker. During the first ten years of my medical residency and practice, I succeeded in giving up tobacco and reducing high-fat foods — but my weight increased to 200 pounds, and I had high cholesterol and blood pressure levels to match. More than simply sedentary, I had remained nearly inert. My medical col-leagues, especially those who knew that my mother and uncles died from heart disease before they were 43 and that my father developed cardiovas-cular disease in his 30s, were concerned, but they were not particularly helpful. I was rescued not by my doctor but by my wife. Today, 15 years after I began to exercise and implement life-style changes, I weigh 165 and have a normal blood pressure and spectacular cholesterol profile. I began today with my customary 12-mile run, yet I have much more energy than I did as a younger man. My professional life remains stressful, but I feel much calmer and happier. With simple preventive life-style changes I am happier and physiologically younger as well as healthier. Do I really look better? You'll have to ask my wife!

■ How to Use This Book

The Ten Commandments for health enhancement and disease prevention are very simple. If you understand and obey them, you don't really need this book. But in my clinical experience successful life-style modification depends on more than broad guidelines: you should understand, not only the big picture and the reasons behind the rules, but also the fine print, the specific practical details that will enable you to live by the rules. I'll try to give you both in the chapters that follow.

The scope of prevention extends to diseases of all severities. The ten rules I've outlined are directed chiefly to the ten leading causes of death; they should improve the quality of your life while helping to prevent these killers. But it won't do you much good to prevent the ten leading causes of death if you succumb prematurely to the eleventh or twelfth. As a result, I'll include information on preventing less common diseases which can threaten your health. Similarly, you won't be able to enjoy fully the quality of life you've achieved through cardiopulmonary fitness if you are plagued by periodontal disease or limited by visual impairment, so I'll take on non–life threatening diseases as well as the killers. But I am not writing a medical text, much less an encyclopedia; in these pages you'll find discussions *only* of diseases that are preventable.

The scope of prevention includes ideas that are old as well as some that are new. The desire to prevent disease is as old as civilization, and probably accounts for many of the taboos, dietary laws, and traditions that have survived for centuries. Whereas some venerable practices have stood the test of time, many have become obsolete. In this book I'll focus on the latest information on prevention, but I'll also include some traditional wisdom that seems sound by modern scientific standards.

The scope of prevention encompasses interventions that depend on high technology at high expense, as well as those that are based on simple life-style changes that carry little or no cost. I will include both ends of the spectrum, but you'll be happy that most of my recommendations are decidedly low tech and low cost. In the final analysis, a pair of running shoes will probably do more for you than a colonoscopy. But even when you need modern technology, your monetary costs will be paid back many times over by your savings in health. Prevention is cost effective. Tell it to your insurance company!

The scope of prevention encompasses the health care system. To make the most of prevention, we need to increase its position in medical research and medical education. But we also need to enhance its place in medical practice. To help you get the preventive services you need, I'll discuss in detail what you should expect from your doctor and how you can utilize medical tests and treatments to prevent disease. You should be able to rely on your doctor for some crucial aspects of preventive medicine, but first and foremost you must be able to rely on yourself.

The scope of prevention includes major changes in health care delivery, funding, and insurance coverage. I'll point out some deficiencies that exist and some of the goals we should work toward. The purpose of this book, however, is not to change the system but to show you how to use the system.

The scope of prevention incorporates scientific advice based on firmly established medical data, but it must include advice based on reasonable probabilities as well. My scientific training and conservative education at mainstream institutions such as Harvard Medical School, Massachusetts General Hospital, and the National Institutes of Health cause me to focus first on scientific certainties — which is the way it should be. But as a practicing internist, and as an individual who has to make health choices for myself and my family, I know that we often have to decide on a plan of action before every single detail is established beyond any scientific doubt. No less an authority than Aristotle reminds us that in areas that demand practical wisdom, we should not insist on the same degree of absolute certainty as we do in pure science.

The scope of prevention incorporates all stages of life. At its best, preventive health care should begin even before conception, with genetic screening and counseling and with family planning to prevent unwanted and adolescent pregnancies. Maternal care is clearly a most important component of optimal preventive medicine, as is pediatric care during the infant and childhood years. Indeed, obstetricians and pediatricians far outstrip most internists in their emphasis on preventive medicine. Even so, many of the chronic diseases that kill and disable in adulthood have their antecedents in childhood; we must do a much better job of medical screening, health education, and life-style improvement during childhood to prevent the diseases that become manifest at maturity. Despite the importance of prevention at these early stages of life, however, my major focus will be on adulthood. Many of my recommendations will be most effective if implemented early in adult life. But it's never too late to change for the better, and I will include some specialized advice for older adults as well.

Finally, the scope of prevention extends to all stages of health. *Primary prevention* is the prevention of disease before it first occurs. *Secondary prevention* is the detection of disease after it has already started, but before it has caused any symptoms or functional impairments. And *tertiary prevention* is the treatment of symptomatic disease to prevent further progression.

The relative roles of the three stages of prevention depend in part on the specific disease in question. For example, we know the major causes of lung cancer, so primary prevention is a realistic goal, requiring the avoidance of tobacco, radon, and certain industrial exposures and pollutants. In contrast, the treatment of lung cancer is poor, even in its early stages, so routine chest x-ray screening does little for secondary prevention. Quite the reverse is true for breast cancer. Primary prevention can help: low-fat diets, alcohol avoidance, exercise, and breast-feeding all play a part. But even with these measures, breast cancer will still occur. Fortunately, secondary prevention for this disease is excellent: mammograms can detect very early breast cancers before they are even large enough to produce a lump, and excellent treatment is available for early disease.

Tertiary prevention requires medical therapy and is largely beyond the scope of this book. Secondary prevention also requires medical screening studies. You'll need your doctor. But you should be an informed consumer, understanding which tests and treatments are helpful and which are not. I'll try to help you with secondary prevention as we go along, so you can best collaborate with your health care providers. But the ultimate responsibility is yours. It's not always easy to shoulder that responsibility. René

Dubois said it best: "To ward off disease or recover health, men as a rule find it easier to depend on the healers than to attempt the more difficult task of living wisely." Difficult or not, the responsibility is yours, the choice is yours, and the possibilities are yours. To help you take responsibility and choose wisely, I'll focus much of my attention on primary prevention, on the things you can do for yourself, on the life-style changes that can prevent you from becoming a patient. Ben Franklin was right: an ounce of prevention *is* worth a pound of cure. Primary prevention is, in fact, the best medicine of all.

■ T W O ■

Preventable Illnesses —
and How to Prevent Them

■ 2 ■
Heart Disease

To stay well, you should start right at the heart of the matter. Heart disease is, after all, the leading preventable disease in the United States today.

Preventing heart disease is our number one priority because cardiovascular disease is our number one killer. Six million Americans have coronary heart disease. There are 1.5 million heart attacks in our country each year; three people have heart attacks every minute. Despite spectacular improvements in the treatment of coronary artery disease, the death toll remains catastrophic: 500,000 Americans will die from coronary heart disease this year, about one per minute.

Preventing heart disease is our number one priority because it affects all Americans. We used to think of heart attacks as a problem of older white male executives. But we now know that atherosclerosis, the disease that leads to heart attacks, actually begins in childhood. Heart disease affects both sexes; although women under 45 are only one tenth as likely to have heart attacks as young men, women over 65 have nearly half the risk of men. And heart attacks strike people of every social class and race: laborers now have more heart attacks than executives, and blacks more than whites.

Preventing heart disease is our number one priority because the disease is so costly. The direct medical care of heart disease victims and their lost productivity cost the United States nearly $110 billion in 1991 — and the tab keeps rising. It is much less expensive to prevent a heart attack than to treat one: each heart attack costs about $50,000 in medical care and lost wages.

Preventing heart disease is our number one priority because of another hidden cost: the medical brain drain. An enormous number of talented doctors and biomedical engineers are devoting themselves to high-tech treatments for heart disease, ranging from angioplasties to bypass operations to transplants and artificial hearts. I am, of course, very grateful to have these treatments for my patients. But with prevention they would be unnecessary — and this marvelous medical talent could be turned loose on problems that can't be eliminated by prevention.

Preventing heart disease is our number one priority because prevention

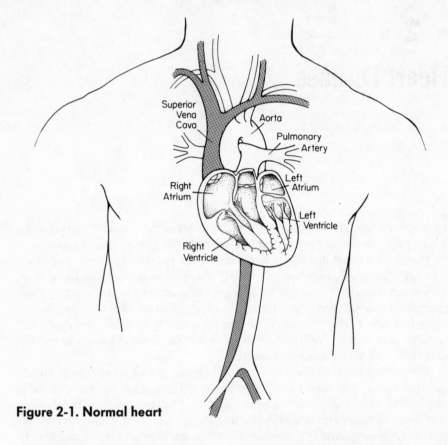

Figure 2-1. Normal heart

works. The mortality from heart attacks has decreased by 44 percent in the past 30 years. About half this progress is due to improved medical treatment, the balance to life-style improvements. But even this progress is not enough. Remember that coronary disease is a new event in human evolution, caused by self-inflicted abuse and disuse of the body rather than by human genetics. When it comes to *your* heart, 44 percent protection is not enough. You should aim for 100 percent protection; and with some surprisingly simple steps, you can achieve this goal of freedom from heart disease.

■ The Healthy Heart

To understand how to keep your heart healthy, you should understand how a healthy heart works.

Your heart is a pump that collects blood from your veins, pumps it through your lungs, where it is enriched with oxygen, then pumps it again throughout your entire body to nourish your tissues (figure 2-1). To do all this, the heart is divided into four pumping chambers, separated from one another by valves that open and close in a precisely timed sequence to keep blood flowing in the right direction.

Your heart is a muscle — a very special and strong muscle. Although no larger than a clenched fist, it beats more than 100,000 times each day, pumping more than 2,000 gallons of blood through some 60,000 miles of blood vessels throughout your body.

Your heart muscle, like all muscles, needs its own supply of oxygen to keep working and stay healthy. All the heart's nourishing blood flows through two small arteries, the right and left coronary arteries, which then divide into successively smaller and smaller arteries that branch out to feed the entire heart muscle.

If you take care of yourself, your heart will do its work without complaint throughout a long and healthy life. But things can go wrong. The heart muscle can be weakened by several preventable problems, including high blood pressure and alcohol abuse. The heart muscle can also be damaged by inflammation, and heart valves can be scarred by rheumatic fever and infections. I'll explain how to prevent these heart diseases toward the end of this chapter. But the most common — and the most preventable — heart disease of all is coronary artery disease.

■ What Is Coronary Artery Disease?

Coronary artery disease occurs when blockages develop in the blood vessels that provide oxygen-rich blood to the heart muscle. Because they are such small arteries, even tiny blockages can cause big trouble.

The Symptoms of Coronary Artery Disease

The most common symptom is chest pain. When your heart muscle is not getting enough oxygen, it generally sends out a painful warning signal called *angina*. Because your heart needs oxygen the most when it's working the hardest, angina is most likely to occur during exercise. Since mental stress raises your blood pressure and taxes your heart, it too can trigger angina. Sometimes a large meal can set off the pain because your heart is doing extra work to supply blood to your stomach and intestines.

Angina is usually felt as a strong pressure deep in the center of the chest. The pain often radiates to the neck and jaw or to the shoulders and arms, especially on the left. But there are variations on this theme. Angina can occur during rest, even during sleep. Sometimes the pain is sharp or burning, and sometimes it's strongest in the stomach or even the back. These variant forms of angina may cause diagnostic puzzles for your doctor. Even more worrisome is painless angina, known medically as *silent ischemia*. We now know that silent angina is actually quite common, and without pain to warn that the heart muscle is in jeopardy, patients may not be able to take medications in time to forestall serious damage.

The Consequences of Heart Attacks

If the heart muscle is deprived of oxygen for long enough, it will die. That's exactly what happens in a heart attack, or *myocardial* (heart muscle) *in-*

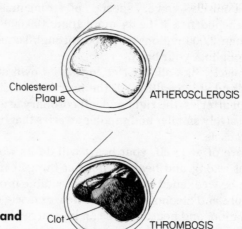

**Figure 2-2.
Atherosclerosis and
thromboses**

farction (tissue death). If the heart attack victim is lucky, the heart muscle will heal and form a strong scar. But if the scar is large, or if recurrent heart attacks produce many scars, the heart muscle will be weakened so it cannot pump blood efficiently. Doctors call this consequence of coronary artery disease *congestive heart failure;* patients recognize it as fatigue and weakness, shortness of breath, and swelling of their ankles and feet.

Angina and heart attacks can cause another major problem — a disorder of the heart's rhythm. Disruption of the heart's pumping sequence can cause symptoms ranging from breathlessness to light-headedness or faintness to collapse and sudden death.

Chest pain, congestive heart failure, disordered heart rhythms: it sounds pretty bad. And it is. Thirty percent of all heart attack victims will die from their first heart attack, and 50 percent will die within ten years.

What Blocks Coronary Arteries?

Blockages in coronary arteries result from two problems: fatty deposits (atherosclerosis) and blood clots (thrombosis). Both can be prevented.

Atherosclerosis is the basic problem in almost all cases of coronary artery disease. Its name is derived from two Greek words: *athere* (porridge) and *sklerosis* (hardening). It's a good name; arteries afflicted by atherosclerosis are hard and stiff on the outside, but their inner linings are coated with soft, mushy debris.

Atherosclerosis develops when cholesterol from the blood is deposited in an artery's wall. At first, only faint fatty streaks are present, but larger *plaques* build up as time goes on (figure 2-2). As the plaques enlarge, they gradually impede the flow of blood. It typically takes years before the narrowing is severe enough to cause symptoms. The slow pace of atherosclerosis means that your doctor can sometimes detect blockages while they're still small, giving you time to prevent them from enlarging. But the steady pace of atherosclerosis means that you had better get started on prevention right now.

The other major cause of coronary artery blockages is blood clotting. When it occurs a clot, or *thrombosis*, narrows the artery's channel, slowing or stopping its vital flow of oxygen-rich blood. Coronary clots develop much more rapidly than fatty plaques. In fact, a clot can produce a lethal narrowing in just a matter of seconds. But these dreadful clots rarely occur in healthy coronary arteries; instead, they arise in arteries already damaged by fatty plaques. So by preventing atherosclerosis, you can help prevent coronary clots as well.

Doctors can treat coronary artery disease with drugs that improve blood cholesterol levels to reduce atherosclerosis. They can use surgical treatments to ream out blocked arteries or to bypass them. They can give medications that dissolve clots. But you can do a much better job by fighting atherosclerosis and clotting before they cause disease. And the tools at your disposal are decidedly simpler.

■ Preventing Coronary Artery Disease

The first step is to understand the ten factors that can increase your chances of becoming another statistic in this twentieth-century epidemic. Table 2-1 lists all ten; three are beyond your control, but you can do a lot to correct the other seven; I don't think it's too far-fetched to expect that if you succeed in controlling these seven, you'll virtually eliminate your risk of coronary artery disease.

Uncontrollable Risk Factors

The older you are, the more likely you are to suffer a heart attack. If heart disease runs in your family, your risk, too, is increased. And if you're a man, you're much more likely to develop coronary artery disease than if you are a woman. Since you can't turn back the clock, trade in your ancestors, or replace your sex chromosomes, there's nothing you can do about these risk factors.

It sounds simple. But is it?

Table 2-1. Coronary Risk Factors

Uncontrollable factors	Controllable factors
1. Age	1. Smoking
2. Family history	2. Cholesterol
3. Gender	3. High blood pressure
	4. Lack of exercise
	5. Diabetes
	6. Obesity
	7. Stress and personality

Let's look at each of these "uncontrollable" risk factors to find out what they really mean.

Age. All people age at the same rate, but not all people develop coronary artery disease as they age. Remember the example of Japan: Japanese live longer than Americans, but they have less heart disease at all ages.

Age does not cause coronary artery disease. Incidence of the disease increases with age in Western societies because of the cumulative damage that arteries suffer over the years. That damage can be prevented; in doing so, we'll be able to remove age from the list of coronary risk factors. It's a heartening goal.

Family history. As a middle-aged man whose family has been decimated by heart disease, I'm particularly glad to report that having a disease-filled pedigree does not mean that you should reserve a bed in your hospital's coronary care unit. Far from it.

It's true that heart attacks tend to cluster in families. In some cases the explanation is truly genetic, with inherited abnormalities of cholesterol metabolism. In these unfortunate families vascular disease often develops before age 30; fortunately such cases are rare. Much more often coronary disease strikes family members who are 40, 50, or 60 years old. Here the problem is not the genes that relatives share but the behavioral patterns they have in common.

In cultures where cigarettes are scarce, saturated fat is not a dietary staple, blood pressure is low, and physical work rather than mental stress is the way of life, coronary artery disease is a rarity. Obviously in such societies *all* families are free of heart disease.

You don't have to look to the Orient to find a heart-healthy society. Just 100 years ago our country, too, was nearly free of heart disease. By returning to the basics, we can remove family history from the list of coronary risk factors.

Gender. Gender, too, could be removed from the role of risk factors. Unfortunately, American women are already closing the heart disease gap by adopting the patterns of tobacco abuse, nutritional neglect, sedentary living, and mental stress that cause the disease in American men. As a result, coronary artery disease causes 27 percent of all deaths in women. Obviously there are better ways to deal with the issue of gender and the heart.

The first, of course, is to protect men from heart disease. It can be done, and this chapter will explain how. If men had no heart disease, gender would not be a coronary risk factor — and men might live as long as women.

The second way is to protect women. Like all men, all women should lead heart-healthy life-styles. But older women should consider extra protection; coronary heart disease is a rarity in young women, but it increases sharply after menopause. Above age 65, in fact, one of every three American women has some form of cardiovascular disease.

Menopause is a complex event. But from the heart's viewpoint it's simple: estrogen levels fall, cholesterol levels deteriorate, and atherosclerosis develops. Estrogen replacement therapy prevents all three; postmenopausal women who take estrogen have better cholesterol profiles, 50 percent less heart disease, and longer life expectancies than those who do not.

Should all women take estrogen after menopause? No. Menopause is far too complex to warrant such a simple answer. Estrogen replacement therapy protects the heart, and it also prevents osteoporosis, but it raises concerns about cancer of the uterus and breast. Each woman will have to weigh the evidence for herself. Chapter 9 presents the evidence and offers guidance for that decision; you'll learn why women who are at low risk for cancer but high risk for heart disease should seriously consider estrogen replacement.

Should premenopausal women take hormones for extra protection? Not at all; in fact, birth control pills produce a slight increase in heart attacks, not because they cause atherosclerosis but because they increase clotting, especially in smokers.

Should men take estrogen to protect their hearts? Again, the answer is no. In fact, men who need these hormones to treat prostate cancer actually incur an increased incidence of heart disease.

All in all, there is good news about all three "uncontrollable" risk factors. And the news about the seven controllable factors is even better.

Controllable Risk Factors

All seven controllable risk factors listed in table 2-1 are important, but some are more important than others. Smoking, cholesterol, high blood pressure, and lack of exercise are the Big Four; let's start with these.

▪ **Smoking.** It's easy to understand how smoking can affect your lungs, but it may be harder to see how cigarettes affect your heart. The explanation, though, is painfully simple.

How Smoking Damages the Heart. Cigarette smoke contains thousands of chemicals, many of which are absorbed from your lungs into your blood. These chemicals are carried to your tissues, where they can produce tremendous damage. Unfortunately, blood vessels are particularly vulnerable to the toxic effects of smoke — and the coronary arteries are no exception.

Nicotine causes all blood vessels to constrict, thus raising the blood pressure and stressing the heart. Just one cigarette will narrow coronary arteries by up to 35 percent for as long as 30 minutes. In addition, nicotine makes the heart beat faster, sometimes inducing irregularities of the heart rhythm. Nor is nicotine the only toxin in smoke. Chemicals called polycyclic aromatic hydrocarbons damage blood vessel walls, initiating the formation of atherosclerotic plaques. The carbon monoxide in smoke lowers blood oxygen levels, further taxing the heart.

Smoking also reduces the levels of "good" or HDL cholesterol in the blood, thus increasing the likelihood of developing atherosclerosis. Finally, smoking increases the stickiness of platelets, the blood cells responsible for clotting. All in all, smoking makes the heart work harder at precisely the time when the arteries are narrowed by atherosclerosis, constriction, or clots — a lethal combination indeed.

Smoking and Coronary Risk. Cigarette smoking is the *most* potent risk factor for coronary artery disease. An authoritative review of risk factors by the United States Public Health Service found that smokers are 2.5 times more likely to develop coronary disease than nonsmokers. The more you smoke, the higher your risk. But even a seemingly innocent amount of smoking is hazardous; women who smoke only four cigarettes per day are twice as likely to have heart attacks as women who don't smoke at all.

And all cigarettes are hazardous. There is no evidence that low-tar, low-nicotine brands are any safer than unfiltered cigarettes. Even passive smoking — inhaling secondhand smoke produced by others — significantly increases the risk of heart disease in nonsmokers.

About 30 percent of adult Americans smoke; at least 93,000 of them die needlessly from heart disease every year. In addition, 37,000 *non*smokers die annually from heart attacks caused by passive smoking, victims of our tobacco-abuse epidemic. Smoking is a tragedy for the heart — and, as we'll see throughout this book, for many other vital organs as well.

In short, the first rule for preventing heart disease is also the most unequivocal: *don't smoke.* People who have never smoked will, of course, find it much easier to follow this mandate than people who are already addicted to nicotine. But if you're a smoker, you should make whatever efforts are needed to quit. Even if you have smoked for years, you can prevent heart disease by quitting; smokers who kick the habit have only half as many heart attacks as people who continue smoking. In fact, if you stay away from tobacco for *three* years, your risk of a heart attack will be about the same as that of someone who has *never* smoked.

As a former cigarette smoker, I understand that it's easier to plan to quit than to achieve your goals. I don't have a magic formula for quitting, but I will review a range of effective strategies in chapter 18.

Is quitting worthwhile? Beyond question, yes. One example: 35-year-olds who stop smoking gain two and a half years of life expectancy — and they'll be much healthier during all their years.

▪ **Cholesterol.** Although cholesterol ranks second on the list of coronary risk factors, it's a close second. In fact, an elevated cholesterol level is nearly as harmful as smoking, increasing your risk 2.4 times. The higher your cholesterol, the higher your risk. Because nearly 50 percent of Americans have elevated cholesterol levels, 300,000 heart disease deaths can be attributed to cholesterol each year.

A high cholesterol level is a major risk factor for heart disease, but it's a risk factor you can do something about: for each one-point drop in your cholesterol level, your risk of heart disease will decline by 2 percent. A two-for-one return is an investment in health that you can't afford to pass up. But before you decide exactly how to improve your odds, you should understand the two types of cholesterol in your blood.

Good Cholesterol, Bad Cholesterol. When it comes to the food you eat, there is no such thing as good cholesterol; all the cholesterol in your diet can add to your risk of heart disease. But the cholesterol in your blood is quite a different matter; it comes in two forms, one bad but the other good.

The good cholesterol in your blood is linked to substances called high-density lipoproteins; hence, the good cholesterol is known as *HDL cholesterol*. It's good to have lots of HDL cholesterol in your blood because the role of high-density lipoproteins is to carry cholesterol away from your arteries to your liver, where it's eliminated from your body. So the more HDL cholesterol you have in your blood, the less you have in your arteries — and the lower your risk of heart disease.

But your blood contains a second type of cholesterol, and it's the villain in atherosclerosis. The bad cholesterol is linked to low-density lipoprotein which deposits cholesterol in arterial walls. The deposits of LDL cholesterol begin as fatty streaks and build up into plaques, eventually producing blockages. The more LDL cholesterol you have in your blood, the greater your risk of developing heart disease.

To prevent coronary artery disease, raise your HDL cholesterol. Exercise, weight loss, and smoking cessation are the best ways.

To prevent coronary artery disease, lower your LDL cholesterol. A diet that is low in saturated fat and cholesterol is the best way; weight loss and exercise are also very helpful.

How, Where, and When to Check Your Cholesterol. To find out if cholesterol is a risk factor for you, you'll have to have your blood checked by a lab. Although your cholesterol can be determined from a simple fingerstick specimen (a particular advantage in children), a venous blood specimen drawn from your arm is much more accurate. You don't have to be fasting for a screening cholesterol test, but if abnormalities are detected it's important to have a repeat test after fasting for 14 hours. A single measurement of your total cholesterol level can give you a crude approximation of risk, but it's far better to have your total cholesterol, LDL cholesterol, and HDL cholesterol checked. Needless to say, it's important to use a high-quality lab. If your results are abnormal or out of line with what you and your doctor expect, have your test repeated using another lab; in general, the labs at university hospitals are a good bet.

How often should your cholesterol be checked? Because atherosclerosis begins in childhood, it seems prudent to check levels in children as young as two if they have parents, grandparents, or siblings with high cholesterol levels or early heart disease. In the absence of these warning signals, the first blood test can be delayed until age 20. But even without a blood test, all children should be taught the importance of prudent diet, weight control, and regular exercise.

All the major medical organizations agree that adults who have normal cholesterol results can safely wait five years before repeating their tests. But if the results are abnormal, or if diet, weight, exercise, or medications change, the tests should be repeated more often. Remember, too, that even without such major changes, a person's cholesterol levels can vary by up to 20 percent from week to week. As a result, I check many of my healthy adult patients every year, but I test patients who are on treatment for high cholesterol every two to six months.

Understanding Your Cholesterol Levels. To interpret your results, you'll have to sort out the relative importance of the various blood fats that have been measured. If you get only a total cholesterol level, interpretation is easy: the higher the level, the higher your risk. The same simple relationship holds for LDL cholesterol. But for HDL cholesterol, high numbers are good news. Finally, most labs will also report your blood triglyceride levels. I have not mentioned triglycerides because they are not strongly linked to heart disease; unless your triglyceride levels are very high, you can overlook these numbers and concentrate on the much more meaningful cholesterol results. And even if your triglyceride levels are very high, don't panic; simply repeat the test after fasting for 14 hours. Since most of the fat in food (like most of the fat in your body tissue) is in the form of triglycerides, this is the one element of your blood lipid profile that's accurate only if it's been measured after fasting.

You've had your blood tests, and you have the numbers in front of you; now, what do they mean? We've agreed to set the triglyceride results aside, so you'll be working with three numbers: total cholesterol, LDL cholesterol, and HDL cholesterol.

There are two ways to evaluate your results. The first uses either total cholesterol or LDL cholesterol, while the second uses total cholesterol and HDL cholesterol.

The first method is easier, and is the one used by the American Heart Association and the blue-ribbon National Expert Panel on Detection, Evaluation, and Treatment of High Blood Cholesterol in Adults. These simple guidelines have been sent to all doctors to establish criteria for treating high cholesterol levels, and you can use them as well (see table 2-2).

Although it's hard to dispute standards established by large committees of genuinely distinguished experts, I am concerned that these guidelines are oversimplified.

First, they may be a bit too lenient. I prefer to call the three categories acceptable, high, and very high rather than to use the committees' gentler terminology; perhaps the experts are going easy because fewer than half of all American adults have "desirable" cholesterol levels. I ask my patients to set their standards a bit higher and get their LDL cholesterol levels a bit lower. In my view a total cholesterol of 180 and an LDL of 120 is truly "desirable."

The second potential defect in these simple rules is that they overlook age: a 20-year-old with an LDL level of 130 or a total cholesterol of 240 has a much greater risk of eventually developing heart disease than a 70-year-old with the same results.

Third, guidelines based on either LDL cholesterol or total cholesterol overlook HDL cholesterol, the good cholesterol in blood. A person with a "high" total cholesterol level of 280 is actually at *low* risk of heart disease if the HDL level is 70.

Because of these reservations, I ask my patients to use the second method of interpreting their cholesterol results, even though it's a bit more

Table 2-2. Blood Cholesterol Guidelines

Result		
Total cholesterol	LDL cholesterol	Interpretation
below 200	below 130	desirable
200–240	130–160	borderline
above 240	above 160	high

Table 2-3. Cholesterol Ratio

Total cholesterol/ HDL	Risk
6.0	high
5.0	higher than average
4.5	average
4.0	lower than average
3.0	low

complex. This method, favored by Dr. William Castelli and his colleagues at the famous Framingham Heart Study, depends on the cholesterol ratio. Many labs will do the math for you; ours doesn't, so I keep a calculator in my desk. If you, too, get only the raw numbers, just divide your total cholesterol by your HDL cholesterol to get your ratio. For example, my total cholesterol is 220 — "borderline" by the official standards. But you needn't worry about me or my ability to follow my own advice. My HDL cholesterol is a spectacularly protective 110. The math for my ratio is simple: $220 \div 110 = 2$. Since ratios below 4.5 are good, I can afford to boast about my results. To see how your ratio translates into risk, just consult table 2-3.

Setting Goals for Your Cholesterol. How low should your cholesterol ratio be? As you can see, there is no "safe" level: the lower your ratio, the lower your risk. Since ratios below 4.5 indicate a lower than average risk, 4.5 is a reasonable target level. But you'll be well served if you can get yours even lower without using medications or adopting an unpleasantly ascetic life-style. Younger people, people with multiple cardiac risk factors, and patients with actual heart disease should be particularly diligent about improving their cholesterol ratios as much as possible.

Whichever cholesterol interpretation method you use, the main question is what to *do* about your results. To answer this vital question, you must remember that cholesterol, though important, is just one component of the risk equation. In fact there are *nine* other heart disease risk factors. If you're free of the other nine, you can be less concerned about your cholesterol results. But if you have two or more risk factors, you should work to improve your cholesterol ratio as much as possible. Needless to say, you should also take steps to correct your other risk factors. And if you already have cardiovascular disease, you should be even more aggressive about correcting all your risk factors.

How to Improve Your Cholesterol Ratio. Comparing cholesterol results is a favorite pastime of many Americans, but acting to improve these results is a pastime of few.

You can improve your cholesterol ratio by lowering your LDL levels and by raising your HDL levels. There are five major ways to do the job: diet, nutritional supplements, exercise, weight control, and smoking cessation. Let's consider each.

First, *diet*. Chapter 20 will tell you even more than you may want to know about a heart-healthy diet. For now, though, we should preview the highlights.

Logic dictates that the best way to reduce your blood cholesterol levels would be to reduce your dietary cholesterol. In fact, dietary fat is more important than dietary cholesterol. Still, a low-cholesterol diet can help.

Cholesterol is not actually a fat but a molecule called a *sterol*. Because it's a component of all cell membranes and of many hormones, some cholesterol is essential for health, but too much cholesterol is a recipe for illness. Cholesterol is present only in animal tissues; foods high in cholesterol include egg yolks, liver and organ meats, other meats, and shellfish.

The average American diet contains more than 500 milligrams of cholesterol per day, more than twice what it should. But even if you limit your cholesterol consumption to 250 milligrams per day (the amount in *one* egg yolk), you are likely to achieve only modest reductions in your blood cholesterol levels. The reason is that your body also makes its own cholesterol. About two thirds of your blood cholesterol comes from your liver, not from your food.

Although your cholesterol intake has only a modest impact on your blood levels, another aspect of your diet has a major influence. The culprit is saturated fat. Saturated fat in your food stimulates your liver to produce more cholesterol; the more saturated fat you eat, the higher your LDL cholesterol level. Most saturated fats come from animal sources, including dairy products, beef, and pork.

Fortunately, however, not all dietary fats increase cholesterol production. Eating *un*saturated fats will not raise blood cholesterol levels. Most vegetable oils, including soybean, corn, sunflower, and safflower, are polyunsaturated; peanut and olive oils are monounsaturated. Fish oils contain a special type of unsaturated fat called omega-3s (see table 20-3). Beware, however, of tropical oils; despite their vegetable origins, palm oil, coconut oil, and cocoa butter are highly saturated. Be cautious, too, about hydrogenated vegetable oils, found in margarine and many baked goods; they, too, stimulate your liver to produce LDL cholesterol.

How strict should your diet be? The average American diet contains about 40 percent of calories from fat, with nearly 20 percent in the form of saturated fat. The American Heart Association's prudent diet recommends 30 percent fat, including 10 percent saturated fat. I think you can do better.

For healthy people who have no cardiac risk factors, the AHA diet is okay, but a target of 20 percent fat would be even better. In the presence of risk factors, high cholesterol levels, or heart disease you should be even stricter; the most successful diets for heart patients, the Ornish and Pritikin plans, provide less than 10 percent of their calories from fat. Even without these problems, you might choose to eat less fat. My diet, for example, averages 15 percent fat with only 4 percent saturated fat. With a lean (some would say scrawny) build, a fine blood pressure, a well-established (some would say fanatical) exercise habit, normal blood sugar, and a cholesterol ratio of 2, I could surely ease up. And I do sometimes eat fatty foods — when nothing healthier is available to quell my very substantial appetite. But my "cheating" is infrequent, not only because I know that the less fat I eat, the lower my coronary risk, but because I vastly prefer bread to cake, bran to bacon, and fish to steak. I wasn't always that way, but my tastes have changed over the years.

Your diet is more than a matter of health; it's also a matter of taste and pleasure. The better your risk-factor profile, the more you can afford to indulge your personal preferences. But if you give yourself some time and make changes gradually but progressively, you can actually change your tastes and come to *enjoy* a low-fat diet.

Second, *dietary supplements.* All the experts agree that the key to lowering your LDL or bad cholesterol is to eat a diet low in saturated fat and cholesterol. They disagree, however, on the pros and cons of dietary supplements. These details, too, are discussed in chapter 20. Still, we should note the key points here.

Unsaturated fats: polyunsaturates vs. monounsaturates. There are legitimate grounds for debate about the relative merits of poly- versus monounsaturated fats. Over the years some studies have demonstrated that a high intake of polys will reduce LDL levels, while others have shown that a high intake of monounsaturates will do the same. Safflower oil or olive oil? I don't think the evidence allows us to choose. But the choice doesn't really matter very much. The important thing is to reduce saturated fat and total fat, not to debate what to use as a substitute.

Dietary fiber: soluble vs. insoluble. Controversy also swirls around the relative merits of soluble or insoluble fiber in the diet. Early in the 1980s a series of studies showed that a high intake of soluble fiber in the form of oat bran or psyllium could lower blood cholesterol levels. Late in the 1980s further studies showed that insoluble fiber in the form of wheat bran was just as effective, but in the early 1990s soluble fiber again emerged as the winner in comparative trials. Oat bran or wheat bran? Again this is a contest without a victor — and without much meaning. The important thing is to eat a high-fiber diet.

Omega-3 fats: fish vs. fish oil. The observation that Eskimos have very little coronary heart disease fueled the hope that fish oil, which contains omega-3 polyunsaturated fats, could lower cholesterol and prevent heart attacks. Studies in the late 1970s and the early 1980s showed that fish oil reduces blood clotting, and that it seemed to lower cholesterol levels. As a result, many people began taking large doses of fish oil capsules. Newer observations show, however, that the effects of fish oil supplements on blood cholesterol levels are both minor and short-lived. In addition, heart patients treated with fish oil have not fared any better than those receiving traditional treatment. But if fish oil supplements have failed, fish has not; several excellent studies of healthy people demonstrate that as few as two to three fish meals per week can reduce your risk of heart attack by 50 percent. And even patients who've already had heart attacks can benefit from eating fish; a study of 2,000 male heart patients found that just two fish meals weekly reduced the rate of recurrent heart attacks by 30 percent.

Niacin: vitamin or drug? Another nutritional supplement that has raised as many questions as answers is niacin, vitamin B$_3$. Niacin is present in fish, poultry, meat, legumes, whole grains, and other foods. It can also be purchased in pill form without a prescription. Niacin tablets can lower LDL cholesterol and raise HDL cholesterol. In addition, niacin treatment has been shown to protect heart patients against recurrent heart attacks.

Despite this good news, I don't think you should rush out to buy a large supply of niacin pills. Although niacin is a vitamin, you should consider it a medication. The recommended daily allowance of niacin is 19 milligrams, but the lowest dose used to improve cholesterol is 750 milligrams — 40 times higher. And many patients need 3,000 milligrams of niacin per day to improve their cholesterol levels. In high doses niacin can produce side effects. Flushing, itching, and headaches, the most common side effects, would be easy for you to detect on your own. But another side effect, liver inflammation, is much more subtle and requires blood testing to be detected in its early stages. In patients with diabetes, niacin can increase blood sugar levels, and in patients with gout, it can trigger painful joint inflammation.

Niacin is a valuable drug to improve blood cholesterol levels and reduce the risk of heart disease. But although you can get it without a prescription, you should use it like other cholesterol-lowering drugs. These drugs should be used only after diet, weight control, and exercise have been fully utilized. Drugs should be used to treat a person, not a lab result. The decision to treat requires an evaluation of all risk factors, not just the cholesterol level. Finally, drug treatment should be closely monitored by a physician, both to be sure the medication is working and to be sure it's not producing side effects.

After putting your best efforts into life-style changes, reviewing all your risk factors, and consulting with your doctor, you may decide that niacin is worth a try. Remember, though, that many niacin preparations are available, and that they are not standardized and monitored like prescription drugs. Unfortunately, niacin preparations vary in their potency and side effects; find a formulation that works for you, then stick with it. In general, sustained-release preparations produce less flushing and itching than immediate-release tablets; sustained-release niacin, however, is more likely to cause liver inflammation and elevated blood sugar levels. New information published in the 1991 *Archives of Internal Medicine* suggests that a wax-matrix form of niacin may be best. I've been switching my patients to this formulation (Endur-acin and other brands) since the report was released; it's another reminder that niacin is a potent drug that should be used only as part of a patient-physician collaboration.

Alcohol: good for cholesterol but not for health. The fifth and final cholesterol quandary involves alcohol — also available in the marketplace, and also a drug. Several studies have shown that alcohol elevates HDL cholesterol levels, others that modest levels of drinking reduce the risk of coronary heart disease. The best — and most recent — of these studies is a 1991 report from the Harvard School of Public Health. Fifty thousand men were followed for two years; the subjects who averaged one to two drinks a day experienced a 26 percent reduction in coronary heart disease.

Before you conclude that you've finally found a cholesterol treatment you can love, however, consider the whole picture: think before you drink. Although alcohol protects against heart attacks, it poses many health risks which far outweigh its potential benefits. All in all, I don't recommend alcohol to prevent heart disease. But if you choose to drink, limit yourself to two drinks a day, a dose that's high enough for your heart but safe enough for your liver. Remember, too, that even low doses of alcohol increase the breast cancer risk for women.

These controversies about nutritional supplements and cholesterol have preoccupied doctors and patients alike. There is an important lesson to be learned from all this: there is no quick fix, no "cholesterol cure." The search for a dietary panacea that will lower cholesterol is doomed to failure. Don't let these cholesterol controversies distract you from the big picture: reducing your intake of saturated fat and cholesterol is essential.

It has been said that you are what you eat. People who love beef and those hooked on broccoli are equally glad that it's not literally true. Still, your diet is the major influence on your blood cholesterol; your diet is important both for what it should shun (saturated fat and cholesterol) and what it should contain (unsaturated fats, fiber, and fish). Without forgetting the importance of diet, remember that there are three other items on the list of ways to improve your cholesterol.

Third, *exercise.* Exercise is the very best way for you to raise your HDL cholesterol levels. It will also help lower your LDL cholesterol. And exercise will help your heart in many other ways, which is why it's discussed later in this chapter and in chapter 21.

Fourth, *weight control.* The lower your body fat, the lower your blood fat. Weight control is an important way to improve your cholesterol. Diet is essential to weight control, but it's not sufficient; instead, exercise is an equal partner. Chapter 12 tackles this weighty problem directly. Later in this chapter I'll review the other ways that obesity affects your heart.

Fifth, *smoking cessation.* I hope you remember all the ways that smoking will damage your heart. But while we're on the cholesterol question, a reminder is in order: smoking lowers your HDL cholesterol levels, but they'll rise again when you quit.

These five techniques — low-fat diet, dietary supplements, exercise, weight control, and smoking cessation — will greatly improve your cholesterol profile. It takes planning and dedication to make these changes, but if you proceed at a slow, steady pace, you'll obtain your goals with surprisingly little sacrifice. Is it worthwhile? Just reducing cholesterol levels from 250 to 200 will add one and a half years to the life expectancy of a 35-year-old. Think it over the next time you set your table.

The most hazardous controllable cardiac risk factors are smoking and cholesterol. But table 2-1 lists five others; let's resume our consideration of each.

▪ **High Blood Pressure.** High blood pressure (hypertension) occupies third place on the risk-factor hit parade. As with the other modifiable risk factors, you can control your blood pressure and reduce your chances of singing the sorry song of heart disease.

High blood pressure increases the risk of coronary artery disease 2.1 times. With 58 million hypertensive Americans, we can calculate that high blood pressure accounts for 195,000 deaths from coronary artery disease in our country each year. The higher your blood pressure, the higher your risk. Still, it doesn't take an astronomical blood pressure to increase risk; a 1990 study found that even mild or "borderline" hypertension can damage the heart. All in all, half of all heart attack victims have high blood pressure.

High blood pressure damages the heart in several ways. It forces the heart to work harder; over the years this produces enlargement and thickening of the heart's main pumping chamber. The hypertensive heart is less efficient and requires more oxygen. In time the heart muscle weakens, resulting in congestive heart failure. And if that were not bad enough, high blood pressure also damages blood vessel walls, allowing cholesterol to enter and build up into atherosclerotic plaques.

The hazards of high blood pressure extend far beyond the heart; it also has a tremendous impact on the risk of stroke and an important role in kidney disease. In chapter 3 we'll consider high blood pressure and blood vessel disease in detail. But from the viewpoint of your coronary arteries (as well as your other blood vessels), the major messages are simple. Live healthfully to reduce your chances of developing high blood pressure. Have your blood pressure checked to detect abnormalities before they cause damage. Work with your doctor aggressively to treat high blood pressure, starting with diet, exercise, and weight control.

Will reducing high blood pressure decrease the risk of heart attacks? Although we've known for many years that blood pressure control provides enormous protection against strokes, we could not say the same for heart disease until 1990, when an international team headed by scientists at Oxford University in England found the answer: yes. To reach this conclusion, these epidemiologists used a new technique called meta-analysis (see chapter 24), which allowed them to combine the results of 14 earlier experiments involving 37,000 patients. For each five to six points that blood pressure is lowered, the risk of heart attack declines by 20 to 25 percent, a result nearly as good as the 30 to 40 percent protection against stroke. What do these percentages mean to you? If you're 35 years old and you reduce your diastolic pressure from 100 (a modest elevation) to 88 (high normal) you'll add two and a half years to your life expectancy.

It took us a long time to prove that hypertension is indeed a controllable coronary risk factor. The obvious moral is that you should be sure your blood pressure is normal. Chapter 3 will tell you exactly what to do. But there is another lesson here. If we had waited for final proof before pursuing an aggressive program of blood pressure control, thousands of people would have died needlessly. In the real world of clinical medicine, we often have to act before all the data are signed, sealed, and delivered. We shouldn't leap blindly onto every new bandwagon, but we should act on the best evidence that's available while we're awaiting final answers to clinical questions.

When we come to the next controllable risk factor, we confront an area in which good evidence has already reached the stage of proof. Yet many cardiologists fail to recognize the importance of exercise for preventing heart disease.

▪ **Lack of Exercise.** It may surprise you to know that sedentary living occupies fourth place on our list of coronary risk factors, and that it's nearly as dangerous as smoking, high cholesterol, and high blood pressure. The importance of exercise, I am sorry to report, also surprises many doctors! For example, the prestigious Federal Expert Panel on Detection, Evaluation, and Treatment of High Blood Cholesterol in Adults did not even include sedentary living on its list of coronary risk factors in its 1988 report to the nation's doctors. In the same year an otherwise excellent 450-page medical text on preventive medicine devoted only *two sentences* to the role of exercise in preventing cardiac disease. Exercise is the best-kept secret in preventive medicine.

Exercise has generated lots of controversy in the general public, largely because its benefits are oversimplified and its risks overstated. Chapter 21 details the pros and cons of exercise. For now, consider just one simple, uncontestable fact: people who are sedentary are 1.9 times more likely to develop heart disease than are people who exercise. In all, lack of exercise is responsible for the heart disease that kills 205,000 Americans every year.

How Exercise Protects Your Heart. Exercise protects the heart and blood vessels in many ways. It increases HDL cholesterol and lowers LDL cholesterol. It's very effective in reducing blood pressure and blood sugar levels. Exercise also burns away body fat and fights obesity. Exercise helps reduce mental stress. In short, exercise improves all the controllable risk factors except smoking. And even when it comes to smoking, exercise can help, since physically active people are much less likely to smoke than couch potatoes. In addition, regular exercise improves the heart itself, making the muscle stronger and more efficient. Last but not least, exercise reduces the stickiness of blood platelets and activates the body's clot-dissolving mechanism, both of which should help prevent clots from clogging coronary arteries.

Exercise and Coronary Risk. With all these benefits, it shouldn't be surprising that exercise helps prevent coronary artery disease. Although often overlooked, the evidence that exercise does just that is beyond dispute.

Animal experiments have demonstrated that exercise prevents coronary artery disease and heart attacks caused by high-fat diets. More to the point, studies of humans have shown again and again that people who exercise regularly have much less heart disease than sedentary people. These studies have been going on since 1953, when Professor J. N. Morris demonstrated that bus drivers in London had twice as many heart attacks as bus conductors, who spent their days climbing up and down the stairs of double-decker buses instead of sitting still behind the wheel. In the past four decades many other population groups have been studied, ranging from Masai tribesmen in Africa to housewives in Framingham, Massachusetts, to longshoremen in San Francisco. The conclusions are the same: sedentary living is a major risk factor for coronary artery disease. And it's a risk factor that you can do something about.

Although regular exercise will reduce your risk of heart disease, it will do even more when it's combined with other preventive measures. In a 22-year study of nearly 4,000 San Francisco longshoremen, Dr. Ralph Paffenbarger found that physical activity cut the heart attack rate nearly in half. Controlling blood pressure and quitting cigarette smoking reduced risk further, providing 88 percent protection. Add cholesterol control, and you'll see my goal of complete prevention of coronary artery disease is not a fantasy.

What Exercise Is Best? Your doctor may not know the answer, but your walking buddies and exercise instructors do: aerobic exercise is best for your heart and your health. Examples include brisk walking, jogging, swimming, aerobic dance, biking, cross-country skiing, and vigorous singles racquet sports; in each you'll be using your large muscles in a rhythmic, repetitive fashion for prolonged periods of time. If you work out at 70–85 percent of maximum intensity, you'll feel comfortable as you build endurance. More important, you'll get the metabolic, vascular, and cardiac benefits that can reduce substantially your risk of heart disease.

Just like diet and blood pressure control, however, exercise must be a regular part of your life to produce its benefits. Still, you do not have to run marathons to improve your health. As little as one hour of aerobic exercise per week will boost your fitness, reduce your risk of heart disease, and increase your life expectancy. But if you can build up to higher levels of exercise, you'll do even better; about three hours of aerobics per week will give you the best return on your investment, adding two hours to your life expectancy for each hour that you exercise.

Is Exercise Safe? The tragic deaths of young athletes like Hank Gathers and of older ones like Jim Fixx remind us that exercise is a serious matter. Still, if you follow the precautions and guidelines detailed in chapter 21, exercise will be safe. In fact, an excellent study from Seattle shows that people who exercise regularly have a 60 percent *lower* risk of sudden cardiac death than sedentary people. The network news won't show you clips of someone who has died from a heart attack while sleeping or watching TV. Man-bites-dog fashion, however, you will be told about the athlete who dies while participating in sports. Don't let these rare events provide an excuse for depriving yourself of the benefits of exercise.

Those benefits are indeed impressive. If you are 35 years old when you start exercising, three hours of aerobics per week will add 13 months to your life expectancy. Almost as important, exercise will add vigor and pleasure to all your months.

Smoking, high cholesterol levels, high blood pressure, and lack of exercise are the four most potent coronary risk factors. But there are three others that you should consider.

▪ **Diabetes.** Although diabetes contributes to coronary artery disease, it's a less significant risk factor than the Big Four. Still, 5 percent of all Americans have diabetes, and 30,000 deaths from coronary artery disease are caused by diabetes each year.

Diabetes is, of course, linked to many complications beyond the heart. In fact, it ranks as the seventh leading cause of death in the United States. You can do a lot to keep your blood sugar normal by using diet, weight control, and exercise; chapter 12 discusses diabetes in detail.

▪ **Obesity.** It's obvious to anyone who has visited a coronary care unit that overweight people have more than their share of heart disease. Even so, doctors have debated the scientific validity of this observation for years. The reason for the debate is that overweight people have an excess rate of high cholesterol levels, high blood pressure, and diabetes; they are also less likely to exercise. Is their excess risk of heart disease due to obesity itself, or is it due to the presence of other major risk factors?

After years of analysis, it's now clear that common sense has carried the day. Obesity, even in the absence of other risk factors, does indeed increase the risk of coronary artery disease in both men and women. Central obesity, the "beer belly," is especially hazardous. All in all, a 10 percent increase in body fat will increase coronary risk by about 25 percent. Losing weight will reduce your risk; for example, 35-year-olds who are only moderately overweight will gain six months of life expectancy by attaining ideal body weight. It's important, though, to keep those pounds off. A 1991 study suggests that yo-yo dieting — weight that fluctuates up and down — also increases coronary risk.

Weight loss may also help reduce stress, the seventh and final controllable risk factor.

▪ **Stress and personality.** Can your emotions be heartfelt — literally? Although there is lively debate about the role of stress in causing coronary artery disease, I believe the evidence suggests there is an important link.

The most famous psychological cause of heartache is the Type A personality. Type A people strive for, and often achieve, success. Ambition and drive lead to impatience and time urgency, to "hurry sickness." Type A traits include abrupt gestures, staccato speech, and hostility.

Many studies suggest that Type A people are exceedingly prone to heart attacks, and that modifying Type A behavior with psychological counseling can help prevent heart attacks. Other studies, however, have failed to support those observations, suggesting instead that free-floating hostility and social isolation are the mental factors linked to coronary artery disease.

More work will be needed to settle these issues. But while awaiting the results, don't lose sight of the simple fact that stress can contribute to heart disease. You'll find more information on stress control in chapter 19. But even before you check these tips, you can start modifying Type A behavior on your own: turn these pages just one at a time!

■ Beyond Life-Style Modifications: Medications That Protect Your Heart

Coronary heart disease is caused by the high-fat, high-calorie, high-pressure, low-exercise, tobacco-using life-style so prevalent in Western societies. The best way to prevent heart disease is also the simplest: change your ways, returning to the good nutrition and physical activity that people were meant to enjoy.

If we led an ideal life-style, we could rely on it alone to prevent heart attacks. Since we don't, we should consider the additional protection that medications can provide.

Fittingly enough, three of the four medications that may help are natural substances. I've already discussed the first two: estrogen, the female hormone, and niacin, a vitamin that is present in many foods and is also manufactured by the human body. Of the two, only estrogen requires a doctor's prescription; still, both medications can have serious side effects, and both should be used only with your doctor's supervision.

Two other drugs may reduce heart attack risk. One, beta carotene, is a vitamin, another natural substance. But since its role is unproven, let's consider first the artificial chemical that can help. It's a drug, but it's the most familiar of all medications. It's aspirin.

Aspirin and the Heart

Aspirin does not lower cholesterol. It has no effect on blood pressure or blood sugar. Don't expect aspirin to help with obesity or stress. And although many athletes take aspirin for their exercise-induced aches and pains, you won't get any cardiac protection from the exercise of unscrewing a bottle cap. How, then, can aspirin possibly protect the heart?

Among its many properties, aspirin has the ability to reduce blood clotting. It does this by diminishing the stickiness of platelets, the blood cells that initiate the clotting process. Remember that coronary artery thromboses — clots — are often involved in heart attacks, and you'll understand the theoretical basis of aspirin's protective action.

Not all theories are valid in practice, but aspirin has found an important place in treating patients with cardiovascular disease. In patients who have had warning symptoms of strokes, for example, aspirin reduces the likelihood of an actual stroke by more than 20 percent. In heart attack survivors, aspirin reduces the likelihood of a recurrent attack by more than 30 percent. Only a little aspirin is needed to produce these big benefits: in fact one tablet a day is the best dose; higher doses tend to produce both less protection and more side effects.

Because of these results, the Food and Drug Administration officially approved aspirin for the treatment of patients with coronary artery disease in 1985. But can aspirin prevent heart attacks if it's started before the disease develops?

Our best information on this subject comes from the U.S. Physicians' Health Study, a large trial in which more than 22,000 healthy male doctors volunteered to take either one aspirin tablet or one inert placebo tablet every other day. Half the subjects got aspirin, while the others took the dummy pill; neither the physician-subjects nor the physician-investigators knew which group took the real thing.

After five years the code was broken. The aspirin group had 44 percent fewer heart attacks, a highly significant result. The protective effects of aspirin were seen in subjects over 50. There was only a very slight increase in stomach irritation in the men taking aspirin; there was also a slight increase in an uncommon type of stroke, but the increase was not scientifically significant.

Should we all take aspirin to prevent heart attacks? Despite the great promise of the Physicians' Health Study, it's still too early for such a sweeping recommendation. Like all medications, aspirin should be discussed individually by patient and doctor. I generally recommend low-dose aspirin prophylaxis for healthy men over 50 and for younger men who have serious risk factors for heart disease.

What about women? Sad to say, women have been grossly underrepresented in many medical studies, including most clinical investigations of heart disease. We don't yet have proof that aspirin protects women as well as men. A large investigation of thousands of women will be needed to obtain that proof; a study of alternate-day aspirin use in female nurses is just getting started. But a preliminary look at 90,000 nurses who took one to six aspirin tablets per week on their own suggests that aspirin may reduce the risk of heart attacks by 30 percent in women over 50. So for now, at least, I think we should do what's right by treating women the same as men.

Needless to say, neither women nor men should take aspirin if they have gastritis or ulcers. Stomach irritation, however, is actually quite uncommon when aspirin is used in very low doses, and it can be minimized by choosing a buffered or enteric-coated aspirin preparation. If you have bleeding problems or if you take other medications that affect bleeding, you should not use aspirin.

Did I volunteer to be a subject in the Physicians' Health Study? No. Do I take aspirin to prevent heart disease? Yes, which is why I was not eligible for the study.

Since the Physicians' Health Study was published in 1989, I've been advising selected patients to "take one aspirin and call me the day after tomorrow." Some people (myself included!) find it embarrassingly difficult to remember which is their aspirin day. If you share this problem, you can take your aspirin on Mondays, Wednesdays, and Fridays or on odd-numbered days of the month (my tactic).

One aspirin every other day is not a panacea, and it should never be a substitute for diet, cholesterol control, exercise, and avoiding cigarettes. But in combination with these other strategies, aspirin can play an important role in preventing heart attacks.

Beta Carotene and the Heart

Can a carrot a day keep heart disease at bay? Perhaps.

We don't have the final answer to this question, nor are we likely to get to the root of the issue anytime soon. In the best modern fashion, the doctors who have been digging for answers are studying not foods but pills. Still, it's a good study, again involving the U.S. Physicians' Health team, and it's evaluating beta carotene, a natural vitamin in pill form. While very preliminary, the data suggest that beta carotene may help. A 1991 study of 333 male physicians with angina found that taking 50 milligrams of beta carotene every other day reduced their risk of heart attacks and strokes by 50 percent.

An even newer study, reported only in preliminary form at the end of 1991, evaluated the effects of vitamins on heart disease and stroke in 87,244 female nurses. Women whose diets provided an average of at least 15 to 20 milligrams of beta carotene daily suffered 22 percent fewer heart attacks and 40 percent fewer strokes than women who consumed less than 6 milligrams of the vitamin each day. Vitamin E, taken in pill form, also appeared protective; women taking more than 100 milligrams daily had 36 percent fewer heart attacks and 23 percent fewer strokes than women who were getting less than 30 milligrams daily.

Should you take vitamins in pill form? Not if you're healthy; the evidence is still too preliminary. Because the data are so scant, I don't even prescribe vitamin supplements for my heart patients, but I have no objection if they decide to take them on their own.

Still, you should eat lots of vitamin-rich vegetables and fruits. Studies of vitamins A, C, and E suggest that low levels may be linked to high blood pressure and blood vessel disease. Another preliminary study suggests that eating root vegetables may boost the body's own clot-dissolving mechanisms.

Chapter 20 explains how to get the vitamins you need the old-fashioned way, in foods.

■ Secondary Prevention of Coronary Artery Disease

Prevention is best when it begins before disease has occurred. This best of all medicines is called *primary prevention*. In the case of coronary artery disease, it should begin in childhood and continue throughout life. But it's never too late to start; people of all ages can benefit greatly from diet, exercise, smoking cessation, and stress control to prevent heart disease.

Prevention may also be helpful even after a disease has begun. *Secondary prevention* is just that, the prevention of a disease after it's already under way, but before it has caused any symptoms. The key to secondary prevention is to detect disease early, in its preclinical or silent stages. Sometimes it's easy — for example, routine blood pressure screening can detect hypertension long before it has caused any damage. But in the case of coronary artery disease, screening is much more complex and much less effective.

The electrocardiogram (EKG) is a simple test that measures the heart's electrical activity. When blood flow to the heart muscle is impaired, the electrical signal can reflect that injury. But in angina this electrical abnormality is transient and resolves when the heart is once again getting enough blood. Because muscle cells actually die, heart attacks produce more enduring EKG changes; the scars that result can leave permanent traces on the EKG. Still, many patients with angina and even heart attacks have normal EKGs. Although simple, this test is just not sensitive enough to screen for coronary disease.

The most widely used screening test is the exercise EKG, the *stress test*. The theory is simple: get the heart working hard so it needs more blood, and you'll be able to detect partial blockages in the coronary arteries. In the stress test you'll be asked to walk on a treadmill while doctors and technicians monitor your symptoms. The treadmill will gradually tilt up, moving faster and faster to make you work harder. You'll be encouraged to keep going until you develop fatigue, chest discomfort, or abnormalities of your EKG or blood pressure. Even after you get off the treadmill, your EKG will be monitored carefully until you've recovered. In variants on the theme, a bike can be used instead of a treadmill or a medication can be given to simulate the effects of exercise while you rest on a table. Sometimes tiny doses of a radioactive chemical called thallium are injected before the test starts, and heart scans are performed along with EKGs during and after exercise.

Exercise tests are most valuable when they are used to help take care of patients with heart disease. They can also be effective for the diagnosis of early disease in patients with subtle symptoms. Even in the absence of symptoms, stress tests may be worthwhile if the patient has risk factors that increase the likelihood of coronary artery disease.

Unfortunately, however, exercise tests are *not* accurate screening tests for healthy people with a low probability of coronary disease. The reason is that even the most carefully performed exercise test can produce falsely abnormal results, EKG deviations in the absence of any heart disease at all. In fact, in healthy people *four out of five* abnormal exercise tests are merely false alarms.

False-alarm stress tests can have damaging consequences. Healthy people can be labeled heart patients, changing their life plans and insurance rates. Medications may be prescribed though none are needed. Not uncommonly the patient can even be subjected to cardiac catheterization, a much riskier and more expensive test.

Exercise tests cost about $250. They are time-consuming and inconvenient, and they pose a slight risk of complications. Although stress tests can be very helpful in the care of patients with heart disease, they should not be used to screen for disease in healthy people who are at low risk.

Although the American Heart Association, the American College of Cardiology, and all other major medical societies discourage the use of stress tests for routine "executive physicals," they are still being done. Chapter 23 discusses the pros and cons of stress tests and other screening procedures.

Scientists are at work developing new cardiac screening tests using high-tech scanning devices. And there is always the gold standard, cardiac catheterization, in which a thin tube is passed into a coronary artery, dye is injected, and x rays are taken to obtain pictures of blockages. But the new scans are not yet reliable, and catheterization should never be used as a screening test because of its expense and potential complications.

Is there *anything* you can do to detect early coronary artery disease? My best advice is to listen to your body so you'll detect symptoms such as chest pain, shortness of breath, or palpitations. If symptoms occur, discuss them with your doctor, even if you think they may be nothing more than indigestion. The dictum I offer to medical students may help you as well: chest pain is the most common symptom of coronary disease, but denial is the second most common. Above all, know your risk-factor profile and institute the changes you need to reduce your risk, preventing coronary disease from occurring in the first place.

■ Tertiary Prevention of Coronary Artery Disease

Even if primary and secondary prevention fail, *tertiary prevention* is still helpful in reducing symptoms, preventing complications, and halting progression of disease.

I'm happy to report that we have many excellent ways to treat patients with coronary heart disease. Some are old: nitroglycerin can help dilate arteries; diuretics can remove excess fluid and lower blood pressure; and digitalis can strengthen the heart's pumping ability. Some treatments are new: beta-blocking drugs lower blood pressure and slow the heart, reducing its oxygen demands; calcium channel blockers prevent spasms of coronary arteries while also reducing the heart's need for oxygen. An old drug, aspirin, has found a new use in preventing clots in coronary arteries, and several new medications are able to dissolve clots in the early stages of a heart attack. And if medication fails, arteries can be opened with balloons or bypassed with surgery; lasers and drills will soon be available to open plugged arteries. As a last resort, some patients with irreversibly damaged hearts can be salvaged by the ultimate high-tech treatment, cardiac transplants.

A wonderful array of treatments: I am delighted to have them available for my patients. But I'm also mindful that these therapies would be obsolete if primary prevention had been used. Second-guessing won't help my heart patients — but a second chance will. The simple strategies of primary prevention can also help in the tertiary prevention of heart disease.

Unfortunately, tertiary prevention is often overlooked by both doctors and patients. Medications or operations offer the hope of a quick fix, a modern, high-tech miracle. Although marvelous, these treatments do nothing to treat the underlying disease, atherosclerosis. Only risk-factor modification can do that. In its absence, coronary artery disease is all too likely to recur and progress, even after a bypass operation.

In 1978 we opened the Harvard Cardiovascular Health Center at Massachusetts General Hospital. Since then we have prescribed exercise, diet, and stress control to treat more than 1,500 patients with heart disease. They are the very same techniques you can use on your own to stay healthy. But the center deals with cardiac patients who require careful medical supervision. The results have been wonderful: relief of symptoms, reduced reliance on medications, weight loss, and better blood pressure and cholesterol levels. After three months of close supervision by doctors, nurses, and nutritionists, our patients are encouraged to continue on their own; they generally do, and are rewarded with continued improvement.

Our experience mirrors the results of many cardiac rehabilitation centers around the world. But happy anecdotes, however numerous, do not answer scientifically the key question: Does tertiary prevention prevent heart attacks and extend life?

We now have the answer. Two independent meta-analyses of multiple cardiac rehabilitation trials have documented that patients treated with rehab enjoy a 25 percent reduction in heart attacks — and a similar decline in death rates — as compared to patients treated only with medications and surgery. If these life-style changes succeed for patients with heart disease, they should surely work for you while you're healthy.

■ Can Coronary Artery Disease Be Reversed?

Rehabilitation is one thing, but regression is another. Can coronary artery blockages actually be reversed without surgery? Conventional medical wisdom says no, but I'm not so sure.

Since 1970 more than two dozen experiments on monkeys have demonstrated that their coronary artery disease can be significantly reversed by low-fat diets, cholesterol-lowering drugs, or both. Although evidence is less secure in humans, several trials of cholesterol-lowering drugs have demonstrated that they can partially reverse coronary artery blockages in more than 15 percent of patients.

Dr. Dean Ornish of the University of California used diet, stress re-

duction, smoking cessation, and exercise to treat cardiac patients. Even
without medication, their blood cholesterol levels improved spectacularly,
falling on average from 213 to 151. More important, catheterizations performed after one year showed that coronary blockages improved in 18 of
the 22 patients who completed the program.

We cannot conclude from only 22 patients that life-style changes reverse atherosclerosis, but there is certainly enough promise to warrant
larger trials. True, Dr. Ornish's diet is demanding. The only animal products it includes are egg whites and one cup of nonfat yogurt or milk per
day. The diet draws only 8 percent of its calories from fat, and at 5 milligrams per day, it's virtually free of cholesterol. But if I had coronary artery
disease, I would try to adjust to a similar diet. Since I don't, I'm content to
eat about two times more fat, still considerably less than the American
Heart Association's prudent diet, and much less than the average American's fat intake. You can decide for yourself.

■ Preventing Other Types of Heart Disease

Although coronary heart disease is its greatest enemy, your heart is vulnerable to many other diseases. Since you have only one heart, you should
strive to protect it from all forms of disease.

Heart Valve Diseases

Four sets of valves divide your heart into separate pumping chambers (see
figure 2-1). Although they're just delicate membranes, your valves must
open wide enough to allow each heartbeat to pump blood out freely, and
they must close tight enough between beats to prevent blood from flowing
backwards. Two problems, rheumatic fever and bacterial infections, can
keep your valves from working properly; both can be prevented.

Rheumatic Heart Disease. Though no longer the scourge it once was,
rheumatic heart disease is still a problem affecting more than 2 million
Americans and killing 6,000 each year. Most victims are older adults; new
cases of rheumatic heart disease are very uncommon.

Rheumatic heart disease begins innocently enough with an ordinary
strep throat. If antibiotics are administered properly, the infection is cured
and there are no further complications. Even without antibiotics, the infection will usually resolve. But a small percentage of untreated children develop acute rheumatic fever about two weeks after their strep throats. By
then the strep is gone, but their body's own immune reaction to the bacteria
produces the fever, joint pains, and rash that characterize acute rheumatic
fever.

One of the most critical events in rheumatic fever is inflammation of the
heart valves. With bed rest and aspirin the inflammation settles down, but
scarring may develop over the years. The result: distorted heart valves that
don't open or close properly. The symptoms: fatigue, shortness of breath,
and swelling of the ankles and feet.

Because distorted valves produce abnormal sounds called *murmurs*, doctors can suspect rheumatic heart disease by simply listening to your heart. But don't be alarmed just because you have a murmur. There are many causes of these sounds, most of which are harmless. If your doctor suspects rheumatic heart disease or other serious valve problems, you'll be asked to have a chest x ray and EKG to see if the valve damage is serious. A newer test that provides even better information is the echocardiogram, a simple and harmless procedure in which sound waves are beamed at the heart to measure its valve function. If serious damage is indicated and surgical valve replacement is being considered, a cardiac catheterization will be required.

Rheumatic fever is now very rare in the United States. Its decline has been so extreme that many experts believe antibiotics don't fully account for it; improved living conditions that limit person-to-person spread of the bacteria may play a role, and the strep itself may have become less dangerous. But several recent outbreaks remind us that rheumatic fever is not a thing of the past.

Preventing rheumatic fever is simple; antibiotic treatment of a strep throat will do the job. Penicillin is the drug of choice, but it must be taken for a full ten days; other antibiotics can be used in penicillin-allergic patients.

The hard part is not *treating* a strep throat but *finding* it. Sometimes a strep throat produces no symptoms at all. When symptoms are present, they include fever, swollen glands, and throat pain — but virus infections can produce exactly the same complaints. A throat culture or a rapid strep test will tell if you have strep in your throat, but even here the issue is complex, since half of all positive strep cultures result from a harmless carrier state rather than true infection.

You don't need to run to your doctor every time you have a sore throat. A culture is not necessary if your pain is mild, or if you have a typical viral cold with runny nose, sneezing, or coughing in addition to a sore throat. But if you have sore throat, fever, and swollen glands, it would be best to get a strep test. Testing is more important for children than adults, since rheumatic fever is rare in adults even if their strep throats are not treated with antibiotics.

I sometimes prescribe antibiotics without a strep test, particularly for young people who've been exposed to the germ; because antibiotics can have side effects, however, I prefer to get a culture first whenever possible. Children who have had rheumatic fever should take preventive antibiotics every day until they reach adulthood; because prevention has so drastically reduced rheumatic fever in the United States, this form of secondary prevention is hardly ever needed at present.

Heart Valve Infections. Although rheumatic fever is caused by a strep infection, the heart valves themselves are not actually invaded by bacteria. Instead, the strep stays in the throat, while the heart is damaged by the body's own immune reactions.

Sometimes, however, bacteria can enter the blood and circulate to the heart, where they may infect and damage heart valves. Called *bacterial endocarditis*, this illness was always fatal in the days before antibiotics; even now it's extremely serious, requiring four to six weeks of hospitalization and antibiotic treatment.

Endocarditis can be prevented. The obvious tactic is to keep bacteria out of your blood; the first requirement is never to inject illicit drugs, which are often contaminated with bacteria.

But every time you have dental work, a few bacteria will enter your blood. Fortunately, these relatively tame bacteria won't harm healthy hearts. But if your valves are abnormal, dental bacteria may produce endocarditis. Antibiotics can prevent endocarditis if they are administered before the bacteria enter the blood.

To prevent endocarditis, everyone with rheumatic heart disease or artificial heart valves should take antibiotics before having dental work or other procedures that could allow bacteria to enter the blood. Even milder forms of heart valve disease warrant antibiotic prophylaxis. The bottom line: if you have any heart murmur at all, check with your doctor to see if you need antibiotics before your next dental or medical procedure.

Heart Muscle Disease

When the heart muscle is damaged, its ability to pump blood is impaired. In most cases the diseased muscle can be assisted by medication, but in severe cases only a heart transplant can relieve heart failure and prevent death.

Heart attacks, heart valve disease, and high blood pressure are the most common causes of heart muscle disease. This chapter and the one that follows are devoted to helping you prevent these problems.

Many of the less common causes of heart muscle disease can also be prevented. Exposure to toxins and chemicals heads the list. In large doses alcohol can damage the heart muscle; so can cocaine, even in small amounts; chapter 18 tackles the difficult question of substance abuse. Carbon tetrachloride, cobalt, and other chemicals that can damage your heart muscles are discussed in chapters 17 and 22.

Nutritional deficiencies, too, can produce heart muscle disease. Fortunately deficiencies severe enough to do so are quite rare in the United States. An exception is beriberi, an advanced deficiency of thiamine (vitamin B_1) that may affect malnourished alcoholics.

Finally, your heart muscle can be damaged by myocarditis, an inflammation often caused by viruses. Although most viral infections cannot be prevented, many cases of viral myocarditis may be avoidable. Scientists have demonstrated that mice with certain viral infections are more likely to get myocarditis if they're forced to exercise while the virus is in their blood. I don't know if these experiments apply to humans, but I do know that myocarditis has been implicated in exercise-related deaths of military recruits and athletes. Such deaths are rare, and it's a long way from mouse to man. Still, I advise against strenuous exercise during serious viral infections.

In practical terms ordinary colds are not a worry, since cold viruses are confined to the upper respiratory passages, far from the heart. But fever and muscle aches may indicate that a virus is headed for your blood; to keep it from your heart it seems prudent to avoid vigorous exercise until you're feeling better. But don't wait too long. Exercise, remember, is one of the four major techniques you should use to prevent coronary heart disease.

■ 3 ■
High Blood Pressure and Blood Vessel Diseases

The heart and blood vessels are inseparable components of a single circulatory system. Not surprisingly, many of the things that cause heart disease can damage the blood vessels. Not surprisingly, too, many of the strategies that prevent heart disease will also keep your blood vessels healthy.

■ The Normal Circulation

More than 60,000 miles of blood vessels are linked together in the human circulatory system. The heart's main pumping chamber delivers blood first into the aorta, the largest and strongest of all arteries (see figure 2-1). Like the limbs of a tree, the aorta divides into arteries that grow progressively smaller as they branch from the main trunk. Although the arterial walls are thinner in successively smaller branches, all have the same three-layered structure, with a smooth inner membrane, a strong middle layer containing muscle, and an outer layer of fibrous tissue.

The smallest branches are the capillaries, tiny vessels that have flimsy walls composed of only one layer of cells. As blood flows through the capillaries, it gives up oxygen to nourish the tissues, and it takes up carbon dioxide and other waste products. Blood flows from the capillaries into successively larger vessels called veins, which eventually merge into the two large veins that deliver blood back to the heart. Blood is then pumped to the lungs, where oxygen is added and carbon dioxide removed, then back to the heart and out to the aorta for another cycle through the body.

Whereas all the energy to send blood out through the arteries is generated by the heart, the energy to return blood to the heart comes from muscles throughout the body. Because the return trip requires much less energy, the pressure in the veins is much lower than in the arteries, and veins have much thinner walls.

Even if they don't have to withstand high pumping pressures, veins do have to overcome a powerful force: gravity. The upright posture requires blood to flow upward against gravity to reach the heart. Leg muscles provide the energy to pump the blood, but to prevent stagnation, veins have one-way valves that permit blood to flow only toward the heart.

The arterial blood pressure is determined by the force of the heartbeat, the diameter of the arteries, and the volume of blood in the system. Blood pressure, heart diseases, and diseases of the arteries are closely linked in both causes and prevention. Structurally distinct, the veins suffer from different ailments requiring their own preventive methods.

■ High Blood Pressure

High blood pressure, or *hypertension,* is the most common circulatory problem in America, affecting one third of all adults. It is equally prevalent in many other industrialized countries. Yet elsewhere in the world hypertension is rare — until the salt shakers, fast-food restaurants, and labor-saving devices arrive. In most cases high blood pressure is caused not by chemical or vascular imbalances but by life-style imbalances. In most cases it can be prevented without renouncing the very real benefits of industrialization.

Hypertension can result in heart attacks, strokes, and kidney failure; yet high blood pressure is not a disease. Instead, it's many different conditions, each of which affects the circulatory system, causing it to increase its pressure. Often, high blood pressure results simply from excesses of the regulatory mechanisms that adjust everyone's pressure. The basic problem is not in the blood vessels but in the way they are treated. Bodily abuse and disuse subject the circulation to stress; the overtaxed circulation often responds to that stress by elevating its pressure.

High blood pressure is a hazard, but blood pressure is a necessity. There is no sharp line separating normal blood pressure from high pressure; instead, blood pressures are distributed along a spectrum from lowest to highest. The lower pressures are linked to health, the higher to disease.

Prevention can lower blood pressure. It's mandatory for people with hypertension, and it's a very good idea for people with normal pressures, too.

What Is Blood Pressure?

Despite the confusing terminology associated with blood pressure, there's really nothing mysterious about it.

With each beat, your heart pumps blood to your tissues. To fill your arteries and reach its destination, your blood must be under pressure. The amount of pressure in the arteries while the heart is pumping blood is the *systolic blood pressure;* this is the higher number that's recorded each time your blood pressure is checked.

In between heartbeats your heart relaxes so its chambers can refill for its next beat. During this phase, called *diastole,* the pressure in the arteries is lower; hence, the *diastolic blood pressure* is the lower number that is measured.

When I was in medical school, I was taught that only the diastolic blood pressure "counted." We now know that the complications of high blood pressure are related to both the systolic and diastolic pressures. It's important, therefore, to know both readings. The systolic blood pressure is given first, then the diastolic. You may be told, for example, that your blood pressure is "one thirty over seventy"; this will be written on your medical chart as 130/70.

How Blood Pressure Is Measured

Although your doctor will call the instrument used to measure blood pressure a sphygmomanometer, it's really a very simple device, nothing more than an inflatable cuff that is wrapped around your arm. Air is pumped into the cuff until the pressure around your arm is higher than the pressure in your arteries. Because the arteries are compressed, blood flow will cease, sometimes producing a slight tingling in your fingers. But the full cuff pressure is maintained only momentarily, so the discomfort is brief, and there is no danger to your arm.

The person taking your blood pressure will gradually let air escape from the cuff, slowly lowering the pressure while listening over your artery with a stethoscope. When your arterial pressure is higher than the cuff pressure, your blood will resume flowing through your arm. As blood flow resumes, it produces a sound with each heartbeat; the number showing on the cuff's meter at this time is your systolic blood pressure. As more air is released, pressure on the artery diminishes to the point that blood flow is entirely unrestricted. When this happens, all sounds disappear; the number registered is your diastolic blood pressure.

It sounds easy, and it is. You don't have to be a doctor, nurse, or medical assistant to measure blood pressure; most people can learn to do it for themselves or their relatives. But it does take practice, and there are some pitfalls. The blood pressure meter must be accurate. The cuff must be the right size: if it's too narrow, the reading will be artificially high, if too wide, falsely low. One size does *not* fit all; thinner arms call for narrower cuffs, and conversely. Finally, the cuff must be placed properly over the artery, and it must be wrapped around the arm snugly.

Practice may not make perfect, but it does help. Medical personnel obtain the most accurate blood pressure readings. But some people's pressures skyrocket at the mere sight of a doctor, a phenomenon called white-coat hypertension. This blood pressure rise is temporary and it's not at all harmful — but it can be misleading. If you're prone to wide swings in your blood pressure, home pressure monitoring makes sense. Home readings can also help doctors adjust medications when drug treatment of hypertension is needed.

You can buy a serviceable blood pressure cuff and stethoscope for as little as $30. But if you find it hard to use a traditional cuff, consider one of the newer electronic varieties. At $50 to $150 they're much more expensive, and they tend to be a bit less accurate, but they are much easier to use. In any case, check first with your doctor to see if you really need to measure your own pressure. If so, bring your monitoring device to the office so you can check your accuracy by comparing your readings with the doctor's.

How High Is High?

Before you attempt to interpret your blood pressure reading, be sure that it's a valid result, truly representative of your usual pressure. Everyone's blood pressure varies during the course of the day; blood pressure is generally lower during rest or sleep and higher during physical or mental work. Stress, excitement, and exercise account for the widest swings in blood pressure, but they are not alone: caffeine, nicotine, and alcohol can also affect your blood pressure, raising a normal reading into the high range, at least temporarily. If your blood pressure is high, have it checked again, ideally on a different day when you're more relaxed. To reduce error you may also want to ask several different people to check your pressure.

Once you have numbers that are accurate and representative, you'll certainly want to know if they are normal. A very good question — with a rather complex answer.

There is no "normal" blood pressure. Each person's blood pressure varies from hour to hour (and sometimes from minute to minute), and the person-to-person variability is even greater. It's very clear that the lower your blood pressure, the less stress on your blood vessels and the lower the risk of heart attack, stroke, and kidney damage. Except during acute illnesses that can lower blood pressure to dangerously low levels (a condition known medically as shock), the lower your pressure the better.

Although there is no controversy about the desirability of low blood pressure, there is room for debate about what constitutes high pressure — and what to do about it. Perhaps the most widely accepted criteria for high blood pressure are those of the World Health Organization:

normal   systolic blood pressure below 140
            diastolic blood pressure below 90

borderline systolic blood pressure 140–160
            diastolic blood pressure 90–95

high   systolic blood pressure above 160
            diastolic blood pressure above 95

Blood pressure rises with age; since children have lower pressures, these criteria apply only to adults over 18.

How Often Should Your Blood Pressure Be Measured?

How can you tell if you have high blood pressure? There's just one way: have your pressure measured.

Most people who have high blood pressure feel perfectly well. Despite the medical term *hypertension*, mental stress and agitation are *not* symptoms of high blood pressure; you can be perfectly calm and happy yet have hypertension. Similarly, many other complaints commonly attributed to high blood pressure are invalid: flushing, headaches, nosebleeds, and fatigue are not reliable indicators of elevated pressure. In most cases high blood pressure is entirely silent until it produces serious damage; it is truly "the silent killer."

All of us should have our blood pressure checked at regular intervals, beginning with pediatric care. Because most cases of hypertension begin between ages 20 and 50, you should have your blood pressure checked every one to three years from age 20 on. But if high blood pressure runs in your family, or if your pressures are borderline high, you should check your pressure at least once a year. If your blood pressure is high, your doctor will want to check it even more often.

It's easy to have your blood pressure checked. Like many doctors, I measure my patient's blood pressure during virtually every office visit, even if it's not a regular checkup. Many dentists also offer blood pressure checks as a convenience to their patients. You can also check your blood pressure at free screening clinics and health fairs. Take advantage of all these services when they're handy. But if you're healthy, you don't have to go out of your way to have your pressure checked more than once every year or two. The damage caused by high blood pressure occurs very slowly, so it doesn't make much difference if you detect early hypertension in January or July. But don't wait until *next* July. Without treatment, hypertension will stress your circulation, exacting a terrible toll over the years.

The Burden of Hypertension

High blood pressure is common; 58 million Americans — nearly one third of the adult population — have elevated pressures, and a similar percentage of adults in other industrialized countries have hypertension. With these huge numbers it can be argued that hypertension is the single leading cause of premature death and disability in the Western world. In America, as elsewhere, high pressure is more common in blacks than whites. It's more common in men than women until age 55, after which women catch up. It's more common in older people, affecting up to 75 percent of people over 75.

High blood pressure is serious. Elevated pressures put stress on the heart and arteries. At first the cardiovascular system absorbs this stress without ill effect. But the stress accumulates over the years, eventually resulting in many illnesses.

One major result of untreated hypertension is coronary artery disease. High blood pressure increases the risk of a heart attack 2.4 times; in all, half of all heart attack victims have high blood pressure. Even mildly elevated pressures increase risk: a 40-year-old man whose systolic pressure is 165 is *20 times* more likely to develop some form of cardiovascular disease by age 50 than if his blood pressure were 140.

Another consequence of untreated hypertension is damage to the heart muscle itself. After years of pumping against high pressure, the muscle becomes enlarged and thickened. Eventually it stretches, weakens, and fails.

High blood pressure can also damage the arteries that supply blood to the brain. The result can be a stroke: two thirds of all stroke patients have hypertension.

Another result of hypertension is kidney damage, which can be severe enough to produce kidney failure. Damage to blood vessels in the eye can cause loss of vision. In fact, none of the body's arteries is safe from damage caused by hypertension.

Damage can be prevented, however, by treating high blood pressure. The results have been most dramatic for stroke. Since the advent of drug treatment for hypertension in the early 1950s, deaths from strokes have declined by more than 50 percent in the United States. We can expect a 25 percent reduction in heart attack deaths from treatment, as well as a major decrease in cases of kidney failure. Overall, detecting and treating hypertension could produce a 20 percent improvement in the nation's death rate.

The Medical Evaluation of Hypertension

In most cases effective treatment of an illness depends first on understanding its causes. In the case of hypertension this is not true — a situation that is frustrating for the scientist but reassuring for the patient. Despite intensive study, the cause of hypertension cannot be found in more than 90 percent of patients with the condition. Still, medications that reduce blood pressure have been available for more than four decades, and more are being developed every year.

Until just a few years ago medical texts advocated detailed testing of every newly diagnosed hypertensive patient. But the body's blood pressure control mechanisms are complex: pressure will rise if the heart is pumping too hard, if the arteries are too narrow, or if the volume of blood in the system is too high. Also implicated are the nervous system, the kidneys, and various hormones. Because so many systems are involved, testing them is time-consuming, complex, expensive — and mostly useless, since a specifically treatable cause of hypertension is found less than 10 percent of the time. If you are found to have hypertension, you should have a careful physical exam. Simple blood and urine tests are also useful, as is an electrocardiogram, but these can be accomplished in a single office visit at a modest cost. I generally recommend more extensive testing only if the initial tests are abnormal, if the blood pressure is very high, or if treatment is unusually difficult.

Even without knowing which basic mechanism is abnormal, we can use medications to modulate any step of the body's blood pressure control apparatus, thus lowering the pressure. Antihypertensive medications have saved many lives. More than 20 million Americans take blood pressure pills, at an average daily cost of $1, not counting the costs that can accrue from side effects. In all, Americans will spend $4.4 billion this year for medical management of hypertension, and another $2.6 billion for the drugs prescribed for treatment.

But medication is not the only way to lower blood pressure. In fact it's not even the best way! Let's explore the nonmedical ways you can keep your blood pressure normal.

■ Keeping Your Blood Pressure Normal — without Drugs

You can help control your blood pressure by making adjustments in six areas: diet, weight, exercise, stress, alcohol use, and smoking.

Life-Style Adjustments

Diet is the key to maintaining a normal blood pressure, and restricting your *salt* intake is the key. The idea that excessive amounts of salt can raise blood pressure is hardly new. Huang Ti, the emperor of China, wrote in 2697 B.C. that "if too much salt is used in food, the pulse hardens." Today we know that salt is composed of sodium chloride, and that sodium is the real culprit. Although salt is the most abundant source of sodium in the American diet, other sources can contribute to hypertension. Emperor Huang's descendants should remember this when they add MSG (mono-*sodium* glutamate) to Chinese food.

Excessive dietary sodium raises blood pressure by increasing the blood volume. Salt in food is absorbed through the intestines and carried in the blood to the kidneys, where most of it is excreted in urine. A portion of the salt, however, is retained by the kidneys; retained sodium brings water along with it, adding to the body's fluids. Some people are very sensitive to sodium, retaining excess salt and water. If their circulatory system gets too full, the pressure in it increases. The result: hypertension.

There is abundant evidence that dietary salt is linked to blood pressure. Remember that hypertension is a "new" disease; in the past, when salt was more expensive and less available, blood pressures were lower. Even today there are many cultures that do not use salt. In these groups, ranging from the Bushmen of Kalahari to Indian tribes in Brazil to Solomon Islanders, hypertension is absent or very rare, as are heart attacks and strokes. Equally impressive, the blood pressures of normal, healthy members of these groups do not increase with age, as they do in all salt-using industrialized societies.

Closer to home, many observations of healthy people in Western societies have shown that the individuals who eat the most salt have the highest blood pressures. That's the bad news. The good news is that this effect is reversible: cutting salt intake in half will lower systolic blood pressure by almost eight points and diastolic pressure by half as much. That may not sound like a lot, but over the years even these reductions will protect the body's arteries from an enormous amount of stress and wear.

The average American consumes more than 10 grams of salt (4,000 milligrams of sodium) per day, the equivalent of more than two teaspoons of table salt! This is three to ten times more than the amount required for health. Where does all this salt come from? Only 10 percent is from the natural salt content of food. Another 15 percent tumbles from the salt shaker during cooking or at the table. An astounding 75 percent of our dietary salt comes from processed foods. For example, just ten potato chips contain more salt than 25 pounds of potatoes, to say nothing of the saturated fat and calories added during processing. Junk foods are well named indeed.

Our affection for salt is an acquired taste; until recently, in fact, salt was even added to baby food, starting the conditioning process in the cradle. Many people who've become hooked on salt find it hard to give up — at first. Fortunately, almost everyone can adapt to a low-salt diet by making changes gradually but progressively. Eventually most people come to prefer low-salt foods for one simple reason: they can taste the food.

You can cut down on salt by following a few simple rules. Don't add salt during cooking or at the table. Avoid obviously salty foods such as chips, pretzels, pickles, bouillon, and salted nuts. Cut down as much as possible on processed foods such as fast foods, cold cuts, catsup and other salty condiments, and canned soups. Always read food labels to see what you're getting. Order carefully at restaurants, and don't be shy about asking the chef to hold the salt, MSG, or soy sauce.

Not all people are equally responsive to salt. In general, though, people who need help the most respond the best: the higher your blood pressure, the more it will fall with salt restriction. Remember, there is no "safe" level of blood pressure; the lower your pressure, the lower your risk of heart attack and stroke. A low-sodium diet can help lower your pressure. And because many processed foods have harmful fats, calories, and additives in addition to salt, the diet will have many benefits beyond blood pressure control.

Salt restriction produces no side effects. All hypertension patients should restrict sharply their dietary sodium. And in my view even people with normal blood pressure should shake the habit. A modest reduction in our average daily salt intake from 10 to 5 grams (reducing sodium intake from 4,000 to 2,000 milligrams) would save more than 12,000 American lives each year.

Although salt restriction is the only dietary intervention that has been proven to reduce blood pressure, the evidence suggests that other changes may help. These include increasing the amounts of potassium and calcium in the diet, substituting unsaturated for saturated fats, and increasing vitamin C intake.

Because *potassium* helps the kidneys rid the body of salt, it has long been suspected that eating potassium-rich foods may reduce blood pressure. The role of dietary potassium in regulating blood pressure was first discussed by Dr. W. T. L. Addison in 1928. Since then, studies in Hawaii, California, and Georgia have confirmed that higher potassium intake is linked to lower blood pressure. Even so, the evidence is not perfect. For one thing, the much-studied residents of Framingham, Massachusetts, do not show this relationship between higher potassium intake and lower blood pressure. Another problem is that people who eat lots of potassium-rich foods often favor low-sodium foods as well, so it's hard to be sure which factor is helping the most. Finally, experiments using potassium supplements to treat high blood pressure have been inconclusive, though most suggest benefit. All in all, there is enough evidence for me to recommend eating potassium-rich foods but not enough proof for me to prescribe potassium supplements for blood pressure control.

Among potassium-rich foods (see table 20-10), bananas and citrus fruits head the list. In addition, it's handy that many salt substitutes are high in potassium. One cautionary note: people with kidney disease should avoid high-potassium foods, as should patients who take medications that limit their kidneys' ability to excrete potassium.

The *calcium* story is newer than the potassium data, and it's very exciting and potentially important. Because calcium in the blood relaxes the muscles in the walls of the arteries, scientists have speculated that adding calcium may help the blood vessels dilate, thus reducing blood pressure. Several studies in rats with high blood pressure suggest that this is the case.

Human population studies are also encouraging. Although your laundry and your hair may not like hard water, which is high in calcium, your blood pressure will; people living in areas with hard drinking water have a lower incidence of high blood pressure and other cardiovascular diseases. The same is true for people who get lots of calcium from their diet. For example, one study from Puerto Rico showed that milk drinkers are half as likely to have high blood pressure as are people eating low-calcium diets. The final source of evidence comes from clinical trials in which calcium supplements were administered to healthy people as well as to patients with hypertension. For example, a 1991 study of healthy pregnant women found that calcium supplements reduced the risk of developing hypertension by about one third. In other trials extra calcium lowered blood pressure, but the effect was generally modest, and not all experiments have confirmed these results.

My recommendations about calcium are similar to my advice about potassium: blood pressure control is one of the many good reasons to eat calcium-rich foods, but I don't prescribe supplementary calcium to treat hypertension. Two caveats: first, people who form kidney stones should limit dietary calcium; second, dairy products are the best source of calcium, but they also contain lots of saturated fat and salt. Low-fat dairy products will circumvent the one problem, but if you need to reduce dietary salt sharply, you'll have to rely on green vegetables and soybeans for dietary calcium. Table 20-11 lists the calcium content of many foods.

Dietary *fat* may also affect blood pressure. We know, for example, that strict vegetarians have lower blood pressure than meat and dairy eaters. Similarly, population groups favoring olive oil (monounsaturated fats) or fish oil (omega-3 polyunsaturates) have less hypertension than groups favoring animal fats (saturated). However, trials involving supplementary monounsaturated, polyunsaturated, and omega-3 fats have had disappointing effects on blood pressure. The bottom line: you should eat more vegetable and fish oils and less saturated fats: your blood pressure may or may not benefit, but your cholesterol will fall, as will your risk of atherosclerosis.

Two other dietary factors deserve mention. Several scientists have noted that patients with low vitamin C levels have higher blood pressure readings and more vascular disease. Much more information will be needed before I'll recommend vitamin pills for blood pressure control. But while you're waiting for that information, it certainly can't hurt to peel a few oranges for yourself. Finally, you may be surprised to learn that I'm not taking away your coffeepot, even though caffeine raises blood pressure. I confess to being an inveterate tea drinker, but I'm not being hypocritical. Although coffee, tea, and other sources of caffeine do raise blood pressure, their effect is only temporary. Two cups of coffee will raise blood pressure by about ten points, but the pressure returns to normal within two hours; even ten cups a day will not produce sustained hypertension. As a group coffee drinkers have the same blood pressure readings as nondrinkers. So live a little; enjoy a cup or two after your dinner of fish, veggies, and fruit.

Weight control is another very important way to keep your blood pressure normal. High blood pressure is a major hazard of obesity. In non-Western cultures, body weight does not increase with age — and neither does blood pressure. In our modern world, so notable for overnutrition and underexercise, increasing body weight is consistently and significantly related to increasing blood pressure. More than 60 percent of people with hypertension are at least 20 percent overweight.

Weight loss is not easy, but it's an extremely effective way to lower blood pressure. As a rule of thumb, two pounds of weight loss can reduce blood pressure by about one point. If we could somehow eliminate obesity from our society, we could cure half the hypertension in whites and a quarter of the hypertension in blacks. A dream, I confess, but it underscores a hard reality: hypertension is a man-made disease, and obesity is a major contributor to this dubious accomplishment of industrial civilization.

Caloric restriction is essential for weight control, but preventing obesity is not strictly a question of diet. If your weight is high, you should limit your caloric intake by avoiding fatty foods and alcohol (both of which can raise blood pressure) as well as sweets. Exercise is of equal importance, and behavior modification may help.

Exercise is another way you can keep your blood pressure normal. Although I'm discussing it third, exercise can be every bit as helpful as diet and weight control. Not all forms of exercise, however, are equally good for blood pressure; some, in fact, actually raise blood pressure.

Resistance workouts are among the most popular exercise routines in America today. Whether done with weights or exercise machines, these workouts involve lifting, pushing, or pulling against weight or resistance. Exercise physiologists call it isometric work; you'll call it hard work, and your circulation will call it high-pressure work. Indeed, your blood pressure may soar during isometric workouts. It quickly returns to normal, but repeated resistance work will have a cumulative effect, leading eventually to enlargement and thickening of the heart's main chamber. Healthy people can tolerate the circulatory effects of resistance training, but individuals with high blood pressure or heart disease would be wise to avoid this form of exercise.

But the other form of exercise is right for almost everyone. It's isotonic exercise, already familiar to you as aerobics. During aerobic exercise your muscles move your body instead of struggling against high resistance. You'll find it more relaxing, and your blood vessels, too, will tend to relax. Because your heart is pumping faster and harder, your systolic blood pressure may rise slightly, but your diastolic pressure will fall. Chapter 21 will show you how to make exercise a safe and enjoyable part of your life.

Stress reduction is the fourth way you can lower your blood pressure. Although stress is much harder to quantify than salt intake, body fat, or exercise, it's clear that mental tension can raise blood pressure. In the psychology laboratory this effect can be proven again and again simply by asking a healthy subject to do mental arithmetic; even the best mathematicians will bump up their blood pressure. To raise pressure to very high levels, just ask the subject to solve a "simple" child's puzzle — which is actually insoluble. A dirty trick, perhaps, but a sure-fire way to produce anxiety, embarrassment — and hypertension.

While these dramatic but brief stress-induced increases in blood pressure are easy to demonstrate, it's harder to prove that daily stress produces sustained hypertension. Even so, most clinicians believe that harried patients have higher blood pressure readings. There is a sound chemical basis for this relationship between the mind and the circulation: stress increases the amounts of adrenaline and cortisone in the blood. Adrenaline makes the heart beat faster and harder while also causing arteries to narrow. Cortisone stimulates the kidneys to retain sodium. Each of these changes will increase blood pressure; collectively their effect can be substantial.

Moving from theory to practice, the most telling argument of all is that relaxation therapy can produce substantial reductions in blood pressure. Although newly popular, these techniques are really quite old, dating back many centuries before being revived in the muscle relaxation therapies of the 1940s. In the 1970s and 80s, many careful trials demonstrated that transcendental meditation, biofeedback, yoga, and other relaxation techniques can lower blood pressure by five to ten points. You can learn more about stress reduction in chapter 19.

Alcohol consumption is the fifth link between life-style and blood pressure. If you find an occasional libation relaxing, I'm all for it. Some studies have even suggested that people who consume modest amounts of alcohol have lower blood pressure readings than teetotalers. But if you average more than two ounces of alcohol daily, the amount present in two glasses of wine, two bottles of beer, or two standard cocktails, you'll be at increased risk of hypertension — to say nothing of other problems. I'll explain the risks of excessive drinking, and what you can do about it, in chapter 18.

Smoking

For years doctors have known that smoking even a single cigarette constricts blood vessels, raises the heart rate, and increases the blood pressure by five to ten points. Yet until 1991 smoking was not on the list of controllable causes of hypertension. The tobacco lobby was not responsible for this omission (though they are responsible for many other health offenses). Instead, it appeared that the effects of smoking were transient; like caffeine, nicotine elevates the blood pressure, but the pressure returns to normal in 20 to 30 minutes. Unless they light up in the waiting room (not in mine!), smokers have the same blood pressure in medical offices as nonsmokers.

In 1991, however, doctors at Cornell Medical Center used special automated devices to monitor continually the blood pressure of smokers and nonsmokers during 24 hours of normal activities. Their results: the smokers' blood pressures averaged five to ten points above the nonsmokers' pressures.

You should not need another reason to avoid smoking — but needed or not, you have one.

In a perfect world we would all adhere faithfully to the six life-style precepts that prevent hypertension, and we would all boast nice low blood pressure readings. In twentieth-century America, alas, quite the reverse is true: because we don't take care of ourselves, hypertension is a very common problem. Still, prevention can help.

■ Treating Hypertension: Secondary Prevention at Its Best

By itself, high blood pressure doesn't make you feel sick; but over the years it can make you very ill indeed. We know that simple, routine blood pressure measurements can detect hypertension before it damages health. We know, too, that treatment can lower blood pressure, preventing that damage.

Drug Treatment

The need for drug treatment depends on the height of the pressure and on the health of the arteries and organs at greatest risk: the brain, heart, kidneys, and eyes. All doctors agree that severe hypertension (diastolic pressure above 115) mandates speedy medical evaluation and prompt drug therapy. Moderate hypertension (diastolic between 105 and 115) is less urgent, but aggressive therapy is still essential. Many medical trials have proven that patients with moderate and severe hypertension benefit enormously from vigorous therapy.

Mild hypertension (diastolic between 90 and 105) is more controversial. Because the risks of mild hypertension are lower and the damage it causes is slower, the benefits of treatment are harder to prove. We do know that the lower the blood pressure the better for health. It would seem logical, then, to give blood pressure pills to all patients with even mild hypertension. Unfortunately, any medication can have side effects; in some cases the treatment is worse than the disease. Still, as the evidence has accumulated, the cut-off point for drug treatment has declined. Most internists will treat patients with diastolic blood pressure of 100, and even levels of 95 can call for treatment if there is evidence of organ damage.

Most criteria for the drug therapy of hypertension depends on the diastolic (lower) readings. For years, in fact, the systolic (higher) number was nearly overlooked in formulating a treatment plan. Recently, however, it has become clear that systolic pressures are also important. For example, a major 1991 study evaluated 4,736 people over 60 who had normal diastolic but high systolic pressures. Over a five-year period treatment reduced the risk of stroke by 36 percent, providing protection against heart disease as well. Side effects were relatively infrequent. In light of these findings — and others — my treatment criteria have changed; your doctor's decisions may also change.

Numerical criteria are essential; still, the decision to treat hypertension should be based not on numbers alone but on a careful, comprehensive medical evaluation. The variability of human biology mandates an individualized decision rather than a cookbook — or even a textbook — approach. This is no less true for the choice of medication: an individualized, stepwise approach is best.

With so many hypertensive patients and so many factors involved in the control of blood pressure, it should not surprise you that there are many medications available to treat hypertension — dozens and dozens, in fact. At times the multiplicity of medicines constitutes an embarrassment of riches. It's all but impossible to master the advantages and liabilities of all these drugs; instead, I try to become familiar with a few representative medications from each family of drugs so that I can use them well.

The oldest effective antihypertensive medications are the diuretics, which rid the body of salt and water. Low in cost, they are the traditional mainstays of treatment. But most diuretics also deplete the body of potassium, and recent research shows that they can increase LDL ("bad") cholesterol and blood sugar levels. While still valuable, diuretics are no longer the automatic first choice for treatment.

Another class of medications are the vasodilators — drugs that act directly on arteries to relax their wall tension, thus opening them up. Some vasodilators are old favorites, others newcomers; all can be very helpful.

The beta blockers were the most popular antihypertensives of the 1970s and early 80s. These agents slow the heart and open vascular channels. Many patients respond beautifully to these drugs, but others note side effects, and these drugs can also raise cholesterol levels.

The most exciting medications for high blood pressure in the late 1980s and early 90s are the calcium channel blockers, which reduce blood pressure by acting on the heart and arteries, and the ACE inhibitors, which block the production of a hormone that increases blood pressure. These medications have fewer side effects, and, despite their greater cost, they are often first off the shelf today.

Each of these drug families contains many individual preparations, and new ones are being developed every year. The relative merit of these many pills is the object of extensive research and the subject of hot debate; combination therapy adds to the complexity and controversy. But amidst all this, many doctors lose sight of an important fact: these marvelous medications are not the only way to treat hypertension — and in many cases they are not the best way.

Life-Style Treatment

The easiest way to treat hypertension is to take a pill; the best way is to achieve life-style modification; diet, weight reduction, exercise, stress reduction, moderation of alcohol use, and smoking cessation should be at the core of every treatment plan. And for many patients with mild or even moderate hypertension, the preventive life-style may be all that's needed to restore blood pressure to normal.

Several recent head-to-head trials prove that life-style modification can reduce blood pressure every bit as well as medication, with fewer side effects and with many other benefits to body and mind. For example, doctors in Maryland compared the results of exercise alone with two of the most widely used antihypertension medications, propranol (a beta blocker) and diltiazem (a calcium channel blocker). The men on medication improved more rapidly, but by the end of seven weeks the men who were being treated simply with exercise had caught up. The average readings in all three groups fell from 145/97 to 131/84; in less than two months, two and one half hours of exercise per week completely controlled hypertension without drugs.

Many other trials of exercise, weight loss, and diet have demonstrated that life-style modification is as effective for treating hypertension as it is for prevention. Despite these results, most physicians neglect nonmedicinal treatment. And it's easy to see why: medical training stresses cure over prevention, the sophisticated over the simple, the doctor's role over the patient's.

If you have high blood pressure, your treatment should be chosen after a careful medical evaluation and a detailed consultation between your doctors and yourself. If your physicians neglect life-style therapy, don't hesitate to remind them. One of the very best things about medical practice is that doctors can learn something from patients every day.

■ Diseases of the Arteries

Your arteries are channels that carry blood from your heart to your tissues. More than passive canals, they have muscle in their walls, both for strength and to allow them to narrow and widen, distributing blood to the tissues that need it most. The middle muscular layer of the arterial wall is surrounded by an outer layer of fibrous tissue, providing additional support and strength.

Although the muscular and fibrous layers are very important, it's the inner layer of the arterial wall that is most vulnerable to disease. This thin, smooth lining is called the *endothelium*. Because the endothelial cells are in constant contact with the blood stream, they can be damaged by harmful elements in the blood; LDL cholesterol and the toxins from cigarette smoke are the leading culprits. High blood pressure, too, can accelerate damage to the endothelial cell walls.

Does this sound familiar? It should. The factors that can damage the arteries throughout your body are exactly the same ones that may damage your coronary arteries, leading to heart attacks. And because your brain depends on healthy arteries to supply its needs, these same factors figure in creating stroke.

Arterial Disease

The major threat to every artery in the body is atherosclerosis. LDL cholesterol enters the artery wall and builds up into plaques. Arteries that have been damaged by high blood pressure, smoking, or diabetes are particularly vulnerable to this process. The diseased arteries are hard on the outside; because they are brittle, they may rupture. On the inside, soft cheesy material lines these arteries; bits of it can break off, traveling downstream to clog smaller channels. The plaques themselves may enlarge enough to block the artery, or they can trigger clots that produce blockages.

Atherosclerotic narrowing of the arteries is, by a substantial margin, the most common of these problems. More frequent in men, arterial disease increases with age, becoming so common that 12 to 15 percent of Americans over 50 have the disease. At first arterial disease produces no symptoms. As plaques enlarge, however, they begin to limit blood flow. Because muscles have a much greater need for blood during exercise, painful muscle cramps can occur during exertion. Since atherosclerosis is much more common in leg arteries, calf cramps during walking are the most common complaints. Called intermittent claudication, these cramps can sometimes affect the thighs or buttocks. In addition, many men with arterial disease develop impotence, also as a result of diminished tissue blood supply.

If atherosclerosis progresses, tissues will begin to feel the lack of oxygen even at rest. Rest pain is bad enough, but because tissue nutrition suffers, the affected leg may become cold and white with thin, shiny skin; eventually the disease can lead to infection and gangrene. In fact, arterial disease in diabetics accounts for half of all amputations.

In some cases the walls of an artery that has been damaged by atherosclerosis can weaken and stretch, eventually ballooning out to form an aneurysm. Patients with high blood pressure are particularly vulnerable to this complication. Although aneurysms cause no symptoms when they begin, they can be painful if they enlarge rapidly or get very large. Aneurysms occur most often in the body's main artery, the *aorta*; the lower aorta is more often afflicted than in the upper part, so abdominal and back pain are more common than chest pain. Unfortunately, the first symptom can be the most disastrous; aneurysms can suddenly rupture, producing shock and death unless expert surgical repair is available immediately.

Preventing Arterial Disease

If you've read chapter 2, you already know how to prevent arterial disease. The same life-style changes that protect you from coronary artery disease can and will prevent arterial disease. These precepts, though simple, are important enough to warrant repetition. Lower your LDL cholesterol by eating less saturated fat and cholesterol. Raise your HDL cholesterol by exercising regularly. Be sure your diet includes lots of vegetables and fruits rich in fiber and vitamins, as well as plenty of fish. Restrict calories, if necessary, to fight obesity. Unless your blood pressure is already low-normal, restrict your salt intake. Don't smoke, ever. Reduce excessive mental stress. If you have diabetes, get treatment to lower your blood sugar.

Treating Arterial Disease

Even if you have vascular disease that has progressed far enough to produce symptoms, you can prevent complications.

Various medicines are prescribed to relax artery walls or to smooth the flow of blood through narrowed passages. They sound great, but they don't work. Even anticlotting drugs don't seem to help for arterial disease. Aspirin is the exception. Its benefits, though, are restricted to the arteries of the heart and brain; it does not seem to protect the body's other arteries.

Narrowed arteries in the legs can be opened physically. First, the narrowing should be documented with Doppler ultrasound tests; angiograms are generally used to confirm the findings. Balloons can be used to compress plaques, opening arteries and restoring blood flow. Lasers show promise in accomplishing the same goal. Finally, surgeons can bypass blockages using vein grafts or synthetic fabrics. But all these treatments can have complications, so they should be used only if symptoms significantly impair the quality of life or the integrity of tissues.

Aneurysms can be treated only by surgical repair. The stakes are high: rupture is often fatal. Unfortunately, the surgery itself is quite risky. In general, small aneurysms (less than five inches in the chest or two and a half inches in the abdomen) are best left alone unless they enlarge or cause symptoms. Ultrasound and magnetic resonance imaging (MRI) techniques provide excellent tools to measure the size of aneurysms and to watch for enlargement.

High-technology surgical treatments have provided enormous benefits to patients with arterial disease. Still, the role of simple nonoperative treatments must never be overlooked. Even something as humble as good foot care can prevent infections, sometimes avoiding the need for surgery. Smoking cessation can actually improve blood flow. And because exercise improves oxygen utilization by muscles, walking programs can reduce the symptoms of arterial disease.

Ultimately, of course, arterial disease is but one sign of a more basic problem — atherosclerosis. So even patients who feel great after their arteries have been bypassed should go back to the basics, to the risk-factor modifications and life-style changes that fight atherosclerosis.

■ Diseases of the Veins

At last we come to a part of the body that's not vulnerable to atherosclerosis. As thin-walled, low-pressure blood vessels, veins are much more prone to mechanical disorders. Though common, unsightly, and uncomfortable, these problems are much less serious than diseases of the heart and arteries; still, some can pose serious, even life-threatening, health hazards.

Several problems can affect veins. Because they are thin-walled and delicate, they can easily stretch out of shape. Veins depend on filmy valves to keep blood flowing in the right direction, toward the heart; when they stretch, their valves no longer close properly. Blood flow slows, overfilling the vein so it balloons out even more. Finally, veins are a low-pressure system that depends on the contractions of muscles to propel blood back to the heart. In the absence of adequate muscle pumping, blood can stagnate and clots can form, producing the most serious of all venous diseases.

The veins in your lower body, particularly your legs, are the most vulnerable to these problems. The reason: gravity. Whether you're standing or sitting, your leg veins have to carry your blood up to your heart against the force of gravity. It's an uphill fight; without proper prevention, your veins can lose the struggle, and your health can suffer.

Varicose Veins

Varicose veins are nothing more than stretched-out veins that have faulty valves and contain excessive volumes of blood. Because they are so visible, superficial varicosities — swollen veins just beneath the skin's surface — get the most attention. Superficial varicose veins are unsightly, and they can cause some mild aching. Even so, varicosities of the deep veins hidden in the calf and thigh are much more risky to health.

You can help prevent varicose veins by promoting the flow of blood in your leg veins.

Increased pressure in the abdomen can slow the flow of blood coming up from the legs, eventually producing varicosities. Pregnancy greatly increases abdominal pressure, which is why varicose veins are more common in women than in men. Obesity, too, increases abdominal pressure, so weight control can help prevent varicose veins. Finally, because straining raises abdominal pressure, a high-fiber diet that prevents constipation can help protect your veins.

Because blood flow in leg veins depends on pumping by leg muscles, exercise also helps prevent varicose veins. From the vantage point of your veins, if not your heart, aerobic intensity doesn't count. Anything that gets your muscles working will keep your blood flowing; walking will do just fine.

Standing also taxes your leg veins. If your job requires prolonged standing, try to walk about as much as possible; just lifting yourself up on your toes can help. It's also a good idea to flex your legs while you're sitting. Good, strong support stockings are another asset, helping your muscles pump blood out of your veins; your heart will get the blood it needs, and your leg veins will stay slender and straight.

Superficial varicosities can be a cosmetic problem; still, serious consequences are rare. If varicose veins are bothersome to you, discuss injections or vein-stripping operations with your doctor. Unfortunately, deep varicosities, which can lead to fluid accumulation and clotting, cannot be repaired.

Leg Swelling and Discoloration

Severely stretched veins, particularly deep varicosities, can allow fluid to accumulate in the legs. This fluid, called *edema*, produces an uncomfortable sensation of pressure and can increase the risk of skin infection. Over time a brown or purple discoloration of the skin may develop; in advanced cases the skin may ulcerate.

To prevent these problems, follow the program designed to prevent varicose veins from occurring in the first place. Several extra measures may also help. If you tend to accumulate edema fluid, put your feet up on a hassock while you're sitting, helping to reduce the pull of gravity. In addition, restrict your salt intake to help prevent your kidneys from retaining fluid. If these measures fail, discuss diuretic medications with your doctor.

Thrombophlebitis

A fierce name — and a fierce disease as well.

In this case the fancy medical terminology is easily deciphered and helps explain the nature of the problem. A thrombus is a clot, *phleb* is the Greek root for vein, and *-itis* simply signifies inflammation. So *thrombophlebitis* is a condition in which clots form in veins, and the veins become inflamed.

Thrombophlebitis is one condition that has received its share of preventive effort by the medical community — with good results. Thrombophlebitis is a major complication of hospital care. Medical patients who are kept at bed rest to treat heart conditions and other problems are at high risk. Surgical patients, particularly those recovering from hip, back, prostate, and gynecological surgery, are at even higher risk. The consequences can be disastrous. Blood clots can break off from the leg or pelvic veins and travel to the lungs, where they produce chest pain and shortness of breath. This complication, called pulmonary embolism, can be fatal.

Treating thrombophlebitis with medications that dissolve clots protects against pulmonary embolism. The trick is to detect thrombophlebitis, and it's a tough trick indeed. Superficial thrombophlebitis produces pain, redness, and swelling, which are easy to discover. But superficial thrombophlebitis is rarely serious, and does not ordinarily lead to embolization. In contrast, deep vein thrombophlebitis is often clinically silent but can lead to embolization.

A variety of medical tests including venograms, scans, Doppler ultrasound, and special compression studies can be used to diagnose deep vein thrombophlebitis, allowing early treatment. But the best treatment of all is prevention. Hospitalized patients are now mobilized as early as possible; the simple process of walking has been a great help in preventing clot formation. For bedridden patients, foot and ankle exercises and high-quality elastic stockings can help. But even these measures are not enough for the patients at highest risk. As a result, doctors now prescribe special pneumatic compression stockings or low-dose anticlotting medications to prevent thrombophlebitis in hospitalized patients at high risk. The results have been excellent; before these preventive measures were available, pulmonary embolisms occurred in 60 percent of patients who died in hospitals, but the percentage has decreased appreciably.

I am, of course, glad to report that the prevention of thrombophlebitis has become a standard part of the care of hospitalized patients. But does this apply to you? Indeed it does. Some of the factors that cause thrombophlebitis in hospital patients can also cause it in healthy people, and some of the same preventive measures can help.

Obesity can contribute to thrombophlebitis, so try to stay lean. Pregnancy is another possible factor. During pregnancy women should restrict dietary salt, keep moving, elevate their legs while sitting, and consider wearing elastic stockings. Oral contraceptive pills have also been contributing factors; the low-estrogen pills are much safer, but women should discuss the pros and cons of alternate birth control methods with their doctors.

The leading cause of thrombophlebitis, however, is immobilization. The classic scenario is the cross-country bus trip that terminates with sudden death caused by a pulmonary embolism. Grim, but not far-fetched. Even in this jet age, prolonged sitting can lead to thrombophlebitis. Don't let it happen to you. Get up and walk in the aisles of your airplane or train. Stop your car every few hours to walk around. While you are sitting, flex and extend your feet every few minutes to keep your blood circulating. Consider elastic stockings if you have to stand or sit still for long periods.

Can aspirin help? I'm not sure. Aspirin is effective in preventing clots in arteries. But in these high-pressure, high-flow vessels, platelets are the key to clot formation, so the clots themselves have a characteristic white appearance and firm consistency. Platelets are not nearly as instrumental in the clots that form in low-pressure, low-flow veins; instead a blood protein called *fibrinogen* starts the clotting process, and the clots that result have a red color and loose texture. Because of these differences, aspirin has not been effective in preventing thrombophlebitis in high-risk hospital patients. But it has helped in low-risk patients. Aspirin has not been studied for the prevention of thrombophlebitis in healthy people; certainly I would not recommend long-term aspirin use for this purpose. Unless you have some reason to avoid aspirin, however, you might consider one tablet a day during periods when you are unavoidably immobile.

Even if you can't count on medication to prevent thrombophlebitis, you can rely on simple common sense measures to keep your veins healthy. Start with a stroll. You *can* walk away from diseases of the veins.

∎ 4 ∎

Stroke and Other Neurological Disorders

Humankind occupies a unique place in the animal kingdom. For millennia, poets, philosophers, and theologians have debated the ultimate source of our singular status, with anthropologists and evolutionary biologists joining the discussion much more recently. Some argue we owe our special place to the soul, while others trace it all to a prehensile thumb. Without venturing to reconcile these camps, I have my own candidate: the brain.

At less than three pounds, this small organ has awesome abilities. And just as humans are unique in the world, so are our brains unique among our organs. The brain is one of our busiest, most metabolically active structures. Although it accounts for less than 2 percent of body weight, the brain accounts for 15 percent of the body's total blood flow, 25 percent of its oxygen utilization, and fully 70 percent of its glucose (sugar) consumption.

∎ The Normal Brain: Vulnerable but Protected

The brain has unique metabolic requirements. Unlike other organs, it cannot store its own supply of energy. Instead it depends entirely on a constant flow of blood to supply it with nutrients. Other organs can metabolize fat or protein for energy, but the brain relies entirely on glucose from the blood. Unlike other tissues that can regenerate and heal after injury, brain cells cannot repair themselves.

This constant reliance on glucose, oxygen, and blood flow, coupled with the delicate nature of brain cells and their inability to repair damage, renders the brain uniquely vulnerable to illness and injury. Fortunately, the body does have some built-in protective mechanisms. The small arteries that supply blood to the brain can widen or narrow as needed to ensure a constant flow of blood. This phenomenon, called autoregulation, means that the brain will receive all the blood it needs, but no more, at blood pressure levels all the way from 50 to 150. The small blood vessels within the brain can also autoregulate the flow to bring more blood to the brain cells that are working hardest. I presume, for example, that my thinking centers are getting a bit more nutrition right now. Similarly, cerebral blood vessels open up to admit more blood whenever carbon dioxide builds up in the circulation, another way to ensure a steady supply of oxygen. Marvelous mechanisms, indeed, but they require healthy blood vessels to function properly.

Since the brain depends on glucose for all its metabolic activities, it has a special apparatus to pump sugar from the blood into the spinal fluid. Because brain cells are so delicate, there is also a functional blood-brain barrier that keeps toxins in the blood from crossing into brain tissue. These protective mechanisms, too, can be thwarted by disease, such as infection. Moreover, we have created many new toxins that did not exist when evolution was engineering the blood-brain barrier.

Because the brain is so vulnerable to trauma and injury, protection is provided in the form of a hard skull. In addition, a layer of spinal fluid surrounds the central nervous system, cushioning it from impact. Here, too, the brain's intellectual achievements have diminished the efficacy of its protective systems; the skull was not designed to withstand the impact imparted by high-velocity vehicles and missiles. Fortunately, we can supplement genetics with helmets, seat belts, and common sense; unfortunately, these preventive measures are frequently ignored just when they're needed most.

■ The Normal Nervous System

The brain is composed of a densely packed network of more than 10 billion nerve cells, along with vital supporting tissues and blood vessels. For proper function each element must be healthy, and all must work together. The existence of a well-coordinated network of nerve cells allows groups of cells to assume specialized functions not shared by other cells. Cells with similar functions are found near one another occupying discrete but very small areas within the brain. Hence, the group of cells responsible for motion are found together in a motion center, the cells for speech in a speech center, and so forth. Because the cells performing a given function are so close together, a very small amount of damage can completely disrupt a particular function. Despite this loss, other functions may remain intact; a stroke victim, for example, may be able to feel pain in the left arm but not move that arm, to read but not count, to breathe but not think. Since brain cells cannot regenerate, the loss of function may be permanent if cell death has occurred; sometimes, though, other cells can learn to take on new roles, particularly in young patients.

The nerve cells in the brain send out long projections linking them to cells in the spinal cord. In turn, nerve cells in the spinal cord send out projections to all the body's tissues, where they control movement, sensation, and other neurological functions. The brain cell projections cross over from one side to the other as they descend to the spinal column; hence, cells on the left side of the brain are responsible for movement and sensation on the right side of the body, and conversely.

Although movement and sensation are equally represented in the two sides of the brain, other functions are not. One hemisphere of the brain is considered dominant because it contains the centers for language and speech. In most people the left hemisphere is dominant, but in some left-handed people speech and language centers are in the right side of the brain.

The nerve cells in the brain and spinal cord constitute the *central nervous system*. Nerve cells in the rest of the body are known as the *peripheral nervous system*. These cells, which can regenerate if their projections are injured, are subdivided into the *somatic nervous system*, responsible for movement and sensation, and the *autonomic nervous system*, responsible for temperature regulation, bowel, bladder, and sexual function, and blood pressure control.

All these neurological details seem terribly complex, but don't let them make you nervous. In fact, although not all neurological disorders are preventable, you can protect yourself from the major diseases with very simple measures.

■ Stroke

Stroke is the most common major neurological disease, affecting 500,000 Americans each year. Your chance of having a stroke before age 70 is one in 20; with prevention, however, you can greatly improve your odds.

Stroke is one of the most serious neurological diseases; one quarter of its victims are dead within a month. In all, stroke kills 150,000 Americans each year, making it the third leading cause of death. Ninety percent of survivors have permanent impairments; in half these are major disabilities. These disabilities impose enormous burdens on family and community; more than $7 billion is spent each year to care for our 2 million stroke survivors.

Though common and serious, stroke is also the most preventable neurological disease. The popular term *stroke* is derived from a Middle English word meaning blow or sudden attack. Indeed, most wreak their havoc very abruptly. Even so, many strokes are preceded by warning symptoms; if these symptoms are recognized in time, medical treatment can often prevent the actual blow from falling.

The medical term for stroke, *cerebrovascular accident*, informs us that disorders of the blood vessels are responsible for stroke, but implies that they are unforeseeable events. On the contrary, strokes are not random events but are predictable; by knowing what causes strokes, you can prevent them. And prevention *does* work: deaths from stroke in the United States have declined by 50 percent since 1972, largely owing to treatment of hypertension. Despite this progress, we still have a long way to go; still, you can take steps to reduce substantially your risk of stroke.

What Is a Stroke?

A stroke results from an interruption of the brain's blood flow. It is thus a manifestation of blood vessel disease, the cerebral equivalent of a heart

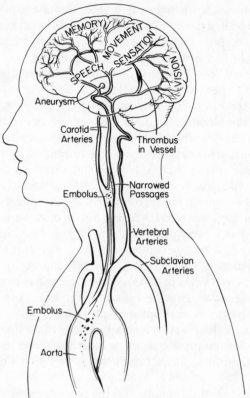

**Figure 4-1.
Brain circulation**

attack. Like heart attacks, which can be signaled by the warning pain of angina, there can be warning symptoms prior to strokes. These are called *transient ischemic attacks* (TIAs) because the culprit is ischemia, or lack of blood flow, and because the interruption of circulation is brief, so that brain cells survive and recover full function within 24 hours. But if the brain's blood supply is interrupted for a longer period, cell death occurs and the loss of function is permanent. This event, whether limited in extent or disastrous in impact, is a stroke.

The blood supply of the brain can be interrupted in either of two ways: by a blockage within an artery or by the rupture of an artery's wall. Hence, there are two main types of stroke (see figure 4-1). Strokes caused by vascular blockage are more common; strokes due to hemorrhage (bleeding) are more serious, with death rates exceeding 50 percent. Paradoxically, patients who survive hemorrhagic strokes often recover function more completely than do survivors of strokes caused by blockages.

Strokes Caused by Blockages

The brain's arteries can become blocked in two ways. More often blockage results from *thrombosis*, or clot formation. Cerebral thrombosis is similar to the coronary thrombosis that causes heart attacks: atherosclerosis damages an artery's wall, producing cholesterol plaques that serve as the focus for clot formation. But clots can also form in blood vessels far from the brain. If a remote clot breaks apart, a fragment can travel to the brain, plugging the circulation. This type of stroke, called an *embolic* stroke, accounts for about 15 percent of all strokes.

Thrombotic strokes occur most often during sleep or first thing in the morning, when the blood pressure is low and the circulation through partially blocked arteries is sluggish. Because the clot grows slowly, the symptoms of thrombotic strokes typically evolve gradually, increasing in a stepwise fashion over several hours. Neurological deficits that begin during sleep don't provide much warning, but TIAs precede about half of all thrombotic strokes, giving hours, days, or weeks of advance warning. And strokes can often be prevented if action is taken during this warning phase.

Embolic strokes typically occur abruptly, generally during the waking hours, when people are physically active. Although embolic strokes themselves are very sudden, warning TIAs precede the stroke itself in 15 or 20 percent of cases. Even without TIAs, cerebral emboli can often be predicted by understanding the underlying causes. Often the cause is heart disease. Heart attacks produce scars that may allow clots to form. A disorder of the heart rhythm, called atrial fibrillation, interrupts the regular contractions of the smaller pumping chambers, allowing blood to stagnate so clots are formed. In addition, disorders of the heart valves can promote clot formation.

The other major source of emboli is the large arteries that lead from the heart to the brain. Here atherosclerosis is to blame; plaques can lead to clotting, or part of a plaque itself can break off, traveling to the brain as an embolus composed of cholesterol particles.

Strokes Caused by Bleeding

Whereas warning symptoms often alert patients that they may be at risk for thrombotic or embolic strokes, no such warnings precede hemorrhagic strokes. Strokes caused by bleeding typically begin abruptly with an extremely severe headache. Within less than an hour major neurological impairments are evident, often including coma. Although hemorrhagic strokes are very serious, medical and surgical treatments are starting to improve the outlook. Because many of the symptoms are caused by brain swelling and pressure on cells rather than cell death, many patients who survive make remarkable recoveries.

Healthy blood vessels do not bleed; before rupturing and causing strokes, they are first damaged by high blood pressure or their walls are weakened by aneurysms. Aneurysms are very hard to predict, but high blood pressure is easily detected, and treatment can prevent many strokes.

Rarer Causes of Stroke

Although the great majority of strokes are caused by thrombosis, embolization, or hemorrhage, there are other, rarer causes of stroke. Like the atherosclerosis and high blood pressure that lead to ordinary strokes, some of these uncommon problems can be prevented. One example is the constellation of migraine headaches, use of birth control pills, and smoking; if all three are present together, young women can suffer strokes. Prevention is straightforward: women with migraines probably should not take the pill, and they surely should not smoke. Other uncommon but preventable causes of stroke include infections and drug abuse.

It's important for doctors to understand all the causes of stroke and to deal with them appropriately. But for you, the important thing is to understand how to prevent the major types of stroke.

TIAs: Warnings That Precede Strokes

TIAs (transient ischemic attacks) are the warning symptoms of thrombotic and embolic strokes.

There are many types of TIAs. When the carotid artery (see figure 4-1) is the source, a common symptom is temporary blindness of the eye on the same side as the blockage. Other patients with diseases of the carotid or the smaller vessels it supplies experience weakness, numbness, and tingling, or even paralysis on the side of the body opposite the blockage. In still other cases, loss of speech is the warning symptom. When the vertebral artery (see figure 4-1) is the source, the symptoms are different and may include dim vision in both eyes, double vision, slurring of speech, loss of memory, dizziness and falling, or loss of consciousness.

In all cases the symptoms of TIAs are brief; many resolve within minutes, most within hours, and all within 24 hours. In fact, if the symptoms persist for more than a day, the cause is a stroke rather than a TIA.

Don't wait to have a stroke. If you think you may be having a TIA, see your doctor at once. Because the symptoms are so variable, you cannot make the diagnosis yourself; often a neurologist is needed and special tests are required to evaluate the arteries and the heart. The stakes are high; about a third of all patients with TIAs recover spontaneously, but another third continue to have TIAs, and the final third go on to have actual strokes. Many of these strokes can be prevented if TIAs are treated properly. Although your doctor will have to direct this treatment, I'll discuss the basic options shortly.

Preventing Strokes

Neurologists have made great strides in understanding how strokes occur. Radiologists have made spectacular advances in their ability to produce images of the brain and its blood vessels. Therapists contribute invaluable skills to the medical and nursing efforts that can rehabilitate many stroke patients. And surgeons are now able to correct some of the blood vessel abnormalities that cause strokes.

All this progress is wonderful. But many of the most accomplished neurologists, neuroradiologists, and neurosurgeons overlook the crucial fact that their sophisticated skills are needed so frequently only because people overlook the simple steps that can prevent strokes.

It may surprise you to learn that the most important predictor of stroke is the presence of coronary artery disease. The reason: both stroke and heart disease are blood vessel diseases, caused by atherosclerosis and hypertension. And so the preventive measures I discussed in chapters 2 and 3 are also the keys to stroke prevention. For good measure, let's review them briefly.

High blood pressure is the most important stroke risk factor, accounting for one third of all stroke deaths. The risk of stroke is directly proportional to blood pressure: the higher your pressure, the higher your risk. We've known for years that this relationship pertains to diastolic blood pressure, and we now know that it's just as valid for systolic blood pressure. In all, if your blood pressure is higher than 160/95, your risk of stroke will increase more than fourfold. Prevent or treat high blood pressure and you'll go a long way toward preventing stroke. Millions have, which is why deaths from stroke have been cut in half since medications for high blood pressure were introduced in the 1950s. Blood pressure pills have been enormously beneficial, but you can do even better by using diet (especially salt restriction and weight reduction), aerobic exercise, and stress reduction to improve your blood pressure.

High cholesterol levels are to blame for many strokes. A recent investigation of more than 350,000 men dramatizes this fact. All were healthy at the start of the study; during just six years of observation, the men with high cholesterol levels had three times more strokes than did men with normal cholesterol levels. Enough said.

Smoking is responsible for nearly one quarter of all strokes. Smoking causes atherosclerosis. It also increases red blood cell counts, blood viscosity (a measure of sluggish flow or blood "thickness"), and platelet stickiness, all of which can lead to clotting. If that were not enough, smoking lowers blood oxygen levels. Each of these factors contributes to stroke; together they explain why smokers have nearly three times more strokes than nonsmokers. Happily, people who quit smoking reduce their stroke risk by 50 percent.

Sedentary living also contributes to the risk of stroke, but as usual it receives much less attention than the other risk factors. Regular aerobic exercise reduces blood pressure and helps prevent atherosclerosis by improving cholesterol levels. Exercise also reduces blood viscosity and platelet stickiness while enhancing the body's clot-dissolving mechanisms. In view of all this, exercise should protect against strokes — and it does. Confirmation comes from the famed Institute for Aerobic Research in Dallas, where more than 8,000 people, both men and women, were studied. The least physically fit subjects had nearly three times the stroke rate as the most fit individuals; intermediate fitness produced intermediate risk. Tennis strokes can help prevent neurological strokes.

In addition to the Big Four of stroke risk, there are other important risk factors, including diabetes, obesity, gender (male), advancing age, and a family history of stroke. A familiar list, because these are just the same factors that predict heart disease. The moral: protect your heart and you'll protect your head!

Another risk factor that you can control is *alcohol abuse*. Drinking increases the risk of thrombotic and hemorrhagic strokes in middle age, probably because alcohol increases blood pressure. Abstinence reduces the likelihood of stroke — one of many good reasons to limit your drinking to two a day or less.

Although the primary prevention of vascular disease is the same for arteries in the heart and the brain, there are some unique issues in the secondary and tertiary prevention of strokes. These are areas of substantial debate and controversy, but in the final analysis my recommendations depend on the basics of atherosclerosis even more than the particulars of neurological disorders.

Secondary Prevention of Stroke

Secondary prevention is the prevention of disease after it has already started but before it produces any symptoms. Secondary prevention for coronary heart disease is difficult because there is no good screening test to detect asymptomatic disease. Secondary prevention for hypertension is easy because blood pressure is readily measured, and abnormalities can be treated effectively long before blood vessels are damaged. Secondary prevention for stroke is much more controversial. Screening is easy, but treatment based on that screening can be difficult.

The carotid artery (see figure 4-1) is at the center of the controversy. You can feel the pulse of blood flowing through the artery simply by placing a finger on your neck over your right or left carotid. Your doctor can listen to blood flowing through this artery just as easily by placing a stethoscope over the artery. And neurologists can measure the diameter of the artery with great precision simply by placing an ultrasound or Doppler probe on the vessel.

Atherosclerosis narrows arteries. Narrowing produces turbulent blood flow. Like white water in a bubbling brook, turbulent flow in a vessel is noisy. Your doctor can hear that noise, called a *bruit*, by listening over your carotid artery. If a bruit is present, as it is in about 1 million Americans, you can have a risk-free ultrasound to find out if the narrowing is severe. If so, you can have an operation called an endarterectomy intended to open the artery so you won't have a stroke.

It sounds simple. It is a common sequence of events in clinical medicine. But it's not really so simple, and, in my view, it shouldn't be routine medical practice.

Listening for a carotid bruit is easy, but it's not a specific predictor of carotid narrowing. In fact, bruits occur about half the time in vessels with good blood flow. But a carotid can be very narrow indeed without producing a bruit.

Measuring the diameter of a carotid artery, in contrast, is very accurate. Many techniques are available. Doppler, ultrasound, and duplex scans are used most often; they are reliable and risk-free. But they cost about $200, and many patients are given the alarming news that these studies show 60 or 70 percent narrowing. In fact, strokes are uncommon unless the channel is narrower than about 1 millimeter. In addition, angiograms are used to confirm severe narrowing, and they are risky, with complications that may include bleeding, kidney failure, allergic reactions, or even strokes.

Surgery is the most controversial procedure of all. More than 100,000 carotid endarterectomies were performed in 1985, making it the third most common operation in the United States. But even in expert hands, these operations are difficult and dangerous, and I'm sorry to say there are probably more endarterectomies done than there are expert hands to do them. Studies evaluating the risks and benefits of carotid surgery have produced conflicting results; the latest studies suggest that surgery is helpful for patients who have had symptoms caused by severe carotid narrowing, but studies of asymptomatic narrowing are still in progress.

Both patients and doctors have been taught to value a complete physical exam. Listening for carotid bruits is a time-honored part of that complete physical. Your doctor has probably listened to your carotids many times over the years. But both the Canadian Task Force on the Periodic Health Exam and the U.S. Preventive Services Task Force recommend *against* this traditional procedure.

Do I listen to carotid arteries? Not routinely. I listen to my patients first, and will listen to their carotids only if they tell me about symptoms of TIAs that suggest carotid disease.

What if I see a patient who has already been found to have an asymptomatic carotid bruit? I don't call a neurosurgeon. I don't even order an ultrasound or Doppler. Instead I view the bruit as just one potential sign of atherosclerosis. I evaluate risk factors and stress primary prevention. I follow the patient closely for emerging evidence of both heart disease and TIAs. And I consider the use of aspirin. I admit that there is no evidence that aspirin is useful to prevent strokes in *asymptomatic* patients, but it does prevent heart attacks even in asymptomatic patients. In addition, aspirin is very useful for preventing strokes in patients who have TIAs.

Tertiary Prevention of Stroke

Tertiary prevention is designed to halt the progression of a disease after symptoms have appeared. Patients with warning symptoms, or TIAs, *can* prevent strokes, as can patients who are at high risk because of heart disease. Because this tertiary prevention requires a doctor's care and individualized therapy, I'll present just the broad outlines here.

TIAs are caused by small clots or emboli that dissolve in time to restore blood flow before brain cells are killed. But about one third of patients with TIAs go on to have strokes, usually within six months of the first TIA. What can be done to prevent this?

If the TIAs reflect disease in the vertebral artery system (see figure 4-1), the only option is medication to reduce clotting. Traditionally patients are hospitalized, treated with injections of heparin, and then returned home to continue therapy with warfarin (Coumadin) tablets. The results are quite good, but warfarin poses an appreciable risk of bleeding, and blood tests must be done every two or three weeks to check on dosage. More recent trials have evaluated aspirin therapy, and the results have been encouraging. Additional studies with aspirin and related antiplatelet drugs are under way, but at present most neurologists recommend simply one aspirin tablet per day.

TIAs related to the carotid artery circulation are more problematic because the options include both medical and surgical treatment. Until recently most neurologists tended to recommend aspirin, whereas most neurosurgeons tend to recommend carotid clean-out operations (endarterectomies). But a careful head-to-head trial of operations versus aspirin treatment now suggests that patients whose TIAs are caused by severely narrowed carotid arteries do better with surgery. In general, surgery will be recommended if the carotid narrowing is severe (70 percent or greater) and the patient is otherwise healthy enough to get through the operation. As a rule, carotid endarterectomies should be performed in specialized centers with lots of experience and complication rates under 4 percent.

The final scenario for tertiary prevention relates not to patients with neurological symptoms but to patients with heart disease. Remember from chapter 2 that the heart has four pumping chambers. The two smaller chambers, the atria, supply only 15 percent of the total pumping power; the larger ventricles must contract regularly to support life, but most patients can get along very well without regular atrial contractions, a condition called atrial fibrillation. But when the atria quiver instead of pumping, clots may build up in the stagnant blood. These clots can break apart, releasing emboli that can lodge in any of the body's arteries. When an artery in the brain is blocked temporarily, the result is a TIA; when the blockage is prolonged, a stroke occurs.

Patients with atrial fibrillation are five times more likely to suffer strokes than are people with normal heart rhythms. It's a big problem: more than 1 million Americans — about 3 percent of all people over 60 — have atrial fibrillation. But even in these high-risk patients, strokes can be prevented.

The standard preventive treatment for patients with atrial fibrillation ("quivering") is warfarin. Warfarin therapy, however, requires careful monitoring to prevent complications. A 1990 European investigation of more than 1,200 patients with atrial fibrillation revealed good results for patients under 75 with another anticlotting medication: yes, it's our old friend aspirin. It's too early to recommend aspirin for every patient with atrial fibrillation, much less add it to the drinking water. But it's a logical treatment, and I have begun to offer it to selected patients as we await more data for head-to-head comparisons with warfarin.

Needless to say, all patients with TIAs and heart disease must also treat their underlying disease, atherosclerosis, with life-style modification and, often, prescription drugs. One precaution: blood pressure control can be tricky. Patients with diseased cerebral arteries can require relatively high pressures to maintain blood flow, but high pressures can cause further damage to the blood vessels and heart. It's a balancing act, which is why patients with this dilemma need to have a good doctor.

■ Other Neurological Diseases

Because of its delicacy, the nervous system is vulnerable to many diseases. Because of its crucial functions, even small insults to the nervous system can have major ramifications. Because of their complexity, neurological disorders are often difficult to diagnose and treat — much less prevent. Even so, prevention can help. And when it comes to your brain (or mine) every little bit of help is welcome indeed.

Trauma

Catastrophic injuries are responsible for more than 2.3 million hospitalizations and 150,000 deaths in the United States each year. Since many of those fatalities involve brain or spinal cord damage, we could argue that trauma ranks just below stroke as the leading neurological killer. And trauma produces many nonlethal neurological injuries, including 325,000 head injuries that consume more than $1 billion in hospital costs annually. More than 40 percent of head injuries are caused by motor vehicle accidents, with falls and assaults in second and third place.

Is trauma a neurological problem? Many would dispute this classification, pointing out that a 2,000-pound automobile is the cause rather than a three-pound brain. My reply: it's true that accidents are caused by primary neurological derangements only rarely. But they are very often caused by derangements of the brain's highest function — human behavior.

Accidents can be prevented. And even when unavoidable trauma occurs, damage to the nervous system (and other body parts) can often be minimized by preventive measures. Chapter 17 deals with these issues.

Infections

The nervous system can be devastated by a variety of infections, many of which are preventable.

Several types of bacteria can produce meningitis, which is always lethal unless appropriate antibiotic treatment is started immediately. All children should receive immunizations to help prevent infection by *Hemophilus influenzae,* the most common cause of childhood meningitis. A vaccine is also available for some types of *Neisseria meningitis,* the leading cause of meningitis in older children and adolescents; this vaccine is recommended in high-risk and epidemic circumstances. Even if you haven't been immunized, antibiotics can protect you from these bacteria if you're exposed to a case of meningitis. Finally, a vaccine is available to help fight the most common cause of bacterial meningitis in adults, *Streptococcus pneumoniae.* The proper use of these vaccines is detailed in chapter 16.

Bacteria can also cause brain abscesses, less common than meningitis but no less lethal. Many of these infections originate from infections in the sinuses, ears, or teeth; preventive dental care may help.

Viruses, too, can cause major neurological disorders. "Childhood" viruses like polio and measles used to head the list, but vaccination has largely eliminated these problems in the United States. Still, travelers, health care workers, and other people at risk must be sure their immunizations are up to date. People living in certain areas, both at home and abroad, should also be prepared to prevent infection by insect-borne encephalitis viruses. Chapter 16 will give you some tips on avoiding mosquitoes and other big bugs that transmit viruses and other tiny "bugs."

Most worrisome of all is the virus that causes AIDS. Human immunodeficiency virus (HIV) can produce severe damage to the brain, but AIDS can be prevented (chapter 16).

Chapter 16 will also tell you how to prevent Lyme disease, tuberculosis, and other infectious diseases that can affect the nervous system.

Toxic and Metabolic Disorders

The nervous system is highly susceptible to damage from toxic substances. Some of these toxins build up from internal sources when the body organs responsible for eliminating metabolic products are diseased. For example, neurological symptoms often result from advanced liver or kidney disease.

Other toxins come from outside the body. Of particular importance is lead. More than 1 million workers are exposed daily; as lead levels build up, symptoms of irritability, fatigue, difficulty in concentration, and arm weakness can develop. These symptoms generally resolve if the lead exposure is ended, but children exposed early in life can experience permanent I.Q. deficits. The Environmental Protection Agency (EPA) has reduced the acceptable blood level to 10 micrograms per milliliter; more than 15 percent of American children, 6 million in all, are at risk for damage from lead levels above this standard. Getting the lead out should be a top priority for American society.

Other toxins with major neurological impact include organic solvents, pesticides, mercury, and methanol. These problems can be prevented entirely by avoiding exposure. Chapters 17 and 22 address household, industrial, and environmental toxins that can damage the nervous system.

Among the toxins that can cause neurological disease, one deserves special mention: alcohol. Acute intoxication causes neurological dysfunction that can be fatal. Chronic alcohol use can produce permanent brain damage. We can prevent those problems by recognizing and treating alcohol abuse.

Another common toxin has been identified as a cause of neurological damage. Tobacco smoke can impair the intellectual development of children born to smoking mothers. Even nonsmokers who are exposed to passive smoke during pregnancy can absorb enough to produce subtle cognitive disabilities in their offspring. It's up to our generation to prevent these problems in the next.

Nutritional Deficiencies

Though rare in this land of plenty, vitamin deficiencies still belong on the list of preventable neurological diseases. Since my practice is confined to urban America, I've dealt with only two nutritional diseases of the nervous system. One, Wernicke-Korsakoff syndrome, results from thiamine deficiency, but its cause goes far beyond a simple lack of vitamin B_1, since these patients are virtually all alcoholics. Vitamin B_{12} deficiency is the other preventable nutritional disorder; although it can cause severe neurological problems, it's better known for its impact on the blood, as reflected in its name: pernicious anemia.

Inherited diseases such as muscular dystrophy and Huntington's disease can also affect the nervous system. Since these diseases are not yet treatable by gene therapy, prevention depends on reproductive counseling.

■ Headaches

At last we come to a common neurological complaint, and to one that can often be prevented at that. The headache for prevention is that there are so many causes of headache. In fact, with 42 million office visits per year, headaches are the seventh most common complaint leading patients to see their doctors.

The most common type of headache is the simple *tension headache*. Often resulting from spasms of neck muscles, tension headaches are typically experienced as tightness and pain at the back of the head and neck. Muscle relaxation exercises, heat treatments, biofeedback, and massage can all help prevent or treat tension headaches. Best of all is to keep your neck muscles strong yet limber with stretching exercises, and to avoid keeping your head in a fixed position over a book or in front of a computer screen.

Emotional tension and *stress* also cause headaches. I doubt the validity of the traditional teaching that there is a "headache personality." Instead, I believe that stress can cause headaches in people of all personality types. My prescription for prevention: learn to recognize stress for what it is, change your life to avoid excessive stress, and learn how to dissipate unavoidable stress.

A variety of head and neck disorders can also provoke headaches. Take care of your *eyes*, your *sinuses*, and your *teeth and jaws* to prevent these problems.

Migraine causes some of the most painful of all headaches, and it has increased by 60 percent over the past decade. More common in women, migraine is classified as a vascular headache, since the pain is thought to result from alterations in blood flow to the brain. But the true cause is unknown; until it's discovered, prevention will depend on avoiding things that trigger attacks. These inciting factors vary widely, and include emotional stress, sleeping later than usual (the "Sunday morning migraine"), missing meals, changes in barometric pressure, excessive alcohol consumption, and bright lights. Two particularly frequent factors are related to hormones and diet. Many women report flares in migraine at the time of menstruation — which is why birth control pills should be used with caution, if at all, by women with migraine (and never by smokers). Finally, many migraine patients report that certain foods trigger attacks. For some it's alcohol, especially red wine. Others get migraines if they have too much — or too little — caffeine. MSG, chocolate, and nitrates are among the items blamed for migraine by other patients.

To prevent migraine, you must first know if your pain is indeed migraine. About half of all migraine patients can recognize the disorder because it has previously affected close relatives. Classic migraine causes severe throbbing pain on one side of the head, frequently accompanied by visual disturbances and nausea. Often there is a milder aura, or warning period, before the attack begins. Sometimes temporary visual loss, tingling, weakness, or even paralysis accompanies the pain. Less often, one or more of these symptoms can occur without any headache at all. Because of this variability, you should ask your doctor for help if you think you may have migraine.

There are two ways to prevent migraine. The best is to identify a triggering factor and to avoid it. But if you have unpredictable or spontaneous attacks, consider taking medications to prevent migraines. The U.S. Physicians' Health Study found that just one aspirin tablet every other day could prevent 20 percent of migraines. And prescription drugs are even more effective, so if aspirin doesn't prevent your headaches, ask your doctor to help. For infrequent attacks, prompt drug treatment is best. But for patients with frequent or disabling attacks, preventive medication with beta blockers, antidepressants, or calcium channel blockers can have marvelous results.

Last but not least, remember that more serious disorders can cause headaches. Don't worry about a brain tumor or aneurysm with every headache; these major problems are really quite rare. But you should consult your physician if your headaches are unusual in severity or in type, if they increase during straining or bowel movements, if they last more than 24 hours, or if they are accompanied by fever or by changes in memory, balance, coordination, vision, speech, or strength. Early diagnosis and treatment may help prevent serious complications from developing.

■ Memory Loss

I discovered a foolproof method to prevent memory loss. But I forgot it.

Memory loss is, of course, no joke. In fact, fear of mental deterioration is one of the most common concerns expressed by older patients. In my experience this concern is so pervasive that it's a more consistent marker of maturity than bifocals; you'll know you're middle-aged when you are more worried about getting Alzheimer's disease than AIDS.

Fortunately, much of this concern is groundless. Most memory loss is mild and nonprogressive, and there are ways to help prevent these commonplace, mild changes in memory that are often age-related. Unfortunately, prevention is not yet effective for the most common major memory loss, Alzheimer's disease. Still, there are treatable and preventable disorders that can mimic Alzheimer's, so we should not forget to consider steps that may help prevent some types of severe memory loss.

Major Memory Loss

Relatives call it senility and doctors call it dementia; by any name it's a tragic, unrelenting deterioration of memory, thought, and emotional function. About 1.6 million Americans are severely demented, and up to 5 million are afflicted with milder cases. Nearly two thirds of our 1.3 million nursing home beds are devoted to the care of demented patients; the annual costs approach $30 billion and are rising fast as our population ages.

Alzheimer's disease accounts for more than half of all cases of dementia. Despite these frightening numbers, the disease is very uncommon in middle age; the prevalence is about 3 percent between ages 65 and 74, but rises to 10 percent between 75 and 84 and to 20 percent beyond age 85. Although progressive memory loss is the main feature of Alzheimer's, it often begins with subtle behavioral changes including moodiness, depression, and decreased sociability and enthusiasm. Memory loss is mild at first, but impairment of memory, thought, and judgment progress to the point of incapacitation over a period of three to ten years. Almost 100,000 deaths are attributed to Alzheimer's disease each year.

We do not know the cause of this dreadful problem. Lacking this crucial understanding, we lack effective means of prevention and treatment. But many things can be done to improve the lives of these patients and their families, so expert care should always be sought.

Although the diagnosis of Alzheimer's disease can be established with certainty only at autopsy, clinical diagnosis is now quite reliable. But it's most important to be sure the patient doesn't have a treatable, even preventable, disease that can mimic Alzheimer's.

The problem that most closely resembles Alzheimer's disease is called multi-infarct dementia. Don't be concerned about your memory if you can't master the name. The important thing to know is that it's a stroke syndrome, so it should be preventable by controlling life-style risk factors, including blood pressure, cholesterol, smoking, and lack of exercise.

This disorder used to be called hardening of the arteries, and indeed atherosclerosis is to blame. But unlike in typical strokes, only small arteries that penetrate deep into the brain are involved in multi-infarct dementia. When they become blocked, only tiny clusters of brain cells are killed. At first these "ministrokes" are difficult to discern; but if they continue to occur, the damage accumulates, often progressing in a stuttering, fluctuating fashion to overt dementia.

Like other strokes — indeed, like all forms of atherosclerosis — multi-infarct dementia can be prevented. In addition, early diagnosis is important because secondary prevention may help. CAT scans and MRI scans can recognize multi-infarct dementia by its small areas of brain damage, called lacunes. Blood pressure control and other measures to treat atherosclerosis can help prevent further damage. Among these, a 1989 study of 70 patients from the Houston VA Medical Center found that aspirin therapy could stabilize or improve brain blood flow and mental function in patients with multi-infarct dementia.

There are many other causes of dementia; some are amenable to prevention and treatment. If you have friends or relatives who may be experiencing symptoms of dementia, be sure that they have detailed examinations. An expert physical exam is most important, but lab tests are also essential and should include a complete blood count, a detailed chemical profile, thyroid function tests, vitamin B_{12} levels, and a blood test for syphilis. In some cases even more tests are needed, including a spinal tap, a brain wave or EEG, AIDS testing, and a toxic screen blood test. It's true that these tests are normal in most cases of severe memory loss; still, it makes sense to test many people if the results will prevent disability in even a few.

Mild Memory Loss

Fortunately, high-tech testing is not needed in the usual case of mild memory disturbance. At one time or another all of us will come home from the market without the thing we wanted most. We'll forget where we put our keys or eyeglasses. Names, faces, phone numbers — nobody can remember them all. Perhaps it's a good thing; there are so many important things to learn and remember that we don't need to clutter our minds with every little bit of information that comes along.

Many people tell me that these little lapses of memory become more frequent as they get older. They worry because they know that Alzheimer's disease is more common in advanced age. True; but 97 percent of forgetful 70-year-olds do *not* have Alzheimer's or other dementing illnesses.

What causes memory lapses? I don't think that it is age per se. Neurobiologists tell us that brain cells do die with age, but only at a rate of 100 per day, a trivial loss in a brain of 10 billion cells. Most often memory lapses reflect simple inattention. But if you are more forgetful than you'd like to be (and who isn't!), consider other possibilities. Depression often causes mental slowness, even without overt feelings of sadness and loss. Sleep deprivation can do the same. Medications used to control blood pressure, allergies, pain, and many other problems can sometimes dull the mind; sleeping pills and tranquilizers are particularly likely to have this side effect. The test and the treatment for this problem is one and the same: stop the medication. But always check with your doctor before you stop any prescription drug, since you may need another in its place. Consider, too, that the chemical most likely to blunt your mental edge is alcohol, particularly if you're also taking certain medications.

Some older people can develop age-related problems that can masquerade as mental decline. Chief among these are impairments of vision and hearing. Your mind may be perfectly fine, but you may have a very hard time making connections if your sensory input is slow or distorted.

If you are worried about your memory, get a competent medical checkup, including evaluation of your eyes, ears, and nervous system. Consider psychological evaluation. Review your medication, alcohol use, and sleeping habits. And fight back.

There are many tricks to help forgetful people function flawlessly. Most are variants on the advice of the eminent psychologist B. F. Skinner: "In place of memories, memoranda." Use a calendar to note appointments and deadlines, as well as birthdays and other events that you want to remember. Carry a note pad to jot down memos to yourself — but don't forget to read your notes! Make little things a matter of routine; if you always put your keys in the same place, they'll be much less likely to wander off. Keep checklists: what to pack for trips, what to bring to appointments, and so forth. Plan ahead, practicing names and faces of people you may meet at a party or gathering. Don't be shy about asking people to repeat names, numbers, dates, and other data. Read important information as often as necessary. Concentrate on learning things that really matter, using the same tricks of repetition, acronyms, and other mnemonic devices that got you through school.

Above all, find the tricks that work best for you, and don't be ashamed to use them. I am delighted when a patient begins our consultation by taking out a list; after all, I begin each appointment by reviewing *my* list of their problems and medication. You can ask my nurse, my secretary, or my wife; the memos and notes that have gone into this book could paper many a room. Since I get lots of ideas when I'm out running, I have even carried a pad to jog my memory from time to time.

These tactics can help win the battle against forgetfulness. But there is much more you can do. You can win the war.

Like most of the body's organs, the brain improves with use. People who stay involved, committed, and mentally stimulated are likely to remain alert, productive, and creative at all ages. When Oliver Wendell Holmes was asked why he was reading Plato at age 92 he replied simply, "To improve my mind." It works. You don't merely have to take the word of a Chief Justice of the United States or read any number of glowing testimonials. Many psychologists and neurologists have studied people of all ages, finding that mental activity enhances mental ability. In laboratory animals mental stimulation even induces longevity!

It's not necessary to read Plato to improve your mind; almost any book will do (even this one, I hope). Plan your own "mental workout" just as you would a physical workout, by finding what suits you best. Take courses, assume new responsibilities, meet new people, travel — anything to stretch your mind. And while you're at it, don't neglect your physical fitness. Evidence is emerging that physical exercise improves reaction time (your reflexes) and even I.Q.

■ ■ ■

Prevention can forestall many neurological disorders, both small and serious. But many others are still beyond our grasp. The old stereotype of the neurologist as a specialist who can diagnose but not treat is no longer valid, if it ever was. Neurological diagnosis and treatment have improved greatly. But when it comes to preventing disorders as severe as epilepsy, Parkinson's disease, and brain tumors, we are hampered by our ignorance of the basic causes of those diseases. More research will be needed to make progress. Knowledge is the key that will unlock the door to prevention.

■ 5 ■
Lung and Respiratory Tract Diseases

With each and every breath, your lungs are providing the oxygen necessary to sustain life. With each breath, your lungs are removing carbon dioxide from your blood, a function no less essential. But with each breath your lungs may be exposed to agents of disease. At 20,000 breaths per day, your lungs are working hard for you. At 8 million breaths per year, your lungs run quite a risk of encountering noxious substances. Still, if you take care of your lungs, they should be good for 600 million breaths during the course of a long and healthy lifetime.

■ The Normal Respiratory Tract

Your lungs are just one part of a complex respiratory apparatus that must work as a coordinated unit to sustain life. Breathing is an automatic function requiring no voluntary effort, but the timing and pace of breathing depends on sophisticated control mechanisms in your nervous system. In healthy people the amount of carbon dioxide in the blood is the prime factor governing the rate of respiration; as carbon dioxide builds up in your blood, it signals your brain to increase the rate and depth of breathing, so you'll blow out excess carbon dioxide. But the power to exchange carbon dioxide for oxygen doesn't come from the lungs themselves; instead, your nervous system signals the muscles of your chest and diaphragm to contract, bringing in fresh air and expelling stale air with each breath.

Air passes through some important structures on the way to your lungs (see figure 5-1). Entering through your nose or mouth, air travels first through your trachea, or windpipe. The trachea divides in midchest, at about the level of your heart, into the two ducts that carry air to the lungs. The air tubes divide in turn into successively smaller passages. Finally, the smallest tubes terminate in the air sacs, or alveoli.

The air sacs are where the actual exchange of oxygen and carbon dioxide takes place. Blood collected from your veins funnels into the two right-side chambers of your heart, which pump it into your lungs. Your blood passes through progressively smaller vessels until it reaches the capillaries. Each capillary passes around an air sac. Because both the capillaries and the air sacs have thin lining membranes, carbon dioxide can pass

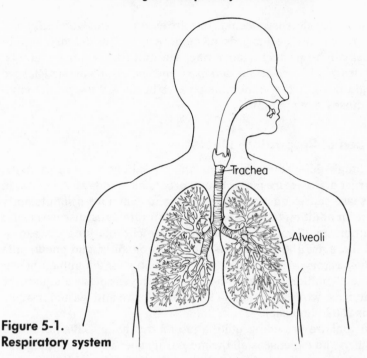

Figure 5-1.
Respiratory system

from the blood into the air as oxygen travels in the opposite direction, from air to blood. Oxygen-rich blood is then collected for return to the left-side heart chambers, which pump it to your entire body.

To sustain life, an average of nine quarts of air pass through the lungs each minute. To accommodate all this air there are an enormous number of air sacs — 300 million to be exact. Collectively these air sacs have a surface area of 75 square yards, making your lungs one of the largest organs in your body. This huge surface area actually provides much more breathing power than you really need. In fact, you could get along perfectly well with just one lung, even getting enough oxygen to play sports.

With such a tremendous reserve capacity it might seem surprising that your lungs are so vulnerable to disease. But they are — and, paradoxically, their huge surface area contributes to their vulnerability. Each breath brings oxygen to the lungs, but harmful substances in the air can be carried right along.

The body has developed many efficient mechanisms to protect the lungs. Foreign particles in the air trigger the cough reflex, generating a tremendous outward rush of air to expel those particles. The windpipe is lined with cells producing mucus which entraps particles and bacteria that sneak past the cough reflex; tiny hairs, called cilia, propel the trapped particles up and out. The air sacs are the most vulnerable to damage, but even here white blood cells are present in the lining membranes, ready to gobble up bacteria, thus fighting infection. Finally, the air sac membranes are protected by a substance that allows the lungs to expand properly, and by proteins that prevent damage by enzymes.

These respiratory defense mechanisms are essential and wonderful, but they are no match for the hazards of modern life. The defense system evolved principally to protect against bacteria. But smoke, air pollutants, alcohol, and drugs all damage our defenses, and the chemical particles we inhale get right down to the vulnerable air sacs because we were not engineered with those toxins in mind.

■ The Burden of Respiratory Illness

Despite the lung's defense mechanisms and their huge reserve capacity, respiratory tract diseases are major health problems in today's America. In fact, lung disease causes one in eight deaths, and contributes significantly to one in four. In addition to this appalling death rate, lung diseases cause enormous suffering: 17 million Americans have chronic lung disease or asthma, and there are 100 million cases of flu, bronchitis, and pneumonia each year. Respiratory tract diseases are responsible for 2.5 million hospitalizations and 25 million doctor's office visits each year. If we add in more than 30 million lost workdays, the bill for medical care and wasted productivity exceeds $50 billion each year.

It is clear that we are doing quite a job on our lungs. This burden of death, disability, and expense is all the more tragic because many lung diseases, including the most lethal and debilitating, are preventable.

There are ten important ways to prevent lung disease. The first nine are to avoid smoking.

In the preceding chapters of this book, cigarette smoking emerged as a critical cause of heart disease, peripheral artery disease, and stroke. But as damaging as smoking is to all blood vessels, there are other risk factors of nearly comparable harmfulness including high cholesterol, high blood pressure, and lack of exercise. When it comes to your lungs, however, smoking stands alone as a hazard to your health and your life. It's no wonder, then, that my First Commandment of Prevention is the shortest: Don't smoke.

Avoiding smoking is essential to preventing lung disease, but it's not the only thing you can do. Smokers and nonsmokers alike should understand the other important ways to prevent respiratory tract diseases.

■ Lung Cancer

Cancer is the second most common cause of death in the United States, and lung cancer heads the list of cancer killers. Long the leading cause of cancer deaths in men, since 1985 lung cancer has been the most common fatal cancer in American women as well. In all, 160,000 cases of lung cancer are newly diagnosed each year; 145,000 patients die from lung cancer annually, accounting for nearly one third of all cancer deaths.

As you can see from these grim statistics, even the most aggressive modern medical and surgical treatments have but a poor chance of curing lung cancer. Despite the enormous progress in medical science over the past 50 years, the five-year lung cancer cure rate increased only from 4 percent in 1940 to 13 percent in 1990. The moral? Yes, we need better treatment, but that's not my point. We shouldn't have to spend our precious medical and financial resources on improving the *treatment* of lung cancer, since the vast majority of these tumors are *entirely preventable*.

Smoking

Lung cancer was not always a major killer; as recently as 1935 it was a rare disease in the United States. What went wrong? In 1915 fewer than 20 billion cigarettes were smoked in the United States. In the 1920s the tobacco industry discovered how to mass manufacture and mass market cigarettes. Sales got rolling — and after 20 years, the time needed for most lung tumors to develop, so did lung cancer. In 1987, for example, there were 575 billion cigarettes sold in the United States and 136,000 lung cancer deaths.

Cigarette use has finally started to decline, but because of the long time it takes for cancer to develop, we are still paying the price. Between 1979 and 1986 lung cancer deaths increased by 7 percent in men and 44 percent in women. Why the disparity? Cigarette use in women continued to increase for at least a decade after men began to kick the habit in the mid 1960s. Women are finally starting to cut down as well, but smoking in minority groups continues to increase, as do their lung cancer rates. In all, about 30 percent of Americans still smoke cigarettes. Even if they had all stopped in 1990, we would face at least 1 million additional smoking-related lung cancer deaths before the new century.

There is absolutely no doubt that cigarette smoking causes lung cancer. The risk of cancer increases in direct proportion to the duration of smoking in years, the number of cigarettes consumed per day, the tar and nicotine content of cigarettes, and the depth of inhalation. In all, the risk of lung cancer is increased about tenfold in light to moderate smokers, and more than twentyfold in moderate to heavy smokers.

The best way to prevent lung cancer is to avoid smoking. Don't start if you've never smoked. And if you've been a smoker, quit and stay quit. The benefits of quitting are enormous: your risk of lung cancer, for example, will decline to the same low rate as for nonsmokers in about ten years. Quit now.

Unfortunately, even nonsmokers must be concerned about the risks of tobacco. Passive smoking — inhaling other people's cigarette smoke — causes 3,700 lung cancer deaths in the United States each year. Add the 37,000 annual heart attack deaths caused by passive smoking, and you'll see why passive smoking is the third leading preventable cause of death in the United States. We need action to protect smokers from themselves and to protect the rest of us from smokers.

Radon

Radiation is a proven cause of cancer, and the source of radiation most likely to cause lung cancer is radon. Doctors have known for years that radon is a major cause of lung cancer in coal miners, but the risk to people who do not work underground was not appreciated until 1985. It's now apparent that radon is our second leading cause of lung cancer. A flurry of publicity followed from this new medical information, generating lots of concern but, I'm sorry to say, very little action. To plan the action that's best for you and your family, you should understand the whole radon story.

Radon is a colorless, odorless gas that is a natural part of the uranium family. Uranium is present in the earth's crust; although some geological formations have much higher concentrations, no area is uranium-free. As uranium breaks down, it releases radon gas, which seeps from soil and rocks into the air. Like all radioactive chemicals, radon is unstable, breaking down in less than four days. But radon's breakdown products are also radioactive; unfortunately, they emit even more high-energy radioactive particles than radon itself.

Because radon is a gas, it quickly dissipates in all outdoor areas. But radon can seep into buildings, entering through cracks in foundations and basement floors, dirt crawl spaces, porous cinder blocks, and loose-fitting pipes, sump holes, and drains. If ventilation is adequate, radon gas can seep out again, and the cancer risk will be very low. But in poorly ventilated areas radon concentrations can mount to dangerous levels. If you spend lots of time in such areas, you'll inhale more than your share of radon; the particles can lodge deep in your lungs, injuring the cells and eventually causing cancer.

You can prevent radon from causing lung cancer. First, find out if your house has excessive radon levels. You can test your own house quite simply with a radon detection kit, widely available at hardware and department stores for about $30, but sometimes provided free by local government agencies. Two types of kits are available — charcoal cannisters that trap radon gas over a three-to-seven-day period, and plastic plates that detect particles during a span of three to twelve months. Both are accurate if used correctly; for best results, choose a kit that has been approved by the EPA. Kits to test drinking water are also available, but their usefulness is not yet clear.

Place your radon test kit in the lowest part of your house, usually the basement or first floor. Even better, use two kits and average the results. Be sure the windows and doors remain closed during the collection period so radon won't dissipate. Then just mail your kits to the lab and wait for the results.

How much radon is safe? Like all radioactive exposures, the less the better. Your risk for developing lung cancer will depend on how much radon is in the air, and how much time you spend breathing that air. The Environmental Protection Agency considers radon concentrations below 4 to be generally safe. The average house has levels of 2 or less, but some have much higher readings, even exceeding levels in uranium mines. You can't predict your levels based on how your house is constructed, where you live, or what your neighbors have found; you must do the test yourself.

Once you know your home's radon level, you'll have to decide what to do about it. And that's where we've been falling short. Thousands of people have tested their houses, but few have taken corrective action. Call a qualified contractor if your levels are high; I'd recommend repairs even with borderline levels if you spend lots of time in rooms that have radon readings of 3 or 4. Repairs amount to sealing basement and foundation leaks to keep radon out, and providing enough ventilation to allow any gas that enters to dissipate. Repairs are usually quite simple, costing $300 to $2,000.

Radon causes an estimated 16,000 lung cancer deaths in the United States each year. They are preventable. About 1 million houses have excess radon levels; few home owners know it, and fewer still have corrected the problem. Every home owner should test for radon; people living in basement or first-floor apartments, row houses, and mobile homes with permanent foundations should do the same. If your levels are high, make the necessary repairs, then retest.

There is one other thing you can do to protect yourself from radon-induced lung cancer: don't smoke. Radon is ten times more dangerous to smokers than to nonsmokers; about 85 percent of radon-related cancers develop in smokers.

Asbestos

Like radon, asbestos is much more hazardous to smokers, but it can cause cancer in nonsmokers if their exposure is intense. About 10 million Americans have been exposed to asbestos. Half these exposures occurred in shipyard workers during World War II, but 300,000 workers are still exposed. People at risk include construction and maintenance personnel working to repair or demolish buildings with asbestos insulation, automobile brake repairmen, and certain industrial workers.

Asbestos was also used to fireproof buildings between 1920 and 1978, when it was banned by the EPA. Asbestos around pipes and in ceilings and walls is not a health hazard, unless the structure is damaged so that asbestos particles enter the air. Programs for asbestos testing and repairs are controversial, and decisions must be individualized. If you think your apartment building or school may pose a risk, check with your local office of the EPA. The Consumer Product Safety Commission Hotline (800-638-CPSC) can also help.

Other Causes of Lung Cancer

Various industrial exposures can lead to lung cancer. The list of hazards includes soot and tar, coke oven emissions, arsenic, cadmium, chromate, and polycyclic hydrocarbons. The principles of occupational health (see chapter 17) can protect you from them.

You may be surprised by an omission from this formidable list of agents that cause lung cancer. I'm surprised by it, too, but at present there is no conclusive evidence that air pollution leads to lung cancer. Still, there are many important reasons for cleaning up the air we breathe.

Diet and Lung Cancer

Another surprise. It's easy to understand that chemicals in the air are related to cancer of the lung, but you may be surprised to learn that chemicals in food can also influence your risk of developing lung cancer. But the news here is all good. At last I'm not urging you to *avoid* something to reduce your lung cancer risk but to *increase* your intake of something to reduce risk. That something is beta carotene.

Beta carotene is a precursor of vitamin A. People who eat little beta carotene have two times more lung cancer than people who eat food rich in beta carotene. This relationship has been confirmed in many population groups around the world, and remains valid whether tested by dietary history or blood carotene levels. One caveat: a high-carotene diet is less protective in smokers than in nonsmokers.

You'll remember from chapter 2 that beta carotene is also showing promise for the prevention of heart disease. How can one chemical fight both cancer and atherosclerosis? We don't know for sure, but it's probably because beta carotene is an antioxidant. Chapter 20 will discuss antioxidants in detail, explaining how vitamins A, C, and E may help protect you from cancer and vascular disease.

Beta carotene is widely distributed in fruits and vegetables. Dark green and yellow-orange vegetables are particularly rich sources (see table 20-8). You don't have to gorge yourself on spinach or sweet potatoes, much less pop megavitamins, to get all the beta carotene you need; the equivalent of one carrot a day will cut your risk of lung cancer in half. A small gain, perhaps, when compared with the benefits of avoiding tobacco smoke, radon, and asbestos. But with this deadly disease every ounce of protection counts. Use some of the money you save from kicking the cigarette habit for a radon detection kit and a generous daily portion of veggies.

Secondary and Tertiary Prevention of Lung Cancer

A fundamental principle of medical practice is that early detection of disease, even before symptoms develop, will allow prompt treatment, prevent complications, and save lives. Lung cancer is the exception that proves this rule.

The problem with secondary prevention of lung cancer is that screening tests cannot detect the disease early enough to make a difference. Two techniques can be used to screen for lung cancer. Chest x rays look for nodules or spots, while sputum cytologies rely on microscopic examinations of sputum specimens, much as Pap smears look for cancer cells. Sputum cytology tests are risk-free, but x rays require exposure to radiation, which can cause cumulative damage if x rays are repeated frequently over the years. Chest x rays are also likely to show spots that are not cancerous, leading to unnecessary tests that are frightening, expensive, and even hazardous.

Even these problems would be acceptable if screening tests could detect lung cancer at a curable stage. Unfortunately, they cannot. Careful studies of tens of thousands of smokers fail to demonstrate *any* survival benefit from routine chest x rays or sputum cytologies, even if both tests are performed by experts every four to six months.

Despite these dismal results, we are still spending $1.5 billion a year on screening chest x rays. With rare unanimity, the American Cancer Society, National Cancer Institutes, Food and Drug Administration, U.S. and Canadian Task Forces on prevention, and World Health Organization all agree that screening chest x rays are not helpful. Even the American College of Radiology — the folks collecting all that money — concurs. We'd get much more value from our $1.5 billion by investing it toward the goal of a smokeless society.

Tertiary prevention is no more encouraging. Lung cancer is a silent disease in its early stages. By the time it has grown large enough to be visible on a chest x ray, it has often spread to lymph nodes, liver, bone, or brain so that surgery can no longer cure it. Spread is even more likely by the time lung cancer produces symptoms such as coughing, bleeding, pain, or breathlessness. Radiation therapy can help control these symptoms, but it cannot cure. Chemotherapy is only partially effective, producing limited benefit only in certain relatively uncommon types of lung cancer.

With the exception of AIDS, I can think of no other disease with such an enormous gap between the results of prevention and treatment. Primary prevention of lung cancer is highly effective, but even the earliest diagnoses and best treatments fail to cure more than 85 percent of the many lung cancer victims. We need to improve therapy. But even more, we need to work as individuals and as the body politic to prevent people the world over from victimizing themselves.

■ Chronic Obstructive Lung Disease

Although it doesn't get much attention, chronic obstructive lung disease is one of the most serious health problems in the industrialized world. An estimated 10 million Americans suffer from this problem, and 1 million new cases occur each year. Some victims are only mildly affected, but others can be completely incapacitated. In fact, chronic obstructive lung disease is second only to coronary artery disease as a cause of social security–compensated disability. Nor does the impact stop with disability; more than 70,000 Americans die from chronic obstructive lung disease each year, making it our fifth leading cause of death. Despite medical advances, deaths actually increased by 33 percent between 1979 and 1986. At a cost in excess of $10 billion per year, chronic obstructive lung disease is a major economic burden as well.

Nearly all this death, disability, and expense is preventable.

What Is Chronic Lung Disease?

You may be asking yourself why you don't know more about such a serious preventable killer. You probably do, but recognize it better by another name — *emphysema*. Emphysema is one of the major types of chronic obstructive lung disease; the other is chronic bronchitis. They are linked together because the central problem in both is blockage of air flow into and out of the lungs, and because most patients with chronic obstructive lung disease have some features of both conditions. The diagnosis of both varieties is best accomplished with chest x rays and lung function tests.

Chronic bronchitis begins with excess mucus production by the glands that line the mid- and large-sized breathing tubes, the bronchi. Many of us have experienced increased mucus production in the course of *acute* bronchitis, but we recover in a week or so with the aid of antibiotics. In *chronic* bronchitis, however, the problem does not go away. Instead, the patient continues to cough and bring up sputum. Over time, the irritated bronchial tubes become thickened and narrowed. Breathing becomes difficult. At first patients huff and puff only on stairs, but if the disease progresses, breathing becomes harder and harder until even getting out of bed is difficult. Blood oxygen levels fall, giving the lips and skin a blue appearance called cyanosis. Often stocky to begin with, patients with chronic bronchitis tend to gain weight as fluid builds up in their legs. Pneumonia is a frequent complication and is hard to treat even with the best antibiotics. Heart failure is often the end result of severe chronic bronchitis.

Patients with pure emphysema tend to be thin, and they are spared from daily sputum production, blue skin, and fluid accumulation. But they are even more short of breath, and often require oxygen treatments in the advanced stages of their disease. Their bronchial tubes don't produce excessive mucus, but they are narrowed. As a result of this narrowing, the air sacs become hyperinflated, much like balloons that are overfilled nearly to the point of bursting.

Chronic bronchitis and emphysema sound very different, but they're actually only extreme forms of a single disease which can cause a wide spectrum of abnormalities. Most patients with chronic obstructive lung disease are in the middle of that spectrum, with mixed symptoms caused by a combination of chronic bronchitis and emphysema.

Cause and Prevention

Chronic bronchitis and emphysema are also united by having a single cause: smoking.

About 90 percent of chronic obstructive lung disease is caused by smoking; it is 30 times more likely to kill smokers than nonsmokers. Not all smokers get chronic obstructive lung disease. Just as with coronary artery disease and lung cancer, however, the more you smoke, the more likely you are to get sick. In all, 15 percent of cigarette smokers develop chronic obstructive lung disease. And if they continue to smoke, they will inexorably get worse and worse. Cigarette smoke damages lung cells and also irritates a type of white blood cell called the macrophage. Angry white blood cells release enzymes that digest the lungs' elastic tissue, creating a vicious cycle of damage and destruction.

Once tissue damage has occurred, there is no way to correct it. But smoking cessation will dramatically reduce the progression of chronic obstructive lung disease. Many forms of treatment can help patients feel and function better and can reduce the risk of infection, heart failure, and other complications. These treatments, too, are much more effective after smoking is halted.

You can prevent chronic obstructive lung disease by not smoking. You can prevent the disease from getting worse by quitting. And even if you have emphysema or chronic bronchitis, you can work with your doctor to prevent lung infection and other complications.

■ Asthma

With 10 million cases in the United States, asthma is just as common as chronic obstructive lung disease. In asthma, as in chronic obstructive lung disease, the main problem is narrowing of the breathing tubes. But that's where the similarities end. In chronic obstructive lung disease the narrowing is permanent, while in asthma the narrowing is temporary. In chronic obstructive lung disease the goal of treatment is simply to prevent complications, but successful asthma treatment can actually prevent obstruction.

Whereas chronic obstructive lung disease is much more common in the elderly, asthma is much more common in children. Despite its favorable response to treatment, asthma is responsible for 100 million days of restricted activity, 6 million lost schooldays, and about 2,000 deaths in America each year. Alarmingly, the asthma death rate has actually *increased* by 30 percent in the past decade. The economic cost is worrisome as well, exceeding $4 billion annually.

What is Asthma?

If American schools still taught classical languages we might not be asking this question, since *asthma* is derived from the Greek word meaning "to pant."

Most people with asthma are perfectly healthy until an attack occurs. Attacks are caused by spasms of muscles in the walls of the bronchial tubes; when these muscles contract, they narrow the air passages, constricting the free flow of air. To force air through the narrow passages, patients with asthma breathe faster and harder — they pant. As air travels through the narrow tube, it produces a whistling, wheezing sound, which may be audible even without a stethoscope. In addition to wheezing, coughing and breathlessness are the major symptoms of asthma. Anxiety and agitation result from the terrible feeling of air hunger.

All bronchial tubes have muscles in their walls; these muscles are important in adjusting the diameter of the breathing tubes so that air flow can be properly distributed within the lungs. All people can be provoked to wheeze under certain conditions. But not everyone has asthma. Far from it. Asthma is a condition in which the bronchial tubes are *abnormally* re-

sponsive to various stimuli; this hyperresponsivity is manifested by contractions of the bronchial muscles and increased mucus production by the
bronchial glands.

Why do some people have hyperreactive bronchial tubes? We don't yet
know the answer, but we do know that asthma is often inherited and that
it's frequently linked to allergies.

Preventing Asthma

You cannot prevent hyperresponsive bronchial tubes. If you've got them,
you've got asthma. But you can help prevent asthma *attacks*. This is tertiary prevention at its best. The trick is to identify the factors that trigger
spasms and attacks.

Most often allergies are to blame. Patients with allergic asthma frequently have relatives with similar disorders. They may notice that their
attacks are seasonal, triggered by the arrival of particular pollens or
grasses. Or they may notice that attacks are provoked by animal hair,
feathers, dust, or other things to which they are allergic. Other allergic
symptoms, particularly nasal congestion, are often present.

Lung function tests can document bronchial hyperactivity, but they
don't distinguish allergic from nonallergic asthma. A simple blood count
can help if a specific type of white blood cell, the eosinophile, is present in
abnormally high numbers. Allergy testing can be very helpful in detecting
the particular items that trigger attacks.

The best prevention is to avoid the substances that provoke allergies
and asthma. It is conceptually easy to find a new home for the family
cat, but theory and practice don't necessarily coincide. Less emotionally
charged items such as feather pillows, down comforters, and shag rugs are
easier to change; dust and molds are excellent targets in many households.
If pollen is the cause of asthma, children should be taught to minimize exposure as much as possible.

If spring cleaning doesn't prevent allergic asthma, consider desensitiz-
ing injections. "Allergy shots" have not been scientifically proven to prevent allergic asthma, but many of my patients have found them helpful
indeed. The next line of prevention is medication. Antihistamines generally
reduce allergic symptoms and may help with the asthma itself. In many
patients, however, medications specifically designed to relax bronchial
muscles are needed. Fortunately, a great variety of these medications is
available; some are administered by inhalation, others in pill or syrup form,
and some by injection.

As a respiratory disease, most allergic asthma is triggered by material
in the air. The source is typically in the home or in nature, but fumes or
particles in the air at work or at school may also be responsible ("Monday
morning asthma"). Air pollution, too, is a factor. A 1991 study from Toronto
found that even ozone concentrations considered "safe" by the EPA double
the likelihood of allergy-induced asthma attacks. But sometimes asthma is
provoked by medications or by substances in food. Aspirin-induced asthma

is the best-documented example. Most common in adults who also have nasal polyps, it is readily prevented by avoiding aspirin and related medications.

Food allergies are greatly overrated as causes of asthma, but two additives can trigger asthma in some sensitive individuals. Sulfites are widely used by the food-processing industry as preservatives. Present in some medications, they are most prevalent in restaurant food and in fruits, wine and beer, shellfish, peeled potatoes, and avocado dip. So if your breathing is labored in a restaurant, don't assume your wallet is the cause; it may be your lungs if you are among the 5 percent of asthmatics who are sensitive to sulfites.

The other additive that's been blamed for asthma is tartrazine, a coal-tar derivative approved by the Food and Drug Administration as Yellow Dye Number Five. Tartrazine sensitivity is quite controversial; some experts make the diagnosis fairly often, while others doubt its existence! My best estimate is that it's quite *uncommon*, occurring almost exclusively in aspirin-sensitive asthmatics. I hope I'm right. Tartrazine is so widely used in food, beverages, mouthwash, and medications that a tartrazine-free diet is extremely restrictive.

Although allergic sensitivity is often the root cause of asthma, many other factors may be responsible for provoking attacks. Infections are high on the list, ranging from simple colds to flu to pneumonia. We still don't do a very good job preventing colds, but all asthmatics should have flu and pneumonia vaccinations to help prevent respiratory infections. Fumes and vapors can also trigger asthma; to prevent attacks, shun tobacco smoke and air pollutants.

Another factor traditionally linked to asthma is stress. It's a bit hard to sort this one out; because breathlessness always causes anxiety, it's difficult to know what factor is the chicken and which the egg. Still, even the skeptics agree that stress may exacerbate asthma, and that it's a major factor in some patients. Psychological interventions are the best way to prevent attacks in these circumstances.

A final type of asthma deserves special mention because it is so different and so common. Exercise can produce asthma in some people, even if they don't have allergies or other underlying conditions. The reason is that exercise causes rapid breathing that can lead to excessive cooling down or drying out of the bronchial tubes. Exercise-induced asthma is most common during vigorous exertion in cool, dry air, but only certain individuals are susceptible. Chapter 21 will explain the prevention and treatment of exercise-induced asthma.

While on the subject of exercise and the lungs, I should pass along some good news and some bad news. The good news is that medical management will allow most people with asthma, of either the ordinary or the exercise-induced variety, to enjoy the benefits of exercise and sports. Swimming is the best sport for asthmatics, but anything is possible; in fact more than 10 percent of America's 1984 Olympic athletes had asthma. The bad news is that the lungs are one of the few organs that don't improve with exercise training. True, when people get into shape, they feel that their "wind" is improved. It is; but the improvement depends on benefits to the heart, blood vessels, and muscles rather than the lungs. The reason is that healthy lungs have such an excess breathing capacity that they don't need to improve to keep pace with the circulation.

Diseased lungs are a different story, because their diminished capacity often limits or prevents exercise. Exercise training will not rehabilitate these lungs, but it may help patients use oxygen more efficiently by improving muscle function. You won't have to worry about pulmonary rehabilitation, however, if you follow the simple steps needed to keep your lungs healthy in the first place.

■ Occupational Lung Disease

A general principle of prevention is that you can avoid many diseases simply by keeping toxins out of your body. In the particular case of your lungs, clean air is the key to respiratory health. By avoiding tobacco smoke, you'll nearly eliminate your risk of lung cancer and chronic obstructive lung disease. But many toxins are pumped into the air by other people; odorless and invisible, they can be difficult to avoid. Because many of these toxins are by-products of industry and agriculture, you should pause for a moment to evaluate the air quality of your workplace.

Occupational lung diseases come in two varieties. In the first, toxic particles produce direct damage to the cells of the respiratory tract. Anyone who is exposed will develop lung damage. The severity of damage is directly proportional to the intensity, duration, and frequency of exposure, but cigarette smoking greatly magnifies the harm produced by toxic particles. Examples include lung tumors in asbestos workers, black lung in coal miners, and silicosis in sand blasters.

In the other variety of occupational lung disease, the particles don't harm the lung directly but instead trigger an allergic reaction. The allergy may be manifested as asthma or, more often, as a type of pneumonia called hypersensitivity pneumonitis. To develop hypersensitivity lung disease, then, you need both the *exposure* to airborne material and an *allergy* to that material.

It might seem that only a few people would meet both criteria, but quite the contrary is true. Occupational lung disease is relatively common because molds and bacteria are widespread contaminants of organic materials. Their tiny spores are readily aerosolized and inhaled, and they frequently provoke hypersensitivity reactions, even in people without other allergies.

The names of these lung diseases testify to the diversity of workers at risk: farmer's lung, furrier's lung, Bible printer's lung, tea grower's lung, and paprika slicer's lung are just a few. Nor are these problems confined to farming and manufacturing. Humidifier–air conditioner lung can arise at home from molds growing in the water reservoirs of devices designed to *improve* air quality. To prevent this ailment, keep your humidifier scrupulously clean. Change the water daily, using demineralized water if possible.

Clean your unit at least once a week with an ounce of chlorine bleach diluted in a pint of water and rinse with fresh water before you resume use. Detergent lung is another home-grown example, an occupational disease affecting one of the most important of all groups of workers. You don't have to switch to paper plates or settle for dirty laundry to prevent detergent lung. Instead, switch to liquid soaps if powdered detergents seem to provoke sneezing, coughing, or wheezing.

To avoid occupational lung disease, learn all you can about the air you breathe. The Occupational Safety and Health Administration is an excellent source of information.

■ Air Pollution

A lifelong New Yorker once expressed great anxiety during a trip to the country. The cause of his distress: he didn't trust air he couldn't see. Unfortunately, he won't be anxious in many places anymore, since the whole eastern half of the United States is under a constant blanket of haze, and much of the West is catching up. In pristine parts of the world 90-mile visibility is still possible, but in the United States 15 miles is the rule — on a good day.

The average person breathes about 35 pounds of air per day. Is it really all air? In 1987 American industry pumped 2.6 billion pounds of pollutants into the air, enough for 10 pounds per person.

Two major groups of atmospheric pollutants predominate in the United States. Fossil fuel combustion releases particles, nitrogen oxides, and sulfur oxides into the air; these contaminants are most concentrated in the industrial centers of the Northeast and Midwest. Motor vehicle emissions are the primary source of the second major contaminant, photochemical pollution or smog. Smog is produced when sunlight acts on the nitrogen oxide and hydrocarbons that spew from tailpipes and factories, forming ozone. Unlike the *upper*-atmosphere ozone, which protects against ultraviolet radiation, *ground*-level ozone (smog) is an irritant that can interfere with lung function, causing wheezing, shortness of breath, and coughing as well as eye and nose discomfort. Most prominent in urban areas, smog is a particular problem during summer; it's the haze that accompanies the heat and humidity.

Surprisingly, although air pollution is often accused of causing lung disease, neither sulfur oxide particulates nor photochemical pollutants seem to damage lung cells permanently. Are they innocent of all charges? Of course not. Patients with chronic obstructive lung disease, asthma, and heart disease can be seriously harmed by air pollution because their lungs don't have the reserve and resilience to combat toxins. The short-term solution for those patients is to stay home with the air conditioner running during summer air-quality alerts. The long-term solution is to clean up our air!

Even healthy people should be concerned about air pollution. Eye and nose irritation are common consequences of contaminated air. Carbon monoxide is produced by all forms of combustion, ranging from cigarettes to charcoal grills to auto engines. Blood carbon monoxide levels are doubled by standing on a New York City street for 30 minutes; jogging near traffic will triple levels in 30 minutes because lungs working hard to take up more oxygen will also take up more of the noxious gas. The EPA considers blood carbon dioxide concentrations of 2 percent acceptable, while the Occupational Safety and Health Administration tolerates 4 percent. These levels may at first seem reasonable since freeway commuting or cigarette smoking produce levels of 4 percent or more. But carbon monoxide displaces oxygen from the blood, and as little as 2 percent can impair the exercise capacity of healthy people, to say nothing of heart patients. Do we need tougher standards? Decide for yourself; then write to your senator.

■ Impaired Breathing Patterns

Most lung problems force patients to breathe abnormally fast and hard. But one unusual lung problem can be caused by breathing that is too slow and shallow.

Normal breathing requires coordinated function of the nervous system and respiratory muscles. Additionally, the upper air passages must be open to allow air to reach the lungs. Even healthy lungs can suffer if these conditions are not met.

Some people temporarily stop breathing during sleep. Although these pauses, called *apneas*, can last a minute or more, most of the 2.5 million people afflicted with the "sleep-apnea syndrome" don't know it's happening. Instead, abnormal breathing at night makes their sleep restless and agitated, resulting in morning headaches, daytime sleepiness, and personality changes. The clue to the correct diagnosis generally comes from a spouse who complains about loud snoring as well as thrashing in bed. Additional clues: most patients with this problem are stocky or obese, and many have high blood pressure.

Ineffective nighttime breathing will lower blood oxygen levels and increase carbon dioxide levels. Over the years this can produce heart and lung disease. You can prevent these life-threatening complications with early diagnosis and treatment.

If you (or your spouse!) think you may have this problem, you can help yourself greatly by losing weight and by avoiding alcohol and other sedatives. Another trick is to sew a pocket on the back of your pajamas or nightgown. At bedtime, put in a tennis ball. It's guaranteed to keep you from sleeping on your back, thus helping to prevent airway blockage. Needless to say, you should also check with your doctor. A sleep clinic may be needed to confirm the diagnosis, but good treatments, ranging from medications to mechanical aids to surgery, are available.

■ Respiratory Tract Infections

About 100 years ago Sir William Oster, the greatest physician of his day, called pneumonia the "Captain of the Ship of Death." Indeed, in 1900 respiratory tract infections (pneumonia, influenza, and tuberculosis) were the leading cause of death in the United States. About 50 years ago antibiotics became available to fight infections, and experts predicted that pneumonia would become a thing of the past. Today pneumonia and influenza rank sixth on the list of leading killers. An improvement? Perhaps — but an illusory one, since infections have descended on the list largely because we've created epidemics of heart disease, cancer, stroke, highway carnage, and chronic lung disease to replace them.

Initial optimism notwithstanding, we now know that antibiotics cannot prevent lung infections. But there are important steps you can take to protect yourself from these problems.

The Common Cold

The most common respiratory tract infection is the ordinary cold. Despite a substantial nuisance value and a sizable economic impact, these pesky infections are not really serious. With cold remedies, or even antibiotics, virtually all patients will recover in seven days; without treatment, in a week.

Although benign and self-limited, upper respiratory tract infections can lead to bronchitis and pneumonia. It would be nice to prevent them. I wish I could tell you how; if I could, you'd have easier winters and I might now be in my hammock instead of at my desk.

Two factors account for our inability to prevent colds. First, they are caused by viruses. Antibiotics are *not* active against these tiniest of microbes, so we can't use pills to prevent or cure the common cold. Second, more than 200 different viruses can cause colds. Vaccines have proved dramatically helpful in preventing many viral infections, but a cold vaccine is nowhere in sight because it's just not possible to develop a vaccine against so many different viruses.

The only way to prevent catching colds is to reduce your exposure to the viruses. You'd have to become a hermit to succeed completely, but you should do your best to shield yourself from virus-laden sneezing and coughing. Remember, too, that these viruses can survive on inanimate objects, so you should wash your hands frequently when handling utensils and dishes used by an infected person.

The Flu

Influenza is also caused by a virus. It's a much more serious problem because it involves the bronchi and lungs as well as the upper respiratory tract. In fact, the flu virus can even spread from the lungs through the blood to infect other parts of the body.

Most common in winter, influenza causes epidemics that claim 10,000 lives in the United States each year — in a good year. During the major epidemics that occur about once a decade, as many as 40,000 people die from the flu and its complications.

The flu begins innocently enough with coldlike symptoms, but in less than a day fever, chills, muscle aches, headache, and cough have arrived. Most people recover in five to seven days, but people with other medical problems can die from influenza, as can healthy elders.

Influenza *can* be prevented! The flu virus has a unique and nasty trick of changing its outer coat, disguising itself from the immune system. Fortunately, we've been able to keep pace by designing new vaccines to match the new viral strains. Each year a vaccine is prepared to fight off the three flu strains that can be expected to spread throughout the United States between November and March. The vaccine is effective, safe, and inexpensive. Why, then, do more than 10,000 people still die from the flu each winter? Because the flu vaccine is not used appropriately. Shockingly, only 20 percent of high-risk Americans who should be vaccinated actually get a flu shot each fall.

All people over 65 should be vaccinated against the flu every year. So too should residents of chronic care facilities and people with heart disease, lung disease, diabetes, kidney disease, and certain other chronic medical conditions.

Do I take the flu shot myself? Yes, even though I'm neither 65 nor chronically ill. Because of heavy exposure, health care providers should also be vaccinated. But I'm happy to give flu shots to anyone who wants one, as long as the supply holds out. The only exceptions are people who are highly allergic to eggs, and pregnant women.

If your doctor doesn't recommend a flu shot next fall, ask why not. You can take your vaccination even if you have a cold; but if you have a fever, you'll be wise to wait until you've recovered.

Can you prevent the flu once you've been exposed even if you didn't have a flu shot? Yes. Influenza is one of the few exceptions to the rule that viruses are not susceptible to medications. A drug called amantadine can prevent the flu if treatment is started promptly after exposure. Although it's not an antibiotic, amantadine is a prescription medicine. Generally safe, it does, of course, cause occasional side effects. If you are exposed to flu, you'll need to ask your doctor about amantadine. Here, too, you'd best initiate the discussion, since amantadine is overlooked and underprescribed by most practitioners.

Pneumonia

One of the reasons why the flu is so serious is that it can lead to bacterial pneumonia. It does this by interfering with the normally effective defense mechanisms of the respiratory tract. The sticky carpet of mucus which should trap bacteria becomes watery and ineffectual, and the tiny filaments that usually expel bacteria lose their oomph. As a result, bacteria can slide down from the nose and mouth into the lungs, where they cause bacterial pneumonia.

It is true that we do a better job curing pneumonia than the sniffles. Antibiotics are effective against bacteria but not viruses. Even so, pneumonia is a very serious infection, causing fever, chills, cough, and often chest pain and shortness of breath. These symptoms resemble the flu, but typically patients with bacterial pneumonia have another symptom that should tip off the diagnosis: they produce large amounts of sputum that is thick, gray-green, or bloody. In fact the sputum, along with chest x rays and blood counts, is the best way to diagnose pneumonia; your doctor should look at the sputum under a microscope, and microbiology technicians should perform cultures and other tests.

Sputum examinations are important because many different bacteria can cause pneumonia. Each requires a different antibiotic. And we'd better get it right, since pneumonia can be fatal if treatment is incorrect. Even with the best treatment, 5 to 10 percent of elderly or debilitated patients who get pneumonia will die from the infection.

Fortunately, one type of bacteria, the pneumococcus, causes about 60 percent of the bacterial pneumonias that begin outside the hospital. Why is this fortunate? Because there is a vaccine that can help prevent pneumococcal pneumonia.

You may not have heard about the pneumonia vaccine, but it's really nothing new. A vaccine was developed in the 1940s, and tests showed that it was very effective. Just at that time, however, penicillin was introduced; because the antibiotic was so beneficial for pneumonia patients, the vaccine was abandoned. It's too bad; even with penicillin, pneumonia is a very serious infection, especially in older patients and those with underlying illnesses.

A new pneumococcal vaccine was introduced in 1977 and was improved further in 1983. But, like the flu vaccine, it is very underutilized, in part because it's a bit controversial. There is no controversy about its safety; everyone agrees that it's very safe indeed. There is legitimate dispute, however, about its effectiveness. Many studies have found that it is about 80 percent effective in preventing pneumococcal pneumonia, but other trials have been much less encouraging. Having reviewed the data, I agree with the United States Public Health Service that the vaccine is effective.

Even granting doubt about the percentage of protection conferred by the pneumococcal vaccine, I recommend it to my patients because it's safe and inexpensive — and because any protection is better than none at all. But not all people need pneumococcal vaccine. I generally offer it to people over 65 and to patients with heart or lung disease, liver disease, impaired immune systems, or certain tumors. It is particularly important to vaccinate patients who have had their spleen removed and people with sickle cell anemia.

Many other bacteria can cause pneumonia; except for the Hemophilus vaccine given to all children, we don't have shots to protect you from them. But you can help prevent pneumonia by keeping your defense mechanisms in shape. Karate lessons are not required. Just keep your teeth and gums healthy to reduce the bacteria in your mouth, and avoid drugs and excessive alcohol, which can depress your cough reflexes, allowing mouth bacteria to sneak down to your lungs.

Tuberculosis

A unique type of lung infection requires special mention. Tuberculosis has been a major human disease since history was first recorded. TB is a dramatic example of the benefits and limitations of prevention.

Most people think that tuberculosis has been all but eliminated in the United States, and that antibiotics deserve the credit. Both assumptions are wrong.

Special antibiotics *are* very effective for treating tuberculosis. For the first time in history, these drugs enable patients with TB to be cured. Since the TB bug spreads from person to person, treatment reduces communicability, thus preventing infection. But the control of tuberculosis in the United States began at the turn of the century, 50 years *before* antituberculous drugs were developed. Prevention was achieved through better social and economic conditions, which decreased crowding and improved nutrition and immunity. Much of the world has not shared in our improved standard of living, which is why TB remains rampant in the Third World. In fact, despite excellent medications, an astounding 50 percent of all humankind is infected with the TB germ. The moral: prevention depends on socioeconomic as well as medical advances.

Even in the United States, TB has begun to increase once again. Two factors are responsible: homelessness and AIDS. We are nowhere near an epidemic of tuberculosis, but with more than 20,000 new cases each year, there is cause for concern.

TB can be prevented. Maintaining good nutrition and general health will help. Avoiding exposure is an obvious goal. But two medical interventions are also available.

A vaccine for primary prevention stops the disease before it occurs. The vaccine, called BCG, was introduced more than 70 years ago, but it remains controversial. BCG trials in Europe have demonstrated good protection, but large trials in India have failed to show any benefit from the vaccine. The European trials seem more relevant to the United States, and I expect the vaccine could work here. Still, it is recommended only under very special circumstances because another strategy for prevention is available.

TB is an ideal disease for secondary prevention for three reasons: asymptomatic infection generally precedes actual disease by many years; an excellent screening test is available; and medical intervention can prevent early infection from progressing.

Here's how secondary prevention can work. Nearly everyone who is infected with the TB germ feels entirely well after inhaling the bacillus. In fact, good immune mechanisms ensure that infected people will continue to feel perfectly healthy. Even so, the TB germ lurks in the lungs or other organs, and can be activated years or even decades later. During this latent period most chest x rays are normal, but infection can be detected with a simple, safe, inexpensive skin test. People with reactive TB skin tests can be given a medication called INH, which usually prevents TB from ever producing disease.

In practical terms, the best way for you to prevent TB is to know your skin test results. If your test is positive, discuss the pros and cons of INH with your doctor. Individual treatment decisions are required; the benefits of INH are well documented, but side effects can occur, particularly in older people and those with liver disease. If your skin test is negative, you have nothing to worry about. But if your test is negative, you should repeat it periodically if exposure is likely. I recommend annual skin tests for health care workers, for certain inner-city residents and minority-group members, for people with impaired immune systems, and for residents of chronic care facilities. I also recommend repeat skin testing two months after travel to any part of the world where TB is common. Most important of all is repeat testing after suspected exposure to TB.

In case you're wondering, my TB skin test is negative, so I have it repeated yearly. If it converts to positive, I'll get a chest x ray and see my doctor, expecting a recommendation of preventive treatment with INH.

Tuberculosis is an ancient disease, but new diseases can also affect your respiratory tract. Two are worthy of mention because they can sometimes be prevented. And this time you can do it yourself.

Upper Respiratory Tract Infections

The modern life-style is responsible for many modern illnesses. High living is to blame for some of these woes, including infections that occur high in the respiratory tract.

Infections of the sinuses or ears can be precipitated by air travel. All commercial flights are pressurized, but cabin pressure is not maintained fully at sea level. Pressure changes occur at altitudes above 22,500 feet. When you ascend to this level, or when you descend from it, pressure changes can block your sinuses or ears. The result can be painful infections, particularly if you have a cold or allergy. You don't need to stay home to prevent this; just take a decongestant tablet or use a nasal spray 30 minutes before ascent and descent. As usual, simple preventive measures can compensate for many of the ups and downs of contemporary life.

■ 6 ■

Diseases of the Stomach and Intestinal Tract

The average American consumes about 80,000 meals during the course of a lifetime, to say nothing of countless snacks and libations. In view of what these meals contain — and lack — it's no surprise that intestinal complaints are among the most common of all medical symptoms. Most are minor, but some are lethal; many could be prevented, particularly by dietary improvements.

Each year, 8 percent of us have gastrointestinal disorders severe enough to restrict activity or require medical attention. The majority of these conditions are temporary, but more than 20 million Americans have chronic digestive disorders, and over 2 million are disabled by these diseases. Responsible for over 50 million office visits and 4 million hospitalizations each year, digestive disorders are also very expensive, costing $17 billion annually in direct medical expenses and twice as much in lost productivity. If we spent a few of our food dollars more wisely, we could save many of these medical dollars.

■ The Normal Digestive System

If you think of the gastrointestinal tract simply as a 25-foot series of interconnected hollow tubes, you'll understand how food gets from the top of the system to the bottom, but you won't appreciate the subtle digestive mechanisms that nourish and sustain life. Far from being a passive conduit for transporting food in and passing wastes out, the intestinal structures are metabolically active tissues with precisely regulated roles.

The central role of the digestive system is, of course, to extract nutrition from food while leaving waste products behind. It's no easy task. The food we eat is composed of large, complex molecules of fat, protein, and carbohydrate. Essential vitamins and minerals are present as well. But these molecules are too large to be absorbed intact. The digestive system must first break them down into smaller subunits and then absorb the nutrients needed for energy and as the building blocks of the body's tissues.

Digestion actually starts in the mouth, where chewing reduces the size of food particles, and salivary juices begin digesting carbohydrates into

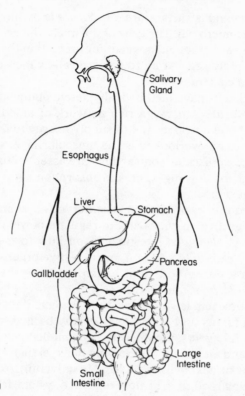

Figure 6-1.
Digestive system

simple sugars, proteins into amino acids, and fats into fatty acids (see figure 6-1). The esophagus, or food pipe, carries food to the stomach, where digestion continues. The stomach contains hydrochloric acid as well as digestive enzymes; its lining is normally tough enough to withstand damage from acid, but tissues of the esophagus are much more vulnerable. Next stop is the small intestine, where the majority of digestion and absorption occurs. The intestinal lining contains its own digestive enzymes, and the pancreas adds many more. The liver and gallbladder deliver bile to the small intestine, allowing fat to be digested and absorbed.

The small intestine does much more than digest foods; it also absorbs the nutrients and water that are released by the digestive process. By the time the intestinal contents get to the colon, most of the usable food molecules have already been extracted. The colon absorbs additional water, concentrating and storing waste material until it is excreted. Colonic contents include countless millions of bacteria which produce enzymes that act on food and fiber residues.

The digestive process may sound easy, but it's a lot more involved than simply mixing food with enzymes and sopping up the products. Many enzymes are needed to do the job right: to date, more than 25 digestive enzymes have been identified. To absorb all the nutrients, the small intestine must have a tremendous surface area; it does this by having innumerable projections called microvilli. The cells of the microvilli are essential for absorption, but they are readily damaged; for protection they secrete mucus, and they also rapidly regenerate to replace cells which die and are shed into the intestinal contents.

The intestinal cells have metabolically active pumps to bring nutrients into the blood. Needless to say, a rich network of blood vessels must be present to absorb the nutrients and to supply energy to the intestinal cells themselves. Not to be overlooked is the muscular layer on the outside of the intestinal tract; muscular contractions are essential to propel food at a pace slow enough to allow digestion and absorption but fast enough to prepare us for the next meal.

All of this requires coordination. The nervous system helps to control the release of digestive enzymes and to regulate bowel contractions. The circulatory system regulates intestinal blood flow to meet the increased needs created by eating. In addition, the digestive organs themselves produce more than a dozen hormones which fine-tune the interactions between intestinal enzymes and motility.

This intricate system is vulnerable to injury and damage. Of particular concern are the toxins and microbes that may be ingested with food. To fight these harmful agents, the digestive system depends on stomach acid to kill bacteria, and on intestinal emptying to expel them. The immune system also helps by attacking microbes and inactivating toxins.

Your well-being requires a healthy digestive system, from top to bottom. In considering disorders of the intestinal tract, we'll start at the bottom because that's where the most serious disorders begin.

■ Cancer of the Colon and Rectum

There is good news and bad news about cancer of the colon and rectum. The bad news is that colon cancer will be diagnosed in 150,000 Americans this year, and that 60,000 will die from the disease. Rare in young people, colon cancer risk increases with age; the average age at diagnosis is 70. Overall, your risk of getting colon cancer at some time in your life is one in 20; only skin and lung cancers occur more often, and only breast and lung cancers kill more Americans. In all, colon cancer accounts for 15 percent of all malignancies.

If that news isn't bad enough, then consider the fact that between 1973 and 1986 the rate of colon cancer *increased* in the United States by 9.4 percent.

Ready for some good news? Despite the increased occurrence of colon cancer, the death rate has gone down by 7 percent. The credit goes to medical progress. We've gotten much better at early diagnosis, which means the disease is being detected when it's much easier to cure. And new chemotherapy programs are making progress even in advanced cases. I anticipate continued improvement in both areas.

But there is even better news about colon cancer: it can be prevented.

Colon cancer is not an automatic part of the aging process. In other parts of the world it's uncommon at *all* ages. In Japan, for example, the rate is only 21 percent of the rate in America, but ethnic Japanese living in the United States have exactly the same rate as other Americans. A similar, but even greater, disparity occurs in blacks: in Nigeria the rate of colon cancer is less than 10 percent of the rate in Afro-Americans.

It is clear that some aspects of the Western life-style cause colon cancer. Let's review what is known about those causes, so you can take steps to protect yourself from this unnecessarily common malignancy.

The Causes of Colon Cancer

Diet is the crucial factor in causing colon cancer. It's not that we eat toxins that directly damage colon cells the way that tobacco smoke injures lung cells. Instead, it's a combination of a lack of some dietary factors (fiber and possibly certain vitamins) combined with an excess of others (fat, calories, and possibly meat proteins). It's not certain just how this combination leads to cancer, but the data suggest that intestinal bacteria are the ultimate culprits. The American diet encourages the growth of certain bacteria in the colon, promotes bacterial production of toxic enzymes, and allows the injurious chemicals to remain in contact with colon cells for an excessive period of time. Over the years, cells that are injured form polyps which can undergo malignant transformation. Genetics, too, play a role; some families are unusually susceptible to colon cancer.

Even though the entire colon cancer equation has not been solved, the individual factors that can help or hurt have been clarified.

Cancer-Protective Dietary Factors

Dietary fiber. Interest in dietary fiber dates back to the observations of Drs. Denis Burkitt and H. C. Trowell more than 20 years ago. Working as medical missionaries in Kampala, Uganda, they noted the rarity of "Western" diseases in their patients. Colon cancer was very uncommon, as were other digestive disorders (constipation, diverticulosis, appendicitis, hemorrhoids, hernias, and hiatus hernia), cardiovascular disorders (coronary heart disease and hypertension), and metabolic disorders (diabetes and obesity). The good doctors formulated the "fiber hypothesis," suggesting that roughage in the African diet was the protective factor. Burkitt stated this hypothesis most simply (and explicitly) by noting that he could predict the number of hospital visits from the size and frequency of his patient's bowel movements, bulky stools indicating less illness. Over the years, the fiber hypothesis has been challenged, debated, and refined, but the basic observation has held up.

Fiber is present in all plant materials, and is therefore a natural part of the human diet. But processing removes fiber; milling of wheat, for example, produces white flour for baking but leaves all the fiber behind in the bran. Unfortunately, the American diet favors highly processed, refined foods at the expense of fiber.

Although the many forms of fiber in vegetable foods are nothing more than carbohydrates, they are different from ordinary carbohydrates because they resist the activity of human digestive enzymes. Instead of being absorbed like other carbohydrates, plant fiber enters the colon unchanged. It has no caloric value, but it has many other benefits. It draws water with it, making the bowel contents much bulkier and softer. The increased bulk serves to dilute potentially harmful chemicals. Fiber can also bind bile acids, reducing their ability to irritate colon cells (and possibly lowering blood cholesterol levels as well). Perhaps most important of all, the bulky, fiber-rich bowel contents stimulate intestinal contractions, greatly speeding the process of elimination. One result is less constipation. Dr. Burkitt's Africans digested and eliminated their meals in less than 12 hours, while the Englishmen he used for comparison took 36 to 60 hours. A more important consequence is that toxins in the stool are rapidly eliminated from the body instead of lingering in the colon, where they can damage cells.

The typical American diet contains only 11 grams of fiber daily, about one third of what it should. You can get fiber supplements at your drugstore to bring up your intake, but it's much better to rely on fiber-rich foods. Choose cereals, breads, and pastas made with whole-grain flours instead of refined flour. Eat lots of fruits and vegetables such as apples, pears, peaches, and potatoes — but leave the skin on, please. Peas and beans, either fresh or dried, are excellent sources of fiber, as are cruciferous vegetables such as broccoli and cabbage. Nuts, berries, figs, and prunes are all high in fiber. Another good source is popcorn, but don't add salt or butter if you want to protect your heart as well as your colon. In chapter 20 I'll try to smooth out the details about dietary roughage.

Can you get too much of a good thing? Yes. In some people fiber can cause bloating, gas, cramps, or diarrhea. You can minimize this risk by increasing your fiber intake gradually, and by experimenting to find the source of fiber that suits you best.

A final tip. To allow a high-fiber diet to do its work for you, it's important to drink lots of water. One of the ways that fiber helps is by drawing water into the intestinal waste, making it soft as well as bulky. It's up to you to provide the fluids that will make this happen.

Vitamins. Certain vitamins may help reduce your risk of colon cancer, but the case for them is not as strong as for fiber.

Vitamin D protects experimental animals from colon cancer induced by toxic chemicals. In human population studies, colon cancer is most common in the geographic areas getting the least sunlight. In a 19-year study of nearly 2,000 men in Chicago, moderate amounts of dietary vitamin D reduced the incidence of colon cancer. More recently, doctors in Maryland studied blood vitamin D levels in 25,000 volunteers, finding that the people with the lowest levels had the highest risk of colon cancer.

The Japan-Hawaii cancer study evaluated vitamin C and colon cancer in 8,000 ethnic Japanese men living on Oahu. Men with the lowest vitamin C intake had nearly two times more colon cancer than men with the highest intake. In other studies beta carotene (vitamin A) has been found protective; vitamin E may also help, but the data are scant at present.

There is certainly not enough data to prescribe vitamin pills to fight colon cancer, much less to support basking in the sun. But there is enough evidence to recommend foods rich in vitamins A, C, and D such as vegetables, fruits, and vitamin D–fortified (but low-fat!) dairy products.

Other protective factors. Several investigators have reported a decreased risk of colon cancer in people eating lots of cruciferous vegetables (cabbage, broccoli, Brussels sprouts), but protection may depend on the fiber in these vegetables rather than on vitamins or other contents. Calcium reduces the proliferation of colon cells in the laboratory; high calcium intake has been linked to low colon cancer risk, but this may be due to the large amounts of vitamin D added to most milk products.

If fiber, vitamins A, C, and D, and possibly calcium may reduce your risk of colon cancer, there are other dietary factors that may increase risk.

Cancer-Promoting Dietary Factors

Fat. As is the case of some other cancers, high-fat diets appear to increase the risk of colon cancer; as for other cancers, saturated fats from animal sources appear to be the culprits.

Dietary fat stimulates the growth of certain bacteria in the colon. These bacteria convert bile acids to potentially carcinogenic chemicals. Perhaps that's why rodents fed high-fat foods develop more colon cancer. More to the point, international human studies have consistently found the highest rates of colon cancer in the countries with the highest dietary fat content. For example, a multinational study published in the 1990 *Journal of the National Cancer Institute* found that saturated fat is strongly linked to colon cancer; the risk of colon cancer doubled with every 10 grams of saturated fat in the daily diet.

Closer to home, a ten-year Harvard study of nearly 90,000 American nurses confirmed the link between animal fat and colon cancer. Women who ate beef, lamb, or pork as a main dish every day had two and a half times more colon cancer than did women who ate such meals less than once a month. Not all animal products, however, were guilty; fish and chicken (*without* the skin) seem to *reduce* cancer risk.

I can't promise that avoiding saturated fat will prevent you from ever getting colon cancer, but it should give you a fat chance for prevention.

Meat protein. Because studies reveal that diets high in meat increase the risk of colon cancer, meat protein has been blamed. Although not a vegetarian, neither am I a great advocate of meat. Still, I'm not sure that we can link meat protein to colon cancer, since diets high in meat are high in fat and calories, and are often low in fiber. Scientists will have to chew over this one before they are sure which factor counts the most.

Calories and obesity. A variety of animal and human studies have linked total caloric intake and obesity to an increased risk of cancer. The evidence with regard to colon cancer is mixed, but staying lean certainly won't do you any harm, and a low-fat, high-fiber diet is an excellent way to restrict calories.

Although diet is the best way to reduce your risk of colon cancer, there is another way that you should not neglect: exercise.

Exercise and Cancer Protection

Seven independent studies, some small but others very large, some from Europe and China but others from California, New York, and Washington State, have explored the link between exercise and colon cancer; all agree that physical activity reduces risk. While not enormous, the magnitude of the protection is impressive: sedentary people are 1.3 to 1.6 times more likely to develop colon cancer than physically active people. The protective effect of exercise may seem surprising, and even unlikely, but there is a good explanation. Physical activity promotes intestinal emptying, thus protecting colon cells from prolonged contact with potential toxins in waste materials. Exercise may also help by fighting obesity, another factor that contributes to the risk of cancer.

How much exercise do you need to reduce your risk of colon cancer? A 1991 report from the famous study of 17,148 Harvard alumni provides an answer. Men who exercised vigorously enough to burn off about 2,500 calories per week experienced a 50 percent reduction in colon cancer — if they maintained regular exercise over the years. Coincidentally, perhaps, this is exactly the same amount of exercise that will provide optimal protection against heart attacks and death from cardiac disease. Chapter 21 will explain how to get your 2,500 calories of weekly exercise safely and enjoyably.

No single life-style change will confer immunity from colon cancer, but collectively they will provide substantial protection. So jog on down to your grocery store, and walk back with an armful of bran and veggies. But don't rely solely on diet and exercise; your doctor can also help, since screening and early detection will save lives if primary prevention fails.

Aspirin and Cancer Prevention

Diet and exercise are well-documented ways to reduce your risk of colon cancer. A 1991 report in the *New England Journal of Medicine* raises the possibility that aspirin may also help. Doctors from the American Cancer Society analyzed aspirin use and colon cancer in 662,424 adults over a six-year period. Aspirin use appeared to reduce the risk of dying from colon cancer by 40 percent. Experiments in animals have reported similar results with several aspirinlike anti-inflammatory medications. Still, more human data will be needed before we can add colon cancer to the list of diseases that may be prevented by low-dose aspirin therapy.

Secondary Prevention of Colon Cancer

For secondary protection to succeed, three criteria must be met. First, the illness must evolve slowly, so there is time to detect latent disease before it causes any symptoms. Second, an effective screening test must be available to detect early disease; ideally the test should be simple and inexpensive as well as sensitive, specific, and safe. Third, an effective medical intervention must be available to prevent the disease from progressing to the stage of symptoms, disability, or death.

Colon cancer meets the first and third criteria with ease; it is slow-growing and highly amenable to cure in its early stages. The problem lies with the second standard: simple screening tests are available, but they are not hugely effective; highly effective tests are available, but they are neither simple nor inexpensive.

Colon cancer grows slowly. In most cases the first abnormality to occur is not even the cancer itself but a benign polyp. Most polyps remain benign; some can bleed, but most are entirely harmless. Nonetheless, a small number of polyps, perhaps 2 percent of the total, can enlarge and undergo malignant transformation. Even this occurs at a leisurely pace, taking at least five to ten years in the average patient. It's not known what makes a polyp enlarge and become cancerous. In an exciting 1989 experiment, however, Dr. Jerome DeCasse of New York Hospital–Cornell Medical Center found that feeding high-fiber diets to patients with polyps actually caused the polyps to shrink.

Even after cancer cells arise in the tip of a polyp, they grow slowly. In the earliest form of colon cancer, called Stage A, the tumor remains confined to the polyp. In Stage B the cancer cells have spread to the wall of the colon, slowly making their way through the wall. By Stage C they have spread to abdominal lymph nodes, and from there, in Stage D, to the liver, lungs, and other distant organs.

Colon cancer is highly treatable. Stage A disease can be cured more than 90 percent of the time, often simply by removing the polyp through an instrument called a colonoscope. Surgery is required for Stage B, but five-year cure rates are very encouraging, approaching 80 percent in favorable cases. Even patients with early Stage C cancers have a 50-50 chance of cure, but the odds drop dramatically once organ metastases have occurred in Stage D.

Early detection is obviously very important. Unfortunately, most colon cancers are clinically silent in their early stages. Even bleeding cancers can be hard to detect because most bleed so slowly that the bowel movements look normal. If bleeding eventually produces anemia, patients may experience fatigue, light-headedness, and rapid heartbeats. Tumors on the right side of the colon are particularly hard to detect because the bowel contents are still liquid in the upper colon and can slide past tumors without causing any sensations of blockage. In contrast, waste material is in solid form when it reaches the left or lower colon, so tumors may produce cramps, constipation, pain on defecation, or visible bleeding. Needless to say, if you develop any of these changes in your bowel habits, you should promptly report them to your doctor.

Since symptoms occur quite late in most patients with colon cancer, we'd like to use screening tests to detect these common cancers when they are localized, small, and curable. Though conceptually simple, screening has a number of practical limitations and is quite controversial.

Perhaps the simplest way to screen for colon cancer is to test samples of bowel movements for trace amounts of blood. Although it's not aesthetically pleasing, it is very simple to collect specimens at home, using a test kit available from your doctor or pharmacy. In practice, to make the test accurate it is important to follow a special diet (no red meat, cauliflower, turnips, horseradish, or cantaloupe) and to avoid certain medications (vitamin C, iron, aspirin, and other anti-inflammatories) for three days before and during the test. Collect two samples from each of three consecutive bowel movements, and be sure they arrive at the lab for testing within six days.

At about $5 per patient, stool testing seems inexpensive as well as risk-free and easy. The American Cancer Society recommends this process for everyone once a year beginning at age 50. But many other authorities, including the U.S. Preventive Services Task Force and the Canadian Task Force on the Periodic Health Exam, disagree. These experts point out the two problems with stool testing: First, many cancers do not bleed and will be missed. Second, 95 percent of patients who test positive don't have cancer at all; hence many people will be put through additional tests, which may be frightening, uncomfortable, and expensive, merely to be told they are okay. And, as Drs. David Ransohoff and Christopher Lang point out in the 1991 *New England Journal of Medicine,* even these seemingly simple stool tests would add up to an enormous national expense: testing all Americans over 50 once a year would add $1.2 billion to our annual health bill. Money can't buy everything; in this case there is no certainty that it would buy health, since it has never been shown that this form of screening for colon cancer saves lives.

An older screening test is the barium enema or "lower GI series." After evacuating the colon with laxatives and enemas, radiologists instill a solution of barium that coats the wall of the colon. When x rays are taken, polyps and tumors can be visualized. Barium enemas are very valuable tests, but they are not suited to mass screening of patients who feel well because they are time-consuming, uncomfortable, and moderately expensive at about $200 each, and because they can miss small tumors. They also involve exposure to radiation, a real drawback for healthy people.

A second traditional screening test with none of these problems is the simple rectal exam. The American Cancer Society recommends this, combined with a stool test for occult blood, annually beginning at age 40. There is little controversy about this procedure since it's normally part of the annual physical exam. But it's a poor screening test for cancer, since only one stool specimen is checked, and since the doctor's examining finger will detect only the cancers that arise in the final three inches of the rectum, amounting to fewer than 10 percent of all colon cancers.

The colon is five feet long. It is possible to look up into it to detect polyps and tumors beyond the reach of a digital exam. The traditional way to do this is by using a sigmoidoscope, a hollow tube introduced into the rectum and then gently advanced upwards. Two types of sigmoidoscopes are available. The older, rigid type can reach only 12 inches, but the newer flexible instruments can go twice as far. Since polyps can often be removed through sigmoidoscopes, these instruments can be used for treatment as well as diagnosis. Sigmoidoscopy can be performed in the doctor's office with minimal preparation; there is some discomfort, but complications are rare. Because of better visualization and less discomfort, flexible sigmoidoscopies are now preferred; they usually cost $100 to $200.

The American Cancer Society recommends that everyone undergo sigmoidoscopy every three to five years beginning at age 50. Again, the U.S. Task Force and many other authorities disagree. Unlike with stool testing, there are few false positive sigmoidoscopies. The drawbacks, though, are expense, discomfort, and especially false negative results, since about half of all colon cancers originate beyond the reach of even the newest flexible sigmoidoscopes. Writing in the *American Journal of Gastroenterology* in 1991, Drs. David Lieberman and Fredric Smith conclude that routine sigmoidoscopies are insensitive tests, detecting only 44 percent of polyps. Still, a 1992 study by Dr. Joe Selby and colleagues found that sigmoidoscopies could significantly reduce the colon cancer death rate; these doctors suggest that a sigmoidoscopy every ten years may be best, but additional studies will be needed to validate this recommendation.

The colonoscope is an instrument that allows visualization of the entire colon as well as removal of polyps and biopsy of suspicious lesions. It sounds like the ideal solution for colon cancer screening — but it's not. Colonoscopy is highly reliable and accurate; the problem is that it requires a specially trained team of doctors and nurses and is performed at a hospital. Patients must follow low-residue diets and then drink four quarts of a rather unpleasant cleansing solution the night before the test. The colonoscopy itself takes only 20 to 30 minutes, but because of sedation the patient loses an entire workday. Sedation minimizes discomfort, but serious complications such as bleeding or intestinal perforation occur in three of each 1,000 examinations. Another side effect is expense: the typical colonoscopy costs $500 to $1,000. Most insurance companies will not pay for colonoscopies that are performed for cancer screening.

Not a mass screening test, colonoscopy is an invaluable tool for evaluating and treating patients who have symptoms or who are at high risk for colon cancer.

With all these options and all this controversy, what should we be doing to screen for colon cancer? We need carefully controlled scientific trials to find out which strategy is really best. Until the results are available, what should we do now?

The choice should be made individually by patients and their doctors. I recommend annual rectal examinations beginning at age 40. I am frankly ambivalent about multiple stool examinations; I don't urge them on everyone, but I am delighted to arrange testing for all patients who want it, as long as they understand the potential limitations as well as the possible benefits. I do not recommend routine sigmoidoscopy or colonoscopy unless special colon cancer risk factors are present. These factors include a previously detected polyp or cancer, colon cancer in a parent or sibling, a family history of a multiple-polyp condition, or chronic ulcerative colitis. If such risk factors are present, I generally refer patients for periodic colonoscopies by specialists.

Much more information about colon cancer screening will become available in the next few years. Until then there is no right way. Discuss the options with your doctor and decide what seems best for you. Above all, remember to practice primary prevention. If everyone followed my guidelines for diet and exercise, the debate about screening and secondary prevention would soon be irrelevant.

■ Diverticulosis

Can a condition that affects 30 million Americans, including 50 percent of all people over 60, be considered a disease? When it comes to diverticulosis, my answer is yes. True, most people with diverticulosis feel fine and don't even know they have it. But diverticulosis can cause problems — enough, in fact, to account for 200,000 hospital admissions each year, at a cost of more than $300 million. If that's not a disease, I don't know what is.

Despite its complex name, diverticulosis is a very simple process, an outpouching of the wall of the colon (see figure 6-2). Some people have only a few diverticula, while others have many. Scant or abundant, they tend to be located at the lowest end of the colon, in the lower left side of the abdomen.

Although most people with diverticulosis have no symptoms, 3 to 5 percent do become ill. Two problems may develop. The more common is bleeding. If blood vessels in the walls of the pouches become damaged, blood will be lost into the intestinal contents. Small amounts of blood will go unnoticed but can gradually cause anemia if the bleeding recurs; small amounts can also show up when specimens are tested for occult blood, confusing the issue of cancer screening. Large amounts of blood are hard to miss: abdominal cramps and red or maroon diarrhea are the typical symptoms. Although diverticular bleeding will often settle down on its own, patients require careful monitoring in the hospital, and may need aggressive medical or surgical treatment.

The second complication of diverticulosis is diverticulitis, which occurs when the pouches become inflamed and infected. The result is fever and abdominal pain and tenderness. Because most diverticula are in the lower left abdomen, this inflammation is often called left-sided appendicitis. Mild cases respond to antibiotic pills, but more severe cases mandate hospitalization and intravenous medications and feedings, with surgery the ultimate treatment for severe cases.

Diverticular bleeding and inflammation are not pretty prospects. Don't

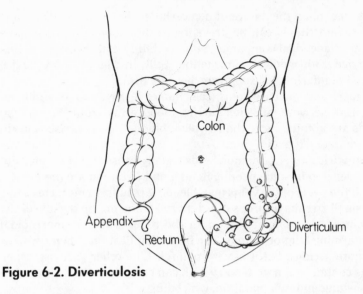

Figure 6-2. Diverticulosis

resign yourself to them. Despite the frequency of diverticulosis in older Americans, it is not a simple consequence of maturity. Diverticulosis is a disease — a preventable disease.

Diverticulosis is so common because of the poor dietary habits of industrialized societies. Unknown in primitive cultures, it results from a lack of dietary fiber. A highly refined, low-residue diet deprives the intestinal contents of bulk. To expel small, hard waste products, the colon must contract and squeeze much harder than it should. All this pressure gradually weakens the wall of the colon, which bulges and then develops outpouches — diverticula.

The primary prevention of diverticulosis is simple: eat a high-fiber diet.

But if you already have diverticulosis, what can you do about secondary prevention to avert bleeding and inflammation? The program is simple: eat a high-fiber diet. Although this advice seems obvious, when I was in medical school I was taught just the reverse, and for years I joined my colleagues in recommending low-roughage food to treat diverticulosis. Perhaps that's why bleeding and inflammation were so common!

Fiber is so important for patients with diverticulosis, in fact, that I often prescribe fiber supplements in addition to bran cereals and fruits and vegetables (see table 20-6). Of the old-fashioned restrictions only one remains: patients with diverticulosis would probably be wise to avoid seeds and nuts.

■ Hemorrhoids

Despite being common enough to spawn a huge (and profitable) branch of the pharmaceutical industry, hemorrhoids are banned from polite conversation. The drug company ads promote ointments and suppositories, but they do little to explain the nature of hemorrhoids. Even worse, they don't explain how hemorrhoids can be prevented. I don't object to reasonable profits for pharmaceutical companies, and I certainly don't presume to mix financial advice with medical information. Still, in this area my advice crosses these boundaries: sell suppositories, buy bran.

If you understand varicose veins (see chapter 3), you understand hemorrhoids. A fine network of veins carries blood away from the rectum. Hemorrhoids are nothing more than swollen blood-filled varicose veins in the lower rectum and the anal canal.

Like other varicose veins, hemorrhoids usually cause no symptoms. But problems do develop in some people. Itching and irritation are the mildest complaints. If the walls of the veins tear, bleeding results; in most cases this amounts to small streaks or drops of bright red blood on the outside of the bowel movement, on toilet tissue, or in the toilet water. Hemorrhoidal bleeding is alarming but not serious. The final complication of hemorrhoids is not any more serious, but it is very painful. Like other varicose veins, hemorrhoids contain stagnant blood which can clot. Thrombosis is accompanied by swelling and inflammation, which hurt.

Just as it contributes to varicose veins in the legs, the abdominal pressure of pregnancy can cause hemorrhoids; obesity can also play a role in both variations on the theme of swollen veins. But the major causes of hemorrhoids are constipation and excessive straining during bowel movements.

Sound familiar? It should. Like the other intestinal disorders I've discussed in this chapter, hemorrhoids are a creation of the industrial revolution, a consequence of the "civilized" refined diet.

You're right: dietary fiber will prevent hemorrhoids. A high-roughage diet is also the key to secondary prevention, but for acute symptomatic flares, stool softeners, sitz baths, and those ointments and suppositories can help. Your friendly rectal surgeon is always available to inject or ligate hemorrhoids that fail to respond to conservative treatment. Remember that the next time you shop for cereal, bread, and vegetables.

■ Hernias

Hernias result when the lining of the abdominal cavity weakens, allowing the intestines to bulge outward. Very common in infancy as a result of developmental abnormalities, hernias are also common in older adults as a result of weakened tissues and excessive abdominal pressure. By now you should certainly understand the chief cause of excessive abdominal pressure: straining to expel fiber-deficient intestinal contents.

There is no doubt that hernias in adults are much more common in Western societies, and that high-fiber diets will help prevent them. But there is some room for debate about the proper management of hernias. Surgical repair is routine for children and was once nearly automatic for adults as well. Surgical techniques have improved since those days but, paradoxically perhaps, we are currently aiming to let patients "live with" hernias if they are not uncomfortable. People with hernias should avoid heavy lifting and other maneuvers that result in straining and increased abdominal pressure. In addition, they must remain alert for pain and tenderness. On occasion the intestines can become trapped and twisted in hernia sacs, causing a surgical emergency. Because of this potential, many patients very reasonably choose elective surgical repair as their means of secondary prevention. I'm all for it — as long as they don't forget that low-tech dietary management can prevent recurrences mandating high-tech surgical treatment.

■ Constipation

Despite its widespread occurrence in Western societies, it has been hard to get the facts about constipation out into the open. Americans who have constipation regard it as a medical problem — enough of a problem to spend $400 million on laxatives annually. Despite laxatives, however, millions of people are plagued by bowel movements that are infrequent and hard; they strain during defecation and often complain of bloating and abdominal discomfort. Their next step is to visit their doctor; more than 2 million office visits are occasioned by constipation every year. But many doctors respond unsympathetically, dismissing constipation as a normal pattern and diagnosing related symptoms as psychosomatic. Even worse, when patients persist in their complaints, they are often rewarded with fancy tests — and sometimes with even more laxatives.

Constipation is extremely common but it's *not* normal, nor is it harmless. We now know that straining at stool predisposes to hernias and hemorrhoids, and that constipation is associated with colon cancer and diverticulosis. Despite widespread use (and abuse!) of laxatives, 2 percent of Americans have fewer than three bowel movements per week, and countless more have milder degrees of constipation. In a minority of cases, constipation is caused by medications, diabetes, neurological disorders, underactive thyroids, or structural problems of the intestines. A simple medical checkup can exclude most of these problems; x rays and sigmoidoscopies are required only for unusual or severe cases. Medical tests are needed so infrequently because in most cases the cause of constipation is not illness but the highly refined Western diet.

Constipation is another disorder of the industrialized life-style. You can prevent it by returning to the basics. A high-fiber diet is the key. If your body is not used to dietary fiber, increase your intake gradually, building up to 30 grams a day over three or four weeks. Don't forget to drink plenty of fluids; without them, fiber may do as much harm as good. And be patient: it may take a month or more for a high-fiber, high-fluid diet to relieve constipation. A final tip: because exercise stimulates bowel motility, regular exercise is an important aid to regularity.

Diet and exercise should prevent you from needing laxatives. But constipation may recur from time to time, especially during trips or illnesses.

Temporary constipation does not require special treatment; just increase your fiber intake, using dietary supplements (bran, psyllium, or methyl cellulose) if necessary. An old standby, prunes, really can help. If you still need an occasional laxative, use an osmotic agent such as sorbitol, milk of magnesia, or magnesium citrate rather than a bowel irritant such as castor oil, phenolphthalein, senna, cascara, or bisacodyl.

Bowel movements are rarely the subject of polite conversation, nor should they become a personal preoccupation. Still, don't be soft on your symptoms. Simple measures can prevent constipation, relieving discomfort and reducing your risk of long-term complications.

■ Irritable Bowel Syndrome

After this one last pitch for a high-fiber diet, I'll get down from my cereal box to discuss other issues.

One of the most common problems in clinical medicine, irritable bowel syndrome differs from the other problems I've been discussing because it has a functional rather than a structural or anatomical basis. The bowel itself is perfectly normal. The problem is that its contractions are irregular and erratic instead of orderly and coordinated. The result: cramps, bloating, and often alternating periods of constipation and diarrhea.

Because blood tests, barium x rays, and even colonoscopies are normal, diagnosis is based on clinical features rather than lab tests. The cause is poorly understood and controversial, probably because there is not one cause but many. I am convinced, however, that lack of dietary fiber is the major contributor to many, if not most, cases. High-roughage diet helps, but fiber supplements are necessary in most patients. I've found that many patients are initially reluctant to try fiber, a reasonable reluctance if they've been experiencing diarrhea and cramps. Fiber, however, is not a laxative that irritates the bowel; by providing bulk and moisture, it helps reduce the need for colonic contractions and pressure. The trick is patience. The fiber should be increased gradually but progressively until the symptoms improve. Very large amounts of fiber are sometimes required. And it's important to include lots of water. Not to be forgotten is another way to promote coordinated contractions of the bowel muscles; regular physical exercise will literally help to keep your gut muscles in shape.

There are, of course, many other causes of abdominal bloating, cramps, gas, and constipation or diarrhea. Some are discussed in the next few pages. But if you don't respond to the programs outlined here, you should have a medical evaluation to be sure your symptoms don't reflect a more serious problem.

■ Diarrhea

The causes of diarrhea are many and varied; the tactics for prevention are no less diverse.

Although most people think of diarrhea in terms of excessive frequency of bowel movements, the actual problem is excessive fluid in the waste contents. The intestinal tract is responsible for absorbing tremendous amounts of fluid every day; the two quarts of liquid in the average diet are obvious, but the digestive system's own secretions contribute a hidden seven quarts more. Diarrhea results if abnormally large amounts of fluid pass through without being absorbed, or if the intestinal tract itself secretes additional fluid into the waste material.

Most often diarrhea is a mild and self-limited problem that you can treat yourself by adopting a low-roughage diet (temporarily!) and by using over-the-counter remedies. But if you have strong cramps or pain, moderate to high fever, severe diarrhea, general weakness, and large amounts of mucus or even small amounts of blood in your stools, you should see your doctor. Diarrhea that persists for more than 10 to 14 days is also an appropriate topic for medical consultation.

To prevent diarrhea, consider its many causes. *Mental stress* is a major factor for many people. *Medications* can also cause diarrhea; laxatives are an obvious cause, but many other drugs may be responsible, with antibiotics high on the list. Excessive amounts of nondigestible carbohydrate or fiber can also contribute.

Another dietary cause of diarrhea which is often overlooked is *lactose intolerance.* Lactose is the principal sugar in milk. To be absorbed, lactose must be broken down into two smaller sugar molecules by an intestinal enzyme called lactase. If not enough lactase is present, milk sugar passes into the colon without being absorbed. It draws water with it, and it feeds the intestinal bacteria that produce gases. The result: abdominal bloating and rumbling, gas, and diarrhea.

Lactose intolerance is often overlooked because milk is a highly valued foodstuff in our culture. In fact, home remedies for abdominal discomfort often include dairy products. Folk wisdom notwithstanding, lactose intolerance is a very common problem; beyond age six, 5 to 40 percent of Americans of Northern European descent are affected, as are 50 to 70 percent of blacks, Asians, Jews, and American Indians.

A genetically determined inherited trait, lactose intolerance varies widely in severity. Some people will develop symptoms only after they consume moderate to large amounts of milk, whereas others feel ill after just a little ice cream or cheese.

Lactose intolerance can be diagnosed formally by measuring blood glucose levels after consuming lactose or by a lactose breath test. But you don't need a doctor or lab to make the diagnosis. Just eliminate lactose from your diet and see how you feel. Remember, though, that milk and milk products can lurk in unexpected places.

Treatment is as simple as diagnosis; a low-lactose diet will do the trick. But you don't have to give up all dairy products, which are excellent sources of calcium, protein, and other nutrients. Many lactose-intolerant people can tolerate yogurt or cheese because they are fermented. Even better, you can buy low-lactose milk or add the lactase enzyme to ordinary milk to digest the lactose for you. You can also buy enzyme pills which you can take in case you are unable to plan your menu in advance. And I am happy to report that low-lactose milk is widely available in low-fat form, so you can get all the nutrition without the saturated fat.

Infections are responsible for many cases of diarrhea. Most often the problem is "food poisoning." Food poisoning typically occurs when food is contaminated with certain bacteria after cooking but is not refrigerated. The bacteria produce toxins that cause diarrhea, and sometimes vomiting, within 6 to 12 hours after the meal. Because the toxins are odorless and tasteless, you won't suspect anything until diarrhea begins. You'll feel miserable for 6 to 24 hours, but you'll recover fully without needing medical treatment. You should suspect food poisoning if others who shared the meal develop similar symptoms, if there is no fever, and if you recover quickly. All you need for treatment is to take enough fluids so you don't become dehydrated. Prevention is not the work of your doctor; the key is appropriate cooking and refrigeration of food as well as hygienic food preparation (see chapter 20 on food safety).

A variety of viruses can also cause diarrhea. These often cause small outbreaks, particularly in children late in the summer and early in the fall. Viral diarrhea may last for a week or so; low-grade fever is common, but there is no bleeding. Complications are rare and recovery complete. For prevention, run away from people with the trots.

Bacterial diarrhea can be more serious, since it can be accompanied by high fever and is sometimes complicated by intestinal bleeding or even bowel perforation. Fortunately, serious complications are rare, and most patients recover without treatment. In fact, some of the stronger antidiarrhea medications can make things worse. Antibiotics shorten diarrhea caused by some bacteria, but may actually prolong the infection caused by other germs. A stool culture will help decide if you will benefit from treatment.

Infectious diarrhea is most common in travelers, especially during trips to tropical, semitropical, or underdeveloped areas. Chapter 16 details dietary precautions and immunizations that can help prevent traveler's diarrhea. But even at home, some precautions can help prevent intestinal infections. Infected people should not prepare foods; handwashing and good hygiene and sanitation are no less important. But nothing is completely safe. For example, apparently pristine mountain streams can be the source of an intestinal parasite called giardia. And if you eat eggs, or even just egg whites, be sure they are cooked to 160 degrees or boiled at 140 degrees for three and a half minutes to kill salmonella, the most common cause of bacterial diarrhea in the United States. A final tip: don't use antacids unless they are really necessary, since stomach acid helps kill bacteria that cause diarrhea.

In many cases you can prevent diarrhea or can simply treat yourself for temporary episodes. But you should remember that serious problems ranging from colitis to tumors can sometimes produce diarrhea; if your symptoms are unusual, severe, or persistent, see your doctor.

■ Gas

I am extremely fond of most of my patients. I must confess, however, that those who are full of hot air can be a nuisance.

Intestinal gas is a frustrating problem for patient and doctor alike. Part of the frustration comes from misunderstanding. Far from being a sign of disease, intestinal gas is entirely normal; perfectly healthy people, in fact, expel nearly a quart of gas per day, on average. It's a good thing that gas is rarely serious, because treatment is mediocre at best; some patients benefit from over-the-counter preparations containing activated charcoal or simethicone, but many do not. Unfortunately, I have nothing better to offer by prescription.

But don't resign yourself to a lifetime of gas. You can often prevent this problem by careful attention to what you eat and how you eat it. Air swallowing owing to rapid eating and poor chewing is the main cause of belching. Anxiety is another cause of air swallowing, and carbonated beverages can also add to stomach gas. Flatulence can be harder to track down. Diet is usually the culprit; often, undigestible carbohydrates or unabsorbed lactose feed bacteria so they produce excessive amounts of hydrogen, methane, and carbon dioxide.

If you are bothered by excessive gas, try to control the problem by adjusting your diet. Eliminate carbonated beverages. Eat slowly and chew carefully. Avoid chewing gum, especially diet gums that contain sorbitol. Reduce or eliminate caffeine and alcohol from your diet. Above all, manipulate your carbohydrate intake. First, try eliminating milk products that contain lactose. If that fails, systematically reduce foods that contain fermentable carbohydrates; common offenders include beans and other legumes, cabbage, radishes, cauliflower, broccoli, onions, oats, and uncooked apples. Many of these foods, though, are valuable sources of fiber and nutrients. If you discover that one or more of these items is responsible for your gas, you can try to retain them in your diet by adding three to eight drops of Beano, a commercially available enzyme preparation, to your first bite of the gas-producing food. If none of this helps, try a gluten-free diet by temporarily avoiding wheat products. And even if flatulence persists, you may be able to reduce its unpleasant odor by eliminating red meat and fatty foods from your diet.

To prevent embarrassment, eliminate suspect items from your diet one by one until the problem is resolved. If all else fails, avoid crowded elevators; walking upstairs will be good for your health as well as your psyche.

■ Diseases of the Pancreas

Located at the rear of the abdomen behind the stomach, the pancreas is an endocrine gland responsible for regulating blood sugar (see chapter 12 on diabetes) as well as a digestive organ that delivers vital enzymes to the small intestine.

Pancreatitis, inflammation of the gland, causes pain, loss of appetite, and fever. Pancreatitis can be mild and self-limited or severe enough to cause shock and even death. It can occur just once or can relapse over and over. Chronic cases can damage pancreatic function, leading to impaired digestion or diabetes.

Among the many causes of pancreatitis, three stand out. All are to a greater or lesser degree preventable: alcohol, trauma, and gallstones.

With a mortality rate of 99 percent, pancreatic cancer is the deadliest of all cancers. Its 25,000 victims make it the fourth most common cause of cancer death in the United States. Early diagnosis is difficult and contributes little to care because treatment is so poor. Since the causes of pancreatic cancer are largely unknown, prevention is also unsatisfactory. Coffee consumption was proposed as a risk factor, but newer research reveals this association to be spurious. We do know, however, that cancer of the pancreas is two to three times more common in cigarette smokers, giving you one more good reason to abjure tobacco.

■ Diseases of the Esophagus

As we near the end of our review of preventable digestive disorders, we return to the top of the digestive tract, to the "foodpipe" leading from the mouth to the stomach.

The most common disorder of the esophagus is known to doctors as esophagitis but to patients as heartburn. In this case, at least, the medical term is better. Heartburn has nothing to do with the heart. True, the typical symptom is a burning pain in the center of the chest, but the cause is inflammation (-*itis*) of the esophagus.

The lining of the esophagus is tough enough to withstand digestive enzymes in saliva, but it's not hardy enough to handle acid. This is not an engineering flaw; the esophagus is not normally exposed to acid. Acid is produced by the stomach, however, and if it finds its way upstream to the esophagus, you'll hear from your foodpipe.

To prevent esophagitis, just remember what your mother taught you. Don't overstuff your stomach or bolt your food; smaller, more frequent meals are much less likely to force acid up into the esophagus. Above all, don't lie down right after a meal; gravity is the esophagus's best friend. Although the role of diet in producing esophagitis is debatable, it is surely prudent to avoid caffeine, alcohol, and spices if they produce heartburn. Garlic, onions, and even chocolate may also promote the backflow of stomach acid. And if the advice of your mom doesn't do the trick, you can listen to your friendly TV announcer — antacids actually do help. Finally, if your treatment of heartburn fails, your doctor can provide very effective (but expensive) prescription drugs for esophagitis.

Whereas some medications prevent and treat esophagitis, others can cause it. If pills are taken improperly, they can lodge in the esophagus for five minutes or more. You won't know it until a particularly nasty form of inflammation, erosive esophagitis, occurs. Any pill can do it, including over-the-counter medications (especially aspirin, iron, and vitamin C) and prescription drugs (especially anti-inflammatories, tetracyclines, and potassium). Preventing erosive esophagitis is so straightforward that I would be reluctant to mention it were it not for the problems I've seen in perfectly intelligent patients. Simply swallow all pills with at least three or four ounces of fluid and remain upright for one to two minutes.

Cancer of the esophagus is another particularly deadly tumor, killing well over 8,000 of the 9,000 cases diagnosed in the United States each year. For reasons that are not clear, esophageal cancer is even more common elsewhere, particularly in parts of Africa, Europe, and the Asian "esophageal cancer belt."

A variety of environmental insults and life-style abuses account for this uneven distribution of esophageal cancer. Cigarette smoking and alcohol abuse explain at least 80 percent of all cases in the United States. Toxins in foods (nitrates, fungal products, and some pickled vegetables) account for a much smaller fraction. Physical damage caused by lye ingestion or possibly even repeatedly drinking extremely hot tea have also been implicated. Dietary deficiency of vitamin A, iron, zinc, or molybdenum are also among the potential risk factors for esophageal cancer. Pay attention to all these things, but remember that they are bit players when compared with smoking and alcohol abuse.

■ Diseases of the Stomach and Small Intestine

Stomach Cancer

At several points in this book I have lauded the Japanese life-style for its low risk of heart disease and colon cancer as well as its superior longevity. But when it comes to stomach cancer, America is way ahead, with less than 25 percent of the rate in Japan. And we're getting better all the time; the incidence of stomach cancer in the United States has declined by more than 75 percent in the past 50 years.

We owe our progress not to Lee Iacocca but to the refrigerator. Before the universal availability of home refrigerators, chemicals were used to preserve many foods. Of particular concern are nitrates, which are converted by bacteria into carcinogenic nitrites and nitrosamines. Still, with nearly 15,000 deaths recorded annually in the United States from stomach cancer, we cannot afford to be complacent. You can help prevent stomach cancer by avoiding habitual consumption of smoked, dried, pickled, and salted foods.

Gastritis and Ulcers

Considering that the stomach produces hydrochloric acid and powerful peptic digestive enzymes with every meal, it's a wonder that we don't all have ulcers. But many of us do. Up to 10 percent of people in industrialized nations will develop an ulcer at some time during adult life, and the majority of these ulcer patients will relapse at least once following treatment. Countless others suffer from gastritis.

With powerful new medications to prevent acid production and others to protect the stomach lining from the effects of acid, we are now very good at treating gastritis and ulcers. The typical gnawing stomach distress and abnormal sensation of hunger respond promptly to treatment. Complications such as bleeding, perforation, and scarring and obstruction have become much less common in the era of modern medicine. Once a common form of therapy, surgery is now rarely needed to treat gastritis and ulcers.

Unfortunately, our progress in treating the ravages of excessive stomach acidity has outstripped our understanding of causes and prevention. Even worse, this is one of the few cases in which the more we learn, the less we understand. Excellent medical studies have cast doubt on many of the factors we've traditionally blamed for ulcers, including mental stress, caffeine, citrus fruits, spicy foods, aspirin and other anti-inflammatories, medications, and even alcohol. Similarly the benefits of the time-honored treatment program of bland diet and dairy products have not been verified. In fact, only one association has held up: smoking predisposes to ulcers.

While leaving us only one villain, recent studies have at least added a new hero. High-fiber diets reduce the risk of ulcer disease and may even accelerate healing.

Exciting new research has also revealed that a unique bacterium, *Helicobacter pylori,* is associated with many cases of gastritis and ulcers. We are not sure if it's the cause of ulcer disease, but if it turns out to be important, a brand-new approach to prevention will open up. Once we learn how to prevent this infection, we may even be able to reduce the risk of stomach cancer, since two studies published in 1991 indicate that *Helicobacter pylori* produces a three- to sixfold increase in stomach cancer.

With everything turned upside down, what can you do to prevent getting an ulcer? Fortunately, the old school and the new agree on the importance of avoiding smoking and excessive alcohol, and of eating a healthful balanced diet including lots of fiber. If you are free of stomach complaints, no other prevention is necessary. But if you have symptoms, avoid the foods, drinks, or stresses that seem to trigger them. For patients with symptoms I confess to siding with the traditionalists, recommending small, frequent, bland meals and avoidance of alcohol, spicy foods, caffeine, and aspirinlike medications. I aspire to practicing the latest scientific medicine, but I, too, remember what my mother taught me.

▪ 7 ▪

Diseases of the Liver
and Gallbladder

The liver is the second largest organ in the human body. It puts its size to good use, serving as the body's metabolic mainstay. The liver is vital for absorbing fats, synthesizing proteins, storing and releasing energy, and eliminating toxins.

▪ The Liver in Health and Disease

The liver is a digestive organ. Located in the upper right quadrant of the abdomen (see figure 6-1), the liver produces bile and delivers it to the gallbladder, where it's stored. When fat enters the small intestine, the gallbladder contracts, emptying bile into the intestines. Bile helps to emulsify fat so it can be absorbed; some elements of bile are themselves absorbed so they can be reused (just one example of the way the body conserves and recycles). If the liver is damaged or if the bile ducts are blocked, bile builds up in the body; the yellow pigment bilirubin is responsible for the yellow jaundice seen in liver disease, and bile salts are responsible for the itching that plagues many patients with liver ailments.

The liver is an organ responsible for the synthesis of many of the body's crucial substances. Like every organ, the liver gets its oxygen-rich blood directly from the heart and arteries. But unlike other organs, the liver also has a second blood supply. A special network of veins, called the portal circulation, brings blood from the intestines directly to the liver. This blood is rich in nutrients that have just been absorbed. The liver uses amino acids to build proteins, glucose (sugar) to make glycogen, and fat to synthesize cholesterol and bile acids. Liver disease impairs all these synthetic activities; as a result, liver patients' protein levels fall, so they bleed easily and become wasted and swollen. They are malnourished.

The liver stores energy and regulates its use. After sugar is absorbed, it is delivered by the portal circulation to the liver, where it is converted into glycogen and stored in the liver cells themselves. When the body needs energy, as during exercise, fasting, or starvation, the liver converts glycogen back into sugar, and it can synthesize additional sugar as well. By delivering sugar to the blood when it's needed, the liver helps maintain the body's energy economy; patients with liver disease are fatigued, and they may be unable to maintain normal blood sugar levels.

The liver also detoxifies many potentially noxious substances, excreting them through the bile into the intestinal contents. When liver disease interferes with this process, toxins from the body's own metabolism build up in the blood, as do estrogen hormones. High blood levels of ammonia and other toxins are responsible for the grogginess and confusion so characteristic of advanced liver disease. Because they are unable to detoxify chemicals, liver patients are unduly sensitive to many medications normally metabolized by the healthy liver.

The gallbladder's role in all this is really quite minor; it simply stores bile for delivery to the intestines when a fatty meal passes through the stomach. This storage function sounds like a good idea, and it does promote efficient fat absorption. But even without a gallbladder, the liver will deliver enough bile to absorb fat; in view of all the trouble caused by gallstones, I sometimes think the gallbladder is more trouble than it's worth.

But there is no mistaking the liver's worth; it's a vital organ, essential for life. To protect life, the body has given us more liver than we really need; there is enough excess capacity to keep us going even if a substantial proportion of the liver cells are damaged. Another protective factor is the liver's extraordinary capacity to heal and regenerate after injury.

Unfortunately, the liver's redundant capacity and repair capability has its limits; a variety of problems can inflict permanent damage. That damage can be severe indeed, which is why liver disease is the ninth leading cause of death in the United States.

Fortunately, much of this liver disease, both mild and lethal, can be prevented.

■ Viral Hepatitis

The 1970s witnessed great progress in understanding the nature of viral hepatitis. The 1980s saw spectacular breakthroughs in the technology needed to prevent the most serious form of hepatitis. Despite these achievements, however, widespread application of these advances has been left to the 1990s; we have the means to prevent hepatitis, but we have not yet utilized that potential to its fullest.

The clinical picture of viral hepatitis is extremely variable. Some patients, particularly children, look and feel entirely well throughout the infection. Others develop fatigue, loss of appetite and weight, yellow discoloration of the skin and eyes (jaundice), dark-colored urine, and light-colored stools. Fever and joint pains may be prominent. Still other patients suffer a fulminant course with confusion, coma, and bleeding. Except for these critically ill people, most patients with hepatitis recover fully, but some go on to develop chronic liver inflammation or even liver cancer.

There are three major types of viral hepatitis, each of which can now be diagnosed with simple blood tests. Each has its distinct patterns of transmission and clinical consequences, and each requires distinct tactics for prevention.

Hepatitis A

Formerly known as infectious hepatitis, hepatitis A is acquired mainly from food or water contaminated by the virus. Patients with hepatitis A shed the virus in their fecal waste for about a month. If even a tiny amount of infected waste material inadvertently contaminates food or water, the virus can be spread to another person. The source of infection may be hard to track down because there is an incubation period of about a month, and because the virus can enter feces even before jaundice and clinical hepatitis appear. Epidemics can occur if infected sewage spills into water supplies. Shellfish exposed to such sewage may harbor the virus, transmitting it to the unwitting hungry.

Hepatitis A occurs most frequently in underdeveloped areas of the world where hygiene is poor. But even in the United States it's a common infection; only 30,000 cases are reported annually, but more than 1 million cases go unrecognized or unreported. Blood test surveys, in fact, show that 45 percent of all Americans have been exposed to the virus. Because hepatitis A is a mild infection with few long-term consequences, most people with positive blood tests don't know that they've ever had the infection! Whether aware of it or not, people who have had hepatitis A are permanently immune to the virus.

Mild or not, hepatitis A should be prevented. Here's how: health departments should monitor all water supplies for fecal contamination. Only shellfish from clean water should be sold, and should always be cooked thoroughly before being eaten; boiling for one minute should do the job. Patients with hepatitis need not be isolated, but they should use separate eating utensils until recovery is complete. Contaminated objects can be cleansed with household bleach diluted 1 part bleach to 25 parts water. Needless to say, hepatitis patients should not prepare food, and all household members should be diligent about handwashing and personal hygiene.

A vaccine for hepatitis A is not yet available. Ordinary gamma globulin, however, can provide protection even after exposure — if it's given early enough. Close household contacts of patients with hepatitis A should ask their doctors about gamma globulin shots, which are safe but painful. Medical care personnel who have been exposed should also receive gamma globulin, but injections are not needed by a patient's casual contacts.

Because hepatitis A is so common in underdeveloped areas, travelers should receive gamma globulin shots to prevent infection. The injections should be given just prior to departure, and must be coordinated with other vaccinations. Even with gamma globulin under your belt, it's important to avoid exposure to contaminated food and water.

Hepatitis B

Although less common than hepatitis A, hepatitis B is much more serious. A safe and effective vaccine has been available in the United States since

1982, but cases continue to *increase* annually; 300,000 people will develop hepatitis B this year, 15,000 of whom will be sick enough to require hospitalization. It's bad enough that 400 of these patients will die from acute hepatitis B, but they are only the tip of the iceberg. At least 30,000 people will become chronic hepatitis B carriers. Carriers can spread the virus. In addition, 1 of every 4 carriers will develop chronic hepatitis or cirrhosis, and 1 in 20 will develop liver cancer.

Formerly known as serum hepatitis, hepatitis B is spread mainly through infected blood. Transfusions were once a common form of transmission, but the routine testing of all blood since 1972 has nearly eliminated this hazard. Why, then, are cases increasing? It doesn't take exposure to whole blood to transmit hepatitis B; even a tiny amount of infected serum can do the job. Sexual contact with patients — or chronic carriers — can spread the virus. So, too, can infected needles; medical personnel are at risk, but drug addicts are particularly vulnerable. Tragically, infected mothers can also transmit the virus across the placenta to their unborn babies.

There are three ways to prevent hepatitis B.

The first and best is to avoid exposure. Medical and dental personnel have become much more careful about wearing gloves and handling blood and body fluids with special precautions. As a result, health care workers now account for only 3 percent of hepatitis B cases. You should also be careful if a household member has hepatitis; never share razors, toothbrushes, or other items that may be contaminated by blood or body fluids. Unfortunately, sexual transmission of the virus continues to increase. Both gay men and heterosexuals with multiple partners are at high risk; condoms and safe sex could prevent hepatitis B (and other sexually transmitted diseases) in these people. Worst of all is the increasing epidemic of hepatitis B in drug abusers, just one of the many tragic medical and social consequences of drugs.

The second way to prevent hepatitis B is to get the vaccine before you are exposed. Three injections spaced over a six-month period are required. The vaccine is safe and effective but is very underutilized, having been administered to only 2.5 million Americans. There are several explanations for this poor record of vaccine use. The first vaccine was derived from human plasma; even though extensive studies proved that it was safe, many people were reluctant to accept the vaccine because of fear of AIDS transmission. Although unfounded, these fears were understandable. But since 1986 the vaccine has been produced entirely in the laboratory without any blood products. A second concern, also understandable, is expense: the three-injection series costs about $120. The third reason for the poor distribution of hepatitis B vaccine is that it is generally recommended only for adults belonging to high-risk groups (health care workers, gay men, drug users, sexual partners of patients, certain immigrant groups, kidney dialysis patients, and residents of chronic care institutions). It is certainly true that people at high risk should be protected first, but now that the vaccine is plentiful, protection should also be made available for others who may be unexpectedly exposed to the virus.

In my view we need a new approach to hepatitis B vaccination. The vaccine is now being produced abroad for a fraction of the American price. If we can reduce costs here as well, universal vaccination should be considered seriously. The U.S. Public Health Service took the first step toward this goal in 1991, recommending routine hepatitis B vaccination for all children at two, four, and six months of age.

There is a third way to prevent hepatitis B. If you are exposed to the virus but have not been vaccinated, you can get a special hepatitis B gamma globulin injection to prevent infection. To be effective, the shot should be administered early after exposure. If you think you have been exposed to hepatitis B, check with your doctor as soon as possible. A simple blood test can determine if you are susceptible to the infection; if so, gamma globulin and vaccine can be used to prevent hepatitis B.

Prevention is also available for a group that can't ask for help — unborn children. I believe that all pregnant women should be tested for hepatitis B. Newborn babies of mothers who test positive can be given hepatitis B gamma globulin and vaccine. Testing would cost $10 to $20 for each pregnancy, but would prevent 3,000 cases of newborn hepatitis B each year. This is not yet national policy, but I think it should be.

Hepatitis C

For a change, medical terminology is right: hepatitis C ranks third among the hepatitis viruses in importance, and was also the third to be discovered. Hepatitis C is transmitted through serum. Because it was not discovered until the late 1980s, prevention is not yet ideal. Hepatitis C may result from contaminated blood transfusion, but universal donor testing is now putting an end to this. Neither a vaccine nor a special gamma globulin is yet available. Until one is, follow the same exposure precautions as for preventing hepatitis B, and get an ordinary gamma globulin shot if you are closely exposed to patients whose blood tests show they have hepatitis C.

■ Liver Cancer

Cancer of the liver is very common in areas of Southeast Asia and Africa, where it affects young people and accounts for up to 50 percent of all malignancies in men. Fortunately, liver cancer is quite uncommon in the United States, where it is chiefly a disease of the elderly.

Liver cancer can be caused by toxins, particularly aflatoxin, which is produced by a mold that can infect food in tropical areas. Vinyl-chloride can also cause a type of liver cancer, but occupational exposure is now uncommon owing to progress made by the American rubber and chemical industries. But in the United States there are still four major causes of liver cancer, all of which are preventable: hepatitis B, hepatitis C, cirrhosis, and long-term use of androgens (male hormones). The first three are discussed in this chapter. As for the fourth, prevention is simple: weightlifters, body-builders, football players, and other athletes should not use hormones in an attempt to build strength; their muscles may grow in size, but a growth in the liver, to say nothing of many other medical consequences, is too high a price to pay.

■ Toxic Liver Disease

One of the liver's important jobs is to deactivate toxins. In so doing it protects the body from injury. Unfortunately, the liver itself can be damaged by a variety of toxins. Carbon tetrachloride and other organic solvents head the list; industrial and environmental exposure must be prevented (see chapters 17 and 22). And industry is not the only thing to worry about; nature can also damage your liver if you are imprudent enough to eat toxic mushrooms or unlucky enough to eat foods contaminated by aflatoxin.

Some other potential liver toxins are close at hand in virtually every medicine chest in the land. Both acetaminophen (Tylenol and many other brands) and aspirin can damage the liver, but only under very special circumstances. Acetaminophen will cause liver disease only if huge amounts are taken, generally the equivalent of 75 tablets; attempted suicide is therefore virtually the only situation in which this medication causes liver disease. Still, patients with chronic liver disease should avoid taking acetaminophen on a daily basis. In the case of aspirin, even small amounts can cause severe liver trouble, but only in young children who have influenza, chicken pox, or other infections. To prevent this uncommon but serious problem, called Reye's syndrome, young children should always be given acetaminophen rather than aspirin to treat fever.

Many other medications can cause liver damage in people who develop drug allergies. Because the reactions often look just like viral hepatitis, these cases can be hard to sort out. The preventive moral applies to all medicines: use them only if you need them, listen to your body to spot side effects, and promptly report possible adverse reactions to your doctor. This advice applies even to vitamins; among other problems, excessive amounts of vitamin A can cause liver damage.

All these liver toxins can cause damage, but they are bit players when placed on the stage with the most destructive liver toxin of all: alcohol.

■ Alcoholic Liver Disease and Cirrhosis

Alcohol causes three distinct types of liver disease. Virtually everyone who drinks heavily will develop a fatty liver; the liver is enlarged because its cells are engorged with fat, but the process will reverse and resolve if drinking stops. About 30 percent of heavy drinkers will develop the second problem, alcoholic hepatitis. The liver is inflamed and tender, causing fever and fatigue as well as jaundice and abnormal blood tests. Many, but not all, cases of alcoholic hepatitis resolve with abstinence.

Occurring in about 15 percent of heavy drinkers, cirrhosis is the most serious liver disease because its scarring is permanent. Abstinence will prevent further damage, but the cirrhotic liver will never fully recover. It's not clear why some drinkers get cirrhosis while others do not. In general, the risk of cirrhosis increases with the amount and duration of drinking, but as little as three and one half ounces of alcohol daily for five years can sometimes produce cirrhosis, especially in men.

Cirrhosis is simply scarring of the liver. Remember that the liver has a great capacity to regenerate after injury. Unfortunately, the process of regeneration can result in scarring instead of healing. In the mildest cases cirrhosis will go unnoticed. But in severe cases the consequences are disastrous. The liver is small and rock hard, but the spleen is enlarged and soft. The abdomen and feet are swollen with fluid. The skin and eyes are discolored by yellow jaundice. The mind is confused and clouded. Violent bleeding into the stomach is a constant risk. All too often this combination of symptoms is lethal. Liver disease is the ninth leading cause of death in the United States; cirrhosis is the most common fatal liver disease, taking more than 30,000 lives annually, many in middle age.

Cirrhosis can be the end result of any disease that injures the liver severely enough to produce scarring. Hepatitis B, for example, accounts for more than 5,000 cirrhosis deaths in the United States each year. Liver damage from toxins, certain parasitic infections, and the inherited disorders that deposit excessive amounts of iron or copper in the liver can all cause cirrhosis. But by far the leading cause of cirrhosis is alcohol.

We can patch up some of the complications of cirrhosis, at least temporarily, but we can't treat cirrhosis itself — except by prevention. Don't abuse alcohol, and you won't get alcoholic cirrhosis. For most people two drinks per day is a safe limit. It's simple in theory, but in our society, sadly, the reality is often complex.

■ Gallbladder Disease

A small organ whose sole function is to store bile so it can be squirted into the intestines to help digest fat, the gallbladder gets no attention when it's working right. Unfortunately, things often go wrong. In fact, about 10 percent of adults in Western societies have gallstones; in the United States there are 5 million men and 15 million women in this category. It's no wonder that removal of the gallbladder is the second most common operation in America, with 500,000 performed each year.

The diagnosis of gallbladder disease underwent revolutionary changes in the 1970s and 80s with the introduction of ultrasound and nuclear scanning techniques. The treatment of gallstones is now undergoing even more dramatic changes with the development of nonsurgical techniques. As in so many areas of medicine, however, prevention has not kept pace with diagnosis and treatment. We can do better.

Gallstones come in two varieties. Pigment stones are composed mainly of bilirubin, the yellow substance in bile. Pigment stones are relatively un-common in the United States, occurring mainly in patients with blood dis-orders that result in high bilirubin levels, in patients with cirrhosis, and in the very elderly. The cause of pigment stones is not clear but appears to depend on infection and slow flow of bile; there is no proven way to prevent these problems or to reduce the formation of pigment gallstones.

The second type of stone predominates in the United States and Europe. These stones are composed of cholesterol. The liver produces large amounts of cholesterol that is then excreted with the bile. Cholesterol has a marked tendency to form crystals that slowly enlarge into stones. Considering this, it's a wonder that we don't all have gallstones! The reason we don't is that bile acids keep cholesterol in solution, preventing stone formation — if conditions are just right. But if there is too much cholesterol in bile, if there are not enough bile acids, or if the flow of bile is slow or stagnant, stones can form. Once started, stones grow very slowly, increasing in size by about 3 millimeters per year.

It would seem logical that diets low in saturated fat and cholesterol would reduce the risk of gallstones by lowering blood cholesterol levels. I'm a great believer in these diets; but we cannot count on them to prevent gallstones. The situation is more complex, and blood cholesterol levels do not accurately predict the risk of cholesterol gallstone formation.

Other factors, however, do predict the risk of gallstones. Some of these are not modifiable: gallstone risk increases with age and is higher in people whose close relatives have gallstones. Race also influences risk: stones are most common in Native Americans, followed in descending order by Mexi-can-Americans, whites, Afro-Americans, and Asian-Americans. Another major factor is gender: gallstones are three times more common in women than men. Because estrogen stimulates the liver to secrete more cholesterol into bile, the gender gap is increased further by pregnancy and estrogen treatments.

Other gallstone risk factors are within your control. Perhaps the most important of these is obesity, which increases the liver's cholesterol pro-duction. A 1989 study of nearly 90,000 nurses confirmed this traditional association; very obese women had a sixfold increase in the risk of stone formation, and even slightly overweight women had nearly double the nor-mal risk. Total calorie intake also predicted risk, but alcohol tended to re-duce risk. You shouldn't plan to drink away your risk of gallstones, how-ever; more information will be needed to establish a relationship between alcohol and stones. And even if drinking reduces the risk of stones, it also causes much more serious problems.

If you are enthusiastic about preventing gallstones, your logical next step might be to lose weight. Weight loss will reduce your risk of coronary heart disease, high blood pressure and stroke, and diabetes. But weight loss can *increase* your risk of gallstones, *if* it is rapid. This is one of the surpris-ing lessons of the current very low-calorie diet craze. In one study from California, an astounding 25 percent of people on a 500-calorie diet developed gallstones in just two months. In some the stones dissolved when a normal diet was resumed, but three needed gallbladder surgery. True, the dieters lost an average of 33 pounds, but gallbladder disease is a high price to pay.

Ultra-low-calorie diets appear to cause gallstones by slowing the flow of bile and by reducing its content of bile acids. It's hard to stimulate the flow of bile without eating more; 500 calories, about one quarter of the normal daily intake, just doesn't give you much room to maneuver. But you can take bile acid pills to keep bile cholesterol in soluble form; in a small preliminary study this approach appeared to protect crash dieters from gallstones. More thought will be needed before supplements are recommended to all low-calorie dieters. In fact, more thought is needed before recommending very low-calorie diet programs in the first place; weight loss is usually temporary, but the gallstones can be forever. See chapter 12 for additional discussion of these diets and their complications.

While in the process of blaming diet clinics for gallstones, I should confess that I, too, have caused gallstones. Gemfibrozil, one of the medications I sometimes prescribe to lower blood cholesterol levels, can cause gallstones. This is not a common side effect, and the medication is generally quite safe and effective. But it's a good reminder that diet and exercise, rather than medications, should always be the first steps to improve blood cholesterol levels.

Is there any way that diet can reduce your risk of gallstones? Gradual but sustained weight loss is the best idea. Another thing that may help is dietary fiber. Fiber tends to bind cholesterol in the intestines and to increase the liver's production of bile acids, both of which should reduce the risk of gallstones. A few preliminary animal and human studies have suggested that high levels of dietary fiber help keep bile cholesterol soluble. More studies will be needed, however, to establish a role for diet in the primary prevention of gallstones.

■ Secondary Prevention of Gallbladder Disease

Twenty million Americans have gallstones. What should we be doing about them?

For most the answer is simple: nothing. Gallstones will not cause any problems for the great majority of people who have them. The stones grow only slowly, generally taking eight years or more to become large enough to cause trouble. But even large stones are harmless in most cases. In fact, the overall risk of developing problems from gallstones is less than 20 percent over 20 years of life with stones. Five hundred thousand operations can't all be wrong — but many are. In my view there is no justification for removing asymptomatic stones; if they don't bother you, don't bother them.

Stones that cause symptoms are another matter, since about half the people who have one gallbladder attack can go on to have additional attacks. Unfortunately, it can be rather hard to determine if their symptoms are actually caused by gallstones, since their complaints are often very nonspecific: crampy abdominal distress can have many other causes, even in patients who have gallstones. Most gallbladder attacks are mild. If patients are determined to avoid treatment, I think it's reasonable to see how they do on a low-fat diet before going further.

But gallstones can also cause serious attacks, blocking the outflow of bile and producing gallbladder inflammation and infection. Patients with these problems need hospitalization and antibiotics. Gallbladder removal has been the traditional treatment, and is still the gold standard. But new approaches are being developed and may have a role in preventing serious attacks in people with symptomatic gallstones.

Gallstones can actually be dissolved by medications. Bile acids can be taken in pill form, and two preparations have been government approved for clinical use. It's surely an attractive concept — but one with many limitations. Only about 20 percent of patients with gallstones are suitable candidates for these pills, which must be taken daily for months or even years while the stones slowly dissolve. At that, only half the stones dissolve, and there are side effects including diarrhea and liver irritation, to say nothing of expense. Most discouraging of all is the fact that many of the stones recur after treatment is stopped. Many patients with gallstones have asked me to prescribe these pills; I have yet to do so.

An experimental approach that generated great enthusiasm in the late 1980s is lithotripsy. High-pressure shock waves can be used to break up kidney stones with excellent results, so gallstones were a logical next step. To date the results have been disappointing. Only patients with fewer than three small stones are eligible for treatment, and some don't respond. Because the shock-wave generators cost $1 million to $2 million each, these treatments are as expensive as gallbladder removal, and patients require anesthesia. New techniques are being developed, but shocking as it may sound, gallstone lithotripsy has not yet arrived.

The hope for the 1990s is a new type of gallbladder surgery. Using a tiny incision, surgeons place a small fiber-optic laparoscope into the abdomen. While watching on a TV screen, doctors use instruments to grasp the gallbladder and pull it to the surface so it can be removed, stones and all. This new approach offers many advantages: a small incision, brief anesthesia, a one-night hospitalization, and a fast recovery.

Like you, I am eagerly awaiting more data to learn if these new techniques live up to their early promise. Meanwhile, I'll do my best to stay lean and follow a high-fiber, low-fat diet. How about you?

■ 8 ■

Musculoskeletal Disorders

When patients ask me how they can stay healthy, they want answers about heart disease, stroke, and cancer prevention. They want to know how to avoid infections, and how to keep their lungs, liver, and kidneys in top condition. All this is, of course, perfectly appropriate; in fact, I wrote this book to help answer such questions. Not appropriate, though, is the general lack of concern about musculoskeletal health. True, disorders of bones and joints are not as likely to be life threatening, but they can cause severe discomfort and disability. And many of these problems are preventable.

■ Bones

Far from being inert supporting structures like the girders in a building, the 206 bones in your body are metabolically active, living tissues. Even after growth ceases in adolescence, bone formation continues. In actuality, bone remodeling is a lifelong process, with continuous resorption of old bone and formation of new bone. About 7 percent of your body's bone is being reconstructed at any given time.

Two types of bone cells maintain the process of bone remodeling; one deposits new bony tissue while the other removes old bone. To keep bones strong, the activity of these two cell types must be balanced and coordinated. The cells also need the raw materials to build bone, including calcium, vitamin D, and the amino acids that are joined together to form bone proteins such as collagen.

The process of bone remodeling must be carefully controlled. The endocrine system is largely responsible for regulating the activity of bone cells, with the parathyroid glands and the sex hormones playing key roles. Not to be overlooked are simple mechanical factors; bone cells respond to the stress of extra work by building extra bone tissue.

Bone is more than hard, calcium-rich tissue. A matrix of protein supports the bone cells, and a network of blood vessels supplies the nutrients and oxygen they need to go on working. Because they are so active, bone cells are vulnerable to nutritional deficiencies and circulatory problems; they can also be damaged by toxins carried in the blood.

■ Osteoporosis

The rate of bone formation and bone removal is not always balanced. In childhood the rate of bone formation exceeds the rate of removal; that's how bones grow. In early adulthood, during the third and fourth decades of life, bone formation and removal are balanced and bones are at their strongest; the average adult has two and one half pounds of calcium, 99 percent of which is stored in the bones. But beyond age 40 or 50 bone tissue is removed faster than it is formed. Even though everyone loses bone calcium, if the net loss is low, bones will stay strong. If too much calcium is removed, however, bone density or mass will decrease to unhealthful levels. The amount of bone that can be lost is staggering; women may eventually lose half their bone mass, and men one quarter. Bones that are deprived of calcium are thin, weak, and easily fractured. The name of this condition is osteoporosis; it's a good name, since bones that lack calcium are indeed porous (see figure 8-1).

More than 24 million Americans have osteoporosis; 80 percent of its victims are women. The consequences of osteoporosis vary greatly. Often, weakening of the vertebral bones in the spine leads to a loss of height and a "dowager's hump" (see figure 8-2). Even worse is the risk of fracture. Osteoporosis is responsible for 70 percent of all fractures in adults over 45; more than 1.3 million Americans suffer fractures because of osteoporosis each year. The spine, hips, forearms, and wrists are most vulnerable. One third of all women will develop vertebral fractures at some time in their lives; the likelihood of a hip or wrist fracture is about 15 percent. Pain and disability are the obvious effects of these fractures. Not so obvious is the risk of death; hip fractures in the elderly have a one-year mortality rate of 20 percent, and 30 percent of survivors require long-term nursing home care. The total economic burden of osteoporosis exceeds $7 billion per year.

Although extremely common, osteoporosis is not inevitable. By understanding the factors that contribute to osteoporosis, you can devise strategies to prevent it. Here is a list of factors:

Factors that increase risk
Age
Female gender and menopause
Heredity
Thin body build
Dietary deficiencies of calcium, vitamin D, or fluoride
Dietary excess of protein, sodium, aluminum, magnesium, or caffeine
Smoking
Alcohol consumption
Sedentary living
Various illnesses and medications
Factors that decrease risk
Dietary calcium, vitamin D, fluoride, and possibly vitamin K
Exercise

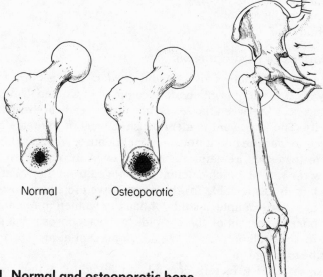

Figure 8-1. Normal and osteoporotic bone

Normal   Osteoporotic

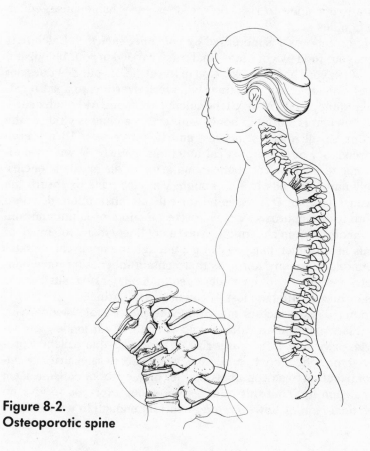

Figure 8-2.
Osteoporotic spine

Estrogen replacement therapy
Pregnancy and lactation
Heavy body build

The Causes of Osteoporosis

The two leading risk factors are *age* and *gender*. The risk of osteoporosis increases with age, and it is much more common in women. Unlike with so many "differences" between the sexes, hormones really are responsible for this disparity. The key event is menopause. Levels of the female sex hormone, estrogen, decline precipitously at menopause, whereas the male sex hormone, testosterone, remains unchanged even in older men. Sex hormones slow the rate at which calcium is removed from bone. Estrogen deficiency is largely responsible for the progressive increase in osteoporosis as women age. For example, a study of healthy women in Michigan found that only about 15 percent of 45-year-olds had osteoporosis, but the prevalence rose to about 55 percent at age 55, 70 percent at age 65, and almost 90 percent beyond age 75.

Another set of risk factors depends on *heredity*. A fair complexion, northern European ancestry, a small body build, and a family history of osteoporosis all contribute to risk. So too does early menopause, which often runs in families.

The risk of osteoporosis is increased by *calcium deficiency*. Calcium is absorbed from your food by your intestinal tract, carried in your blood, and finally deposited in your bones or excreted in the urine. If your diet does not contain enough calcium, your intestines will work overtime to absorb calcium, and your kidneys will retain all the calcium they can. Although nearly all the body's calcium is stored in bones and teeth, calcium is vital for the normal function of all muscles, nerves, and blood vessels. To preserve these vital circulatory and neurological functions, your body will eventually have to remove calcium from bone to make up for dietary deficiencies.

Eating calcium-rich foods is not enough; you also have to absorb the calcium. Because *vitamin D* is essential for calcium absorption, deficiencies contribute to osteoporosis. Yet excessive amounts of aluminum and magnesium impair calcium absorption. You're not likely to get too much of these minerals in your diet, but you can get enough to impair calcium absorption by taking too many *antacids* that contain magnesium or aluminum. Excessive intake of another mineral, sodium, may also contribute to osteoporosis by accelerating the loss of calcium in the urine.

Several other dietary factors may influence the risk of osteoporosis, though to a lesser extent than calcium and vitamin D. An *inadequate intake of calories or vitamin K* increases risk. Whereas adequate dietary protein is essential for bone growth, *excessive protein* accelerates urinary calcium loss, contributing to osteoporosis. Rather high doses of *caffeine* seem to increase calcium loss, but this effect is not enough for you to give up coffee. Three final factors, however, are important enough to warrant lifestyle changes.

Smoking is a leading cause of osteoporosis. You may have noticed that chapter 7 was the first one in this book that did not implicate smoking as a cause of disease. Never fear, I'm back at it again: To reduce your risk of osteoporosis, don't smoke.

Excessive alcohol intake also increases the risk of osteoporosis, probably by damaging the cells that make bone. It's not clear if these cells will be injured only by large amounts of alcohol or if even small doses can be harmful over the years. Until we know more, moderation is the best advice; my usual two-drink-a-day rule of thumb seems reasonable.

Smoking and alcohol abuse are familiar stalwarts in the "don'ts" of preventive medicine. An equally familiar "do" will go a long way to preserving bone calcium and strength. *Exercise* is a very important stimulus to bone formation. Like so many of the body's organs, bones improve with use. But not all forms of exercise are equally beneficial for bones; weight-bearing exercise is best. One caveat: a very high level of exercise can actually contribute to osteoporosis in women *if* it produces the marked weight loss and temporary loss of menstrual periods experienced by some highly competitive female athletes.

Finally, a variety of *medical conditions and treatments* can cause osteoporosis. Although they are responsible for only a small number of the many cases of osteoporosis, it's important for your doctor to think about diabetes, overactive adrenal, thyroid, or parathyroid glands, and chronic liver or intestinal diseases that impair calcium absorption. Certain prescription medications, including some used for seizures, fluid excess, and tuberculosis and other infections, will also accelerate calcium loss, contributing to osteoporosis. So, too, will excessive doses of thyroid hormones. Prednisone and related steroids are the greatest offenders among medications.

Factors That Protect against Osteoporosis

On the other side of the ledger there are some factors that reduce the risk of osteoporosis. Surprisingly, *obesity* is one of these, possibly because of the extra work load it puts on bones and the higher estrogen levels that result from excess body fat. Another surprise: *pregnancy and nursing* each reduces the risk of osteoporosis despite the calcium that is diverted into the baby's bones and the mother's milk. Hormone levels may explain this as well.

Diet can also reduce the risk of osteoporosis. Adequate supplies of calcium and vitamin D are of prime importance. Another mineral that may do some good is fluoride; women living in communities with fluoridated water have a reduced risk of osteoporosis.

Risk factors are valid predictors of osteoporosis in large population groups. Let's see how they can be put to practical use for you.

Preventing Osteoporosis

The prevention of osteoporosis is a rapidly evolving, often controversial area. Let's begin with the basics before turning to the areas of contention.

Diet. Because calcium deficiency clearly increases the risk of osteoporosis, calcium supplements to prevent osteoporosis were heavily promoted by doctors, nutritionists, and manufacturers in the mid-1980s. This enthusiasm reached its peak in 1984, when the National Institutes of Health recommended calcium supplements for all postmenopausal women. All this optimism — my own included — was blunted in the late 1980s by several studies which suggested that calcium supplements would not by themselves prevent osteoporosis. But the wheels of science continue to turn, if slowly and erratically. A 1990 study from Tufts University showed that calcium supplements *can* slow bone loss in postmenopausal women.

Divergent findings notwithstanding, all the experts agree that calcium *is* important — not only for bones but also for proper function of muscles, nerves, and blood vessels. Dietary calcium may even reduce the risk of high blood pressure and colon cancer. But don't overdo it, since very high dietary calcium levels may contribute to kidney stones.

How much calcium do you need, and what's the best way to get it? The United States Recommended Daily Allowance (U.S. RDA) for calcium is 1,200 milligrams per day, but many authorities recommend daily intakes of 1,500 milligrams for postmenopausal women. There is no proof that even this much will prevent osteoporosis, but combined with exercise and possibly estrogen, calcium will reduce the risk of fractures. There is little to lose and much to gain, so I go along with the 1,500-milligram target. In fact, it seems to me that it's also very important to be sure that *premenopausal* women get enough calcium when they need it to build bone strength for the years ahead. Unfortunately, 25 percent of American women get less than 300 milligrams per day, and the average for postmenopausal women is less than 600 milligrams daily, very low by any standard.

The best way to get your daily allotment of calcium is by eating calcium-rich foods. Dairy products will give you the largest amount. An eight-ounce glass of milk contains 300 milligrams, and an eight-ounce cup of yogurt has 400 milligrams. They are both available in low-fat varieties, unlike most cheeses, which will give you the saturated fat you don't need along with the calcium you do need. Many nondairy foods are also good sources of calcium, including canned sardines (250 mg per portion) or salmon (250 mg), broccoli (200 mg), and spinach (250 mg). Chapter 20 details the calcium content of selected foods (see table 20-11).

If you can't bring your diet up to par, you can consider taking calcium supplements. Many formulations are available at drugstores without prescription; some are synthetic whereas others are made from oyster shell or bone. They vary in price, in convenience, and in the amount of calcium that can be absorbed from each tablet. If you choose to take calcium supplements, you can experiment to find the preparation you like best; if it's a tablet, check to see if it will release the calcium you need by placing a pill in a glass of white vinegar to be sure it breaks up within 30 minutes. Better still, pick a preparation that meets the standards of the U.S. Pharmacopeia, a nonprofit testing lab that sets drug standards.

Although the scientific data are incomplete, I generally recommend calcium supplements for women who do not average 1,500 milligrams per day from dietary sources. The cost is low, the risks are few, and the potential benefits are many. The only complication of calcium supplements is constipation, which is occasional, and kidney stones, which are rare. Dietary fiber and exercise will help prevent constipation, and a high fluid intake will help prevent both side effects. Many of my patients prefer their calcium supplements in the form of chewable calcium-carbonate antacid tablets; Tums, for example, contain 200 milligrams of calcium per tablet. Calcium is not a total solution to the problem of osteoporosis, but it certainly won't hurt.

To help prevent osteoporosis, your diet should also contain sufficient amounts of two vitamins. *Vitamin D* is essential because it allows calcium to be absorbed from the intestines, and it enables bone cells to produce new bone. Vitamin D is synthesized in skin in response to sunlight (the "sunshine vitamin"). Only a few minutes of sunlight is needed, but many people don't get enough sun in the winter, and I certainly don't recommend supplementary ultraviolet exposure (see chapter 15 on skin cancer). All in all, diet is the best source of vitamin D. Fortunately, it's easy to get enough since most dairy products are fortified with vitamin D, and fish also provides it. The RDA of 400 units per day will do the trick; there is no evidence that higher doses of vitamin D will provide additional help. And even if you take vitamin supplements, you should never take more than 50,000 units twice a week, because higher doses can raise blood calcium to dangerous levels; as in so many areas of nutrition, a little vitamin D is good for you but a lot is *not* better.

The other vitamin to consider is *vitamin K*. There is no controversy about vitamin D, but the role and dose of vitamin K is not yet settled. Doctors from the Netherlands administered vitamin K in doses of 1 milligram per day to both pre- and postmenopausal women. The calcium balance in younger women was unchanged, but postmenopausal women with the highest calcium wastage reduced their urinary calcium losses by 33 percent. The dose used was about ten times the U.S. RDA for vitamin K. Even though there is no known toxicity from these higher doses, I'd like to see confirmatory studies before recommending vitamin K supplements to every postmenopausal woman. Leafy green vegetables and members of the cabbage family provide plenty of vitamin K, which is also made by intestinal bacteria, so deficiencies are rare.

To help prevent osteoporosis, be sure your diet contains sufficient amounts of calcium, vitamins D and K, and fluoride. Be sure, too, to avoid excessive amounts of the dietary factors that promote calcium loss: alcohol, sodium, and protein. The hazards of excess alcohol and sodium are well known, but high dietary protein is often mistakenly equated with good nutrition. In fact, high-protein diets increase urinary calcium loss; every time dietary protein is doubled, urinary calcium levels increase by 50 percent.

Exercise. Diet is important to prevent osteoporosis, and it has gotten the attention it deserves. Equally important, but not equally promoted, is exercise.

Throughout life, bones need exercise to stimulate calcium deposition and new bone formation. Without exercise, bones lose calcium and become osteoporotic; bed rest reduces bone density by nearly 1 percent *per week*, and recovery takes up to four months.

It has been known for years that athletes have denser bones than sedentary people. True, athletes may eat differently, and they tend to smoke and drink less. But exercise rather than diet, life-style, or genetics is the thing that strengthens the athlete's bones. Tennis players, for example, have 30 percent more bone mineral in their racquet arm than in their opposite, less exercised arm.

You don't have to star at Wimbledon to build strong bones with exercise; recent studies prove that ordinary people can benefit as much as athletes. Every little bit of exercise helps; one study of female nursing home residents with an average age of 82 showed that even minimal amounts of activity slowed bone loss. But until you are 82 you should not settle for minimal exercise programs. In another study, three hours of aerobics per week *increased* bone mass by 5 percent in just over a year. Not so coincidentally, three hours per week is also the ideal exercise "dose" for cardiovascular health.

Exercise must be sustained to protect your bones; if you stop exercising (heaven forbid!), your bones will again begin to lose calcium. Whereas all forms of aerobic exercise are equally good for your heart and circulation, weight-bearing exercises are best for your bones. Walking, jogging, aerobic dance, skiing, skating, and racquet sports are examples. You can find the details about safe and enjoyable exercise programs in chapter 21.

A small cautionary note about exercise is in order. Competitive female athletes who work out at very high levels can lose their menstrual periods. This problem, called athletic amenorrhea, is only temporary; normal periods, and fertility, are restored when the intensity of exercise is reduced. But these women athletes do have low estrogen levels, bone calcium loss, and an increased risk of fractures. Several studies to determine how best to prevent osteoporosis in these athletes are under way. Because I have a number of patients (and a daughter) with this problem, I've been prescribing high calcium intake and low-dose estrogen replacement until the results are available.

Estrogen Replacement. The role of calcium in preventing osteoporosis is much discussed, the role of exercise little discussed. I recommend both to every woman. Estrogen replacement is also much discussed, but recommendations must be individualized.

There is no doubt that estrogen replacement prevents postmenopausal osteoporosis. Estrogens reduce the activity of the cells that remove bone; they may also enhance the absorption of calcium from the intestines. Because estrogens slow bone loss rather than stimulating bone formation, they are most effective when started early. If estrogens are to be used to prevent osteoporosis, they should be started at the time of menopause or shortly thereafter; studies have shown good results even if replacement therapy is delayed for three to five years after menopause, but the results are poor if replacement is delayed for six years or longer. Estrogens are very effective at preventing postmenopausal osteoporosis, but they are much less useful to treat osteoporosis once it has occurred; prevention is, as usual, the best medicine.

Estrogens are available in many forms. To date, only the tablets have been shown to prevent osteoporosis. I can see no reason for the newer estrogen patches to be less effective, but we'll have to await results of trials to be sure. The estrogen preparation most widely used is conjugated estrogen (Premarin); a dose of .625 milligrams per day is needed to prevent osteoporosis, but recent data suggest that as little as .3 milligrams may work if combined with daily calcium supplements. An alternate estrogen tablet, ethinyl estradiol, seems just as effective if taken in doses of 25 micrograms per day.

You must continue taking estrogens to protect your bones; once therapy is discontinued, bone loss resumes. Long-term observations have proven that estrogens will continue to prevent bone loss during at least the first six years of treatment. As more observations come in, we'll learn if estrogen replacement will continue to be effective at ten years and beyond.

The benefits of estrogen replacement have been demonstrated in two ways. First, bone density is 20 to 50 percent higher in postmenopausal women who take estrogens than in women who do not. Second, and even more impressive, estrogens reduce the fracture rate in postmenopausal women by 50 to 60 percent.

Should every postmenopausal woman take estrogens? If our only concerns were osteoporosis and fractures, the answer would be a resounding yes. But estrogens have many other effects; some are potentially beneficial (preventing heart disease, lowering cholesterol levels, raising overall life expectancy, controlling menopausal symptoms), others deleterious (increasing breast and uterine disease, raising blood pressure, causing gallstones and other side effects). The decision is complex and must be individualized. In the next chapter I'll detail the pros and cons of estrogen replacement so you can draw up your own personal balance sheet.

Medications. As new ways to prevent osteoporosis become available, there will be alternatives for women who do not take estrogens because of their medical status or personal preference. At the present time only one other drug, *calcitonin*, has been approved by the Food and Drug Administration for clinical use in the United States. Calcitonin is a natural hormone produced by cells in the thyroid gland; the therapeutic preparation is made from salmon. Like estrogen, calcitonin reduces bone loss but does not stimulate new bone formation; like estrogen, therefore, it's much more effective when started early for prevention, and it must be continued to maintain its benefit. Although an intranasal spray is being studied, only an injectable form of calcitonin is now licensed. The drug is safe, with itching the only side effect, but injections are inconvenient, and at $2,500 per year it's very expensive.

A promising new drug on the horizon is *etidronate*. Exciting studies have shown that etidronate prevents bone loss and reduces the fracture rate in postmenopausal women with few side effects. Although not yet FDA approved for osteoporosis, etidronate is already licensed for treatment of another bone disease.

We'll need more experience before we can say that etidronate is the best way to prevent osteoporosis. It's humbling to remember that the last great hope, fluoride, has not lived up to its promise; it increases bone density but does not reduce fracture rates. Etidronate is more promising, and it has the advantages of being suitable for administration in pill form for 14 days each month at moderate cost. But until more results are in, the basics will do nicely: high calcium intake, exercise, and individualized decisions about estrogen replacement therapy.

Secondary Prevention of Osteoporosis

It's a happy truth that not all women are alike. Instead of prescribing the same primary prevention of osteoporosis for all women, should doctors screen women to find out who actually has osteoporosis, so that more intensive treatment can be made available for these individuals?

Screening for osteoporosis is neither easy nor inexpensive. We used to rely on a simple spine x ray; unfortunately, we've learned that bone density cannot be determined reliably from ordinary x rays. Instead, sophisticated tests ranging from single-photon absorptiometry to quantitative CAT scanning and dual energy x-ray absorptiometry are required. You're right; tests with such fancy names require specialized facilities and have price tags to match, often exceeding $400. Most insurance companies don't pay for screening; I can understand their viewpoint on this one, since studies have not yet discovered whether routine screening leads to treatment that actually prevents osteoporosis and fractures.

For the present it seems best to institute primary prevention for all women at the time of menopause, and use screening tests for those who are at high risk for osteoporosis.

Fractures

Osteoporosis accounts for 70 percent of all fractures in adults over 45; using the math made famous by Yogi Berra, I must point out that the remaining 100 percent is explained by trauma.

Behind every good fracture is a bad accident. Far from being random events, many accidents are predictable and therefore preventable. It is, of course, important to prevent osteoporosis. But to keep their bones healthy, people of both sexes and all ages must also prevent trauma. Chapter 17 will tell you how.

■ Joints

Bones provide the rigid support for the body, joints the flexibility that makes movement possible.

Placed at the junction of two or more bones, joints have a difficult job to do: they must be supple enough to permit flexibility and motion yet strong enough to provide support and stability. Although these roles seem mutually contradictory, healthy joints are equal to the task. To allow smooth movement, the ends of the bones are coated with a slippery tissue called cartilage. The entire joint is surrounded by a membrane, the synovium, which produces a watery fluid that cushions the joint, absorbing shock and lubricating it. Because cartilage is one of the few human tissues that does not have its own blood supply, the joint fluid is also responsible for providing oxygen and nutrients to the cartilage. For additional support and strength, most joints are surrounded by tough fibrous tissues called ligaments; the muscles and tendons that provide the power to move joints offer a final source of external support.

The body has dozens of joints, ranging from tiny ones in the fingers and toes to large, strong joints like the hip. Some (like the hand) are engineered for fine motion, others (like the knee) for large movements, and still others (like the sacroiliac) for strong support but little motion. All will function automatically in health, but all are vulnerable to disease.

Arthritis, or joint inflammation, is one of the leading causes of disability and discomfort in the United States. Twelve percent of American adults have some form of arthritis. Although it's often mild, arthritis can be severe enough to produce partial or complete disability; more than 3 million people are seriously impaired by arthritis, accounting for 15 percent of all chronic disability in the United States. The costs are enormous, exceeding $35 billion annually in direct health care and lost productivity.

The causes of most types of arthritis are unknown. In part because of this ignorance, cure is not possible. Still, progress in treating arthritis has been impressive; powerful new anti-inflammatory drugs and, as a last resort, complete surgical replacement of severely arthritic joints with artificial substitutes have provided comfort and good function to millions of patients.

Granting that artificial joints are great achievements, preventing arthritis would be even better. Unfortunately, we don't yet know how to prevent the most common types of arthritis. Why, then, have I included these pages on arthritis? I have two reasons. First, to dispel some common myths about arthritis prevention. Second, to provide a few tips that may help reduce your risk of developing some joint diseases.

Arthritis is not one disease but many. Osteoarthritis is by far the most common, affecting many times more people than all other types of arthritis combined.

Although anyone can get osteoarthritis, some risk factors do predict vulnerability. Age is by far the most powerful; rare before age 25, osteoarthritis increases steadily in prevalence with advancing age, so that x rays can detect the condition in up to 85 percent of people over 75. Heredity is a much weaker risk factor, but osteoarthritis of the hands can run in families. A final risk factor is obesity, applying mainly to osteoarthritis of the knees.

Osteoarthritis, also called degenerative arthritis, begins in the cartilage, with slow, progressive deterioration before the joint lining and bones are ever involved. It's widely believed that osteoarthritis results from excessive wear and tear. The logical preventive measure would be rest. Many people accept this logic; even after I convince patients that exercise will protect their cardiac and circulatory systems, many cite arthritis as an excuse for remaining sedentary.

This is the prevention myth I would like to dispel. Far from causing osteoarthritis, exercise may even help prevent it.

Our understanding of the interaction between joint use and joint disease comes from three areas. Laboratory experiments are the first. Animals that are forced to use joints don't develop arthritis any faster than animals whose joints are protected from motion and stress.

The second line of evidence comes from human industry. Workers do not get arthritis from repetitive use of their joints. Good news for all of us: I'm personally relieved that my right hand is no more likely to get arthritis than my left because I'm writing this book with a pencil instead of on a computer.

The third and most dramatic evidence that arthritis is not caused by overuse comes from observation of athletes. Runners in particular pound their hips and knees, generating forces eight times greater than their body weight with each stride. In just one mile runners will have to absorb more than 100 tons of impact force on *each* ankle, knee, and hip. If overuse caused arthritis, long-distance runners would be the first to show it. They don't. Six careful studies from Finland, Massachusetts, Florida, and California have evaluated runners' joints, comparing them with swimmers' and with sedentary people's. Whether evaluated by arthritic symptoms, physical examinations, or x rays, runners don't have more arthritis — even if they've run more than 50,000 miles (another personal relief, since that's my lifetime total thus far). Runners do get tendinitis, bursitis, and other soft-tissue complaints, but a Stanford University study revealed the surprising fact that runners actually have *fewer* musculoskeletal complaints than do sedentary people. Runners in this study also had 40 percent more bone mineral, so their exercise protected against osteoporosis without producing arthritis.

Can exercise help prevent arthritis? There is no scientific proof of this possibility, but there is theoretical reason for hope. Remember that joint cartilage is one of the few human tissues without its own blood supply. Cartilage depends on joint fluid, not blood, for its oxygen and nutrients. How does the fluid get into the cartilage? It enters when cartilage is compressed, when joints are used. It is possible that exercise can help keep cartilage healthy by promoting nutrition. Time will tell. I hope you'll spend some of that time exercising, since we know already that exercise will protect your heart without causing arthritis.

With our present state of knowledge (or ignorance!) about the causes of osteoarthritis, there is little else you can do to prevent it. Since obesity is linked to knee arthritis, it seems wise to stay lean as well as active, but there are no guarantees that the combination will prevent osteoarthritis.

There are no sure-fire methods for preventing the most crippling form of arthritis, rheumatoid arthritis, which is caused by inflammation originating in the joint membrane rather than the cartilage. But some types of arthritis are initiated by infections; here, prevention does have an important role. Chapter 16 provides tips for avoiding Lyme disease and preventing rubella and mumps.

A much more common form of arthritis, gout, is caused by the buildup of uric acid crystals in joints. Affecting more than 2 million Americans, gout causes painful joint swelling and redness which is abrupt in onset but usually responds well to treatment. The traditional image of the fat, rich epicure with a swollen great toe has for generations implied that a rich diet causes gout. While hardly advocating rich foods, I must report that even the most abstemious diet has only a minor role in preventing gout. But you should prevent the one excess that can trigger an attack of gout: alcohol. And people whose metabolism predisposes them to recurrent attacks of gout because of high blood levels of uric acid should consult their doctor; excellent medications are available for the secondary prevention of gout.

Not to be forgotten in this litany of arthritic conditions is trauma. Physical injury is a common cause of arthritis, which may be acute or chronic. Many cases of joint trauma can be prevented, including those caused by accidents or violence and sports.

■ Muscles, Tendons, Ligaments, and Bursas

Despite being the first word in *musculoskeletal*, muscles and their related structures are unlikely to cause major illness.

Muscles provide the power to move the body. Tendons are fibrous bands that attach muscles to bones, transmitting force to them. Ligaments are fibrous bands that help support joints, while bursas are the fluid-filled sacs that help cushion all these structures. Life-threatening diseases of those tissues are extremely rare, but uncomfortable, sometimes disabling conditions are very common — and are often preventable.

Muscles suffer from strains, ligaments from sprains, and tendons and bursa from "itis," or inflammation. Although there are differences among these conditions, pain and stiffness are the major symptoms; often these are mistakenly self- (or physician-) diagnosed as arthritis. Frequently related to overuse or overstress, these ailments are most often caused by physical exertion. But you can learn to exercise safely, preventing many of these problems. Chapter 21 details prevention through warm-up and cooldown exercises, stretching for flexibility, and appropriate equipment and technique. Common sense and a keen ear for the messages from your own body are no less important; chapter 21 also details warning symptoms and outlines the things you can do to prevent small problems from becoming big ones.

■ Low Back Pain

What better way to conclude a review of musculoskeletal problems than with a discussion of low back pain. It involves bones, joints, muscles, ligaments, and nerves. It is common, nearly to the point of universality. It can be severe enough to disable, thus having a significant socioeconomic impact. It is mysterious. And, at least in part, it is preventable.

It is hard to overestimate the prevalence of low back pain. About 10 percent of all American adults have at least one bout of back pain each year; the lifetime risk for back pain is an astounding 60 to 90 percent. Many of these episodes are brief, half resolving in less than a week and three quarters within a month. Unfortunately, however, many episodes of low back pain recur, and some become chronic. Low back pain disables 5.4 million Americans; it is the leading cause of work loss before age 45 and the third leading cause above that age, accounting for more than 2.7 million lost workdays each year. Bad business for insurance companies paying out more than $1 billion in worker's compensation annually, low back pain is good business for orthopedists, who record some 25,000 office visits for this complaint each year. But at an annual cost of $5.4 billion, low back pain is actually bad business for all of us — for patients, doctors, employers, and insurers alike.

Because of the widespread occurrence of low back pain, it's almost impossible to sort out meaningful risk factors. Various studies have implicated heavy lifting or prolonged sitting, obesity or tallness, smoking, alcohol abuse, depression, trauma, metabolic abnormalities, and, of course, age.

The causes of low back pain are every bit as hard to pin down. In a small minority of patients a discrete anatomical diagnosis can be discovered; included in this group are herniated discs, spinal stenosis, infections, and bona fide arthritis. But in the vast majority of cases the true cause remains unknown. Not content to admit uncertainty, practitioners have a panoply of diagnoses on hand to explain the pain, including sciatica, sacroiliac sprain, degenerative disc disease, arthritis, myositis, fibrositis, and lumbago. No happier about my ignorance, I prefer the diagnosis of low back syndrome.

Common, painful, and obscure: *of course* there are innumerable tests for low back pain. Unfortunately, low-tech tests such as ordinary x rays are rarely helpful; fortunately, high-tech tests such as CAT scanning and magnetic resonance imaging are rarely necessary. There are almost as many treatments for back pain as there are patients. Medical studies have compared various programs without demonstrating the superiority of any, or even proving that any has real value. Tests and treatments must of course be individualized. Some cases of low back pain are caused by serious problems that require prompt diagnosis and specific therapy. But for "garden-variety" low back syndrome I generally rely on a simple history and physical exam for diagnosis, and for treatment I suggest aspirin or other anti-inflammatory drugs, heat, and progressing from rest to mobility to back exercises as rapidly as possible. My results are no worse than anyone else's.

With back pain so widespread, it is tempting to assume it's an inevitable part of the human condition. Indeed, the upright posture which elevated bipeds above quadrupeds puts the human back at a unique mechanical disadvantage. But don't be too fast to criticize human engineering. My theory is that the back is as well constructed as the rest of the body, but that it suffers because of the disuse and abuse associated with industrial civilization.

If this theory is correct, we should be able to prevent low back pain with exercise and other life-style changes. No scientific studies have yet supported (or refuted) this hypothesis. But a 1985 study of more than 1,600 firefighters gives me hope: the men who succeeded in achieving fitness through diet, blood pressure control, smoking cessation, aerobic exercise, and special back exercises had much less back pain and disability.

To take care of your back, take care of your health with the cardiovascular conditioning, weight-control, nutrition, and stress-control measures advocated throughout this book.

To take care of your back, take care of your back — and your abdominal and leg muscles. Tables 21-6 and 21-7 list exercises for back strength and flexibility, abdominal muscle strength, and hamstring flexibility.

To take care of your back, listen to your mother: good posture, proper body mechanics and lifting techniques, a firm mattress, and supportive chairs can only help.

I can't guarantee that this program will prevent all low back pain. But it will enhance your health. As in other areas of prevention, the best approach is simply back to basics.

▪ 9 ▪
Disorders of the Breast and Reproductive Systems

Although not essential for the life of the individual, the breast and reproductive organs are nevertheless vital for the life of the species. And since there is much more to life than mere survival, these organs assume a personal importance for most people that rivals their biological importance for all people.

The principal diseases of the reproductive organs fall into two broad categories. In younger people disorders arise from reproductive activity — sexually transmitted disorders and complications of pregnancy. Paradoxically, perhaps, the most serious disorders — malignancies — occur in older people when reproductive function has ceased. Clearly related to human behavior, the first group of disorders should be preventable. Although the second group may seem to be inevitable consequences of reproductive obsolescence, there are effective preventive interventions for these diseases as well.

▪ Disorders Affecting Women

The Breast

The breast is an organ with one function; its ability to provide milk following pregnancy begins at puberty and continues until menopause. Estrogens stimulate the glandular tissue of the breast; when estrogen levels decline after menopause, breast tissue atrophies. Even so, the major breast disease, cancer, is much more common in the postmenopausal years.

The most common breast "disease" is not a disease at all. Until recently, many women were labeled with the diagnosis of "fibrocystic disease of the breast" because they had dense breast tissue and cysts. We now know that these women are perfectly healthy, that dense tissue and cysts represent merely one end of the spectrum of healthy breasts. In fact, the only diagnosis now applied to these women is "lumpy breasts," a term surely less elegant and aesthetic but also less frightening and more accurate.

Lumpy breasts can be painful, particularly when cysts fill with fluid as the menstrual period approaches. We do not know how to prevent lumps and cysts; earlier beliefs that caffeine was responsible have not been confirmed. But the most important fact about lumpy breasts is that they do *not* increase the risk of breast cancer. They do, however, make breast evaluation more difficult.

When women worry about their breasts, their concerns, of course, are not about cysts but about cancer. Unfortunately, that concern is justified.

▪ **Breast Cancer.** Breast cancer is the most common malignancy in women living in Western industrial societies. In American women breast cancer has only recently fallen to second place behind lung cancer as the leading cause of cancer deaths. This change in status does not signify a decrease in breast cancer, however, but marks an increase in lung cancer caused by smoking.

About 175,000 new breast cancers will be discovered in American women this year. Despite major advances in diagnosis and treatment, nearly 45,000 patients will die from breast cancer. Prevention could save many of these women; life-style modification can reduce the risk of breast cancer (primary prevention), and early diagnosis can lead to curative therapy (secondary prevention).

In all, one of every nine American women will develop breast cancer, and if present trends hold, the toll will continue to rise. The risk of breast cancer, however, is not equally distributed in all women, nor is it uniform at all stages of life. By understanding the risk factors that predispose to breast cancer, you can design a program to help prevent this dreadful disease:

Factors that increase risk
Family history
Advancing age
Early onset of menstruation
Late menopause
No pregnancies
Dietary fat
Obesity
Alcohol consumption
Prolonged estrogen use (unproven)

Factors that decrease risk
Early pregnancy
Exercise
High-fiber, vitamin-rich diets (unproven)

Breast Cancer Risk Factors. *Family history* and *age* head the list of non-modifiable risk factors. Breast cancer is rare but potentially very aggressive in premenopausal women; the risk increases progressively with advancing age. More than half of all women who die from breast cancer are 65 or older. Unfortunately many older women, not recognizing this fact, resist mammography just when they need it most. Although no woman is safe from breast cancer, women whose mothers and sisters have had the disease are two to three times more likely to develop cancer themselves.

Their risk is particularly increased if cancer developed in more than one first-order relative, if it occurred before menopause, or if it was bilateral (occurring in both breasts). Women who have had cancer in one breast also have an especially high risk of developing it in the other.

Since breast tissue is so sensitive to estrogens, it is not surprising that the risk of breast cancer is affected by hormonal factors. *Menstrual history* is one such factor; early onset of menstruation (before age 12) and late menopause (beyond age 50) both increase risk. Pregnancy has the opposite effect. Women who have *never* been pregnant have a higher risk than women who have been pregnant; a late first pregnancy (after age 30) is less protective than an early first pregnancy. *Lactation*, especially if prolonged, appears to reduce the risk of breast cancer, but more studies will be needed to confirm this observation.

The theme that explains how menstrual history, pregnancy, and lactation can affect risk is that prolonged, uninterrupted estrogenic stimulation increases the incidence of breast cancer. It is important to point out, however, that not all hormonal stimulation can be blamed. For example, it's quite clear that oral contraceptive pills do *not* increase risk. Similarly, fetal exposure to DES (an estrogen used by some pregnant women years ago) does not increase risk. In postmenopausal women, too, the use of conjugated estrogens such as Premarin for replacement therapy does not predispose to breast cancer. A 1989 study of more than 23,000 Swedish women, however, found that nine or more years of replacement therapy with *un*-conjugated estrogens (the form prescribed much more often in Europe than in the United States) increases risk nearly twofold. Even more worrisome, the concomitant administration of a second hormone, progesterone, appeared responsible for an additional doubling of risk. More study will be needed to learn if the currently widespread American practice of prescribing cyclic conjugated estrogen-progesterone hormone replacement should be modified.

Every woman will have to decide the question of postmenopausal estrogen for herself. I provide some guidelines to help with that decision later in this chapter. With the still controversial exception of postmenopausal estrogens, the other risk factors I have discussed thus far are hard to modify. But there are important risk factors that every woman can — and should — alter to reduce her chances of getting breast cancer.

Dietary factors are significant contributors to the risk of breast cancer. Much of our information in this area comes from international cross-cultural comparisons. For example, the risk of breast cancer is five to six times greater in American than in Japanese women. On average, American women consume 1,000 more calories each day as well as two to three times more fat. As a result, women in America have more body fat, and they begin menstruating at a younger age than in Japan. But when Japanese women move to the United States and assume a Western diet, they gain weight, increase body fat, begin menstruating younger, and, in the course of two to three generations, increase their risk of breast cancer to the average American level.

The relationship between diet and breast cancer has been compared in more than 40 countries. In every case, ranging from the very low risks of breast cancer in Thailand to the ten times higher risk in Denmark, societies with high dietary fat intakes have a high risk of breast cancer.

International studies consistently confirm that the more dietary fat, calories, and body fat, the higher the risk of breast cancer. In approximate terms, doubling dietary fat doubles the risk of breast cancer. A 1990 report in the *Journal of the National Cancer Institute* explains why low dietary fat is protective: women who switched to low-fat diets dropped their blood estrogen levels by 17 percent. The results of dietary surveys in American women are inconclusive, but in Canada women who consume more than 100 grams of fat per day have a 35 percent higher rate of breast cancer than women who eat less than 50 grams daily. All in all, I believe the overwhelming weight of evidence adds breast cancer to the list of reasons for following a low-fat diet.

Another dietary risk factor that has been appreciated recently is *alcohol*. This link is particularly disturbing because even very modest amounts of alcohol appear to increase risk. Doctors at Harvard Medical School report that three to nine drinks a week increase risk by 30 percent; higher amounts may increase risk by as much as 60 percent. With all due respect for my colleagues at Harvard, I think it is necessary to confirm this observation in other population groups; indeed, a 1991 study in the *International Journal of Cancer* reports similar findings for Russian women.

Should all women give up alcohol to reduce their risk of breast cancer? It's still too early to make such a sweeping recommendation, but I do suggest that women consider reducing their alcohol consumption as much as possible, particularly if they have other breast cancer risk factors. Chapter 18 reviews the many ways in which alcohol affects health.

If alcohol and dietary fat increase breast cancer risk, are there any nutritional changes that may decrease risk? There is evidence that women who eat fiber-rich diets have a reduced risk of breast cancer, but this link is clouded by the fact that women who eat more fiber also tend to take in less fat and fewer calories. Dietary fiber binds estrogen, thus accelerating fecal loss and lowering blood estrogen levels. Thus there is a biologically sound reason for fiber to help protect against breast cancer, and there are certainly many other reasons to eat lots of fiber-rich foods. The same is true for vitamin A: women whose diets are high in vitamin A seem to get less cancer, but this may be due to their preference for low-fat, low-calorie, high-fiber foods rather than vitamin A itself. Finally, women living in sunny climes appear to have less breast cancer than women who get less sunlight, presumably because sun increases vitamin D levels.

A last note about diet and breast cancer: widespread rumors notwithstanding, coffee will *not* increase your risk.

The Harvard study of diet and breast cancer may have given us some bad news about alcohol, but another investigation from Harvard provides good news: *exercise* reduces the risk of breast cancer. Dr. Rose Frisch and her colleagues evaluated exercise habits and cancer risk in more than

5,000 American women. Women who began to exercise early in life, during their college years, had only half as much breast cancer throughout life as did their sedentary peers. This very powerful protective effect may be explained by the tendency of regular exercise to reduce body fat and lower estrogen levels. Like so many other observations about exercise and health, this one is sadly overlooked; like so many others, it should provide powerful evidence that exercise belongs in every woman's life.

Secondary Prevention of Breast Cancer. Low dietary fat, abstemious alcohol intake, and regular exercise can all reduce the risk of breast cancer while helping to prevent many other diseases. But unlike many other diseases, breast cancer is also well suited for secondary prevention since it can be detected early, before symptoms develop, and treated effectively.

There are three ways to screen for early breast cancer: self-examination, medical examination, and mammography (breast x ray). Mammography is the most effective and sensitive of the three, but the advantages of mammography should not cause you to neglect the simpler techniques.

Breast self-examination is universally available and cost-free. Despite these advantages, it's not sensitive enough to be relied on as your only breast cancer screening test. Untrained women detect only about 25 percent of breast lumps; training improves results to 50 percent. When it comes to breast cancer, however, half a loaf is not enough. Self-examination is not accurate enough to be your *sole* screening test, but it is an excellent supplement to mammography. Women who practice self-examination tend to have smaller cancers at the time of diagnosis — and better results from treatment. You have little to lose and much to gain. Learn to examine your breasts (see figure 9-1), and check yourself monthly, right after each menstrual period. Don't panic if you find a lump; most are benign, but all should be evaluated by your doctor.

Medical examination is the second way to screen for breast cancer. Breast examination by a physician or nurse is more reliable than self-examination, and should be part of every regular checkup, once a year beyond age 40. You don't have to schedule extra breast exams if you don't have any symptoms, but be sure your breasts are examined during routine physicals, even if you check yourself and have periodic mammography.

Routine mammography is the key to the secondary prevention of breast cancer. It has been estimated that our breast cancer death rate could be reduced by 30 percent if all American women followed current guidelines for mammography. Mammograms are accurate, detecting very early breast cancers that are still too small to feel up to 90 percent of the time. Mammograms are safe, quick, and only minimally uncomfortable; new techniques have reduced the radiation dosage to extremely low, nontoxic levels. Mammograms are moderate in expense; charges average $100 to $125, but in many areas excellent mammograms are available for half as much. In all but 13 states insurance payment is mandatory, and Medicare began paying for mammograms in 1991.

Although details vary, every major health organization endorses periodic mammography for every American woman. As techniques and inter-

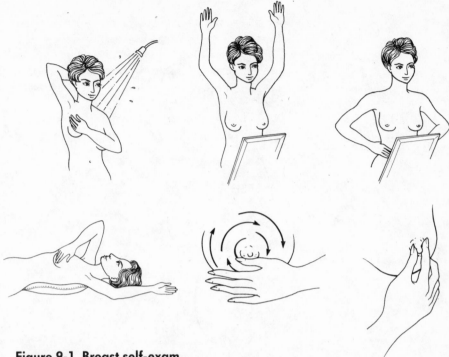

Figure 9-1. Breast self-exam

pretation improve further, expense declines, and experience accumulates, these recommendations will continue to evolve. At present the National Cancer Institute guidelines seem best: a baseline mammogram between ages 35 and 40, with repeat studies every year after age 40. Women with serious risk factors, particularly a mother or sister with premenopausal breast cancer, should move their baseline mammography to age 30. Needless to say, if abnormalities are detected, more frequent mammograms may be necessary; suspicious lesions require expert evaluation, often including biopsy.

It is, I think, the fear of an abnormality that causes so many women to neglect these guidelines. As of 1990 the National Cancer Institute reports that fewer than one third of American women over 40 were following the guidelines for screening mammography. Is it any wonder that deaths from breast cancer continue to increase in the United States? While supporting intensive research into the causes, diagnosis, and cure of breast cancer, we should also greatly intensify our efforts to educate American women (and their doctors) about the benefits of breast examination and mammography. The lives of one out of every nine American women are at stake.

The Female Reproductive System

Popular conceptions notwithstanding, the female reproductive system is not restricted to the pelvic organs. Rather, it's a complex network involving the central nervous system and the pituitary gland as well as the ovaries

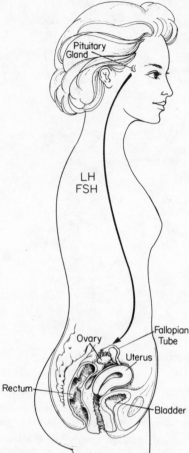

Pituitary
Gland

LH
FSH

Ovary

Fallopian
Tube

Uterus

Rectum

Bladder

Figure 9-2.
Female reproductive system

and uterus (see figure 9-2). All these elements must function with precise coordination to maintain normal menstrual and reproductive function. The interactions are so intricate that the ordinary menstrual cycle, to say nothing of a successful pregnancy, represents a triumph of human engineering.

The Normal Female Cycle. Parents, educators, nurses, and physicians often tell young people to use their heads in regard to reproductive behavior. Good advice — even more accurate, perhaps, than it appears. The driving force controlling reproductive hormones is actually in a part of the brain, the hypothalamus. Shortly before puberty the hypothalamus begins to produce a small protein called *releasing hormone*. Releasing hormone is carried to the pituitary gland, the "master gland" of the endocrine system, which is also located in the brain. Stimulated by releasing hormone, the pituitary gland in turn secretes two additional hormones, FSH and LH, which are carried by the blood to the ovaries.

The central nervous system hormones are vital to stimulate the ovaries, but it is the ovaries that produce the more familiar female sex hormones, estrogen and progesterone. Estrogen stimulates the breasts, uterus, and genital tissues; it also signals the pituitary, influencing the timing and release of LH and FSH. Estrogens are produced by the ovary, and they also act on ovary, causing egg cells to develop. Ovulation occurs at the midpoint of the menstrual cycle. In the second half of the cycle the ovary produces large amounts of progesterone, which allows the lining of the uterus to proliferate. If a fertilized egg is implanted in the uterus during this time, estrogen and progesterone levels remain high, allowing the uterus to enlarge to support the pregnancy. But without a pregnancy, estrogen and progesterone production decrease, and the lining of the uterus is shed. After menstruation estrogen levels start to rise again, repeating the entire cycle.

The female reproductive cycle begins with puberty and ends with menopause. Puberty is initiated by the brain, as the hypothalamus begins to produce releasing hormone. Menopause is caused by the ovaries, which lose their ability to produce estrogen. Estrogen deficiency, in turn, is responsible for the familiar changes in every woman's tissues and metabolism.

Disorders of the Reproductive Cycle. With so many hormones and organs involved in the menstrual cycle, it's not surprising that disorders of the cycle can occur. In some cases the cycles just never get started, usually because of genetically determined disorders of the hormones or ovaries. Much more frequently cycles get started normally enough but become irregular, or stop altogether, in early adulthood. There are many causes of this problem, called secondary amenorrhea, and some are preventable. The most common preventable cause (aside from pregnancy) is mental stress, which affects the hypothalamus and pituitary. Very intense exercise can also produce secondary amenorrhea by affecting the hypothalamus and by reducing body fat. Finally, severe caloric restriction interferes with menstrual function by a combination of mechanisms involving the hypothalamus and body fat.

The obvious consequence of amenorrhea is infertility. Fortunately, the common causes of secondary amenorrhea are reversible; with resumption of menstrual cycles fertility is restored. But if stress, exercise, or caloric deficiencies are not corrected, estrogen levels remain low, mimicking a premature menopause. Hormone therapy should be considered in these circumstances.

A Word about Pregnancy. The entire reproductive cycle, in all its elegant complexity, is designed for just one purpose: pregnancy. Preventable, perhaps, pregnancy is surely not an illness. It is included briefly here, however, because of two implications for preventive medicine.

The first issue is unintended pregnancy. Although precise data are lacking, it is reliably estimated that about one third of all pregnancies in America are unintended. The majority of these occur in adolescents. There are about 1 million teenage pregnancies each year; 40 percent are terminated, the remainder carried to term. More than two thirds of our teenage mothers are unmarried. And the problem is getting worse; the birth rate among 15- to 17-year-olds increased 10 percent between 1986 and 1988.

Unintended pregnancies, particularly in teenagers, have medical as well as social consequences. Prenatal care is often deficient and maternal health habits poor. The result: premature and low-birth-weight infants, with an increased risk of medical and developmental problems. An unstable family environment and substandard pediatric care all too often compound the difficulties facing these children. In addition to the increased burden of illness thrust upon the offspring of teenage pregnancies, a financial burden of $13 billion a year is thrust upon society as a whole. Worst of all, the cycle of unintended pregnancy, deficient health habits and medical care, abnormal development, illness, and social instability is often recapitulated in the next generation.

Although adolescent sexual activity is comparable throughout the industrialized world, teenage pregnancies are four times more common in the United States than in any other developed country. We must do better. Improvements in public education and in the availability of family planning and health care service are essential. Counseling should be intensified. Incentive systems designed to improve motivation and compliance should be studied. Last but not least, medical and social research in this area should be bolstered.

Unintended pregnancy is reaching epidemic proportions in the United States. Although we lead the industrial world in these sad statistics, the population explosion in the Third World poses an even greater long-term threat to global health, nutrition, and environmental quality. Without apology for editorializing, I believe that our role as a world leader in so many areas should obligate the United States to assume a leading role in addressing this problem as well. It is, after all, a small planet; efforts to improve global health are in our own best interests.

Unintended pregnancies illustrate deficiencies in our systems of health care delivery, education, and social support. In contrast, ideal prenatal care represents prevention at its best, setting standards for all areas of health care.

Obstetricians and pediatricians have long been leaders in preventive medicine. Routine prenatal care involves education and counseling, nutrition, good maternal health habits, and carefully considered medical screening studies. These low-cost, low-technology interventions have proven to be effective in preventing disease. To back them up, research in prenatal medicine has developed a wonderful array of treatments to attack fetal disease at the earliest possible stage. At its best, prenatal medicine is a paradigm for all prevention. Each person should be as diligent about nutrition, exercise, stress, and exposure to toxins, chemicals, and drugs as the best-motivated pregnant woman. The medical establishment should be as diligent about planning and providing preventive services to all people as it is to the pregnant. And society should be diligent about facilitating and rewarding these efforts on behalf of all its citizens.

Toxic Shock Syndrome. Another example of prevention at its best.

Toxic shock syndrome was unknown until 1979; within about a year, however, more than 1,000 cases were reported, nearly all in menstruating women. Women with toxic shock syndrome are acutely ill with low blood pressure and shock, high fever, severe rash, diarrhea, and abnormalities of liver, kidney, and nervous system function. Even with the best of treatment, many women die from toxic shock.

Our treatment for toxic shock syndrome has not improved substantially, yet very few women now die from it. The reason is prevention: in 1980 there were 890 cases with 35 deaths, but in 1989 there were only 61 cases with no deaths.

The control of toxic shock syndrome is worth considering as an example of successful prevention. The first step was to determine the cause of this mysterious and previously unknown illness. The scientific discipline of epidemiology was crucial. Investigations quickly found that toxic shock syndrome occurred principally in menstruating women using a new, extraordinarily absorbent tampon. But the tampons themselves did not cause any unusual inflammation or signs of illness. How, then, could they be the cause of this terrible epidemic? The next step forward came from laboratory scientists who found that the tampons allowed the growth of a particular strain of bacteria, *Staphylococcus aureus,* which produces a toxin. The toxin in turn enters the blood, causing all the symptoms of toxic shock syndrome.

Antibiotics can kill the staph germ. But by the time the toxin is in a woman's blood, it's too late for antibiotics to work. And so the third crucial step in controlling toxic shock syndrome involved nonmedical resources. Publicity and education were the keys to prevention, informing women of the risks and persuading them to change to tampons that were safer, if less convenient. The federal government coordinated much of the research and the educational campaign; it also mandated the elimination of superabsorbent tampons made from polyester foam and carboxymethylcellulose in favor of safer cotton-rayon tampons. In addition, all tampons are now packaged with warnings and instructions for safe use. I'm happy to say that the tampon industry and the mass media have cooperated fully with these efforts.

Although it's now rare, you should still take measures to prevent toxic shock syndrome. First, use the least absorbent tampons that are comfortable (as a result of the lessons from toxic shock, all tampons are now standardized and marketed with absorbency ratings ranging from 6 to 15). Second, change tampons as often as possible, omitting them for part of the day if you can. Third, listen to your body; be alert for symptoms, and report them promptly if they occur.

A frightening illness with a happy ending, toxic shock syndrome illustrates beautifully the value of prevention. Like so many of the diseases covered in this book, it was caused by well-intentioned new technology which produced unforeseen consequences. As with many illnesses of the modern world, its causes were uncovered first by epidemiologic studies and then by experiments in the basic science lab. Finally, prevention was achieved by a combination of education, government regulation and industrial cooperation, and behavioral change. Unfortunately, it is this last process that holds back our efforts to prevent many of the diseases of industrial societies; we understand what needs to be done but have not made the changes that are required. I hope you will help achieve our very realistic goals of preventing many major illnesses by making changes to protect yourself, and by mobilizing society to achieve reforms that will benefit us all.

Cancer of the Cervix. Cervical cancer is another success story, but it's a story in progress that has not yet reached a completely happy ending. It could.

Deaths from cancer of the cervix have declined by 75 percent in the past 40 years. That's the good news. The bad news is that 7,000 American women still die from the disease each year. The vast majority of these deaths could be prevented.

Although the precise cause of cervical cancer is unknown, it is clearly linked to sexual activity. The risk is higher in women who begin to have sexual intercourse at an early age, and in women who have multiple sexual partners. Conversely, the risk is extremely low in women who have never been sexually active. It seems likely that cervical cancer is actually a sexually transmitted disease; although proof is lacking, the papilloma virus has emerged as the likely cause.

Another risk factor for cervical cancer is exposure to cigarette smoke — either by active smoking or by passive or secondhand exposure. A final, less powerful risk factor is oral contraceptive use. This association may be partly artifactual, since women on the pill are more likely to be sexually active; they are also more likely to have gynecological exams, so their increased incidence of cervical cancer may be partially explained by better diagnosis.

Changes in sexual behavior and in smoking could reduce dramatically the incidence of cervical cancer. These changes have not occurred, yet deaths from cervical cancer have declined substantially. The reason is early detection and treatment — secondary prevention.

A screening test for cervical cancer was devised by Dr. George Papanicolaou in the 1930s and was introduced into widespread use a decade later. The test involves scraping cells from the cervix at the time of a pelvic exam, fixing them on a slide, and sending them to a lab for microscopic examination by a cytologist. The Pap test is quick, painless, and extremely safe. It is also inexpensive. The smear itself costs just a few dollars; the entire process averages about $60 — still a bargain for what it can achieve. Best of all, the Pap test is accurate, with an overall reliability of about 90 percent.

The Pap test is able to detect cervical cancer in its earliest stage. Each year about 50,000 cases of this very early "carcinoma-in-situ" are discovered; virtually all can be cured by a simple office procedure, either cone biopsy or cauterization.

About 13,000 cases of more advanced invasive cervical cancer are also diagnosed each year. Early invasive cancer has an excellent outlook; various combinations of hysterectomy and radiation cure 80 percent of these women. But if diagnosis is delayed until late (Stage IV) disease, survival falls to 10 percent.

Why do 7,000 women die from cervical cancer annually? The answer is both simple and sad: delayed diagnosis because they have not had their recommended Pap smears.

Every sexually active woman should have routine Pap smears; all the experts agree with this proposition, but they do differ a bit in the details (see chapter 23). A reasonable consensus calls for the first smear when sexual activity begins or at age 18. Smears should be repeated at regular intervals. Some authorities recommend yearly smears, whereas others advise that every three years is often enough. Fortunately, a recent study by Dr. Kirk Shy and his colleagues in Washington State splits the difference, indicating that every two years is best. The differences in outcome are small. I'd suggest that you go along with your doctor's routine as long as the smears are done no more than three years apart. If all your smears have been negative, you may safely choose to discontinue them at about age 65; most of my patients, however, prefer to continue routine Pap smears, which is also extremely reasonable.

Endometrial Cancer. Cancer of the endometrium, the lining of the uterus, is common; 34,000 cases are discovered in the United States each year. Treatment can save about 70 percent of women who are diagnosed early.

Like the breast, the endometrium is a hormonally sensitive organ. Many predisposing risk factors are shared among these cancers, including early puberty, late menopause, never having been pregnant, and a high-fat diet. Obesity predisposes women to both cancers, tripling the risk of endometrial cancer. Birth control pills do not increase the incidence of either breast or endometrial cancer. But the risk of endometrial cancer *is* increased by postmenopausal estrogen replacement therapy; lower-dose estrogen therapy and the addition of progesterone diminish the endometrial cancer risk of replacement therapy.

Occurring most often between ages 50 and 70, the first symptom of endometrial cancer is usually postmenstrual vaginal bleeding. The diagnosis is generally established by a surgical procedure, the dilatation and curettage (D and C).

Unfortunately, we do not have a good screening test for endometrial cancer. A simple Pap smear, so valuable for cervical cancer, is not reliable for endometrial cancer. A reliable test, the D and C, is not simple enough for mass screening.

In the absence of a suitable screening test, we do not have an effective strategy for the secondary prevention of endometrial cancer. In any case, primary prevention is the most desirable approach. The same Harvard study which showed that exercise protects against breast cancer revealed

that women who began exercise during their college years also enjoyed a
50 percent reduction in endometrial cancer. Weight loss and a low-fat diet
have not been studied as carefully, but they seem to be reasonable and desirable; endometrial cancer is five times more common in America than in
Japan, suggesting that life-style changes *can* make a difference.

Endometriosis. Endometriosis occurs when cells from the lining of the
uterus travel up the fallopian tubes and become implanted in the abdominal cavity. The aberrant endometrial cells grow in response to estrogenic
stimulation, causing pelvic pain, intestinal complaints, or urinary symptoms around the time of menstruation. In severe cases scarring can lead to
adhesions that may interfere with bowel function or cause infertility.

We need better ways to diagnose and treat this common disorder that
plagues up to 3 percent of American women during their reproductive
years. But you don't have to wait for medical progress to help yourself.
Researchers at Harvard Medical School have found that regular, vigorous
aerobic exercise can reduce the risk of endometriosis by up to 80 percent.
But to get this benefit exercise must be started before age 26. Endometriosis
is another good reason to exercise early and often.

Cancer of the Ovary. Ovarian cancer, the deadliest malignancy of the
reproductive tract, takes the lives of about 12,000 American women each
year. It's most common over age 60 and in women with a family history of
ovarian cancer. Prolonged ovulatory activity is another risk factor; ovarian
cancer is more common in women who have never been pregnant or who
have had a late first pregnancy, but is less common in women who have
used oral contraceptives.

For the purposes of primary prevention, it's important to note that life-
style factors must also have a role: the disease is rare in Japan but common
in Japanese women who have migrated to the United States. The basic
modifiable risk factors are shared by other estrogen-sensitive cancers; like
breast and endometrial cancer, ovarian cancer is more common in women
who have diets high in animal fat and who lack exercise. The use of cosmetic talc appears to be a unique risk factor in ovarian cancer.

At present, most ovarian cancers are not detected until they have enlarged enough to cause symptoms. It would be much better to detect the
disease early, when treatment is most likely to succeed. Unfortunately, a
suitable screening test for ovarian cancer is not yet available. Pap tests,
frequent pelvic examinations, ultrasound studies, and CA-125 blood tests
have all been studied; none leads to earlier diagnosis or improved survival.

The prevention of ovarian cancer, then, resembles the approach to endometrial cancer. Since secondary prevention is not yet possible, you must
rely on a low-fat diet and on regular exercise for risk reduction. More research is needed to improve the diagnosis and treatment of both malignancies. But even when these gains have been achieved, it will be important for you to continue the healthful life-style that can assist in primary
prevention.

Cancer of the Vagina. Vaginal cancer is a unique situation. It is so rare
that no special approach to prevention or detection is necessary — except

for one group of women. Between 1940 and 1960 DES (diethylstilbesterol, an estrogen) was prescribed for about 6 million women with high-risk pregnancies. Daughters of these women have an increased risk of vaginal cancer. The risk is still very small — about one in 1,000 — but women whose mothers took DES or any other estrogen while pregnant should be sure to get special gynecological follow-up tests.

Menopause. It's not a disease, but every woman gets it. It's entirely natural, but every woman worries about it. It's much researched and discussed, but it's still controversial.

Reproductive cycles begin at puberty at the behest of the hypothalamus. The hypothalamus and pituitary gland continue to secrete their stimulating hormones throughout life; menopause is caused not by the brain or pituitary but by the ovaries. The ovary is unrivaled among human organs in planned obsolescence, and this is one type of obsolescence that's every bit as common in Tokyo as in Detroit. At birth the ovaries have more than 7 million follicles which are all capable of producing estrogens. At the time of menopause, 99 percent of these follicles are used up. The result is a nearly complete halt in ovarian estrogen production — menopause.

Menopause is inevitable, but its timing is variable. The contemporary American life-style, with its overabundant nutrition and increased body fat, has increased the average duration of menstrual cycles. American girls begin menstruating earlier than did their grandmothers, probably contributing to an increase in breast, ovarian, and endometrial cancers. Menopause also tends to occur later in the United States than in other countries, now at an average age of 51.

Menopause is an entirely natural process. In most women menstrual periods slowly become scanty and irregular before stopping altogether. Some women experience increased bleeding in the year or two before menopause; this, too, can be perfectly normal, but endometrial disorders should be ruled out by gynecological examination.

Many women do not experience either physical or psychological distress at menopause; it is, after all, a normal process. But in some women bothersome symptoms can occur. The most common symptom is hot flashes — warm feeling with flushing of the skin, especially on the face, neck, and upper chest. Hot flashes last only a minute or two, but they can occur up to ten times a day and they may interrupt sleep. Estrogen replacement therapy will control hot flashes, but even without treatment flashes tend to diminish in severity, disappearing altogether within a year or two.

Another common symptom of menopause is vaginal dryness, which can produce complaints ranging from mild vaginal irritation to urinary burning to pain and even bleeding during sexual intercourse. Whereas hot flashes occur early in menopause, vaginal dryness usually does not become a problem until five or more years after periods stop. But if present, dryness continues as a lifelong complaint. Mild dryness is often relieved by vaginal lubricants, but estrogens are needed for more troublesome cases. The response to estrogens is gradual, typically taking many months for complete relief of symptoms. Estrogen vaginal creams will work as well as pills or patches; remember, though, that the hormone is absorbed from the vagina into the blood, thus affecting the entire body.

A third potential symptom of menopause is bladder dysfunction. Without estrogenic stimulation, tissues of the lower urinary tract can become dry and thin. Most often these changes are of little consequence, but sometimes urinary burning, bleeding, infections, or incontinence can result. Estrogen replacement therapy can be very helpful if these symptoms are indeed caused by menopause.

Most of the other symptoms attributed to menopause are minor, or even unsubstantiated. Singers may notice slight problems with upper-register notes resulting from changes in their vocal cords. Some degree of skin dryness and breast softness may be attributed to menopause, but estrogen replacement will *not* prevent normal aging of the skin or breasts. Although depression and irritability are often blamed on the "change of life," there is little hard evidence that these midlife phenomena are actually caused by estrogen deficiency. However, a 1991 study from California reported that estrogen therapy improved psychological function and mood in a small group of postmenopausal women who were free of psychological complaints. Finally, menopause does *not* cause a decrease in sex drive. Libido in women is dependent not on estrogens but on low levels of androgens (male hormones), which are maintained long after menopause.

If that were all there was to menopause, the medical issues would be simple: doctors would prescribe estrogen replacement only for women with troublesome symptoms. But menopause causes changes in every woman's body that she cannot see or feel — unless they lead to medical problems, which may be quite serious. The two areas of concern are the cardiovascular system and the bones.

Heart attacks are rare in premenopausal women, but they increase progressively with each year after menopause. As I detailed in chapter 2, estrogens benefit the heart and blood vessels by increasing blood levels of the protective HDL cholesterol. After menopause, HDL cholesterol levels decline and cardiovascular risk increases. Estrogen replacement therapy preserves high HDL levels without causing deterioration in other cardiovascular risk factors; therapeutic doses of estrogen do not increase the "bad" (LDL) cholesterol, the blood pressure, or the blood sugar levels.

It's nice to know that estrogen replacement therapy improves cardiovascular risk profiles, but it's much more important to realize that treatment actually decreases the rate of heart attacks experienced by postmenopausal women. The magnitude of protection is very impressive. Careful studies have shown that estrogen replacement reduces the number of heart attacks by one half to two thirds. By protecting blood vessels, estrogens also reduce the occurrence of stroke by about 50 percent — major gains indeed.

The second problem caused by postmenopausal estrogen deficiency is osteoporosis. As we saw in chapter 8, bone density begins to decline at the time of menopause, and calcium loss progresses with each passing year. As a result, women have a 30 percent lifetime risk of suffering a vertebral fracture and a 15 percent risk of hip fracture. Estrogen replacement therapy preserves bone calcium and reduces the risk of fractures by 50 to 60 percent. To be effective, though, estrogen must be started within five to six years of menopause.

Control of symptoms, improved cholesterol levels, less heart disease and stroke, prevention of osteoporosis, and protection against fractures: estrogen replacement sounds great. But don't rush to your doctor for a prescription without giving it a little more thought. As with all medications, there are potential problems with estrogen treatment.

The greatest concern is endometrial cancer. Estrogen stimulates the lining of the uterus. If that stimulation is continued without interruption after menopause, the risk of endometrial cancer increases. Various studies have placed the magnitude of increase between two and ten, with most at about five. But there are ways to protect against estrogen-induced endometrial cancer. Interrupting estrogen therapy by taking the pills for only the first 25 days of each month is one tactic. Even better is adding progesterone for days 15 to 25 of each month, stopping both hormones at the end of each month. Cyclic estrogen-progesterone replacement mimics the body's natural menstrual cycle and largely counteracts the increased risk of endometrial cancer. Because it mimics the normal cycle, however, this procedure produces menstrual bleeding at the end of each month. Bleeding is scant, however, and cramps do not occur. Needless to say, women who have had hysterectomies have no worries about endometrial cancer, and can take estrogen replacement daily without progesterone.

The other great area of concern about estrogen replacement therapy is breast cancer. Despite many studies of this question, the actual risk of estrogen replacement remains uncertain. Many studies conducted in the mid-1980s showed that estrogen replacement does not increase breast cancer risk. In fact, a careful study of female military dependents at the Wilford Hall U.S. Air Force Base demonstrated that estrogen replacement actually *reduced* the risk of breast cancer by more than 50 percent.

Most doctors were very sanguine about estrogen replacement and breast cancer until 1989, when a Swedish study reported that nine or more years of replacement therapy with unconjugated estrogens doubled the risk of breast cancer, and that concomitant progesterone therapy produced an additional doubling of risk.

In an attempt to resolve the uncertainties about estrogen replacement and breast cancer, two groups of scientists turned in 1991 to the technique of meta-analysis, in which the results of many small trials are combined in a single, more powerful analysis. Drs. William Dupont and David Page analyzed 28 previous studies that met their standards for scientific accuracy. Their conclusions: postmenopausal replacement therapy with conjugated estrogens (Premarin) at a daily dose of .625 milligrams or less does *not* increase the risk of breast cancer. In smaller analyses of 16 studies, however, Dr. Karen Steinberg and her colleagues found that prolonged use of unconjugated estrogens (such as estradiol therapy for 15 years or more) did produce a modest increase in breast cancer risk.

When studies contradict one another, the next step is obvious: more studies. But until the results are available, which will take years, the effect of postmenopausal estrogens on breast cancer will remain uncertain. Despite legitimate grounds for disagreement, it would seem prudent to use conjugated estrogens (Premarin) in the lowest effective dose if replacement is elected.

The major risk of estrogen replacement is endometrial cancer; progesterone treatment neutralizes that risk but may increase the risk of breast cancer. Besides these central concerns, there are less consequential drawbacks to estrogen replacement. Vaginal bleeding is one. In addition, about 10 percent of postmenopausal women experience side effects from estrogen, which may include nausea, fluid retention, weight gain, and breast fullness. In most cases these side effects are mild and can be controlled by changing the estrogen dose or preparation. Some women with migraine experience increased headaches during estrogen treatment. Finally, estrogens increase the risk of gallstones and may possibly predispose toward thrombophlebitis.

The fundamental goal of preventive medicine is to extend the duration of life while enhancing its quality. To see how the pros and cons of estrogen replacement measure up to this standard, let's review the causes of disability and death in women who do not take postmenopausal estrogens.

Imagine 2,000 women who are healthy at age 50. In each postmenopausal year:

- 20 will develop heart disease; 12 will die of it
- 11 will develop osteoporosis; 1 will die of it
- 6 will develop breast cancer; 2 will die of it
- 3 will develop endometrial cancer; 1 will die of it

As you can see, heart disease is so much more common than breast and endometrial cancer combined that estrogen therapy should produce a net gain of major proportions for postmenopausal women. And you don't have to imagine those results; direct observations have demonstrated that women who take postmenopausal estrogens do in fact live longer.

In 1991 doctors from the University of California published the results of their seven-and-a-half-year study of 8,881 postmenopausal women. Estrogen replacement therapy produced a significant decrease in the death rate from all types of coronary artery disease and stroke. The death rate from breast cancer and all other cancers was also lower in women who took estrogens, but this reduction was not statistically significant. Overall, estrogen replacement therapy produced a 20 percent reduction in mortality — a highly significant benefit indeed. Also important, the study found that the women who had been taking estrogens the longest experienced the greatest benefits; for example, women who had used estrogen replacement therapy for 15 years had a 40 percent lower death rate than women of the same age who had never taken estrogens. Nor do these important findings stand alone; a 1991 Harvard study of 48,470 nurses confirms that postmenopausal estrogen replacement reduces the rates of heart attacks and overall mortality.

Every woman will experience menopause. Every woman should consider hormone replacement. But not every woman is the same; each must consult her doctor to decide if estrogen replacement therapy is best. To help with that decision, you can construct your own hormone replacement balance sheet:

Factors that favor estrogen replacement therapy

Troublesome menopausal symptoms (especially hot flashes and vaginal atrophy)

Risk factors for cardiovascular disease and stroke (especially unfavorable cholesterol, smoking, high blood pressure, lack of exercise, and diabetes)

Risk factors for osteoporosis (especially European ancestry, small build, lack of exercise, smoking, low dietary calcium intake, alcohol use, and a family history of osteoporosis)

Having had a hysterectomy

Availability of good medical follow-up (including annual mammograms and gynecological exams, possibly including endometrial biopsy)

Factors that discourage estrogen replacement therapy

Risk factors for breast cancer (especially mothers or sisters with breast cancer)

Risk factors for endometrial cancer

Fibroids or endometriosis

Uncontrolled hypertension

History of deep vein thrombophlebitis (especially multiple episodes)

Risk factors for gallstones

Active migraine headaches

Factors that preclude estrogen replacement therapy

Breast cancer

Endometrial cancer

Acute or chronic liver disease

Draw up your own balance sheet carefully, considering both pros and cons. And remember to factor in the most important elements of all: your own personal instincts and the advice of your physician.

If you decide to take estrogens, you and your doctor will still have to consider the type of replacement therapy that's best for you. Here, too, there are many options and little proof that any one program is superior. See what your doctor thinks. For estrogen replacement I usually pick conjugated estrogen (Premarin), prescribing either .3 milligrams with 1,500 milligrams of calcium or .625 milligrams. Women who have had a hysterectomy can take the estrogen daily. For the majority who have not, there are two options. First, use estrogen alone, taking the pills for the first 25 days of each month. Because of the risk of endometrial cancer, I usually recommend yearly gynecological exams for women taking estrogen alone; although proof of benefit is lacking, many gynecologists perform endometrial biopsies at the time of those exams. If vaginal bleeding at the end of each month isn't a nuisance, however, I prefer to add 10 milligrams of progesterone (Provera) per day for days 16 to 25 of each month, thus eliminating the need to consider endometrial biopsies. In either case, annual mammograms are important — just as they are for postmenopausal women who do not take estrogens.

If you decide to take estrogens, when should you start? Finally a question with an easy answer: as soon as possible after menopause, but in any case within five to six years. How long should you continue treatment? Another tough question! In fact, there is no good answer to this one. Ten years, or until your mid-60s, seems about right — but keep alert for changes in your body that may cause you to reevaluate treatment. You've signed on for only one day at a time, and you can always change your mind. In fact, we can all anticipate changes in the guidelines for estrogen replacement as new data become available.

Ledger sheets, risk factors, pluses and minuses, and calls for new data — it sounds as if I'm hedging. In fact I agree with all the major health organizations that it's still too early to make a sweeping recommendation for all women. But I do have to take a stand for my patients. In the absence of major concerns about endometrial and breast cancer, I generally favor estrogen replacement because of its protective effects on the heart and bones.

If you've been with me for these first nine chapters of *Staying Well*, you know that I am entirely committed to prevention, but that I greatly prefer simple life-style changes to preventive medication. Estrogen replacement does not change my stand. Even if you take estrogens in your postmenopausal years, you must still continue the basics: a diet low in saturated fat and high in fiber and calcium, regular exercise, abhorrence of smoking, and moderation of alcohol use. These measures will do even more than estrogen to prevent heart disease and osteoporosis — and they'll also reduce your risk of breast and endometrial cancer.

■ Disorders Affecting Men

The male reproductive system is every bit as vital as the female system for the survival of the species; in this regard, at least, one plus one equals three. Although the male system is simpler, it too may be the site of major disease.

The Normal Male Reproductive System

As in the female reproductive system, the signals that awaken the male organs at puberty and maintain their activity throughout life originate in the brain (see figure 9-3). The hypothalamus produces releasing hormone,

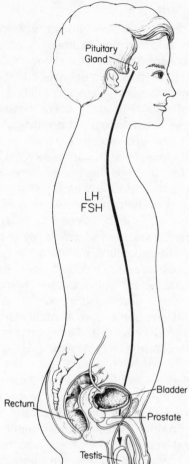

Pituitary
Gland

LH
FSH

Rectum

Bladder

Prostate

Figure 9-3.
Male reproductive system

Testis

which causes the pituitary gland to secrete LH and FSH, the very same hormones that stimulate the ovary. In men, of course, LH and FSH act on a different target, the testicles, causing special cells to produce the male hormone testosterone. In turn, testosterone acts on another set of testicular cells to stimulate sperm production. Testosterone enters the blood and is carried by the circulation to the entire body. As a result, testosterone stimulates sensitive tissues to develop characteristic male traits including deep voice, muscle bulk, facial and body hair, and in some men (I am sorry to say) male pattern baldness.

Testosterone is also responsible for the sex drive and for potency. Male potency is a complex process. Insofar as mental factors influence arousal, the brain is again in the act. Penile erection also requires the coordinated action of blood vessels and nerves in the penis; as a result, the vessels become engorged with blood, producing the erection. At the time of ejaculation, the prostate gland discharges fluid which helps carry sperm.

Sexual Dysfunction

With so many tissues and control mechanisms involved, it's not surprising that erectile dysfunction is common. A majority of men experience transient episodes of impotence. In some cases, however, erectile dysfunction can persist. I've found that many men delay or altogether avoid discussing such problems with their doctors — which is too bad, since frustration and unhappiness can be alleviated in many cases. Among the most common causes of impotence are medications. Many drugs, including those prescribed to treat high blood pressure, anxiety, depression, and ulcers, can have this side effect; happily, the difficulty resolves when the medication is changed. Remember, too, that you don't need a prescription to suffer from drug-related impotence; alcohol is a chemical that can have this effect. In other men abnormalities of the pelvic nerves or blood vessels are responsible. Particularly common in diabetics and smokers, these problems are more difficult to resolve. Testosterone deficiency is rather rare, but since it's a correctable cause of impotence, it should always be tested for; blood tests should also be used to measure levels of three pituitary hormones (LH, FSH, and prolactin). Last, but far from least, psychological factors are often responsible for impotence — and they *are* treatable. A simple way to screen for this is to find out if erection occurs at night. Most men get nocturnal erections when their bladders are full; if a man has normal nocturnal erections but sexual dysfunction, psychological factors are likely to be the cause of impotence.

Many men experience a gradual decline in sex drive beyond age 50. A male counterpart to menopause has been postulated, but it's not that simple. Unlike the ovaries, which lose their ability to make estrogen, the testicles continue to produce testosterone throughout life. In most older men who experience decreased libido, then, hormones are not to blame; medication, diabetes, vascular disease, neurological disease, and — above all — psychological difficulties should be considered. But in a small group of men testosterone levels do fall with age, and a trial of testosterone therapy may be worth considering. Long-term treatment should not be taken lightly, though, because of potentially serious side effects and generally disappointing results.

Testicular Cancer

I don't know any way to prevent testicular cancer. But I do know a simple, effective way to screen for the disease. This technique permits early detection, leading to permanent cure in the great majority of cases. The screening test is free of side effects and free of cost. In short, it's an ideal tool for secondary prevention. Despite all those advantages, however, it is sadly neglected, possibly because it is so very simple. The technique is self-examination.

Testicular cancer is diagnosed in 5,700 American men each year. It's a relatively uncommon malignancy, but since it occurs most often between the ages of 20 and 35, it is actually the most common cancer in young men, much more common in whites than in blacks. The causes of testicular cancer are unknown. It is known, however, that a developmental abnormality in which the testicle fails to descend into the scrotum during fetal life does increase the risk of testicular cancer. To prevent this malignancy, male infants who have an undescended testicle should have corrective surgery before age two.

Testicular cancer can cause pain, heaviness, or swelling. Much more often, however, the disease in its early stages causes nothing more than a painless lump. Because there are no other early warning symptoms, the only way to detect very early testicular cancer is to feel the lump. And prompt detection is very worthwhile; up to 99 percent of men who are diagnosed early can be cured.

The U.S. Preventive Service Task Force argues that because there is no proof that self-examination will save lives, there is no reason to recommend it routinely. But since self-examination is so simple, I can see no reason to wait for proof. Most men learn the technique easily; false alarms are rare, and are easily resolved by a physician's exam or ultrasound test.

I recommend that all men between the ages of 20 and 35 perform testicular self-examination. Since it's so much easier to remember something that is regular and routine, I advise my patients to check themselves on the first day of each month. I can't prove this advice will save lives, but there is nothing more than a few seconds each month to lose.

Disorders of the Prostate Gland

Situated at the base of the bladder (see figure 9-3), the prostate gland makes its presence known by producing urinary symptoms. Indeed, prostate diseases are generally treated by urologists. But since the prostate's main function is to provide fluid for ejaculation, I've included it here rather than in the chapter on urinary tract disorders. Its location in the book is less important than its location in the body, which accounts for the symptoms of prostate disease.

The prostate gland begins to enlarge at the time of puberty, when testosterone levels rise. After reaching the size of a small walnut in early adulthood, the prostate remains stable in size until the fifth decade, when, for reasons that are obscure, it begins to enlarge once again.

Benign Prostatic Hypertrophy. Middle-aged and older men are often troubled by prostate enlargement, known medically as benign prostatic hypertrophy, or BPH. The prostate enlarges in virtually all men; there is no way to prevent it. Try diet, try exercise, try even prayer — but be prepared to feel the pinch of an enlarged prostate.

And a pinch it is. The enlarged prostate is painless and harmless unless it pinches the urethra, slowing the flow of urine from the bladder. The symptoms are easy to imagine (if difficult to experience): slow urinary stream, incomplete emptying of the bladder, frequency and urgency of urination, and urination at night.

I cannot help you prevent BPH. But I hope I can help you prevent unnecessary treatment.

First, don't fall for vitamins, amino acids, or other over-the-counter remedies. They just don't work. Your money may flow freely, but your urine won't.

Second, don't rush into surgery. Although BPH can be treated with a relatively simple operation, you can safely wait until your symptoms become troublesome to you. Only you can decide when you are ready for surgery. It's not the number of times you get up at night but how tired or refreshed you feel when you start your day.

About 400,000 American men undergo prostatectomies annually at a total cost of nearly $4 billion. The federal government's Agency for Health Care Policy and Research suggests that up to 75 percent of these operations may be unnecessary. Surgery will not prevent prostate cancer. Surgery can prevent complete blockage of the bladder, but this complication is not common enough to warrant preventive surgery. Prostatectomies usually do an excellent job of relieving symptoms, but although they are generally safe, there can be complications such as bleeding, infection, retrograde ejaculation, impotence, and urinary incontinence. True, most men don't have these complications. But they are common enough for me to suggest that when your urine is slow, you should go slow, discussing your options carefully before agreeing to surgery.

You can also help reduce the symptoms of BPH with a few simple tricks. Drink less fluid, particularly after dinner. Reduce your intake of alcohol and coffee, both of which increase urine flow. And, if all else fails, always know the location of the nearest men's room.

Prostate Cancer. Prostatic enlargement is nearly universal in older men. Prostate cancer, occurring principally in the same age group, is not universal but it is distressingly common. In fact it's the most common cancer in American men and is the third leading cause of cancer death. In this year alone we can expect prostate cancer to be diagnosed in 100,000 men and to take nearly 30,000 lives. The risk of prostate cancer begins to increase at about age 50 and continues to rise throughout life.

Conventional wisdom holds that there is no way to prevent prostate cancer. I can't argue with the facts, but I can offer a theory. Prostate cancer is 15 times more common in America than in Japan. Multinational studies provide an explanation for this cancer imbalance: the risk of prostate cancer is lowest where fat consumption is lowest, and it rises steadily with increasing fat intake. Moreover, saturated fat is particularly linked to the risk of prostate cancer; men who eat the most meat, eggs, and dairy products have the highest incidence of the disease.

Another life-style factor may be linked to prostate cancer. A 1991 study of nearly 250,000 U.S. veterans found that cigarette smoking significantly increased the risk of prostate cancers. In all, heavy smokers had 50 percent more prostate cancer than nonsmokers.

I can't prove that a low-fat diet and smoking cessation will reduce your risk of prostate cancer — but they can't hurt. And, of course, they will provide many proven health benefits.

Can secondary prevention work for prostate cancer? It's much easier to treat early disease than advanced cancer. As usual, the key to secondary prevention is early detection by a screening test suitable for mass use. The acid phosphatase blood test can quantify advanced prostate cancer but cannot detect early disease, so it fails as a test. A newer blood test, the prostate-specific antigen (PSA), shows more promise but is not yet suitable as a mass screening test. Transrectal ultrasound tests are under study; still experimental, they appear most useful when combined with the PSA blood test. Even the PSA-ultrasound combination, however, leaves much to be desired. And so we are left with the old standby, an ordinary digital rectal exam.

Using the same accurate mathematics and sound logic as for testicular cancer, the U.S. Preventive Services Task Force points out that there is no proof that routine rectal exams will save lives. Using the same logic, I prefer not to wait for proof positive. In addition to checking the prostate, rectal exams screen for rectal cancer and bleeding. They are quick, only minimally uncomfortable, and free of side effects, and they do not add to the cost of a physical exam. I recommend an annual rectal for every man over 40.

■ Disorders Affecting Men and Women

Owing, no doubt, to the undiminished popularity of their mode of transmission, *sexually transmitted diseases* are on the rise in the United States. The figures are staggering: each year there are 3 million to 4 million chlamydial infections, 2 million cases of gonorrhea, 270,000 cases of genital herpes, and nearly 50,000 cases of syphilis. In addition to these classic venereal diseases, hepatitis B can be transmitted sexually as well as through blood and body fluids. These multiple routes of transmission apply also to the most terrible of all sexually transmitted diseases, AIDS.

The prevention of sexually transmitted diseases is medically easy (see chapter 16); we have not made much progress, unfortunately, because the behavioral changes that are needed have been difficult to achieve. As for so many diseases that plague us today, human behavior, not medical technology, is the key to prevention.

▪ 10 ▪
Disorders of the Kidneys and Urinary Tract

The kidneys are often thought of as very simple organs that rid the body of waste products. In actuality they are very complicated organs that rid the body of waste products — and do much, much more.

▪ The Kidneys in Health and Disease

Located deep behind the abdominal structures at the midportion of the back (see figure 10-1), the kidneys are first and foremost excretory organs. Blood enters the kidneys and is divided into small arteries which lead into tiny vascular tufts called *glomeruli*. Each of the 2.5 million glomeruli is a miniature filter; blood is returned to the veins, but the waste-containing urine is filtered off, passing next through a series of small tubules. In the tubules the composition of urine is fine-tuned to meet the body's needs. Most of the fluid is returned to the blood to prevent dehydration, and other chemicals are also returned to the circulation to maintain the body's balance of these elements.

During its passage through the tubules, the urine becomes progressively more concentrated. Eventually the tubules join together, and the waste-filled urine collects into the center of the kidneys, flowing next down long tubes called *ureters*. The ureters are passive conduits that simply carry the urine without adjusting its composition. This is true also of the next stop, the bladder, where the urine is collected and stored until it is expelled through the final tube, the *urethra*.

Urine contains waste products of the body's metabolism, including urea, creatinine, and acids. If kidney function fails, these toxins build up in the blood, producing uremic poisoning. The first job of the kidneys, then, is to excrete waste.

Each of us can attest to the fact that the rate of urine flow can vary widely. If you are dehydrated, urine forms slowly and is dark and concentrated because your kidneys return fluid to meet your body's needs. By contrast, if your fluid intake is abundant, urine is formed rapidly and is clear and dilute. Healthy kidneys, in fact, can function perfectly well while producing as little as two pints or as much as four gallons of urine a

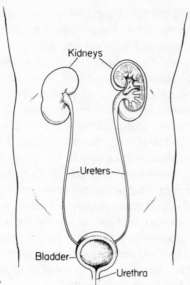

Figure 10-1.
Kidneys and bladder

day. The second job of the kidneys, then, is to regulate the body's fluid balance.

A third function is to regulate the composition of body fluids. Normal kidneys have an extraordinary ability to cope with huge variations in the amounts of sodium (salt) and potassium in the diet. If your diet is low in sodium (as it should be), your kidneys will avidly retain sodium so that your body will have all the salt it needs; if your diet is high in potassium (as it should be), your kidneys will be able to excrete any excess to prevent blood levels from becoming too high. The kidneys are unmatched in their ability to regulate minerals and acids; in this respect they are the best nutritionist your body could have.

The kidneys also have a major role in regulating blood pressure. For one thing, excreting excess salt and water helps keep blood pressure from rising. In addition, the kidney produces a hormone that helps control the constriction of arteries. But it's a two-way street: although healthy kidneys help keep blood pressure normal, diseased kidneys can produce hypertension. In addition, high blood pressure can damage kidneys, eventually leading to kidney failure in severe cases.

In addition to the hormone that controls blood pressure, the kidneys produce another hormone which stimulates the bone marrow to produce red blood cells. Diseased kidneys produce less of this hormone, which is why anemia is a universal feature of kidney failure.

Another task performed by healthy kidneys is the conversion of vitamin D into an active hormone which helps regulate calcium balance, maintaining bone strength. Patients with kidney failure often suffer bone disease caused by a lack of this hormone.

Excretory organs, yes. But the kidneys are also essential in regulating the body's fluid balance, chemical composition, and acid content. And, acting as hormone-producing endocrine glands, the kidneys also help regulate blood pressure, red blood cell production, and bone calcium content. In addition to being complex, all of these functions are vital to life.

To protect these indispensable functions, the body has endowed us with two kidneys. As is the case with other paired organs such as the lungs, there is safety in numbers; each kidney has more than enough glomeruli and tubules to maintain our health. Despite this tremendous reserve capacity, however, diseases of the kidney can damage and destroy these organs.

We have made spectacular progress in treating kidney disease: 90,000 Americans currently depend for their lives on dialysis by artificial kidneys, and another 10,000 undergo kidney transplants each year. These high-tech medical marvels have helped remove kidney failure, which was responsible for more deaths than cancer in 1900, from the list of leading killers. But these life-sustaining treatments come at a heavy price; patients and their families endure great physical and emotional burdens, and society contributes more than $2 billion each year. It is clear that preventing kidney disease is a high priority for American health.

■ Kidney Function, Aging, and Diet

Although each person is born with 2.5 million kidney units, or glomeruli, kidney function does not remain constant throughout life. Instead, our glomeruli begin to "drop out" at about age 40; this loss of functioning kidney units is a slow process, but it continues progressively throughout life. Because there is so much extra capacity to begin with, people who remain healthy will never notice the change. But blood and urine tests can detect a decline in kidney function with age. More important, this decreased function leaves the kidneys with much less reserve capacity to cope with disease.

Is declining kidney function an irreversible consequence of normal aging, or is it preventable?

Like you, I'm not getting any younger. Like you, I'd like to know the answer to this important question. Like you, I'll have to wait for the results of studies which are now in progress to be sure. But I can propose an interesting theory which may offer you a way to preserve kidney function throughout life.

The first body of evidence comes from animal experiments. Rats who are fed high-protein diets undergo changes in kidney structure and function. Kidney blood flow increases, as does the pressure behind that flow. Later, the glomeruli themselves enlarge. But in this case increased blood flow and structural enlargement is not a sign of health. Instead, if these animals continue to eat large amounts of protein, some of their glomeruli become scarred, and kidney function declines. Healthy rats can tolerate this decreased kidney function. But if other diseases are superimposed, animals who have been fed high-protein diets suffer an abnormally high rate of kidney failure.

The second body of evidence comes from observations of humans. We don't yet know if high dietary protein can damage healthy kidneys. But we do know that protein restriction slows the progression of advanced kidney disease; in fact, protein restriction is an important part of the medical management of patients with kidney failure. And a 1991 study from Dallas demonstrated that dietary protein restriction can retard the progression of kidney failure in diabetics.

We have all been taught to value high-protein foods. This sacred cow of nutrition dates back to the ancient Greeks, who believed that high-protein foods would build up high-protein tissues — muscles. Two millennia later this belief is still fundamental to the dietary habits of many competitive athletes. Popular belief notwithstanding, we know that extra protein will *not* produce either extra strength or better health; muscles do not benefit from high-protein diets, and kidneys may suffer over the years.

As the structural building blocks of all human tissues, proteins are of course essential for life. To maintain the body's tissues, protein is a vital part of the diet. But a muscular 150-pound man has only three pounds of protein in his body, and the average diet contains much more protein than is needed to maintain the body's balance. Healthy, active adults need only .36 grams of dietary protein per pound of body weight; for a 150-pound person this amounts to about two ounces of protein each day, the amount contained in two cups of cottage cheese, or four cups of beans, or nine ounces of fish or poultry. As a rule of thumb, you only need 15 percent of your daily caloric intake in the form of protein, or about 225 protein calories per day. Chapter 20 details the protein content of various foods, and also discusses the quality of dietary protein (see table 20-7).

Today's standard medical and nutritional advice holds that dietary protein in excess of the established requirements is wasteful but not harmful. I don't have facts to refute this wisdom, but I suspect that before too long excessive dietary protein may be implicated in the kidney dysfunction now attributed to aging. Until the proof is in, I'll hold my average protein intake to about 15 percent of calories. I'll lose nothing, and I can enjoy lots of carbohydrate-rich foods to make up the difference.

Some doctors may consider this recommendation premature, and indeed it may be. But it relies on a basic principle of prevention: for protein, as for so many other things, the fact that a little is essential for health does *not* necessarily mean that more is better.

■ Vascular Disease and the Kidney

We are not sure if dietary protein can harm healthy kidneys. In contrast, it *is* clear that excessive dietary salt and animal fat can contribute to kidney disease — not by directly damaging the kidneys but by increasing the risk of high blood pressure and atherosclerosis.

High blood pressure is extremely dangerous to the kidneys. In the days before medications to control blood pressure were available, hypertension was a leading cause of kidney failure. Cases of acute kidney failure caused by abrupt, severe hypertension (aptly called malignant hypertension) are now rare. But hypertension is still a major cause of chronic kidney failure. To protect your kidneys, to say nothing of your heart and brain, follow the blood pressure program detailed in chapter 3.

Like all arteries, the kidney's vessels are vulnerable to atherosclerosis. One way to prevent cholesterol deposits from damaging your kidneys is to keep your blood pressure down. Equally important are smoking cessation, cholesterol control, and regular aerobic exercise. If you need a refresher, return to chapter 2; all your blood vessels will thank you for getting it right.

■ Kidney and Bladder Cancer

Like the lungs and the stomach, the kidneys are internal organs which encounter more than their share of toxins from the outside world. The lungs and stomach meet these toxins on their way into the body as contaminants in air, water, and food. Because of its role in excreting toxins, the kidney encounters these toxins on their way out of the body; the bladder's potential exposure is even greater since it stores urine for hours. It's not surprising, therefore, that toxins contribute to many urinary tract diseases, including cancer.

Twenty-three thousand cases of kidney cancer are diagnosed in the United States each year, and 10,000 people die from this malignancy. Twice as common in men as in women, kidney cancer peaks at age 60. The most common symptoms are bloody urine, flank pain, or an abdominal mass. Once the disease is suspected, diagnosis is usually straightforward, depending on x rays, ultrasound examinations, or CAT scans, and examination of the urine for cancer cells. But cancer of the kidney can produce unusual symptoms ranging from fever to elevated red blood cell counts to hormonal abnormalities; diagnosis can be very tricky in these cases.

Instead of challenging your doctor with unusual symptoms, do what you can to prevent kidney cancer. The most important step may surprise you: don't smoke. It may seem a long way from the lungs to the kidneys. Remember, though, that toxic chemicals in smoke enter the blood and circulate through the whole body; the kidneys do their best to excrete the toxins, but in doing so they may suffer damage that can eventually lead to cancer. In the same way, kidney cancer is more common in workers with occupational exposure to asbestos or cadmium.

Much the same scenario applies to bladder cancer. Although it's twice as common as kidney cancer, bladder cancer causes only the same number of deaths because treatment is more successful. Like kidney cancer, bladder cancer occurs most often in older men. Bloody urine and frequent or painful urination are the typical symptoms. Diagnosis is readily accomplished by urologists, who can use instruments called cystoscopes to look directly into the bladder. Early diagnosis is very important, since small bladder cancers can be cured with simple cystoscopic treatments, but more advanced tumors may require surgery, chemotherapy, or even complete removal of the bladder.

Tactics to prevent bladder cancer involve some facts and some theories. The key fact is that cigarette smoking triples the risk of bladder cancer. The disease is much more common in industrialized countries (especially Sweden), suggesting that environmental factors play a causal role. Those factors have not yet been identified, but occupational exposures are responsible for an excess risk of bladder cancer in aniline-dye, rubber, textile, and leather-finishing workers. Prolonged, excessive use of phenacetin can also lead to bladder cancer; fortunately, this drug, once included in many over-the-counter painkilling medications, is no longer available.

Those are the facts. There are also some theories about preventing bladder cancer; all three involve diet. First, there is some evidence that vitamin A may reduce the risk of bladder cancer. You don't need vitamin supplements to get enough vitamin A, but lots of deep green and yellow veggies are a good idea.

The second theory involves artificial sweeteners. Large doses of cyclamates have been linked to bladder cancer in experimental animals. Although there was no evidence that cyclamates caused human disease, the Food and Drug Administration acted prudently and withdrew the product. New data, however, may soon restore cyclamates to the market; in the meanwhile, America's artificial sweet tooth is being satisfied by aspartame. Although some consumer groups are concerned that history will repeat itself again, aspartame appears safe for the bladders of both mice and men. Still, except for diabetics, there is little to recommend aspartame for health. If you choose to use aspartame, just let moderation be your guide.

The final theory of bladder cancer prevention is the simplest but the most conjectural. If toxins cause this cancer, diluting the urine by drinking lots of water may reduce risk. A reasonable but unproven approach. Try it if you like, but don't float away; two or three quarts of water each day should be more than enough. Be sure, though, that your drinking water is safe; chapter 22 will tell you how.

■ Toxic Chemicals

Some chemicals that injure the urinary tract cause cancer; others damage kidney function. Less dramatic, perhaps, but advanced kidney failure can be just as debilitating and deadly as cancer. Although not a common problem, toxin-induced kidney dysfunction is entirely preventable. Avoid unnecessary exposure to toxic chemicals; metals such as lead, mercury, chromium, cadmium, and gold head the list of kidney toxins. Volatile hydrocarbons such as carbon tetrachloride and trichlorethylene can also cause kidney disease. Workers with industrial exposure are the only people likely to have problems with these compounds; chapter 17 outlines prevention through the principles of occupational health.

■ Medications and the Kidneys

All physicians should pause, at least briefly, and think about the kidneys before signing their prescriptions. Many medications can interfere with kidney function; while these side effects are usually mild and temporary, they can sometimes be severe and permanent. Even drugs that are themselves safe for the kidneys can require some thought because they may accumulate to dangerous levels in patients with kidney diseases that reduce the excretion of drugs.

Your doctors and pharmacists are responsible for protecting your kidneys from their drugs. But even in the age of computerized drugstores, your health care providers can use your help. If you have kidney disease or if medications have caused problems in the past, remind your doctor about these events before you start a new medication.

Not all the responsibility for preventing drug-induced kidney damage belongs to your doctor; nonprescription drugs can also harm your kidneys. Americans spend more than $1 billion annually on painkillers, at least one quarter of which is used to purchase acetaminophen. Long considered safe for our kidneys, acetaminophen generated new concerns in a 1989 study from North Carolina. While confirming that ordinary use of this drug is indeed safe, the study reported that long-term, high-dose, daily use of acetaminophen was linked to chronic kidney dysfunction. I cannot tell you how much acetaminophen you can use before you start to run a risk of kidney damage, but you should not simply treat yourself with daily painkillers. Instead, discuss both the problem and its treatment with your doctor.

In addition, you should take all over-the-counter medications seriously, reading the package inserts, and following the directions carefully. If you have kidney disease, be even more cautious about all medications. Always listen to your body for possible side effects; if possible symptoms develop, discuss them with your doctor or pharmacist, stopping the medicine in the interim. Above all, remember that when it comes to self-medication, *less* is generally *better*.

Exactly the same advice applies to ibuprofen, another over-the-counter medication that can affect the kidneys. Ibuprofen is a valuable drug belonging to the family of nonsteroidal anti-inflammatory agents. Aspirin is the oldest member of this family; because these drugs are so useful for treating fever, inflammation, and pain, no fewer than a dozen similar medications are now available. Apart from aspirin, however, ibuprofen is the only one that can be purchased without a prescription.

Doctors have long known that virtually all nonsteroidal anti-inflammatory drugs can impair kidney function. But a 1990 medical study of 12 patients who experienced reversible kidney dysfunction due to ibuprofen received widespread publicity in the popular media, raising public concerns about the safety of the drug. Kidney dysfunction is a legitimate concern, but this side effect is seen almost exclusively in elderly people, especially those who already have kidney disease. In the great majority of cases, blood tests return to normal promptly after the medication is stopped.

Occasional use of ibuprofen is safe for your kidneys; in fact, stomach irritation is a much more likely side effect. But if you are over 65 and use ibuprofen on a daily basis, you should check with your doctor, asking for periodic monitoring of your kidney function. Working together, you can get the benefits of ibuprofen while preventing its side effects.

■ Kidney Stones

Unless you belong to a family with a high rate of kidney stones, you don't have to spend much time thinking about stone disease. Although kidney stones are among the many diseases related to the Western life-style, your lifetime chance of developing a kidney stone is only 2 in 100. But if you are one of the unlucky people who develop a stone, do spend some time thinking about prevention; without it your chances of forming another stone are 15 percent within one year, 35 percent within five years, and 50 percent within ten years.

Kidney stones are formed when certain chemicals in the urine become too concentrated; instead of staying dissolved, these substances precipitate, producing crystals that gradually enlarge to form gravel and then stones. There are many types of kidney stones; specific dietary restrictions can help reduce each by decreasing the chemicals excreted in the urine. But one dietary factor can help prevent all types of stones. You won't need a calculator or food chart to figure out this one: it's water. By drinking copiously, you will keep your urine dilute, enabling minerals to stay where they belong, in solution. In the absence of other medical conditions that require fluid restriction, all stone formers should drink enough water so that their urine output is at least three quarts per day. Taking in all this water is harder than it sounds. To do it, keep a pitcher of water on your desk at work and on your table at home — and empty it early and often. Never pass a water cooler without sampling its contents. Drink a tall glass of water at bedtime — and another when you wake up to urinate. If there is any question about how much you are drinking, just measure your urine volume to be sure it's adequate; your doctor can also give you a simple device to test your urine to be sure it's dilute enough.

Two thirds of all kidney stones are composed of calcium in the form of calcium oxalate. In addition to increasing your water intake, the logical preventive measure is to decrease your calcium intake. Indeed, most patients with calcium stones respond very well to the substitution of water for milk and the avoidance of other dairy products. Because dietary protein increases urinary calcium, avoiding excess protein may also help. But even with the best of diets, some patients continue to excrete excessive amounts of calcium. If you continue to have stones, your doctor should check your urine calcium levels; if they remain high, preventive medications such as a thiazide diuretic or allopurinol should be considered.

Another common type of stone is composed of uric acid, the same chemical that causes gout. Dietary restrictions won't do much to reduce uric acid excretion, but sodium bicarbonate can help by reducing urine acidity, thus keeping uric acid in a harmless, soluble form. If water and bicarb don't do the trick, your doctor may choose to prescribe allopurinol, which prevents the body from producing uric acid.

■ Urinary Tract Infections

Urinary tract infections are so common that they've earned their own medical shorthand; in the era of rapid medicine we treat not urinary tract infections but UTIs.

Infections can strike any portion of the urinary tract, from top to bottom. In actuality, most infections start at the bottom, where bacteria can enter the urethra and bladder. Infections that remain confined to these lower portions of the urinary tract can be very uncomfortable, but they are rarely serious. Infections that ascend the ureters to involve the kidneys, however, can be very serious indeed. It's important, then, to prevent bacteria from entering the bladder; failing that, it's important to prevent them from reaching the kidneys.

Infection of the bladder is perhaps the most common of all bacterial infections, accounting for 6 million office visits in the United States each year. Lower urinary tract infections, called cystitis, produce burning and pain on urination as well as urinary urgency and frequency. Fever is usually absent or low grade. The urine may be clear, malodorous, cloudy, or even bloody. Microscopic evaluation of the urine disclosing pus cells, and urine cultures yielding bacteria, are the simple but effective ways to diagnose cystitis. Nine times in ten, the bacterium responsible is *E. coli.*

Cystitis is principally an infection of women, who are 50 times more likely to develop it than are men because the much shorter female urethra allows bacteria to creep up into the bladder. Bacterial ascent is greatly facilitated by sexual intercourse. Cystitis is not a communicable or sexually transmitted disease, but the pressure generated by sexual intercourse can force bacteria from the vagina, where they are harmless, up into the urethra and bladder. Other risk factors for cystitis include the use of a diaphragm with spermicidal jelly or the use of spermicidal foam with condoms. At the other extreme pregnancy, too, increases the risk of cystitis. In men, enlargement of the prostate is the usual culprit. Finally, diabetes has been linked to urinary tract infections in both men and women.

Because women are so often troubled by cystitis, they have evolved a series of preventive strategies. Many of my patients tell me that they've changed from tub baths to showers, from nylon undergarments to cotton, and from orange juice to cranberry juice in an effort to prevent cystitis. They often adopt the practice of wiping from front to back after bowel movements and urination. I have no idea if these folk remedies are helpful because they've not been scrutinized scientifically. In fact, I've often scoffed at one of them, demonstrating to my microbiology students that bacteria can grow happily in urine that contains cranberry juice. In 1991, however, scientists from Israel found another way to look at the question.

They agreed that cranberry juice won't kill bacteria in urine, but they found that it contains a chemical that prevents germs from sticking to the bladder wall, an essential step in producing cystitis. Score one for popular wisdom — and for the scientists who took a fresh look at an old custom.

Several other traditional stratagems may help prevent cystitis. Although their merits have not been proven scientifically, I recommend them to my patients and to you. Drink lots of water to keep your urine dilute. Empty your bladder frequently instead of holding your urine. Urinate before and after sexual intercourse — then drink more water to keep your urine flow high. Finally, if you use a diaphragm, consider switching to another means of contraception — or, at the very least, don't leave your diaphragm in place any longer than necessary.

If primary prevention, whether using patients' tactics or mine, fails, secondary prevention can help. The first priority is adequate treatment of the initial cystitis; although kidney infection can be difficult to treat, bladder infections respond beautifully to antibiotic programs as short as one dose or as long as one week. But without prevention, recurrent infections are very likely. Antibiotics can help, but they should be reserved for women who've had multiple episodes. Low doses of certain antibiotics can be given at bedtime every night to prevent recurrent cystitis. Another very effective way to prevent "honeymoon cystitis" is to take these medications immediately after intercourse. Finally, women who are not happy about taking antibiotics when they feel well may be happy to have a prescription for self-treatment at the first sign of the characteristic symptoms of cystitis.

Unfortunately, self-diagnosis and treatment have no place in the management of kidney infections or pyelonephritis. Bacteria that invade the upper urinary tract cause potentially serious infections; fever, flank pain, weakness, and nausea are usually even more prominent than urinary symptoms. And if bacteria get from the kidney into the blood stream, much more severe problems can result, including shock and even death.

Though much more serious than bladder infections, kidney infections are much less common. Still, about 300,000 people each year are treated for pyelonephritis. But patients with kidney infections are quite different from patients with cystitis. Much older, they belong to both sexes about equally. In addition, unlike the healthy young women who get cystitis, many patients with kidney infections have underlying medical conditions. In fact, a large number of those infections occur as complications of hospitalizations and medical treatments. Your doctor will have to take the lead in preventing these infections by using urinary catheters as little as possible, and by caring for them meticulously when they are unavoidable.

■ Screening and Secondary Prevention: The Urine Analysis

There are two ways to screen asymptomatic people for disorders of the kidneys and urinary tract. Blood tests (the BUN and creatinine tests) can be used to evaluate kidney function. Although they are not required at every physical exam, it is reasonable to check these tests periodically. As a practical matter I often check them at the same time that I send blood to the lab for cholesterol determinations. But patients who have high blood pressure or diabetes should be tested more often, as should patients taking medications that can affect the kidneys.

An even simpler way to screen for urinary tract disorders is by analyzing a urine specimen. Until recently a routine urine analysis involved a series of chemical tests and a microscopic examination. Though simple enough to be done by a medical student (however grumpily), these techniques have been largely replaced by an even easier screening test. A single dipstick can be used to screen for the presence of protein (seen in many kidney diseases), glucose (diabetes), white blood cells (infections), and red blood cells (infections, tumors). Costing only a few dollars, these tests are rapid and accurate.

Despite these advantages, there is currently a lively debate about how often routine urine testing should be performed. On one side of the debate are doctors who point out that because asymptomatic urinary tract disorders are uncommon, the great majority of routine urine tests are normal. Moreover, even though they are inexpensive individually, collectively they add $150 million to the nation's annual health care bill. Proponents of testing point to occasional patients who have benefited from early detection and treatment because of screening.

I suggest compromise. Routine urine analyses seem most useful for preschool children, pregnant women, and people over 60 — all of whom are at increased risk of silent, still treatable urinary tract disorders. Because of the increased risk of bladder cancer, I also perform routine urine analyses on all of my patients who defy reason by smoking. Finally, I like to check urine specimens at the time of a college entry or sports participation physical.

Most patients have come to expect a urine analysis at the time of each and every complete physical exam. The presence of urinary tract symptoms is a sure reason to have one performed. In the absence of symptoms, I regard this test as optional — medically unnecessary but often personally reassuring.

Above all, don't get too preoccupied with the issue. While not exactly a tempest in a teapot, the urine analysis brouhaha is not far from it.

Diseases of the Blood
and Immune System

In the first ten chapters of this book, I have repeatedly referred to the blood as a transport system that carries oxygen and nutrients to the tissues while removing carbon dioxide and wastes for disposal by the lungs, liver, and kidneys. The blood does all this, and very much more; far from being simply a passive transport mechanism, the blood is a complex network with many important functions.

■ The Normal Blood

The average adult has five to six quarts of blood, which is about 60 percent fluid and 40 percent cells. The fluid, or *plasma*, looks watery, and it is mostly water. But it also contains vital chemicals including sugar, calcium, sodium, and potassium. In addition, the plasma contains many proteins that are no less essential for health, including albumin, which prevents fluid from seeping into the tissues, clotting proteins, and the gamma globulins of the immune system. Nutrients, hormones, and even medications are carried in the blood plasma, partially transported in the water phase itself and partially bound to proteins. To keep your plasma healthy, you need enough water to prevent dehydration. Needed, too, are good nutrition and a healthy liver to maintain the proteins.

Three types of blood cells are present in the circulation. By far the most numerous are the *red blood cells*, well named because they contain hemoglobin, which looks bright red when it's carrying oxygen from the lungs to the tissues. Red blood cells are manufactured in the bone marrow; they survive for two months in the blood before being removed by the spleen, so the bone marrow must constantly produce new cells to maintain a normal count, preventing anemia.

The smallest blood cells are the *platelets*. Made in the bone marrow, platelets are actually small cell fragments. Small or not, they have a big job: they are crucial for the normal clotting of blood. Because they survive only days in the blood, the marrow must constantly deliver new platelets to the circulation.

The third type of blood cells are the *white blood cells*. There are actually three types of white cells. *Polys,* the most numerous, are the first line of defense against infection; they rapidly home in on bacteria that penetrate into the body and, if all goes well, gobble up and digest the germs to keep you healthy. *Monocytes* complement polys by killing certain dangerous microbes that evade polys. *Lymphocytes* are the key cells in the immune system; they recognize infectious agents and tumor cells, and they coordinate the fight against microbes and cancer. One group of lymphocytes, called B cells, are responsible for making antibodies, the gamma globulin proteins that are essential to fight infection. The other lymphocytes, T cells, are responsible for coordinating the entire immune system. One variety, helper or CD4+ cells (the cells destroyed by the AIDS virus), boost immunity; another, suppressor or CD8+ cells, prevent the immune response from becoming overstimulated.

■ Anemia

Anemia is simply a decrease in the number of red blood cells in the circulation. Although most people think of anemia as a single disease, it's actually a general term that applies to many diverse disorders. Anemia can result from insufficient production of red blood cells in the bone marrow, from premature destruction of red blood cells within the body, or from loss of red cells through internal or external bleeding. In many cases anemia is a secondary phenomenon, occurring as a reaction to diseases of various organ systems; in others the anemia is itself the primary problem.

Among the numerous causes of anemia, many are uncommon, some rare, and others downright exotic. But one group of anemias is common — and preventable. In these disorders the bone marrow can't produce enough red blood cells because it lacks the nutrients it needs to keep its blood cell factory working. Iron deficiency is far and away the most common of these nutritional anemias; in occasional patients deficiencies of vitamin B_{12} or of folic acid can also be involved.

Iron-Deficiency Anemia

Iron is essential for the structure and function of hemoglobin, the pigmented protein that gives red blood cells their color and, more important, carries oxygen to the tissues. Iron is absorbed from food by the intestinal tract; next it's carried in the blood to the bone marrow, where it is stored until it's used to make hemoglobin for red blood cells. After red blood cells finish their two months of life in the circulation, their iron is reclaimed and returned to the bone marrow for reuse in new red cells. This elaborate recycling mechanism shows that iron is indeed a valuable commodity.

Despite the importance of iron, the body doesn't store very much of it. The average adult has only 4 grams of iron, about the weight of a five-cent coin. Some iron is lost every day in sweat, sloughed skin cells, and intestinal wastes, but this totals only a very small amount, averaging about 1 milligram per day. People who take aspirin tend to lose iron into the intestinal tract; even the low-dose, every-other-day schedule I've recommended to prevent heart disease can triple the usual iron losses. Some athletes, particularly long-distance runners, may also lose iron at a faster than normal pace. A much more significant route of iron loss is ordinary menstrual bleeding. Most women lose much less blood than they imagine, amounting to three or four ounces a month; still, this equals an average iron loss of 1 milligram per day.

Since iron is lost from the body, it must be replaced to prevent anemia. Since the losses are slow and small, it doesn't take much iron to keep the body in balance. The only exception is in menstruating women — which is why 9 percent of young American women are anemic. Because pregnant women must supply iron to their babies, pregnancy is particularly likely to produce anemia. Very young children may also develop mild anemia from a lack of dietary iron. In contrast, iron-deficiency anemia occurs in less than 1 percent of American men; men who are anemic should always be investigated for hidden causes of blood loss, particularly stomach ulcers and intestinal tumors.

Most people with mild iron deficiencies don't even know they are anemic, but blood tests will show that their red blood cells are smaller, paler, and fewer than normal, and that their blood iron levels are low. If the anemia becomes more severe, however, it will produce pallor, fatigue, cold feelings, lack of energy, and even shortness of breath during exercise.

Patients who are anemic should have simple tests to be sure that iron deficiency is the cause. If so, the need for further studies depends on the circumstances; women with mild to moderate iron deficiency don't require additional testing, but men should always be evaluated for abnormal bleeding.

Iron deficiency is quite easy to correct with iron supplements in pill or liquid form. While safe and inexpensive, iron therapy can cause intestinal upsets. The best plan of all is to prevent iron deficiency from occurring in the first place.

To prevent anemia, the diet must replace enough iron to keep the body in balance. Since even menstruating women lose only 2 milligrams of iron per day, you'd think that your nutritional requirements should be equally small. They're not. The reason: iron absorption is inefficient, ranging from 5 percent (when the iron is in grain products) to 35 percent (when the iron is in animal tissues in the form of hemoglobin). Vitamin C improves iron absorption, but tea and coffee reduce it. Because of this inefficiency, men should take in 10 milligrams of iron per day, women 50 percent more.

The average American diet contains 6 milligrams of iron per 1,000 calories — more than enough to prevent anemia. Paradoxically, however, the healthiest diets are often the lowest in iron; red meat, while the best source of iron, contains saturated fats and cholesterol that can contribute to atherosclerosis. Fortunately, fish and poultry also contain iron, as do deep green vegetables, beans, and peanuts (see table 20-12). In addition, for the past 50 years Food and Drug Administration regulations have mandated the addition of small amounts of iron to flour, cereals, and grain products, which is why they are described on the label as "fortified." Infant cereals and formulas are also fortified with iron. A nice example of successful public policy, iron fortification has substantially reduced the prevalence of anemia in our country.

A well-balanced diet should provide all the iron you need; chapter 20 details the iron contents of representative foods, so you can see for yourself. Iron supplements may be prudent for pregnant women, breast-fed infants, and certain other people. In particular, women with heavy menstrual periods may need extra iron to prevent anemia, particularly if they eat little red meat.

Iron tablets are available without prescription. The two most popular preparations, ferrous sulfate and ferrous gluconate, are equally effective. The usual practice is to take three capsules a day, each containing 300 milligrams of iron, before meals for about two months. Iron is also available in combination with vitamins, in sustained-release capsules, and in liquid form.

Short-term administration of iron, even in these large doses, is safe; many patients complain of mild intestinal upset, but this can usually be alleviated by building up the dose slowly or by using a liquid preparation. Long-term administration of iron, however, can cause harmful tissue excesses. Moreover, treating anemia without diagnosing its underlying cause may produce a dangerous delay in detecting a treatable disease.

Because of these reasons I caution you against self-diagnosis and treatment, even with over-the-counter iron tablets. Prevent iron deficiency with a balanced, healthful diet. Have your blood count measured during your periodic checkups. If you feel well, it's not necessary to have any extra checks for anemia. But if you have symptoms that suggest anemia, don't simply treat yourself; instead, get a checkup to determine the diagnosis and plan its treatment.

Vitamin-Deficiency Anemias

Two vitamins are also vital for red blood cell production. Deficiencies of either can cause anemia. Except in certain population groups, however, such deficiencies are rare.

Vitamin B_{12} (cobalamin) is present in all animal tissues. The recommended daily allowance of B_{12} is only 6 micrograms, and lots of the vitamin is stored in your liver to carry you over fallow periods. Nutritional lack of vitamin B_{12} is very rare, except in *strict* vegetarians, who should take supplementary doses to prevent anemia. But the stomach and intestines must be intact to absorb vitamin B_{12}; patients with pernicious anemia require B_{12} injections, as do some patients who've had intestinal diseases or surgery. While these circumstances are uncommon, they must be treated properly, since B_{12} deficiency causes neurological and psychological symptoms in addition to anemia.

Over the years many doctors have administered B_{12} shots to treat fatigue, infections, impotence, depression, and many other conditions. In addition, countless people have taken B_{12} supplements in tablet form. The only effect of "therapeutic" B_{12} is disappointment. You need only a well-balanced diet to prevent B_{12} deficiency anemia. Cases of pernicious anemia should be detected by routine medical screening.

Folic acid is also required for red blood cell production. It is present in green vegetables, legumes, fruits, grains, meat, and other foods. The daily requirement of folic acid is only 200 micrograms. Except in alcoholics and other malnourished individuals, deficiencies of folic acid are rare. Patients taking certain antiseizure medications may also need extra doses of folic acid. With these exceptions, the only thing you need to prevent folic acid–deficiency anemia is a healthful diet. And I'm happy to say that for this blood-building nutrient, veggies will do the job beautifully.

Sickle Cell Anemia

Prevention is most effective when applied to diseases that we bring on ourselves. In a very real sense, the major strategy for preventing these diseases of self-abuse is simply a return to the basics — a modern re-creation of the life-style our bodies were designed for. If we are born healthy, we can remain healthy simply by living naturally.

Sickle cell anemia is different. It's a genetic disease, inherited from previous generations. Children with sickle cell anemia are born *un*healthy; even with the best treatment they are destined to suffer through many episodes of pain, infection, and weakness, and to die well before their time.

Can sickle cell anemia be prevented? Not in the usual sense, although spectacular advances in molecular biology are bringing genetic therapy from the realm of fantasy to the threshold of possibility. But we don't have to wait for the twenty-first century to prevent suffering from sickle cell anemia. Even though we cannot yet replace defective genes, we can detect them and provide reproductive counseling to prevent disease.

Carriers of the sickle cell gene can be diagnosed with a simple blood test called a hemoglobin electrophoresis. Before they have children, they can learn if their spouse also has the gene. If so, they may still choose to have children; the odds are that three out of four children will be healthy, though two will carry the sickle cell gene. But one child in four will have the disease, still a terrible risk. Fortunately, prevention can help here as well. A pregnant woman who is at risk can choose to undergo an amniocentesis, permitting an accurate prenatal diagnosis of sickle cell anemia and allowing an informed parental choice about the pregnancy.

Sickle cell anemia is a serious problem in America; about 2 million people are carriers, and 50,000 have the disease. But the sickle cell gene is not distributed uniformly throughout society; instead, it is most common in blacks. Eight to 10 percent of Afro-Americans carry the gene; one of every 150 black couples is at risk of giving birth to a child with sickle cell anemia. There are 3,000 such pregnancies in the United States each year, and one of every 625 black infants born here has the disease.

Sickle cell anemia can be prevented. Genetic screening and counseling are the key. Screening could be accomplished at several stages of life. It could be performed at birth, either on all babies or just on those at risk. Testing could also be performed in early adolescence, before the start of reproductive behavior. Finally, even early pregnancy is not too late for sickle cell screening to prevent disease.

It's unfortunate that many people who are at risk are not being tested. We need a public education campaign to close this gap. As in so many other areas, knowledge is the essential element in preventing disease.

Thalassemia

Thalassemia is an uncommon but serious hereditary anemia. The carrier state is present in 1 to 2 percent of Afro-Americans, 3 to 4 percent of Italian-Americans, 2 percent of Greek-Americans, and 3 to 9 percent of Southeast Asian Americans. Whereas these low frequencies may not justify universal screening, I do recommend a simple hemoglobin electrophoresis screening test for members of these ethnic groups.

■ Toxins

The bone marrow, like most body tissues, is susceptible to harm from chemicals and toxins in the blood. But the bone marrow is unique in its vulnerability. In order to produce the requisite supply of red blood cells, white blood cells, and platelets, precursor cells in the bone marrow must continuously divide and multiply, giving rise to daughter cells that mature in the marrow before entering the circulation. Rapidly dividing cells are particularly susceptible to certain toxins, so the bone marrow is at high risk for chemical- and radiation-induced injury.

The bone marrow can respond to toxins in only two ways. Most often cell division slows or stops. The result is a fall in the number of circulating red blood cells, white blood cells, or platelets. Fortunately, such toxic marrow suppression is usually mild and temporary; when severe, however, it can be lethal. The other bone marrow response to toxic injury is to increase the rate of cell division; if cell division becomes uncontrolled and self-perpetuating, the result is a life-threatening situation — leukemia.

The most widespread bone marrow toxin in the United States is *lead*. Prolonged exposure to lead can produce anemia or neurological abnormalities; kidney damage is less common. About 2 percent of all Americans have elevated blood lead levels. Toxic levels above 10 micrograms per milliliter are found most often in children between the ages of six months and five years; more than 6 million are affected. Permanent intellectual impairment can be a tragic result of childhood lead toxicity.

The key source of lead is paint, usually found in dilapidated houses built before 1950. Plaster, dust, and dirt in these homes become contaminated with lead; young children who ingest this material can build up toxic lead levels. Children living in poor urban areas are at greatest risk; in some communities more than 20 percent of children have toxic lead levels.

We've taken the lead out of new paint, but we've not taken our children away from old paint. Until we do, children at risk should be screened for lead toxicity by checking their blood levels even before anemia develops. Children who live in or frequently visit dilapidated housing should have this simple blood test once a year between the ages of nine months and six years; so, too, should children who live near busy highways or lead-processing plants. Adults with occupational lead exposure should also be screened. Drinking water can also be a source of excess lead; chapter 22 will tell you how to be sure your water is safe. Finally, certain food containers may subject you to excess lead (for details, see chapter 20). Even with screening, blood tests, and precautions for food and water, true prevention of lead toxicity must await improved social and economic conditions that will end exposure.

Many industrial chemicals are also toxic to blood cells; protect yourself by avoiding *cadmium, mercury, hydrocarbons*, and *benzene*. It's just as important for you to avoid voluntary self-exposure to other chemicals that can injure your bone marrow, including *alcohol* and *tobacco smoke*.

Small doses of alcohol don't affect the bone marrow, but large doses will produce anemia; the marrow will recover from alcohol — if the drinking stops. Although smoking doesn't produce anemia, it's hardly safe for the blood. In fact, smoking can cause an *over*production of red blood cells, resulting in excessively viscous or "thick" blood that may contribute to strokes, heart attacks, and other vascular blockages. Smoking has also been linked to leukemia and myeloma, dreadful diseases resulting from malignant overproduction of white blood cells.

■ Leukemia and Lymphoma

Leukemia is a malignant proliferation of white blood cells in the bone marrow. Lymphoma is a malignant proliferation of white blood cells in the lymph nodes, spleen, or bone marrow. There are many varieties of leukemia and lymphoma. All are serious, killing more than 30,000 Americans annually, but all are treatable, and some curable. Few are well enough understood to allow effective primary prevention.

External factors are probably responsible for many of these malignancies; exposure to benzene and to radioactivity are among the well-documented toxic causes of leukemia and lymphoma. Viral infections can also produce these disorders; the AIDS virus is one that can be prevented. Finally, some of the powerful drugs that are so beneficial to cancer and organ transplant patients have a most unfortunate propensity to increase the likelihood of leukemia or lymphoma years after treatment.

Most cases of leukemia and lymphoma occur in patients who don't have any known risk factors. Some of these cases are clustered in geographic areas or family groups. Intensive research will be needed to discover the

causes of these terrible illnesses so that we can make progress in prevention as well as treatment.

■ A Word about Blood Transfusion

Blood transfusion represented a historic advance in medical therapeutics.
The many benefits of transfusions were apparent immediately; indeed, the
lives saved by transfusions are quite literally numberless. As in so many
areas of medicine, however, the risks of transfusions have been recognized
more slowly than the benefits. In some cases, unfortunately, the results of
transfusion treatments have been worse than the diseases being treated.

Having acknowledged the potential hazards of blood transfusions, let
me assure you that the *vast* majority of them are entirely safe. Don't take a
transfusion unless you absolutely need it; but if you do need transfusions,
remember that the numbers are on your side. About 10 million pints of
blood are transfused in the United States each year. Only a small fraction
of this large number results in immediate problems, including perhaps
2,000 allergic reactions and a similar number of fluid overload cases. Blood
banks do a wonderful job of reducing the risks of allergic reactions by meticulously matching the donor's and the recipient's blood. Doctors have
learned to use transfusions only when absolutely necessary and to give the
smallest possible amount to prevent fluid overload.

The major worry about transfusions is, of course, infection. This risk,
too, has been minimized by screening donors and by testing blood before
it's used. Testing has virtually eliminated the risk of syphilis, hepatitis B,
and — as of 1990 — hepatitis C. Testing has also greatly reduced the risk of
acquiring AIDS from blood transfusions; even in American urban areas
at the center of the AIDS epidemic, the risk is no greater than one chance
for every 51,000 transfusions, and may well be as low as one per 300,000
transfusions.

A final word about transfusions. Old Polonius got it only half right when
he cautioned Laertes in *Hamlet* "Neither a borrower nor a lender be." Do
your best to stay healthy so you won't have to become a blood borrower.
But if you are healthy, think seriously about becoming a blood lender.
Fewer than 5 percent of eligible Americans donate blood. Donation is extremely safe; you'll have your blood pressure and hemoglobin checked be-
forehand, and you'll be rewarded afterward with a snack. Much more important, you'll know that you've helped a fellow being in need.

■ Disorders of the Immune System

Excessive activity of the immune system can cause disease by turning
against healthy body tissues, causing inflammation.

Disorders of immunological deficiency are even more dramatic, often
resulting in life-threatening infections and malignancies. Unfortunately,

only one major immunological abnormality can be prevented, but it is one of the most severe: AIDS (see chapter 16).

■ Immunological Myths and Realities

Although AIDS is the only immunological disorder that can be prevented, popular lore holds that the immune system can be affected, for good or ill, by three personal interventions: diet, mental activity, and exercise. There is some truth to each of these claims, but there is also much misinformation. Let's examine these three beliefs about the immune system to see what is fact and what is fantasy.

Myth number one: Your diet can boost your immune system.

Nutrition is, of course, crucial for health; people who assert that you are what you eat are not far off the mark. But not all the body's systems are equally affected by nutrition. Is it true that you can eat your way to immunological health?

Unfortunately, no. But it is easy to see how this myth got started, since its converse *is* true: malnutrition does impair immunity and increase susceptibility to infection. The catastrophic epidemics that decimated humanity over the centuries, including plague, smallpox, tuberculosis, dysentery, and typhus, flourished in times of famine and war. Indeed, for the 10,000-year span of the agricultural era, infectious diseases were the major human killers. Undernutrition (as well as crowding and poor hygiene) played a big role in allowing those infections to spread. Infectious epidemics decreased dramatically when humanity progressed from the agricultural to the industrial era, owing in part to improved nutrition. Paradoxically, we are now vulnerable to diseases caused by *over*nutrition, including coronary heart disease, high blood pressure, diabetes, obesity, and some cancers. But immunological and infectious diseases are not among those contemporary diseases of bodily abuse, disuse, and nutritional excess.

Even in the United States today, malnourished people are at increased risk of infection. This is a particular problem for people who have serious illnesses that produce weight loss and wasting. Elsewhere in the world malnutrition is still a major cause of defective immunity and excessive infection; the terrible measles susceptibility of Third World children who are low in vitamin A is but one example. Good nutrition boosts the immune systems of all sick patients. But for healthy people, neither diet nor nutritional supplements can add to the healthy body's immune power.

I hope you're not confused by conflicting opinions about diet, immunity, and infection. Although the facts are now clear, controversy persists from the old days. More than 100 years ago Henry David Thoreau gave voice to the debate: "There are sure to be two prescriptions, dramatically opposite. Stuff a cold and starve a cold are but two ways."

Myth number two: Mental stress can impair immunity, but mental power can be harnessed to boost immunity and fight disease, including cancer.

Although I've labeled this a myth, I think there is something to it. The problem is that we don't yet know just how much of the speculation is accurate. A brand-new field, psychoneuroimmunology, is starting to study the interactions between the mind, the nervous system, and the immune system. It has already been shown in laboratory animals, and to a lesser extent in humans, that mental factors can affect immune cells. But it's not yet clear if these changes are functionally important.

It will take years for science to find answers to these fascinating questions. Until then you should certainly take full advantage of your mind's ability to improve your health. Chapter 19 explores the proven ways in which stress contributes to heart disease, as well as the ways meditation and biofeedback can be used to prevent and treat medical conditions such as hypertension.

To prevent disillusionment — or even worse — we should try to put some of the current popular beliefs about the mind and the immune system into perspective.

I am strongly in favor of a positive mental attitude to fight disease. Call it faith, optimism, love, positive thinking, humor, or even plain old-fashioned grit, the will to recover does seem to aid recovery.

I have no objection to imaging, a new technique in which patients conjure up mental pictures of the cancer cells or other diseases that afflict them, trying to use mind power to ward off the disease. Many people feel better in the belief that they are assisting their treatment. If so — great. But the efficacy of imaging is entirely unproven, and it should *never* be a substitute for established medical therapies.

I am not enthusiastic about faith healing. As a scientist I must say that I discern no biological reason for it to work. Indeed, there is no evidence that it helps. Even worse, some people turn to faith healers instead of doctors, delaying or avoiding medical treatments that might be crucial. But if patients are willing to accept medical therapy, I certainly have no objection to *supplementary* psychological or religious efforts of any kind. In fact, when it comes to human health, I'll take all the help I can get.

Myth number three: Small amounts of exercise boost immunity, but large amounts impair the immune system.

Like the other myths, this one is based on legitimate scientific observations — observations, however, that have been blown up out of all proportion.

The first study of exercise and immunity dates back nearly 100 years, when Dr. R. C. Larrabee found that white blood cell counts rose dramatically in four men who completed the 1901 Boston Marathon. Since then, many experiments have confirmed that exercise boosts the number of polys in the blood. Exercise can increase poly counts by as much as 300 percent. Polys fight infection. Doesn't it follow, then, that exercise fights infection? No, it doesn't, because the rise is very brief, lasting less than an hour in most cases.

Lymphocytes are also affected by exercise. Percentagewise, however, the changes in lymphocytes are much smaller than the changes in polys. They are also more contradictory, with some studies showing that exercise increases helper lymphocytes that boost immunity while others show an increase in suppressor lymphocytes that reduce immune activity. However contradictory, the studies do agree on one thing: the changes are brief in duration and small in magnitude. By the time you've finished cooling down and you are showering, your lymphocytes will be back to normal.

The story is much the same when it comes to the proteins of the immune system. Exercise can increase two of the proteins that boost immunity, but the increase is brief. And gamma globulins, the protein antibodies that fight infection, are affected only by prolonged exercise in the cold, which decreases only the antibodies in nasal secretions.

There is a larger object lesson in all this. Intelligent and well-meaning individuals have built whole theories about exercise and immunity from just one set of experiments. Those experiments are perfectly valid, but a full picture requires consideration of many other experiments as well.

Like Thoreau's dietary regimens for infection, athletes are evenly divided into those who insist that exercise prevents infection and those who are sure that working out reduces resistance. The best evidence we have suggests that both are wrong: exercise has little net effect on immunity.

Why is this? For the answers to this question we can look back from the research of the 1980s to the insights of the 1850s, when Dr. Claude Bernard introduced the concept of the *milieu intérieur,* now known as homeostasis. The theory of homeostasis explains that the body's wisdom enables it to resist changes that upset the delicate balance in its organ systems and function. This is certainly true of the immune system, which has very elaborate control mechanisms that work to counteract imbalances in immunity just as soon as they start to occur.

Viruses, medications, and malnutrition can all produce profound and lasting suppression of the immune system. But, popular beliefs notwithstanding, diet, mental stress, and exercise are unable to upset the immunological apple cart. You may not be able to use these life-style changes to prevent disease, but by understanding how the immune system works, you can prevent myths from turning into missions impossible.

In the final analysis, Dr. Bernard was right: the wisdom of the body will prevail. Understand your body to use it wisely and keep it healthy.

▪ 12 ▪

Metabolic Disorders:
Diabetes and Obesity

Each and every one of our physical and mental functions involves the body's metabolism.

In its broadest sense, human metabolism serves to extract energy and nutrients from food and to harness that energy for four purposes: to sustain vital functions, to reproduce and grow, to replace cells and repair damaged tissues, and to perform work, both physical and mental. Your body's metabolism powers every heartbeat, stores energy in fatty tissue, adds 500 million new cells to your skin each day, and gives you the mental energy to read these words. To fill these diverse roles, the metabolism has evolved a specialized network of enzymes, hormones, and nerve cells that must interlock with precision to function properly.

It sounds complicated — and it is. But let's simplify things by considering just the key elements of the body's metabolism.

▪ The Normal Metabolism

An elevator is a complex machine, but it has just two fundamental phases: up and down. The metabolism is a complex system, but it too has just two essential phases: energy storage and energy utilization. From the moment of conception to adult life, the net direction of the metabolism is "up"; energy is stored and used to build tissues, allowing growth. Once growth has ceased in adulthood, energy storage and utilization should be balanced; imbalances in the "up" direction lead to obesity, in the "down" direction to weight loss and malnutrition. Your diet provides the energy and building blocks to set your metabolic elevator in motion; your hormones and nervous system regulate its speed and tell it when and where to stop.

Each day is also divided into much briefer cycles of energy storage and utilization. Every meal sends the metabolism in the "up" direction of energy storage; the hormonal "elevator operator" for this phase of energy storage is insulin. Between meals the elevator pauses and then starts down; exercise sets energy utilization into high gear. The hormones that regulate energy mobilization and utilization include adrenaline, glucagon, and growth hormone.

Energy Storage

Your energy elevator starts up with each meal. Food contains a mix of carbohydrates, fats, and proteins. But your metabolism needs simple molecules to fuel it. Your stomach and intestines make it all possible by digesting carbohydrates into simple sugars, fats into smaller fatty acids, and proteins into amino acids. These key nutrients are then absorbed into your blood stream, traveling first to your liver and then to your other organs and tissues. Your intestinal tract also absorbs the water, vitamins, and minerals that are vital for a healthy metabolism.

Eating starts the process of energy storage, but a full belly will not by itself push your metabolic "up" button. Instead, the signal to start energy storage comes from your blood sugar levels. After each meal your blood sugar levels rise. High blood sugar levels signal your pancreas to pump insulin into your blood. In turn, insulin is the hormone that sets the process of energy storage into motion.

Insulin allows sugar to move from your blood into your cells. About 60 percent of the blood sugar is taken up by liver cells, which convert it to glycogen and fat for storage. Muscle cells also take up sugar, burning some for energy and storing the rest for future use, also in the form of glycogen. Fat cells, too, respond to insulin, converting sugar from the blood directly into fat, and also storing fat produced by the well-fed liver.

Insulin and sugar are the key elements in energy storage, but they are not the whole story. After a protein-rich meal, amino acids enter the blood and travel to the liver, to muscles, and to other tissues, where they are reassembled into proteins. Fat, too, is absorbed from food and is transported throughout the body, where insulin stimulates its storage in fat cells.

Energy Utilization

What goes up must come down.

For the first few hours after each meal, your body is busy absorbing nutrients and storing excess energy in the form of glycogen, fat, and protein. But when your blood sugar levels return to normal, your insulin levels fall and energy storage comes to a stop. Still, your tissues need fuel; exercise burns up a lot of energy, but even at rest your body requires a constant source of power. In the hours between meals that energy comes from the body's own energy stores. Your blood sugar levels start down, your insulin levels fall, and your metabolism begins to burn the energy it has stored up for this very purpose.

The liver is the first source of energy. Glycogen is converted back into sugar, which enters the blood, maintaining normal sugar levels even during prolonged fasting or intense exercise. But the liver has only a limited supply of stored glycogen; when supplies get low, liver cells actually manufacture new sugar molecules from fat, lactic acid, and especially from amino acids.

Most of the body's stored energy is in the form of fat. The average adult has 140,000 calories stored in fat, 24,000 in protein, but only 300 in glycogen. For many people body fat represents more of a problem than a solution; indeed, your body can have too much of a good thing. But when your metabolism needs energy, some fat *is* a good thing: fat is broken down into smaller fatty acids that enter the blood and travel to your liver for conversion into sugar and to your muscles, where they're burned for energy.

The primary disorder of energy metabolism in our affluent society is obesity. But in less fortunate cultures energy deficiencies can pose major problems. When the body uses up its fat stores, it has to turn to muscle tissue for energy. The end result of this self-cannibalism is starvation, literally wasting away. But starvation is not confined to the Horn of Africa. Here at home, poverty, hunger, and malnutrition still exist. In addition, patients with eating disorders such as anorexia nervosa can develop similar problems. And patients with advanced cancer also waste away; their problem, called cachexia, results from excessive production of tumor necrosis factor, a hormone that switches the metabolism into a persistent "down" phase.

How Metabolism Is Controlled

Your body's metabolism is, of course, much more complicated than the simple elevator model would suggest. And a healthy metabolism requires many factors to keep it in balance, preventing excesses of energy storage (obesity) and utilization (starvation).

A healthy energy balance requires appropriate building blocks from a sound diet.

A healthy energy balance requires healthful behavior, matching energy intake (diet) to energy use (exercise).

A healthy metabolism requires a healthy intestinal tract to absorb food and a healthy liver to store energy in times of plenty so it can be mobilized in times of need. A healthy family tree will also help, since genetic factors control many aspects of the metabolism.

Finally, a healthy metabolism requires hormones to regulate the entire process. The pancreas produces insulin to stimulate energy storage and glucagon to mobilize energy. The pituitary gland produces growth hormone, and the adrenal gland secretes adrenaline, both hormones of energy utilization. But in addition to these major hormones, dozens of others are essential to fine-tuning the body's metabolism.

Of all the body's metabolic hormones perhaps the best known is the thyroid hormone, thyroxine. Thyroid hormone is essential for all of the body's metabolic process. If the thyroid gland is underactive, the metabolism slows and excessive energy is stored as fat. If the thyroid is overactive, the metabolism races and energy is burned in excess.

Despite its importance and its repute, the exact way thyroid hormone controls the metabolism is still a mystery, locked deep in the most basic functions of the human cell. But you won't have to grapple with the mysteries of cell biology to keep your metabolism healthy. In fact, apart from getting proper amounts of iodine in your diet and avoiding excessive exposure to radiation, there is little you can do to prevent thyroid disease.

There are many ways to prevent diseases of your metabolism. Let's explore the most important of these disorders, diabetes and obesity.

■ Diabetes

What Is Diabetes?

In its full-blown form, diabetes is starvation in the midst of plenty. Blood sugar levels are high — excessively high — but the sugar can't get into the cells that need it for energy and nutrition. Instead, the sugar is spilled into the urine and lost from the body. The result is a medical energy crisis: cells switch over to a starvationlike metabolism because they cannot get enough sugar to fuel normal metabolism.

Why does this happen? The main problem is that the controlling hormone, insulin, does not function properly. Without effective insulin action, sugar cannot enter cells and cellular metabolism will not be stimulated to store energy.

Although all diabetics suffer from insufficient insulin action, there are actually three rather different forms of diabetes.

Type I diabetes. Patients with Type I diabetes produce too little insulin; in advanced cases, in fact, they produce almost none. The pancreas is at fault. In patients with Type I diabetes the pancreatic beta cells that normally produce insulin are severely damaged or destroyed. There are at least three explanations for this damage. The first is genetic; many patients with Type I diabetes have close relatives with the same problem. The second factor is inflammation caused by excessive immune cell function. Many patients develop Type I diabetes because their immune cells turn against their own bodies, damaging beta cells; sometimes other endocrine glands are damaged as well, producing multiple hormone deficiencies. Third, the pancreas can be damaged by viral infections or chemical toxins. Infections or toxins are rarely the sole cause of diabetes; but in patients with genes for Type I diabetes they can sometimes trigger inflammation of the pancreas, thus activating the immune system, which ultimately damages and destroys beta cells.

Type II diabetes. Type II diabetes is a complex, heterogeneous disorder. As in the other forms of diabetes, genetic factors often contribute to its cause. Most patients with Type II diabetes have plenty of healthy-looking beta cells in their pancreas. In fact, they generally have good amounts of insulin in their blood — sometimes even *more* than normal. But their insulin does not function properly, chiefly because their liver and muscle cells are abnormally resistant to the action of insulin.

Diabetes of pregnancy. This relatively mild form of diabetes develops in about 3 percent of all pregnancies, usually occurring in the third trimester. The complex hormonal and metabolic changes of pregnancy are blamed for this type of diabetes. It usually clears up promptly after delivery, but a substantial fraction of these women go on to develop Type II diabetes later on in life.

Manifestations of Diabetes

Because the two major forms of diabetes have different causes, they have different symptoms, different preventions, and different treatments.

Type I diabetes begins early in life, usually before age 40 and often before age 20. Most patients have normal body weight before the disease starts, but many lose weight rapidly when they become ill. In general, Type I diabetes begins quite abruptly. Excessive urination is a key symptom; patients drink abnormally large volumes of fluids but they still feel terribly thirsty and often become dehydrated. Despite excessive hunger and voracious eating, weight loss is common. So, too, are weakness, fatigue, blurred vision, and an acetone-like odor on the breath. Because patients with Type I diabetes have little or no insulin, they depend on daily insulin injections for survival.

Type II diabetes is very different. More common in older adults, it begins gradually and is often present for years before it causes any symptoms at all. When symptoms occur, they are usually mild: increased thirst, excessive urination, and fatigue are most common. Infections and periodontal disease may be the first clues to the diagnosis. The vast majority of patients with Type II diabetes are overweight to begin with, and many report an additional 10- or 20-pound weight gain shortly before their diabetes becomes evident.

The Impact of Diabetes

Diabetes is the seventh most common cause of death in the United States.

Type I diabetes affects about 1 million Americans. Ten million have Type II diabetes, but only half know they have it. In all, about 5 percent of adults in the United States are diabetics.

Diabetes is directly responsible for 37,000 deaths in the United States each year — nearly 2 percent of all deaths. In addition, the complications of diabetes contribute to another 100,000 deaths each year. The life expectancy of diabetics at the time of diagnosis is one third shorter than it is for nondiabetic people of the same age.

As a chronic condition diabetes also causes substantial suffering. Diabetics are four times more likely to suffer heart attacks and strokes than nondiabetics. Diabetes leads to nearly half of all nontraumatic leg and foot amputations in the United States. The primary cause of visual loss between ages 20 and 74, diabetes accounts for 5,000 cases of blindness each year. Last but not least, diabetes is responsible for 25 percent of the causes of severe kidney failure in America; nearly one in every ten diabetics will eventually require dialysis or kidney transplantation.

The economic costs of diabetes are also substantial. Each year we spend nearly $7 billion to care for diabetes and another $5 billion to treat its medical complications. Diabetics are four times more likely to become disabled than are nondiabetics; more than a million are completely disabled, costing our society about $8 billion annually.

Preventing Diabetes

I'm sorry to report that there is no way to prevent Type I diabetes — yet. Now that we know the body's immune system contributes significantly to many cases of Type I diabetes, doctors have begun preventive experimentation with medications that suppress immunity and fight inflammation. Preliminary results are encouraging, but it's far too early to consider these medications for widespread use.

If there's bad news about preventing Type I diabetes, there is good news about forestalling Type II diabetes. Although it's far less serious than Type I diabetes, Type II is ten times more common — and there are many things you can do to protect yourself against it. Moreover, patients with *both* types of diabetes can make simple life-style changes that will substantially reduce their risk of complications and decrease their need for medication.

It is true that diabetes tends to run in families. Obviously you can't trade in your grandparents to prevent inheriting a diabetic tendency. Still, even if you have diabetes in your family, you can — and should — take steps to protect yourself. The primary prevention of diabetes has three key elements: weight control, diet, and exercise.

Weight control. At least 75 percent of patients with Type II diabetes are substantially overweight. Indeed, weight loss should always be the first step in treating diabetes in obese patients. Diabetics who attain ideal body weight are often able to maintain good blood sugar levels without the use of medication. Many times, in fact, their blood sugar levels return to normal, even if their levels were initially quite high. If weight loss is so effective for the *treatment* of Type II diabetes, it should also be effective for *prevention* — and it is. Preventing obesity could reduce the occurrence of Type II diabetes by a full 50 percent, preventing 300,000 cases in the United States each year; diabetes of pregnancy could be reduced by 33 percent, preventing 30,000 cases annually.

Preventing diabetes is only one of many important reasons to avoid obesity. But weight control is a complex problem for doctors to understand and a difficult goal for patients to achieve. I discuss obesity in detail later in this chapter, and chapter 20 gives you practical tips for healthful nutrition.

Diet. Do patients with diabetes require a special diet? The obvious answer is yes — but the details may surprise you.

Diabetes is a disease of sugar metabolism. It's only logical, then, that regulation of carbohydrate intake has long been considered the key to dietary management of diabetes. Logic notwithstanding, however, controversy has dogged recommendations for diabetic diets for nearly 4,000 years. Even today there are grounds for debate as scientific uncertainties persist.

Patients with uncontrolled diabetes have high blood sugar levels, and they spill sugar into the urine, eliminating it from their bodies before it can contribute to nutrition. The earliest Egyptian, Greek, and Roman physicians recognized this; in fact, they diagnosed diabetes based on the sweet taste of patients' urine! Those ancient doctors reasoned that since sugar was being lost from the body, patients should be treated with a high-carbohydrate diet. We've come a long way in the diagnosis of diabetes. But even though the 3,500-year-old taste test has not been revived (fortunately!), we are actually returning to the wisdom of the ancients for the dietary treatment of diabetes, though for better reasons, I trust.

But the diabetic diet has gone through many twists and turns before coming full circle. In 1797 John Rollo, an English army surgeon, reasoned that a high-carbohydrate diet would merely raise the blood sugar higher, exacerbating diabetes. He recommended "animal food . . . with an entire abstinence from every kind of vegetable matter" — a low-carbohydrate, high-protein, high-fat diet. Indeed, severe carbohydrate restriction became the mainstay for the treatment of diabetes.

Insulin was discovered in 1921, revolutionizing the therapy of diabetes. Patients were no longer doomed to suffer from uncontrolled diabetes leading to coma and death. But if insulin could control blood sugar levels, it did not prevent diabetics from dying prematurely from complications of their disease. Heart attacks became the leading cause of death in diabetics; still, low-carbohydrate, high-fat diets were widely recommended despite emerging evidence of their harmful effects on blood cholesterol levels. In fact, it was not until 1971, 50 years after the discovery of insulin, that the American Diabetes Association recommended low-fat diets for the management of diabetes.

Although there is still plenty of controversy about the best dietary approach to the prevention and treatment of diabetes, there is universal agreement that fat intake should be reduced. The current American Diabetes Association guidelines correspond closely to the American Heart Association's recommendations for nondiabetics: reduce total fat to 30 percent of calories, with no more than 10 percent of calories coming from saturated fat. Dietary cholesterol, too, should be reduced, ideally to less than 300 milligrams per day.

It's hard to argue with official guidelines. But if you have diabetes, I think you should consider even more stringent restrictions on your fat and cholesterol intake. I recommend that you limit your dietary fat intake to no more than 20 percent of calories, and that you keep your cholesterol quota below 200 milligrams per day. My reasoning is simple: since diabetics have an increased risk of heart disease, it's particularly important that they do everything possible to reduce that risk. At the very least, dietary fat intake should be tailored to produce the best possible blood cholesterol profile.

To prevent and treat diabetes, reduce dietary calories to attain ideal body weight and cut dietary fat and cholesterol to attain optimal blood cholesterol levels. But what can you substitute for the fat in your diet?

Protein would seem a logical choice. But here, too, logic is suspect. For one thing dietary protein, like dietary sugar, requires insulin for its metabolism. More important, a high protein intake can accelerate the progression of kidney disease in diabetics. In chapter 10 I recommended moderation in dietary protein for everyone to help prevent kidney dysfunction, but I admitted that scientific proof for this suggestion is lacking. When it comes to diabetics, however, that proof *is* available. A 1991 study by Dr. Kathleen Zeller and her associates from Southwestern Medical Center demonstrates that protein restriction slows kidney disease in patients with diabetes. Diabetics should limit their protein intake to no more than .36 grams per pound of body weight per day up to a maximum of 50 grams for women and 63 grams for men. It's sound advice for all of us, diabetic and nondiabetic alike; chapter 20 will explain how to translate grams of protein into choices for your menu.

While avoiding fat and restricting protein, diabetics must surely eat something. That something is carbohydrates. Although severe carbohydrate restriction was the watchword for diabetics during most of the modern era of medicine, even the conservative American Diabetic Association now recommends a *high* carbohydrate intake, amounting to 55 to 60 percent of total dietary calories.

Controversy persists, however, as to which carbohydrates are best. Most experts agree that complex carbohydrates (starches) raise the blood sugar less rapidly than simple carbohydrates (sugars). While agreeing on the merits of complex carbohydrates, however, some authorities would place few restrictions on sugar intake, while others still recommend reduced dietary sugar. Here I side with the traditionalists. Sugar provides an astounding 25 percent of the calories in the average American diet. Sugar contributes significantly to obesity but has no nutritional benefit aside from its caloric content. In less "developed" societies sugars and other refined carbohydrates are used only sparingly — and diabetes and obesity are rarities. To prevent diabetes, eat lots of complex carbohydrates and do your best to avoid refined sugars.

A special form of carbohydrate deserves special mention. Fiber is plant carbohydrate that is not absorbed and has no caloric value. High-fiber diets reduce both blood sugar levels and pancreatic insulin secretion. Fiber, especially soluble fiber, also helps improve blood cholesterol levels and fights obesity. To help prevent diabetes, eat lots of fiber — 30 to 35 grams per day.

A few other dietary tips may help in the treatment, if not the prevention, of diabetes. Alternative sweeteners, such as aspartame, are acceptable, but because long-term human safety studies are lacking, they should not be overused. Alcoholic beverages add "empty" calories and should be restricted, especially in overweight diabetics; they can sometimes elevate triglyceride levels and may reduce blood sugar levels to a harmful extent in undernourished people. Finally, because of the risks of hypertension most diabetics should limit their sodium intake to no more than 1 gram per 1,000 calories, up to a daily maximum of 3 grams.

Exercise. Exercise is the third major way to prevent diabetes. Like weight control and diet, exercise is helpful not only in preventing diabetes but also in treating patients with the disease and in reducing their risk of developing complications.

Exercise is beneficial in three ways. First, it's very helpful for weight control: exercise burns calories and reduces body fat, both of which diminish the risk of diabetes.

Second, exercise in and of itself improves sugar metabolism. When muscles exercise, they require sugar for fuel. But exercise does more than just burn up sugar; it actually helps sugar molecules get from the blood into muscle and liver cells. Exercise does this by improving tissue sensitivity to insulin. So if you exercise regularly, you'll actually need *less* insulin to maintain a normal blood sugar level. If you put some serious miles on your shoes, bike, or rowing machine, you'll get much more mileage from your pancreas's insulin supply.

Third, exercise helps protect against the complications of diabetes. If performed regularly, exercise improves blood cholesterol levels, lowers blood pressure, and improves the body's ability to fight blood clots or thromboses. The net effect is a dramatic reduction in the risk of heart attacks and cardiac death. Exercise is clearly beneficial for all of us. But since 75 percent of deaths in diabetics are related to cardiovascular abnormalities, exercise assumes added importance in this setting.

Weight control, increased insulin activity, and reduced complications — exercise is surely a good *treatment* for diabetes. Common sense dictates that exercise should also help *prevent* diabetes. But although medical science verified the therapeutic value of exercise years ago, its preventive value wasn't proven until 1991. In a 14-year study of 5,990 men, Dr. Ralph Paffenbarger and his associates found that regular exercise actually reduced the occurrence of diabetes; for each 500 calories of exercise per week, the risk of diabetes declined by 6 percent. In sum, the most active men enjoyed a 50 percent reduction in diabetes — and the men at highest risk because of obesity and a family history of diabetes experienced the greatest benefit of all. Even more recently an 8-year study of 87,253 women found similar results, confirming that regular exercise can help prevent diabetes.

What kind of exercise is best to prevent diabetes? Because it has the most beneficial effect on blood sugar, blood cholesterol, and blood pressure, aerobic exercise is the key. Three to four hours a week is ideal, but as little as one hour a week is helpful. Chapter 21 will show you how to develop a safe, enjoyable exercise program tailored to your individual needs.

Diabetics who exercise must take special precautions. Coronary heart disease tends to be common in diabetics, and it's often clinically silent. Hence, patients with diabetes require a careful cardiovascular evaluation before they begin an exercise program. Because exercise improves blood sugar levels, diabetics should monitor themselves carefully as they get into shape, anticipating a decrease in their medication requirements. A light snack prior to exercise helps to avoid an excessive drop in blood sugar levels; I generally recommend skim milk. Even with a snack, it's wise for diabetics to wear a medical alert bracelet and to carry sweets when they exercise strenuously. Diabetics with active eye disease should avoid intense sports and trauma; for example, swimming, biking, or walking would be preferable to running. Finally, if diabetes is complicated by diminished feeling or impaired circulation, meticulous foot care is mandatory.

Is exercise beneficial enough to warrant all these precautions? Yes! Medical studies have shown that diabetics who exercise regularly require less medication but still have improved blood sugar levels. They achieve increased aerobic work capacities and fitness levels. And, most important of all, they have less heart disease.

Exercise, of course, will provide these same benefits to nondiabetics. And nondiabetics will gain an additional benefit: they'll be less likely ever to develop diabetes.

Screening for Diabetes: Secondary Prevention

Everyone should follow a program to help prevent diabetes. People who are at high risk because they are obese or they have close relatives with the disease should be particularly careful to control weight, exercise regularly, and eat a diet low in fat and simple sugars, moderate in protein, and high in complex carbohydrates and fiber.

All of us should be alert for the symptoms of diabetes so we can get prompt and proper treatment at the first sign of this common disease.

But should everyone undergo medical screening tests to detect early diabetes *before* symptoms appear? The U.S. Preventive Services Task Force and its Canadian counterpart say no, arguing that there's no scientific evidence that early treatment produces better results than treatment that's delayed until symptoms occur. After reviewing the evidence, I must conclude that these expert panels are right — in regard to early *drug* treatment. But I've found that diagnosing early, presymptomatic diabetes can be a powerful tool to motivate patients to embrace *life-style* treatment that can help prevent the progression of diabetes and the occurrence of heart disease and other complications. This is secondary prevention at its best. Moreover, screening is simple, accurate, and inexpensive. All in all, even taking expert panels into account, I still believe in periodic screening to detect early diabetes.

If you and your doctor agree with me, what screening tests can be considered?

The traditional screening test is the simple urine analysis. Since most patients with diabetes spill sugar into the urine, where it can be detected easily, it's a tempting possibility. Tempting or not, a simple urinalysis won't do as a screening test because many nondiabetics also have sugar in their urine from time to time.

Blood tests can detect diabetes; abnormally high sugar levels are all we need to make the diagnosis. But even with blood tests, there are two tricky issues.

First, blood sugar levels rise after meals, both in healthy people and in diabetics. In diabetics, however, the sugar levels rise higher and stay up longer. At the very least, your doctor must know when you last ate in order to interpret your blood sugar results. Even better, your screening test can be done after fasting or at defined times after a sugar-rich meal. Best of all, you can have both a fasting blood test *and* blood tests after drinking a standard dose of sugar — the oral glucose (sugar) tolerance test. Since the glucose tolerance test requires several hours at the lab and a series of blood tests, however, I generally reserve it for patients with major diabetes risk factors, with symptoms, or with borderline results from my basic screening tests, fasting, or post-meal blood sugar determination.

The second complicating factor is that blood sugar tests can be abnormal without indicating diabetes. In fact, there is a third group of people whose blood sugar results are midway between normal and diabetes. These people are healthy but have impaired sugar tolerance. Impaired sugar tolerance is more common with advancing age. Many people with this metabolic condition remain healthy, but some do go on to develop diabetes, so they should be extra careful to do everything possible to improve their sugar metabolism and prevent heart disease.

With these two qualifications, you can interpret your blood sugar results to find out if you have diabetes (see table 12-1).

Note that diabetes of pregnancy is a special situation, with its own criteria for diagnosis. Although diabetes of pregnancy is a mild condition that usually resolves after delivery, early diagnosis is very important, since treatment cuts the rate of fetal complications and death. Hence, even the most conservative authorities agree that all women should have a simple glucose tolerance test between weeks 24 and 28 of pregnancy.

How often should nonpregnant adults be tested for diabetes? As you can tell, there is no consensus on this question — so I'll give you my personal recommendations. Think them over, and if they make sense to you, discuss them with your doctor.

I don't ask healthy people to make special trips to the lab for blood sugar testing. But I do request blood sugar tests at the same time that I order routine cholesterol determinations. This approach to diabetes screening does not require any extra time or discomfort, and it adds only a modest expense — generally about $6 per test. People at high risk should, I think, be tested more often, probably at every routine physical. Needless to say, abnormal screening results or suspicious symptoms mandate a detailed evaluation.

Finally, you should know that a new test of glucose metabolism has been developed. Despite its formidable name, glycosylated hemoglobin, it's really a very simple procedure, requiring only a single blood sample. It has the advantage of allowing your doctor to calculate your *average* blood sugar level for the preceding *30 days*. Like most physicians who treat diabetes, I've found the glycosylated hemoglobin test an invaluable aid to *managing* diabetes. Unfortunately, standards are not available to use this

Table 12-1. Criteria for the Diagnosis of Diabetes

Diagnosis	Test result		
	Fasting blood sugar	Blood sugar 30, 60, or 90 min. after eating a sugar-rich meal or drinking a test dose of sugar	Blood sugar 2 hours after food or the test sugar dose
Healthy	less than 115	less than 200	less than 140
Impaired sugar tolerance	115–140	over 200	140–200
Diabetes	over 140 (on more than one test)	over 200	over 200
Diabetes of pregnancy	over 105	over 190 (at 60 minutes)	over 165 at 2 hours or over 145 at 3 hours

test to *diagnose* diabetes. Stay tuned, though, for new developments in this area. A simple one-step test would be sweet indeed.

Preventing the Complications of Diabetes: Tertiary Prevention

Even if blood sugar tests show that you are one of the 11 million Americans who have diabetes, you should not give up on prevention. Quite the contrary. It may be too late to prevent diabetes, but you *can* reduce your risk of complications. And since doctors can achieve excellent control of blood sugar levels with insulin injections or sugar-lowering pills, complications have now emerged as the chief causes of disability and death in diabetics. But tertiary prevention in diabetes involves much more than your doctor's prescription for insulin or pills; it requires you to monitor your sugar levels, to adjust your medication according to your doctor's directions, and — above all — to make the life-style changes that are the keys to prevention.

The leading complications of diabetes are heart attacks, which account for up to 60 percent of deaths in diabetics, and strokes, which contribute to an additional 25 percent of deaths. Another major complication is peripheral vascular disease or narrowing of the arteries, particularly in the legs and feet. While rarely lethal, diabetic peripheral vascular disease leads to more than 30,000 amputations in the United States each year.

Heart attacks, strokes, and peripheral vascular disease are all caused by atherosclerosis, which is much more common in diabetics than in nondiabetics. For example, diabetes doubles the risk of heart disease in men and quadruples risk in women.

That's the bad news. The good news is that atherosclerosis can be prevented, even in diabetics. With optimal prevention, diabetic heart disease could be reduced 45 percent, peripheral vascular disease by 60 percent, and stroke by 85 percent. There is nothing magical about achieving these wonderful gains. In fact, it's back to basics.

There are three other major complications of diabetes. Kidney disease occurs in 10 percent of diabetics; advanced kidney failure is 15 times more likely in Type I than in Type II diabetes, but all diabetics should do everything possible to prevent this complication. Simply controlling high blood pressure could cut the rate of diabetic kidney failure in half. Exciting new research suggests that a particular group of antihypertensive medications, the ACE inhibitors, are particularly effective in preventing kidney damage in diabetics. Restricting dietary protein can also help.

Blindness is another serious complication of diabetes. Most often severe visual loss is caused by damage to retinal blood vessels, but cataracts and glaucoma are also more common in diabetes. Chapter 13 details the prevention of eye disease. Patients with diabetes should be absolutely certain to have eye exams by an ophthalmologist (physician eye specialist) at least twice a year; early laser and photocoagulation could prevent half of all diabetic blindness.

The final major complication of diabetes is nerve damage, which can cause diminished sensation, pain, or both. Rarely lethal, diabetic nerve damage can lead to traumatic injuries, infections, or persistent pain. Unfortunately, neither the treatment nor the prevention of diabetic nerve damage is very effective. But there is emerging evidence that tight control of blood sugar levels may help.

Good control is an important strategy to help prevent all the complications of diabetes. To achieve it, diabetics will have to work closely with their doctors to monitor sugar levels and adjust medications. But they will also have to practice the essentials of prevention for themselves: diet, exercise, smoking cessation, cholesterol control, and weight control. All in all, prevention for diabetics involves the same basics as prevention for the rest of us — but because of the potentially serious complications of diabetes, it's even more important.

■ Obesity and Weight Control

Although I'm genuinely happy to see my patients, I must confess that some are not quite so happy to see me. These less-than-enthusiastic patients come in for their checkups or treatments with ambivalence, reluctance, or downright apprehension. There are, of course, many legitimate reasons for these emotions. Very often, however, the single greatest cause of their mental discomfort is just a simple piece of office equipment: my scale.

To say that we live in a weight-conscious society is to understate the situation. Few other issues in medicine generate such concern and consternation in the public, and few produce such controversy and contradiction in the scientific community. Despite its prevalence, obesity remains a mysterious area, with more questions than answers, more theories than facts.

In spite of all the heat, we are finally starting to shed some light on obesity, gaining insights into its causes, consequences, and correction. As a physician I grapple with these problems daily. As an individual I have had the all-too-common experience of a 30-pound weight gain between ages 20 and 35 — and the all-too-rare experience of a 30-pound weight loss that has been sustained throughout the subsequent 15 years. Both perspectives give me the courage to plunge into this weighty subject.

Body Fat

Whether your priority is health or aesthetics, the real issue is not body weight but body fat. Weight watching is a code name for fretting over fat.

Fat is, of course, not always a villain. A perfectly normal part of the human body, it's absolutely necessary for health. Fat is the body's major storage depot for energy; without sufficient energy stores, we wouldn't have the reserve to carry us through times when food is scarce, much less the energy to survive the stress of exercise, illness, pregnancy, or growth. In addition to storing energy, body fat also provides a reserve for many vitamins. It's an excellent insulator, protecting us from climatic stress. Fat is also essential for the proper metabolism of sex hormones; women who have too little body fat have low estrogen levels, causing them to develop osteoporosis and run the risk of fractures. Finally, fat helps to cushion the internal organs against the stresses of physical trauma.

The Impact of Obesity. Although a little fat is good for health, a lot of fat is not. Excess body fat produces its own stresses and contributes to many serious disorders. Heart disease and other manifestations of atherosclerosis are the best-known examples. Obesity also increases substantially the risk of related conditions such as high blood pressure, high cholesterol levels, and Type II diabetes. Overweight people have more arthritis, and are more likely to develop gallstones. Certain lung disorders are found only in obese patients. Cancer, too, is linked to excess body fat: overweight men are unduly prone to prostate, colon, and rectal cancer, while obese women are at extra risk for cancers of the breast, ovary, uterus, cervix, and gallbladder. In all, obesity increases the risk of dying from cancer by 1.5 in women and 1.3 in men. And if all this were not bad enough, overweight people suffer from more than their share of job discrimination, social isolation, and psychological difficulties.

Weight loss can prevent all these problems — if it's sustained. The yo-yo approach — lose 12 pounds, then gain a dozen — will do you little good. What's worse, continual fluctuations in weight may even add to cardiac risk. Doctors from the Framingham Heart Study reported in the 1991 *New England Journal of Medicine* that fluctuations in body weight produced even higher rates of heart attacks and deaths than sustained obesity. The moral: it's best to shed these excess pounds and to keep them off.

The Forms of Fat. All fatty tissue is composed of adipose cells, simple cells that store up fat molecules in the form of triglyceride. About 40 billion fat cells are distributed throughout the body, with the greatest amount in the abdomen, breasts, buttocks, and thighs. Fatty tissue is also present deep in the body's interior, being especially prominent around the heart, intestines, and kidneys.

Not all fat cells are created equal. Fat cells around the belly, sides, and back are metabolically more active than are the fat cells of the buttocks and thighs. Abdominal fat cells have more lipoprotein lipase, the enzyme responsible for storing fat in cells. As a result, they're the first cells to enlarge when the body has an energy surplus. But upper-body fat cells are also much more responsive to adrenaline, which causes them to mobilize fat, releasing it into the blood. Hence, they're the first cells to shrink during weight loss. In contrast, fat cells in the buttocks and thighs are more responsive to female sex hormones.

Women have more lower-body fat; in an evolutionary sense it's an advantage for them, allowing increased energy storage for pregnancy and breast-feeding. Men have more abdominal fat, possibly because they evolved the ability to mobilize fat for quick energy in response to adrenaline, the stress hormone.

The good news for men is that abdominal fat is more readily mobilized; it's easier to lose a beer belly than to slim down abundant thighs. The bad news for men is that excess abdominal fat is much more likely to cause heart disease and stroke, exactly because it can be mobilized into the blood where it can damage vessels, leading to atherosclerosis.

What Is Obesity?

Like so many questions, this one has two answers, one simple, the other complex.

Simply put, obesity is an excess of body fat.

Like blood pressure, however, there is no single dividing line between the normal and abnormal. And so we need a long answer, too.

When fat cells store energy, they increase in size, accumulating ever-larger droplets of triglyceride. With increased storage, the cells will swell remarkably, growing to ten times their own size. Fat cells make fat people.

When a fat cell is maximally laden, it doesn't simply stop accumulating triglyceride. Instead, it may divide into two cells, each of which can resume storing fat. Extra cells, too, make people fat.

Even in this day of modern technology, however, we can't count or measure individual fat cells. Instead, we weigh and measure whole people. Obesity is defined as a 20 percent excess in body weight. Clearly arbitrary, this definition does not account for many people who are unhappy about less drastic accumulations of body fat. Arbitrary or not, it's a useful definition, since the medical consequences of excess fat begin to increase at the 20 percent level, continuing to mount with each extra pound.

Obesity in America

If you are overweight, it may be of small comfort to know that you are not alone. Far from it! Thirty-four million Americans meet or exceed the medical definition of obesity. Although it can be present from infancy onward, obesity is more common in older age groups. Body fat tends to increase most rapidly in the 20s and 30s — and then keeps right on increasing. Women are more likely to be obese than men; some surveys have shown that one in four American women and one in seven men are at least 20 percent overweight.

But obesity is not equally distributed in our society, any more than fat is equally distributed around the body. Paradoxically perhaps, obesity is linked to poverty, being six times more common in the lowest socioeconomic class than in the highest. Members of certain ethnic minority groups also have an increased risk of obesity.

Obesity is linked to poverty in America, but the reverse is true around the world as a whole. Obesity is much more common in industrialized societies. Leading the way in affluence, America also occupies first place in corpulence.

What Causes Obesity?

Obesity is an excess of body fat. There is only one way that excess fat can accumulate: there must be a positive energy balance, with caloric intake exceeding caloric expenditure. The net result is an excess of energy, which is stored in the body as fat.

But what causes the caloric equation to become imbalanced, creating an energy surplus? Despite intensive research, scientists have produced more theories than facts. To understand their postulates, let's return to our metabolic elevator analogy. In this model a positive energy balance would push the elevator too high, storing the excess as fat, producing obesity. The theories of obesity can be divided into two broad groups. The behavioral theories tell us the fault lies with the elevator operator, who sends the elevator too high by taking on excess fuel or by burning off too little energy. In contrast, the biological theories assert that the fault lies with the elevator's mechanism itself so that it goes up more easily than it comes down, even if the operator tries to adjust the control switches.

The behavioral theories attribute obesity to overeating and under-exercising.

Overeating certainly has a role in obesity; in a sense all people who are obese overeat, since they consume more calories than they need for a normal energy balance. But does overeating depend on psychological factors? In an affluent society sustenance is rarely the motive for eating. Food provides taste and pleasure, solace, relief of stress, and a break from boredom. Meals are social occasions, but even when we're alone we often eat out of sheer habit rather than because of hunger.

These observations produced the *psychological theory* of obesity, which holds that a particular personality type or a special set of emotional problems cause some people to overeat and grow fat. But this hypothesis has not been verified. On the whole, in fact, obese people do *not* eat more calories per pound of body weight than thin people. Obese people have the same psychological responses to food as lean people. Finally, there is no such thing as an "obese personality type." Overweight people do tend to be more depressed, but in most cases depression is the result of the social and economic disadvantages that our culture imposes on fat people rather than the cause of obesity.

Underexercise surely has a role in obesity; as a group overweight people certainly are more sedentary than thin people. But sloth alone cannot account for obesity. Quite the reverse. Being fat is often the cause of inactivity, slowing people down and making exercise difficult and sports frustrating. Although few athletes are fat, many lean people are sedentary. Exercise is important in the treatment of all cases of obesity, but inactivity alone cannot explain excessive fat storage in many people.

The behavioral theories of obesity have an important drawback: they blame the victim. Many of the social biases and barriers faced by obese people result from the belief that obesity stems from personal flaws, from defects in discipline and determination. True, we must take individual responsibility for our bodies, and will power is essential to correct obesity. But new research shows that obese people have a much harder task than thin people; though still incomplete, the biological theories of obesity demonstrate that many overweight people have abnormal metabolic mechanisms.

There are many biological theories of obesity.

Genetic theories attribute obesity to heredity. For centuries philosophers and theologians have told us that destiny shapes man's ends; geneticists now tell us that destiny shapes our middles, too.

A look at your family tree may convince you that heredity does influence body type and body fat. If your family tree has a thin trunk, you are likely to be thin. Alas, the converse is also true: if you have one obese parent, your risk of obesity is 50 percent, and if both parents are overweight, your risk is 63 percent.

Behaviorists argue that obesity runs in families because fat parents teach their offspring to overeat from early childhood on. But it's not that simple. Children who are raised from infancy by adoptive parents have body builds like their biological parents' rather than their adoptive parents'. Similarly, twins separated into different households early in life grow up to resemble each other despite altogether different family environments.

Hormonal theories have been unsuccessful in explaining obesity. Many overweight people blame their "glands" for their problems, but detailed studies cannot detect endocrine abnormalities in most obese people.

Metabolic theories are making some progress. Early attempts to show that obese people burn fuel abnormally were not encouraging, but newer studies suggest that there *are* differences; they are subtle, and they're a long way from explaining all cases of obesity, but they do reveal the importance of metabolic factors in obesity.

Set-point theories begin with the observation that most people, whether fat or thin, tend to maintain a remarkably constant body weight over the years. True, there are fluctuations; for example, weight often declines with illness, but it is rapidly regained with recovery. And it's also true that many people slowly gain weight as they age, particularly during their middle years. All in all, however, the stability of body weight is much more impressive than its rate of change. Consider that only 100 extra calories per day would produce a ten-pound weight gain in a year. It's very easy to take in 100 extra calories — a single cookie will do the trick.

How is the energy equation kept so well balanced? We don't know, but it's clear that the balance is automatic, entirely independent of mirror and scale. A 1991 study examined the daily energy intake of children between the ages of two and five. All the kids were allowed unlimited access to whatever foods they wanted. Their caloric intake varied widely from meal to meal. But when the daily figures were tallied up, the totals were remarkably stable from day to day. As parents we often put great effort into regulating what our children eat. But it's wasted effort, since even in your children the set-point mechanism is strong enough to regulate the energy equation without a guiding hand.

The set-point theory says that the body automatically adjusts itself to maintain energy equality. It adjusts energy intake to compensate for illness or exertion, and modulates energy output to correct for Thanksgiving. According to the theory, obese people differ only in having a higher set point, so their control mechanisms work to keep their body fat stores high.

The set-point theory does explain the stability of body weight and its resistance to change. But no scientist has ever measured a set point, and the theory doesn't explain how the control mechanisms work.

Obesity in Perspective

Each theory of obesity contains a kernel of truth, but none is entirely correct. In fact, obesity is not a single disorder but a family of disorders. Although all obese people have excess body fat, their basic problems vary widely: some have predominantly genetic obesity, others metabolic derangements; some overeat, others underexercise; most have more than one factor at work. When it comes to obesity (or, more precisely, to the *obesities*), there is more than enough blame to go around.

Let me offer my own perspective. Obesity is a modern disorder. Rare before the industrial revolution, obesity as we know it today first began to appear in the English upper classes in the eighteenth and nineteenth centuries. With industrialization obesity spread down through society until it is actually most prevalent today in the poorest segments of Western society. Even today, however, obesity is relatively uncommon in underdeveloped countries.

What accounts for these shifts? Obesity has its behavioral and psychological explanations. It has its metabolic and genetic causes. But it also has important cultural and historical determinants.

Like so many of the preventable illnesses that fill the pages of this book, obesity is a disorder of bodily abuse and disuse. Both are culturally determined. The abuse is dietary, not only in how many calories we eat but in *what kind* of calories we eat. The disuse is physical, reflecting how little we do with our bodies.

Human genetics evolved to cope best with a diet low in fat and high in fiber. Societies that have retained that diet have remained lean. But societies that have switched to refined foods high in fat and sugar have grown corpulent. Fat is the most calorie-dense food, containing 9 calories per gram. In addition, it's easier for the body to store calories from fat than from other sources. Only 3 percent of the calories in dietary fat are burned when it's metabolized to triglyceride for storage in fat cells. But the process of converting dietary carbohydrate into body fat uses up 23 percent of its calories. Not all carbohydrates, however, are equally "safe." Refined, sugary foods with lots of simple carbohydrates are much more calorie-dense than foods composed of complex carbohydrates; sugary foods, too, contribute to obesity.

Human genetics evolved to cope best with a lifetime of physical work. Labor-saving devices have changed our ways: mental work has replaced physical labor. Many benefits have accrued from this progress, but despite all our marvelous technology, health has in many ways suffered, in no small part because body fat has burgeoned.

You don't have to look into prehistory to document these changes, nor do you have to study tribes deep in the rain forest. Our own recent experience tells the tale. In 1900 30 percent of the energy used by American factories and farms was supplied by human labor; today manpower accounts for less than 1 percent. In 1900 the proportion of fat in the American diet was 27 percent; it's now about 40 percent. In 1900 most Americans were lean; now 20 percent are obese. We've become lazy, we've grown fat, and we have created an epidemic of new diseases brought on by our bodily abuse and disuse.

Our genetics have not changed in just 100 years. Metabolic defects cannot be so much more prevalent now than in our great-grandparents' day. Humankind has not changed, but our world and our habits have changed — drastically so.

Obesity has only one really effective long-term treatment. Like so many other aspects of prevention, it's simply a matter of going back to basics. In twentieth-century America that's easier said than done. But you can lose weight — if you need to. How can you tell if you are actually overweight?

Evaluating Your Body Weight and Fat

Are you too fat? There are many ways to get an answer. Health care professionals can give you an extremely accurate response by measuring your skin-fold thickness or by using bioelectric impedance (a newer and better test) to calculate your percent of body fat. Or you could go whole hog and have the Cadillac of tests (at a luxury-car price), a magnetic resonance image, which can measure your internal fat as well as your skin fat. But you can also evaluate yourself, using three much easier tests.

The traditional method is the simplest, but it is the least accurate.

Height and weight tables have guided us for decades. The Metropolitan Life Insurance Company's charts have set the standard since 1949. Revised in 1959 and 1983, they derive "ideal" or "desirable" body weight figures from reams of actuarial data that evaluate longevity as a function of height and weight. The major drawback to these statistics is that they depend on body *weight* instead of body fat. Still, the Metropolitan Life tables can be useful. They're easy to use, and they'll certainly give you a ball-park evaluation of where you stand. You can evaluate yourself by comparing your height and weight with the standards in table 12-2.

A better way to evaluate your body composition is to use the Body Mass Index, but it involves math as well as measurements. Here's the formula:

$$Body\ Mass\ Index = \frac{body\ weight\ in\ kilograms}{(height\ in\ meters)^2}$$

Don't panic — the formula isn't as formidable as it looks. Let's go through it step by step.

A. First, weigh yourself without clothing. Next, divide your weight in pounds by 2.2. The result is your weight in kilograms.

B. Now measure your height without shoes. Next, divide your height in inches by 39.4. The result is your height in meters. To square this number, just multiply it by itself.

C. Finally, divide A by B. The result is your Body Mass Index.

As an example, we can calculate my Index. I weigh 166 pounds. Dividing by 2.2, I find that I weigh 75.4 kilograms. I am 6 feet 1 inch tall, which equals 73 inches. Divided by 39.4, my height is 1.85 meters. The square of 1.85 is 3.42. My weight, 75.4, divided by 3.42 = 22, my Body Mass Index.

Twenty-two is just a number; does it mean that I am lean or that I am hefty? Let's compare it with the standards derived for healthy young adults by the Second National Health and Nutrition Examination Survey (see table 12-3).

In chapter 2 I confessed to being thin (some would say scrawny); now you can see that I wasn't kidding.

For ease of use the Metropolitan Life tables are fine. For precision the Body Mass Index is best. But for evaluating your health risk, I urge you to use another evaluation technique, the waist-to-hip ratio. Both the measurements and the math are easy. Using an ordinary tape, measure your waist at the navel, where it is narrowest, and your hips at the bony prominences, where they are widest. Then simply divide the numbers:

$$ratio = \frac{waist\ size\ in\ inches}{hip\ size\ in\ inches}$$

The calculation is easy enough that I won't bother you with my figures. The calculation is important enough that you should determine your own ratio.

This simple ratio is important because it evaluates the distribution of body fat. Not all fat is equally hazardous to health; remember that abdomi-

Table 12-2. Ideal Weight (in pounds)

MEN

Height		Small Frame	Medium Frame	Large Frame
Feet	Inches			
5	1	112–120	118–129	126–141
5	2	115–123	121–133	129–144
5	3	118–126	124–136	132–148
5	4	121–129	127–139	135–152
5	5	124–133	130–143	138–156
5	6	128–137	134–147	142–161
5	7	132–141	138–152	147–166
5	8	136–145	142–156	151–170
5	9	140–150	146–160	155–174
5	10	144–154	150–165	159–179
5	11	148–158	154–170	164–184
6	0	152–162	158–175	168–189
6	1	156–167	162–180	173–194
6	2	160–171	167–185	178–199
6	3	164–175	172–190	182–204

WOMEN

Height		Small Frame	Medium Frame	Large Frame
Feet	Inches			
4	8	92– 98	96–107	104–119
4	9	94–101	98–110	106–122
4	10	96–104	101–113	109–125
4	11	99–107	104–116	112–128
5	0	102–110	107–119	115–131
5	1	105–113	110–122	118–134
5	2	108–116	113–126	121–138
5	3	111–119	116–130	125–142
5	4	114–123	120–135	129–146
5	5	118–127	124–139	133–150
5	6	122–131	128–143	137–154
5	7	126–135	132–147	141–158
5	8	130–140	136–151	145–163
5	9	134–144	140–155	149–168
5	10	138–148	144–159	153–173

Modified from data of the Metropolitan Life Insurance Company

Table 12-3. How to Interpret Your Body Mass Index

Result	Body Mass Index	
	Men	Women
Average	24.3	23.1
Overweight	above 27.8	above 27.3
Severely overweight	above 31.1	above 32.3

nal and upper-body fat is much more likely to cause heart disease than is buttock and thigh fat. Women with a waist-to-hip ratio higher than 0.8 have an increased risk of death from heart attacks and strokes; men with ratios above 1.0 are also at risk. And the risk is substantial: men with ratios above 1.0 have twice the death rate of men with ratios below 0.85.

If your ratio is above the danger line, you should begin a program to prevent illness by controlling obesity. For that matter, if your Body Mass Index or Metropolitan Life table tells you that you are too heavy, you should also take action to improve. Even a flunking grade on the simple mirror test is a good reason to reform. Feeling good about your body will help motivate you to take good care of it. It's worth the effort. If you reduce your weight by 10 percent, you'll reduce your risk of cardiovascular disease by 20 percent.

Preventing and Controlling Obesity

If the evaluation of obesity sparks controversy, its treatment starts wars.

Were there a foolproof method to control weight, there would be no dispute — nor would there be any fat people. I don't have any secret formulas; if I did, I too would probably become a fat cat. But as a thin doctor I can offer a sound plan for weight control and health. Far from being a secret, it actually involves the same basic program for prevention that I've used throughout this book.

The human body follows the laws of nature, including the law of thermodynamics. Discounting temporary shifts in body water, your body weight — and body fat — depends on a simple immutable equation:

$$body \ weight = energy \ consumed - energy \ expended$$

Let's examine *both* parts of the energy balance equation; you'll read about them one at a time, but when you begin balancing your own equation, you should get to work on both at once.

Reducing Energy Consumption: Principles

1. *Reduce your caloric intake.* To help plan your menu, you should have a realistic target. Even though each person is different, you can estimate your caloric needs from table 12-4. To lose weight, reduce your caloric consumption below the number listed for your weight. To lose one pound a week, which is what I recommend, reduce your daily intake to 500 calories below

Table 12-4. Average Daily Caloric Requirements for Healthy Adults

Weight	Sedentary		Moderately Active		Very Active	
	Men	Women	Men	Women	Men	Women
100	—	1,300	—	1,800	—	2,700
120	1,800	1,560	2,520	2,160	3,600	3,240
140	2,100	1,820	2,940	2,520	4,200	3,780
160	2,400	2,080	3,260	2,880	4,800	4,320
180	2,700	2,340	3,780	3,240	5,400	4,860
200	3,000		4,200		6,000	
220	3,300		4,620		6,600	

the level that keeps your weight constant. As you can see by looking at the right-hand column, the more you exercise, the easier it is to achieve a negative energy balance of 500 calories a day.

You can turn to table 20-2 to find the caloric content of the foods you eat. Keep a record for several days, then total it up. Even better, simply weigh yourself weekly; if you are not losing a pound each week, reduce your caloric intake *and* increase your caloric expenditure until your energy balance is negative.

2. *Eat less fat.* Many diet plans understand that calories do count; few understand that the *type* of calories you eat is also very important.

There are three important reasons to reduce the fat content of your diet. First, at 9 calories per gram, fat contains more energy than proteins or carbohydrates, which have only 4 calories per gram. Second, your metabolism is more efficient at converting the energy from dietary fat into body fat than it is at storing away calories from carbohydrates or protein. Third, a low-fat diet is excellent for your overall health. And in the final analysis it's even more important to *be* healthy than merely to look healthy.

How much fat should you eat? The answer depends on your goals. In chapter 2 I explained that a 30 percent fat diet is officially recommended for cardiovascular health, but that I recommend 20 percent as a more healthful target. For weight reduction 30 percent is a maximum, but to lose faster you may want to eat less fat, possibly much less. Expert panels are reluctant to endorse a very low-fat diet, but I hardly regard it as a radical recommendation since the *average* American diet in 1900 contained 27 percent fat. Remember, too, that the most healthful diets for heart patients contain less than 10 percent fat.

Chapter 20 details the fat content of common foods and explains how to read food labels. You'll also learn how to calculate the amount of fat, carbohydrate, and protein that you should eat to help prevent disease. Most important of all, you'll learn exactly how to translate grams of nutrients into portions of food — and how to enjoy those foods. But for now table 12-5 can help you estimate the amount of fat you should eat.

The closer your diet matches the top of the left-hand column of table 12-5, the faster you will lose weight. Remember, though, that very low-fat diets are restrictive; most people will have to adjust to them slowly by gradually reducing dietary fat. And before going on any very low-calorie diet, you should have a medical evaluation.

To prevent cardiovascular disease you should be careful about the kind of fat you eat; saturated fat has the greatest risk because it raises blood cholesterol levels. But for weight reduction all fats are equally troublesome, containing 9 calories per gram whether unsaturated or saturated. Still, if you care about your heart as well as your belly, you'll limit your saturated fat intake to one third of your total fat consumption.

3. Eat more complex carbohydrates and fewer simple carbohydrates. Carbohydrates should be the mainstay of your diet, accounting for at least 60 to 65 percent of your calories. Just as there are differences in fats, however, there are differences in carbohydrates. Complex carbohydrates are the starches found in bread, pasta, potatoes, and the like; simple carbohydrates are the much smaller sugar molecules found in candy and other sweets. Because simple carbohydrates do not need to be digested before they're absorbed, they will raise your blood sugar more rapidly, and they will stimulate your pancreas to produce more insulin, the hormone that directs your metabolism to store fat in your cells.

The average American diet currently gets 25 percent of its calories from sugar. No wonder we're overweight!

4. Eat more fiber. Dietary fiber is found in foods containing various plant carbohydrates. Unlike ordinary carbohydrates, however, fiber is not digested by the human intestinal tract. High-fiber foods, therefore, are filling yet low in calories. While helping to make you slender, generous amounts of dietary fiber will also help prevent many serious illnesses, ranging from heart attacks to colon cancer.

To lose weight, and to stay well, your diet should contain at least 30 grams of fiber per day. In our culinary world of refined foods, it's not easy to get enough fiber. But it can be done. Once again the trick is returning to basics with bran, vegetables, and fruits. Chapter 20 will explain the facts about fiber (see table 20-6).

These four simple principles are all you really need to reduce your en-

Table 12-5. Your Daily Fat Intake, in Grams of Fat per Day

Your calories per day	If your dietary fat percentage is:				
	10%	15%	20%	25%	30%
1,000	11	17	22	28	33
1,200	14	20	27	33	40
1,500	17	25	33	42	50
1,800	20	30	40	50	60
2,000	22	33	44	56	66

ergy consumption for weight loss: eat fewer calories, eat less fat, eat more complex carbohydrates but fewer simple sugars, and eat more fiber. A fifth principle is no less important: eat a balanced, healthful diet; good health is more important than slim hips. The weight of the evidence, though, suggests that you can have both.

Reducing Energy Consumption: Practical Tips

1. *Don't diet.* No need to worry — I'm not tempting you with a "get thin quick" scheme. Quite the contrary. I'm asking you to *resist* all such schemes. Almost any diet will work — temporarily. It's relatively easy to lose weight, especially when you're motivated by an upcoming wedding or beach vacation. But it's even easier to regain the weight you've dieted away, and almost all dieters do just that.

Diets are temporary. I'm asking for more — for a permanent change in your eating style *and* exercise patterns. You'll find that slow, progressive changes are easier and more durable than radical diet programs. By making them an enjoyable part of your daily life, your rewards will be permanent.

People who go on diets are doomed to repeat them. You can do better.

2. *Change gradually.* By age 40 the average person has eaten more than 40,000 meals, to say nothing of countless snacks. Eating habits are deeply ingrained; the best way to change them is to target one objective at a time, moving on to the next after it has been achieved.

For example, I often suggest that my patients start with breakfast. Those who don't eat breakfast should. It's an ideal way to increase dietary fiber by eating bran cereal (be sure, however, to read the box carefully so you can pick a brand that really has lots of fiber). Substituting cereal for traditional breakfast foods such as eggs and bacon will reduce your intake of cholesterol, saturated fat, and calories. Switching from doughnuts to whole wheat toast will do the same. Use margarine instead of butter, but use it sparingly. Fruit will enrich your diet with vitamins and other nutrients, and switching from whole milk to skim milk will save you saturated fat and calories. You may not like skim milk at first, but if you gradually change to milk with a 2 percent fat content and then 1 percent, you'll become very satisfied with the taste and texture of low-fat dairy products.

3. *Keep records.* Weigh yourself weekly, and keep a diary of your diet and exercise schedules.

4. *Set realistic goals.* Remember, your aim is to be healthy for a lifetime, not svelte for a month. A pound a week will get you there; losing more than two pounds weekly will increase your risk of recidivism.

5. *Understand your eating patterns.* For most of us hunger is the *least* important trigger for eating. Instead, we eat to release tension, obtain pleasure, or participate in social encounters. Eating is a perfectly acceptable way to relieve stress — unless you need to lose weight or correct an unhealthful diet. If anxiety or depression contributes to your eating problems, deal with them directly instead of using food for temporary relief; chapter 19 will introduce you to some techniques.

6. *Eat regularly.* The wall of my den is graced by a slogan embroidered by my mother: "Never Eat on an Empty Stomach." Her intent may have been humor, occasioned no doubt by my voracious appetite and love of good food. Irony notwithstanding, Mom was right (as usual!). If you don't have a schedule, you're more likely to snack. If you put off a meal until you're starving, you're more likely to gorge. And medical studies have suggested that more frequent eating requires less insulin and is better for blood sugar and cholesterol levels.

7. *Shop prudently.* Plan your menus in advance, and buy only what you should be eating. If a high-fat tidbit makes it to your pantry, it will be dangerously close to your lips. Shop from a list, but never when you're hungry. If your list includes calorie-dense foods for skinny household members, store them in a special place out of your usual kitchen browsing patterns.

8. *Cook only what you actually plan to eat.* Eat only at your table, and eat slowly. Don't leave serving dishes on the table. If your portions are small, serve them on small plates; your eye can help trick your stomach. If you feel hungry after finishing your meal, wait at least 15 minutes before you eat any more; it takes time for food to satisfy your appetite.

9. *Beware of "junk food."* A fast food lunch of a burger, fries, and shake can easily give you more than 1,500 calories, 70 grams of fat, and 2 grams of sodium — more than you need for a whole day. Most commercial snack foods are equally undesirable. Learn to like cut-up carrots instead of chips, air-popped popcorn (without salt or butter) instead of candy, and low-cal beverages instead of alcoholic brews or soft drinks.

10. *Plan in advance* for holidays, parties, and for eating away from home.

11. *Don't get down on yourself if you "cheat."* Nobody is perfect. Don't feel guilty and defeated if you deviate from your plan. Instead, be sure that your plan is realistic, and begin again with renewed enthusiasm and optimism. Allow for ups and downs, but stay pointed in the right direction.

12. *Get help if you need it.* Nutritional counseling, support groups, and weight-loss plans can help. Psychological interventions may be important; in particular, behavior modification (see chapter 19) is one of the most successful medical approaches to obesity. But if you enroll in a plan, be sure it's responsibly administered and nutritionally sound.

13. *Don't try to ignore food.* On the contrary, you'll do best if you think about your food. A diet low in fat and high in complex carbohydrates and fiber can be extremely enjoyable as well as healthful, even if it's low in calories. Take it as a challenge. Learn to cook in new ways. The results can be delicious. Select substitute ingredients that are tasty as well as healthful. Artificial sweeteners are acceptable if they fit into your overall prevention program.

14. *Avoid diet pills, expensive weight-loss plans, and radical remedies.* There are a few exceptions to this rule — but only a few. In *Hamlet* Shakespeare tells us that "diseases desperate grown / by desperate appliances are relieved / or not at all." *Extreme* obesity may require radical remedies. Very low-calorie diets are one option. The "liquid protein" diets of the early

1970s were abandoned because of significant complications, including at least 60 deaths due to cardiac disturbances. Newer low-calorie liquid diets appear safe if they are used for periods of up to three months under the careful supervision of experienced medical teams. They do work, but rebound weight gain is a very common problem, as indeed it is with any rapid weight-loss program. Still, patients who are very obese (more than 60 percent overweight) and have failed with less drastic treatments may wish to discuss very low-calorie diets with their physicians. The most radical remedy of all is surgery. Intestinal bypass operations have been all but abandoned because of complications. Operations that bypass the stomach or restrict its capacity are now being studied. They are still considered experimental, and their utility will probably be quite limited. Surgery is the last resort for extreme obesity.

There is no quick fix.

Health should be near the top of humanity's priority list. But there is more to life than just preventing disease. With thought and planning, a healthful diet can provide plenty of variety and pleasure. You can have your muffin and like it, too.

Increasing Energy Expenditure: Exercise

It seems self-evident that the fattest people eat the most calories. It's self-evident, but it's not true. In fact, numerous studies from around the world demonstrate that the *thinnest* people eat the most calories. For example, the Chinese eat 20 percent more calories per pound of body weight than we do, yet they have 25 percent less body fat. The reason is not all genetic: Asians who move to the West add body fat as their diet changes. Diet is part of the answer: although the Chinese diet has more calories, it has much less fat (15 percent versus 44 percent) and much more complex carbohydrate (77 percent versus 25 percent) and fiber (33 to 77 grams per day versus 11 grams). But the other major difference has nothing to do with diet: it's physical work. Exercise is the secret ingredient that allows the thinnest people to eat the most calories.

It seems self-evident that the fattest Americans spend the most time watching TV. Here the evidence supports the obvious: studies from the University of Arizona reveal that men who spend more than three hours per day in front of the tube are twice as likely to be tubby as men who spend less than one hour each day viewing TV. Sedentary living (and munching) will increase your risk of obesity.

How Exercise Fights Obesity

The most important contribution of exercise is that physical work burns calories. At rest an average 150-pound person burns 70 calories per hour, but vigorous exercise can produce a tenfold increase in caloric expenditure. In chapter 21 you'll learn how to compare the energy consumption of many forms of exercise (see table 21-2).

Exercise burns fat. When performed regularly, aerobic exercise will reduce your body fat content. As a result, you'll look (and feel) better even before your scale shows major progress.

Exercise helps you lose weight by keeping your metabolic rate high even after you finish your workout. By itself, caloric restriction actually *decreases* energy expenditure; in effect, losing weight by dieting alone causes the body to fight against further weight loss by burning up less energy. Exercise helps counteract this resistance by consuming more calories during, and even after, exercise.

Many patients tell me that they are reluctant to exercise because they fear it will stimulate their appetite. It's a logical concern, but it's really not a problem. In fact, exercise can actually reduce appetite — another asset if you're trying to lose weight.

Exercise also helps psychologically. You'll feel better about your body as your physical capacity improves during a continuing program. As your self-image improves, you'll find it easier to make the changes needed to lose weight (and to prevent disease). Nothing succeeds like success.

There is a final way in which exercise may help fight obesity; the evidence is preliminary, but my clinical and personal experiences have made me a believer. Remember that most people, whether obese or lean, tend to maintain a surprisingly constant body weight over the years. Although I don't understand all the mechanisms involved, I do believe that there is a "set point" for body weight, an accurate and powerful internal scale that registers our weight and body fat and then causes us to consume or reject calories, bringing our weight up or down to a predetermined point.

Diets fail in the long run because they don't change the set point; it's easy to lose weight at first, but sooner or later the pounds creep back on. Although I can't prove it scientifically, I believe the weight of the evidence suggests that a regular exercise program *can* alter the set point, reducing it so it won't drive you to nibble your way back to obesity despite your best intentions.

What Kind of Exercise Is Best?

Although it may be hard to fathom all the ways that exercise helps to fight obesity, it's easy to understand what kind of exercise is best. Aerobic exercise is the most beneficial for the body's metabolism, burning fat and calories while improving cholesterol levels and reducing blood sugar and insulin levels. Not coincidentally, it is also aerobic exercise that protects against heart attacks and strokes, lowers blood pressure, lowers the risk of certain cancers, and extends life itself, while improving the quality of those extra years. In chapter 20 you will find detailed instructions for starting an exercise program that is effective, safe, and enjoyable.

A Balanced Energy Equation

For effective and sustained weight control, there is just no substitute for a balanced energy equation. Decreased energy consumption and increased energy expenditure are both necessary. Plan a healthful diet with a reduced intake of fat and calories. Plan a sound exercise program emphasizing aerobics. Plan to achieve both through slow but steady change.

For lasting results, your energy equation should remain balanced throughout your lifetime. It will yield more than simply weight control, producing good health, good fun, and a long life — all reasons why a balanced equation is indeed worth its weight in health.

■ 13 ■

Disorders of the Eyes and Ears

Vision and hearing stand out among humankind's five senses. They're our windows to the world, crucial links between the inner world of the human mind and the external world around us. Healthy eyes and ears are important for success at work and at play, for productivity and pleasure. Diseases that impair vision and hearing cause distress and disability; they may also lead to problems elsewhere in the body by contributing to accidents, dysfunction, and even depression.

Medical specialists can do a lot to treat eye and ear diseases. You can do even more by preventing loss of vision and hearing. It's not difficult; a few guidelines and a little common sense will go a long way toward protecting your senses.

■ The Normal Eye

The eye is a complex apparatus packed into a small space (see figure 13-1). Light enters the eye by passing through a clear protective membrane, the *cornea*. A diaphragm, the *iris*, can open to admit light or narrow to screen out harsh rays. The eye's *lens* focuses the light, transmitting it backwards through the *vitreous*, fluid that is normally clear and transparent. Next, light waves arrive at the *retina*, where special cells translate the energy of light into electrical impulses. The *optic nerve* carries the impulses to the brain, where they are finally decoded into the images we call vision. A set of ocular muscles moves the eye and sharpens its focus.

As if in recognition of the importance of vision, the body has taken steps to protect the eye. In the blink of an eye, the lids can close to exclude foreign bodies or dangerously strong light. Tears keep the cornea moist, washing away tiny objects that could injure it and providing antibodies and chemicals to fight infection. The pressure in the eye's fluid-filled chambers is carefully regulated to prevent damage. A network of blood vessels in the retina provides oxygen and nutrients while removing toxic wastes. And the entire eye is surrounded by the *orbit*, a strong set of bones that protect against trauma.

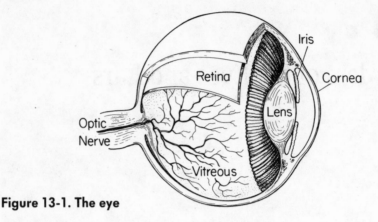

Figure 13-1. The eye

Unfortunately, even these elaborate protective mechanisms sometimes fail. But you can bolster them to prevent eye disorders and visual loss.

■ Eye Disorders

Eye Trauma

It doesn't take a speeding truck or a heavyweight's punch to cause serious eye injury; a fleck of metal or a tennis ball can do plenty of damage.

Two and one half million Americans suffer eye injuries each year; 50 percent occur at work, 25 percent at home. Although many of these injuries are mild, 30,000 are severe enough to require hospitalization. Even with hospital treatment, eye injuries can be very serious: at least 1 million Americans suffer permanently impaired vision in one or both eyes because of accidents and trauma. Don't join their ranks. Simple measures will go a long way toward preventing eye injuries.

Eye injuries come in many forms. Small objects, ranging from a fragment of glass or metal to a fingernail, are able to cause corneal abrasions, or scratches. Although these injuries usually heal well with treatment as simple as an eye patch, scars may result, especially if recovery is complicated by infection. Corneal scars can produce permanent visual impairment. Another common result of trauma is a laceration, or cut, of the eye. Even blunt trauma can cause bleeding into the eye's internal structure, called a hyphema. Both lacerations and hyphemas require surgical treatment. Specialized surgery is also required for one of the most serious of all eye injuries, a retinal detachment; unless the repair is prompt and expert, a retinal detachment can produce blindness. Finally, trauma can break the strong bones of the orbit (the "blow-out fracture") and injure the muscles and nerves that control eye motion.

The most common cause of eye trauma is violence, especially in men younger than 30. Assault and other forms of violence are difficult to prevent. Workplace injuries are easier to anticipate and avoid; in fact, industrial safety standards have reduced substantially the number of occupational eye injuries. Unfortunately, there are no regulations requiring home carpenters, painters, and gardeners to take similar precautions to prevent eye injuries, which still complicate hobbies and work around the house at an alarming rate. Not to be overlooked are sports injuries. The National Society to Prevent Blindness reports that there are more than 25,000 sports-related eye injuries severe enough to require emergency medical treatment every year; racquet sports head the list, with squash and racquetball the most hazardous for your eyes.

You can prevent many injuries by anticipating accidents before they occur, then taking steps to prevent them. In the case of eye trauma, protective glasses or goggles are the extra ingredient that can save your vision.

Ordinary eyeglasses won't do the job; they may even make things worse by giving you a false sense of security. The best safety glasses are made of polycarbonate plastic. They come in varying thicknesses; 3 millimeters is best, but you can get fair protection from the 2-millimeter variety. Be sure to pick a sturdy sports frame, and wear side shields or wraparound goggles if you are working with chemicals or power tools.

Polycarbonate safety lenses can be made to match most corrective eyeglass prescriptions. But if your prescription is one of the few that defy the available optics, try CR-39 plastic, again selecting the 3-millimeter thickness in a sports frame. Plastic lenses won't break easily, but they will scratch; for about $10 an antiscratch coating can help protect your investment in safety glasses.

Wear safety glasses whether or not you need corrective lenses. You are wearing them to protect your vision, not just to correct it. Wear safety glasses or goggles for carpentry, home repairs, and for work with chemicals, solvents, and caustics. Wear them, too, for sports. They are a must for squash and racquetball. Most tennis players do not wear goggles, but they are making a mistake; if you don't believe me, just ask New York Mayor David Dinkins, who was hit in the right eye by an errant ball hit by the mayor of Newark in July 1990. Bicyclists, too, can benefit from safety glasses. You should even consider wearing goggles for basketball — it may be the only way you can be right up there with Kareem Abdul-Jabbar.

Safety glasses are the best ways to protect your eyes from traumatic injuries. A little common sense and care at work and play won't hurt either. And when it comes to sports, a touch of old-fashioned courtesy will complete your prevention program.

All in all, planning and foresight will protect your sight.

Ultraviolet Radiation

Eye trauma lurks behind every racquet on the court, every workbench in the basement — and every cloud in the sky. Some forms of trauma are obvious, while others are insidious and invisible but damaging nonetheless. Ultraviolet injury is an example of hidden trauma.

Sunlight is nature's source of ultraviolet radiation. As we will see in chapter 22, sunlight contains three forms of radiation. The most potent, ultraviolet C, is screened out by the atmosphere. Ultraviolet B also contains lots of energy; because the stratospheric ozone layer is being depleted by man-made pollution with chlorofluorocarbons (CFCs), more and more ultraviolet B rays are reaching our earth — and your eyes. More ultraviolet A rays are also getting through, but they pack the least punch of all.

When it comes to health, ultraviolet B rays are the villains. They carry enough energy to disrupt DNA, the human cell's genetic material. Fortunately, they can't penetrate deep into the body. Unfortunately, they can go deep enough to injure the skin (see chapter 15) and the eye.

The most superficial portion of the eye, the cornea, is the most vulnerable to ultraviolet injury. Even a few seconds of exposure will produce injury if the ultraviolet radiation is very intense. Because welding generates such intense ultraviolet radiation, special goggles are mandatory to prevent "welder's flash."

Even ordinary sunlight can injure the cornea, causing photokeratitis ("sun blindness"); because snow reflects back 80 percent of sunlight's ultraviolet energy, sun injury is a greater risk on a bright winter day ("snow blindness") than in the haze of August. Whether in winter or summer, the result is the same: ultraviolet damage to the cornea produces pain and redness in the eye, usually accompanied by light sensitivity, excessive tearing, uncontrollable blinking, and a gritty or sandy feeling. The symptoms usually begin 4 to 12 hours after exposure. Because the cornea has a wonderful capacity for self-repair, the damage generally resolves in one or two days, even without special treatment.

Because the cornea is so thin, ultraviolet rays can pass right through it to the lens. The lens, however, absorbs the remainder of the ultraviolet energy, transmitting only visible light to the retina.

Does ultraviolet radiation damage the lens? The traditional answer was no. But new research has shed a different light on the question. Unlike the cornea, the lens lacks the capacity for self-repair, so even minimal ultraviolet damage persists. Repeated sun exposures cause additional damage, which accumulates. Over the years sun injury can make the lens opaque, forming a cataract.

You don't have to stay in the shade to prevent photokeratitis and cataracts; you can wear shades. Now faddishly fashionable, sunglasses actually *do* have an important role in preventing ultraviolet eye injuries.

You might think you can get maximum protection simply by choosing the darkest possible glasses. But it's not necessarily so; lens color does not predict ultraviolet absorbency. Even mirrored lenses vary unpredictably in their ability to screen the eye from ultraviolet radiation.

Fortunately, a new rating system will make it easy for you to pick the sunglasses that are best for you. "Cosmetic" lenses are the least protective, absorbing only 70 percent of ultraviolet B, 20 percent of ultraviolet A, and 60 percent of visible light. "General purpose" lenses are the best buy for most outdoor activities, absorbing at least 95 percent of ultraviolet B, 60 percent of ultraviolet A, and 60 to 90 percent of visible light. For intense exposures, such as bright sun reflected off snow or sand, wear "special purpose" lenses; they absorb more than 99 percent of ultraviolet B.

Even if you don't like wearing dark lenses, you can still get protection from ultraviolet rays; clear lenses can be specially coated to screen them out. But you don't need to use coated lenses for protection indoors; although fluorescent bulbs, TV screens, and computer screens do produce ultraviolet rays, they do not emit enough energy to damage the eye.

For outdoor protection, large lenses are best. Choose a frame that places the lens close to your eye. The frame should be comfortable and should fit well — the goal, after all, is to protect not your forehead but your eyes.

Protect your eyes from the sun. It's the bright thing to do.

Cataracts

Cataracts are the leading cause of impaired vision in older Americans. Beginning with mild clouding of the lenses, cataracts progress slowly over the years. As the lenses become more opaque, vision becomes progressively blurry; at first only night vision is affected, but eventually even bright light won't penetrate dense cataracts.

Eye surgery can do wonders for cataracts, removing damaged lenses and replacing them with clear plastic implants. About 1.2 million cataract operations will be performed in the United States this year, at a cost of $3.4 billion. But you can do even better by taking steps to keep your natural lenses clear.

There are two ways to prevent cataracts. The first is already familiar: protect your lenses from ultraviolet radiation by wearing appropriate sunglasses. The second may be a surprise: you may be able to keep your lenses healthy by eating a healthy diet.

Two 1991 studies, both by scientists in Boston, suggest that vitamins may help prevent cataracts. A study of 1,380 adults found that diets low in vitamins increased cataract risk, and that supplementary vitamin pills reduced risk by 37 percent. A smaller study found that people who ate the smallest amounts of fruits and vegetables were six times more likely to develop cataracts than people who ate lots of vitamin-rich foods.

It's too early to recommend daily vitamins to prevent cataracts; we'll need additional studies to confirm these initial observations and to tell us which vitamins to take and when to start taking them. But it's not too early to recommend eating plenty of vitamin-rich foods.

Amblyopia

If you can read these words, you don't have to worry about amblyopia. But if you have young children, you should think about it, since amblyopia is a preventable cause of visual loss in early childhood.

We have two eyes but only one brain. The motion of both eyes must be perfectly coordinated so the brain will get just one image. In addition, the lenses of both eyes must focus similarly, so that the two images will be congruent.

A mature brain is able to cope with two disparate images, temporarily suppressing one and interpreting the other as total vision; nearsighted adults can even wear one contact lens focused for reading while the other is adjusted for distance without confusing their brain.

Young children, however, handle mismatched images differently, suppressing one of the two so completely that one retina loses its ability to transmit clear images to the brain. Fortunately, the other eye retains normal vision, but the eye that does not have an adequate visual experience during early childhood can suffer a permanent loss of visual acuity.

Amblyopia, or "lazy eye," occurs when a young child's eyes transmit different images. This may be caused by markedly unequal focusing or by an imbalance of the eye's muscles. Early detection and treatment can help. If your child seems to be having eye problems, have an ophthalmological evaluation as early as possible; children born prematurely may benefit from an examination as young as six months of age. But even children with apparently normal vision should have an evaluation at about age three. Many abnormalities can be treated effectively with measures as simple as eyeglasses, eye patches, or eye exercises; advanced problems may require surgery, but permanent visual impairment can be prevented if corrective steps are taken before age five.

Glaucoma

Affecting nearly 1.5 million Americans, glaucoma is a common disease. It's also a serious disease, causing 5,000 cases of severe visual loss each year; in all, some 70,000 people in this country are legally blind because of glaucoma. Early detection and treatment would have preserved vision for most of these patients.

The chambers of the eye are filled with fluid (see figure 13-1). Produced in the eye itself, this fluid must be renewed constantly to provide nutrients to the eye's tissues. The fluid drains out near the front of the eye, taking waste products with it. Normally the rate of fluid production and removal are balanced. But if the drainage is too slow, excess fluid builds up in the eye. The extra fluid increases the pressure within the eye; glaucoma is nothing more than high pressure in the eye.

Severe pain will result if the eye's pressure shoots up abruptly. But in most cases of glaucoma the pressure increases only slowly, so there is no discomfort of any kind. At first vision is entirely normal, but over time the optic nerve is damaged by excess pressure, causing vision to deteriorate. Even this visual loss can be hard for a patient to recognize, since it starts with peripheral vision and progresses very gradually. Eventually, however, central vision is also compromised. By then it's too late to restore sight; the optic nerve damage is permanent, and there is no way to reverse it or improve vision.

Glaucoma can be treated. Most often, simple drops will reduce the eye's pressure to normal. In some cases pills are also needed; in others eye surgery may be required. Whatever method is used, treatment halts optic nerve damage, preventing visual loss.

Rare before age 40, glaucoma is progressively more common with advancing years; as many as 3 percent of all persons over 65 are affected. In addition to age, factors that increase the risk of glaucoma include a family history of glaucoma, previous eye trauma, diabetes, and nearsightedness. Glaucoma is more common in blacks than whites.

Glaucoma cannot be prevented; but its consequence, blindness, can be avoided by early treatment. Successful secondary prevention depends on detecting the disease early, before there are symptoms of optic nerve damage. There are three ways to screen for glaucoma.

The first is simply to look at the optic nerve. It's easier than it sounds. You can see out of your eye, and I can see in by using an instrument called an ophthalmoscope. Glaucoma produces an asymmetry between the two optic nerves; the nerve most affected by pressure will look notched or irregular and deeply cupped. I look at the optic nerves of all my patients during their comprehensive physical exams, and your primary care doctor should check yours. The problem with this test, though, is that it detects glaucoma only *after* the optic nerve is damaged, at least to some degree.

Another way to screen for glaucoma is to evaluate vision — not just visual acuity using a normal eye chart but also peripheral vision. But this test, too, detects glaucoma only after it has started to injure the nerve. There should be a better way — and there is.

The gold standard of glaucoma screening is tonometry, a test that directly measures the eye's pressure. First, drops are used to anesthetize the cornea. Next, the tonometer is placed gently on the eye to read the pressure. Pressures higher than 22 are generally considered abnormal, but many people with mildly elevated pressures will escape optic nerve damage even if they are not treated. Tonometry was used to detect President Bush's early asymptomatic glaucoma, which appeared at age 65 in April 1990.

Tonometry is quick and safe. It is also easy — if you know how to do it. When I began in medical practice, I set out to screen my patients for glaucoma with tonometry. My patients and I rapidly concluded that the job would be better done by a friendly eye doctor. Indeed, I think eye care specialists are best equipped to screen for glaucoma, and ophthalmologists are the only people who should treat the disease.

How often should you be checked for glaucoma? The exact guidelines are debated. I think it's reasonable to have an initial evaluation at age 40, to repeat the process every two to three years until 50, and to be checked every one to two years thereafter. If your exams are abnormal or if you have glaucoma risk factors, you will benefit from more frequent exams at intervals determined by your doctor.

Diabetic Retinopathy

Patients with diabetes are at risk for developing blood vessel abnormalities. Unfortunately, the blood vessels of the retina are frequently affected. Diabetes is responsible for 35,000 cases of blindness in this country. Photocoagulation and laser treatments can slow the process, often preventing blindness. All patients with diabetes should be under the care of an ophthalmologist.

■ Ear Disorders

The ear has two important functions. One is highly publicized, the other often overlooked. We all credit the ear with the sense of hearing, but few of us realize that it's also crucial for the sense of balance.

A highly specialized structure, the ear is divided into three parts (see figure 13-2). Sound waves first enter the *outer ear*, which is little more than a passive sound-collecting channel. Next, the waves strike the eardrum, or *tympanic membrane*, causing it to vibrate. The vibrations are transmitted through the *middle ear* along a short chain of three small bones, the hammer, anvil, and stirrup. Finally, in the inner ear these vibrations reach the *auditory nerve*, which translates them into electrical signals for transmission to the brain. The inner ear also contains three semicircular canals which function as a gyroscope, controlling the body's balance.

I can't tell you how many Americans are out of balance, but I can tell you that over 28 million suffer some hearing impairment. Most serious in children but most common in the elderly, diminished hearing is often blamed simply on old age. Indeed, older people are more likely to be hard of hearing; impairments are present in 23 percent of people between the ages of 65 and 74, 33 percent of those aged 75 to 84, and 48 percent of individuals who've made it past 85.

More than an inconvenience, impaired hearing can produce sensory isolation and contribute to accidents, psychological difficulties, and neurological disorders. Hearing aids can help, but they can be cumbersome, unsightly, expensive, and difficult to use properly. Is there a better answer? Perhaps not at age 80 when the world is already a whisper. But many cases of adult hearing loss are not simply the inevitable consequence of age. Although you don't hear much about it, up to a third of these problems are at least partially preventable. Far from being a secret, one culprit is loud and clear throughout the industrialized world: noise.

Acoustic Trauma

The eyes are designed to admit light but can be damaged by ultraviolet radiation from the sun. The ears are designed to admit sound but can be damaged by excessive sound; far from being celestial in origin, however, the excess emanates from our fellow humans and the machines at their disposal. Acoustic trauma is a twentieth-century man-made disorder.

More than 20 million Americans are exposed recurrently to noise levels that are strong enough to damage hearing; more than 70 million have substantial permanent hearing impairment as a result.

Loud noise damages the most sensitive part of the ear, the auditory nerve. Unfortunately, the nerve is also the part of the ear least able to repair

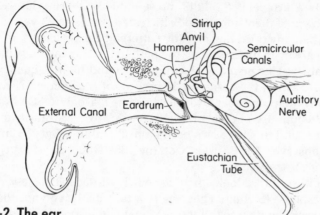

Figure 13-2. The ear

itself. Mild acoustic trauma can produce blurry sounds, buzzing noises, or hearing deficits that improve in time. But more severe acoustic trauma actually kills nerve cells, resulting in permanent hearing loss, particularly for upper-register sounds.

How loud is loud? Damage to the ear depends on the intensity of a sound and the duration of exposure.

Intensity is measured on the decibel scale. Zero is the threshold of hearing; 30 is exemplified by a whisper; 60 by normal conversation; 90 by the sound of a lawn mower, shop tools, or heavy traffic; 100 by a chainsaw or snowmobile; 110 by sand-blasting equipment, the blare of a car's horn, or a "good" rock concert; and 140 by a gunshot, jet engine, or siren.

The spoken voice may not always be pleasant; it may give you a headache, but it won't damage your ears because sounds below 75 decibels are harmless. But sounds of only 85 decibels can cause hearing loss if your exposure is prolonged — perhaps two hours daily. And louder sounds will damage your ears much more quickly. At 100 decibels even 15 minutes a day can be harmful, and at 140 decibels even a single exposure can cause deafness.

Occupational exposure is the most common cause of noise-induced hearing loss. Construction workers, factory workers, policemen, firefighters, military personnel, farmers, and truck drivers are at risk. And yes, musicians are also vulnerable. Noise is noise, no matter what it sounds like.

Workers should be protected by noise abatement standards; sadly, the EPA abandoned its Office of Noise Abatement and Control in 1982. Routine hearing tests and protective devices can also protect workers. But the rest of us are on our own.

Unfortunately, most people neglect to protect their ears. Teenagers are a particular concern. Personal headphone stereos can easily generate sound levels of 100 decibels, comparable to the volume of a pneumatic drill. And rock concerts often generate sounds (or may I say noise?) at the 115-decibel level.

Formerly a problem of adults, noise-induced hearing loss is increasingly a problem of the young. One British study of 15- to 23-year-olds found that more than one third had already suffered hearing loss! And the youth of America are even further along the path to hearing loss: a study of 1,410 freshmen at the University of Washington found high-frequency hearing loss in 73 percent of the men and 52 percent of the women. Acoustic self-mutilation by the young seems to have become a tribal rite. Dr. Walter Brattain laments "the use of solid-state electronics by rock musicians to raise the level of sound to where it is both painful and injurious." Hardly a disinterested observer, Dr. Brattain won the 1956 Nobel physics prize for his invention of the transistor.

The auditory future looks grim for our high-decibel society. And since the usual response to blunted hearing is to turn up the volume, the problem is likely to reverberate into the future. What can be done to prevent it?

First and foremost, turn down the volume. Audiologically speaking, at least, the spoken voice is no threat. But amplified music can be. Learn to enjoy it at reasonable levels. You can turn down the volume knob at home, but you'll need some help to control your exposure to loud sounds at work. This is one issue, though, that you should speak up about. The Occupational Safety and Health Administration established hearing conservation standards in 1983, and they should be enforced. But acoustic trauma is a risk far beyond the concert hall, the home, and the workplace. Many potentially traumatic sounds emanate from our increasingly mechanized environment, and community action will be needed to turn them down. Noise pollution is everywhere, but like other forms of pollution, it can be cleaned up. Our ears should be protected from excessively noisy airplanes, trucks and buses, automobile horns, sirens, construction sounds, and the like. Together we should invite the Environmental Protection Agency back into the noise-control business, enlisting state and local authorities as well. We should also find a way to encourage our kids to turn down the volume on their portable amplifiers; I fear this will require the intervention of an authority even higher than the EPA.

The second way to protect your ears from acoustic trauma is to listen to your body — literally. If loud sounds make your ears ring or hurt, you may be suffering from acoustic trauma. An even more worrisome symptom is partial deafness after exposure to loud sounds; even if you recover within a few hours, you should certainly avoid repeated exposures to loud sounds. The most troublesome symptom of all is high-frequency hearing loss, which may first produce problems understanding a female voice on the phone or detecting differences between words that have similar high-pitched sounds (s, f, sh, h, soft c). Don't ignore these warning signals — the next signal may be harder to hear!

The third step you can take is to wear hearing protectors. You don't need a sound meter to know what noises are worth muffling. If a sound is so loud that you'd have to shout to make yourself heard over it, it's loud enough to cause acoustic trauma. To protect yourself, don't just stuff cotton balls or wads of paper into your ears; they are poor sound insulators, reducing noise by only 7 decibels, and you run the risk of damaging your eardrum any time you introduce a foreign body into your ear. But you can buy efficient ear plugs, which can even be custom fitted. If you find ear plugs uncomfortable, consider protective earmuffs. Plugs and muffs can reduce sound levels by up to 30 decibels; if you're exposed repeatedly to sounds louder than 105 decibels, you should consider wearing both. Don't worry about aesthetics — just think of hearing protectors as sunglasses for your ears.

A fourth way to prevent noise-induced hearing loss is worth considering, even though its efficacy is unproven. A recent study in guinea pigs demonstrated that vitamin A deficiency greatly enhanced susceptibility to acoustic trauma. We don't yet know if a good diet can help protect human hearing, but given our teenagers' proclivity for both loud music and junk food, I hope they won't turn a deaf ear to the possibility.

A final, more serious note about noise pollution: recent human studies suggest that the hazards of exposure to excessive sounds may extend far beyond the ear itself. In Germany children exposed to noise from low-flying jet planes were found to have abnormally high blood pressure levels as well as high-frequency hearing loss. In Israel elderly nursing home residents increased their blood pressure levels by an average of 18 points in response to the noise from low-flying jets. Noise pollution is a problem for people of all ages in all parts of the industrialized world, and it has the potential to affect many parts of the body.

Physical Trauma

The ear is as vulnerable to mechanical trauma as acoustic trauma. Your ears will benefit from everything you can do to prevent head trauma and accidents. You can also protect your delicate eardrum by obeying the obvious rule that you should never put a foreign object in your ear canal (your mother was right, again!). Finally, consider this jarring note: a preliminary 1990 study by Dr. Michael Weintraub suggests that extended periods of high-impact aerobics may injure the inner ear, causing temporary dizziness, buzzing sounds, or muffled hearing. Much more data will be needed to evaluate the significance of this observation. Until it's available, it's surely advisable for you to stay tuned for messages from your ears, exercising restraint if they complain about aerobics.

Ear Infections

Although much less serious than in the days before antibiotics, ear infections are still common and troublesome. They may involve any of the three portions of the ear (see figure 13-2). Preventive measures are often effective for external ear infections, sometimes helpful for middle-ear infections, but only rarely useful for inner-ear infections.

Infections of the external ear have much in common with skin infections. The ear canal normally harbors a variety of bacteria and fungi. These microbes are harmless unless the skin of the ear canal is injured, allowing the bugs to gain a toehold. The most common predisposing factor is moisture, which macerates the skin, providing an unfortunately hospitable environment for infection. This sequence may sound familiar to you even if you've never had an external ear infection because these same events lead to athlete's foot. It's no coincidence, perhaps, that the common name for external ear infection is swimmer's ear.

Swimmer's ear is not a serious infection, but it can be very uncomfortable. The ear canal becomes crusted and irritated; although the eardrum is normal, enough debris can accumulate in the ear canal to muffle hearing. Swimmer's ear is itchy, sometimes maddeningly so, and it can be quite painful when the ear is tugged or moved.

Despite its name, swimmer's ear is not confined to aquatic athletes. All it takes to produce an external ear infection is moisture retained in the ear canal. Bathing, showering, or even a good old-fashioned scrubbing can do the job.

Prevention is simple: keep your ears scrupulously clean and dry. But swimmers should also consider wearing ear plugs, particularly if they've had this infection in the past. Finally, if you are plagued by recurrent swimmer's ear, you can use eardrops to prevent relapses; ask your doctor for Corticosporin or VoSol, the medications that are used to treat external ear infections.

Unlike external ear infections, middle-ear infections are often accompanied by fever and intense pain. Antibiotics will control the process, but they must be administered in pill form rather than in eardrops. Without antibiotic treatment, middle-ear infections can produce hearing loss, chronic infection, and other complications.

The middle ear is connected to the back of the throat by the eustachian tube, which must be open to prevent pressure from building up in the ear. An open tube is also important to prevent infection. The eustachian tube is narrow in children, so it tends to block up, trapping the bacteria that cause middle-ear infection.

Middle-ear infections are less common in adults precisely because the tube is wider. But allergies or viral upper respiratory infection can narrow the tube. You can't do much to prevent these problems, but you can take steps to prevent the third situation, which can close the tube: barotrauma. No, it's not a form of noise injury inflicted by a baritone; it's an abrupt change in barometric pressure that closes the eustachian tube, allowing fluid to build up. The fluid in turn causes discomfort, dulls hearing, and provides a safe haven for bacteria. To help prevent middle-ear infections, use decongestants before airplane trips or scuba diving.

The inner ear is a world of its own. Infections and inflammation here don't cause pain or fever; instead they produce buzzing and dizziness, sometimes accompanied by nausea and vomiting. Usually caused by viruses, these infections generally resolve on their own in less than a week. Antihistamine-like medications can lessen the dizziness, but they won't speed recovery. Nor is there any way to prevent these pesky, sometimes debilitating inner-ear problems.

Hearing Tests

We all hear a lot about screening tests to detect early disease in the hopes of preventing progression and complications. Hearing tests are widely recommended and are very useful when ear symptoms are present. But should hearing tests be part of your preventive maintenance routine?

The answer is no; but there are two exceptions. Good hearing in childhood is essential for the acquisition of speech and language. It would seem logical, then, to recommend hearing tests for all youngsters. It is logical — but it's not practical. Routine hearing tests are just not accurate in infancy, when hearing defects do their real harm. To evaluate hearing very early in life, a sophisticated test called the auditory brainstem response is needed. Because this test requires special equipment and is expensive, it can't be performed on every child. Instead, it should be reserved for young children who seem to lag in development and for those at high risk of hearing impairment (family history of deafness, prematurity, certain early childhood infections, and birth defects).

Hearing tests are not necessary for older children and adults unless they are exposed to acoustic trauma or have symptoms of hearing loss. But there is a second exception, applying not to the young but to the elderly. Older people may develop a nonspecific problem called failure to thrive; symptoms include social isolation, depression, weight loss, and apathy. Sensory deprivation can contribute to this problem. Older people may be unaware that the world around them is muffled and dim, so they should have tests to evaluate both hearing and vision.

There are legitimate grounds for debate about routine hearing tests, but I hope you'll find these guidelines sound. Doctors who disagree are entitled to sound off, but I hope they'll also join me in listening carefully for new developments.

■ 14 ■

Disorders of the Teeth, Mouth, and Throat

Oh, those pearly whites.

Most visible in a brilliant smile, your teeth are every bit as important for your health as they are for your appearance. Your teeth are highly specialized structures that are essential for the proper processing of solid food. The digestive process starts not in your stomach but in your mouth — and strong teeth begin the entire procedure when food is chewed into small pieces that can be mixed with saliva and swallowed. Healthy teeth are also important for interpersonal relationships, influencing speech as well as appearance.

Teeth are the only human structures that are completely replaced during normal growth and development. Children develop a complete set of 20 deciduous or "baby" teeth which are shed and replaced by a set of 32 secondary or "permanent" teeth. Unfortunately, adult teeth are often permanent in name only; without proper preventive care, dental decay and periodontal disease often produce tooth loss. Pain, unsightliness, inconvenience, and expense are the usual consequences of tooth disease, but malnutrition and infection can be even more serious results. All of this is preventable; by taking proper care of your teeth at home and getting good preventive care, you'll keep your teeth and gums healthy throughout life.

■ Normal Teeth

Like the tip of an iceberg, the enamel-covered crowns of your teeth are the visible portions of deep and complex structures (see figure 14-1).

Teeth are anchored deep in the jaw, where they are surrounded by a special type of bone, called *alveolar bone*. Alveolar bone forms the sockets that support teeth, but the relationship is one of mutual dependence; if teeth are diseased or lost, alveolar bone thins and weakens.

Although healthy bone is essential to support the teeth, it does not have to do this important job all alone. The supporting cast also includes the *cementum* (a special calcium-rich tissue that surrounds the tooth root), the *periodontium* (soft connective tissue that encircles the cementum and joins the tooth root to its bony socket), and the *gingiva*, or gums (soft tissues that cover alveolar bone and surround the crown). The supporting tissues are

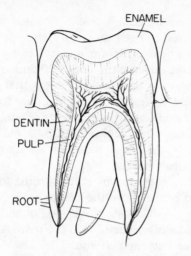

Figure 14-1. Tooth

essential for dental health; because they are metabolically active tissues with rapidly renewing cells, they depend on sound nutrition and good general health as well as on oral hygiene to function optimally.

The teeth themselves are composed of roots and crowns. The roots extend deep into the jawbone, where they attach firmly into the sockets. But the roots are more than simple anchors; they also contain the blood vessels that nourish teeth, the nerves that sound such piercing alarms of dental disease, and the tooth pulp. All of this is capped by the tooth crown, which is composed of an inner layer of *dentin* and an outer layer of tough, white, calcium-rich *enamel*. Dentin and enamel depend on the body's nutrition and health until the crowns erupt from the jaw; this means that dietary deficiencies and excesses can harm the enamel from before birth to adolescence, when the wisdom teeth finally emerge. But once the crowns have erupted, enamel depends for its health on local conditions in the mouth instead of relying on the whole body's nutrition and metabolism.

■ Dental Diseases

Two major problems affect the teeth: tooth decay and periodontal disease. Together they have a substantial impact on health and productivity. An estimated 10 percent of American adults have lost all their teeth; in the elderly the figure is 40 percent. Each year in the United States dental diseases account for 1 million lost schooldays, 2 million lost workdays, 4 million days of bed disability, and 11 million days of restricted activity. Dental expenses exceed $30 billion annually, and even this staggering figure does not include the burden of pain and worry caused by dental conditions — most of which are preventable.

Tooth Decay

Tooth decay, or dental caries, begins on the outside surface of the enamel but can progress to destroy the entire tooth. Decay is caused by bacteria.

An invisible film of bacteria, called dental plaque, coats the teeth. When these bacteria are allowed to feast on sugars, they produce acids that eat into dental enamel, removing calcium and softening the tooth. Without treatment, decay burrows through the entire thickness of enamel. Because the underlying dentin is softer than enamel, decay that penetrates deep into the tooth extends rapidly, undermining enamel until it collapses. Tooth decay usually goes unnoticed until this stage; it is painless and subtle until the enamel collapses to create a visible cavity. But even though cavities may seem to appear suddenly, the decay has been eating away at enamel and dentin long before symptoms occur.

Unfortunately, tooth decay doesn't stop with the formation of a cavity. Instead, it continues to burrow into the dental pulp. Now, in proximity to the nerve, dental decay produces sensitivity to hot and cold foods and beverages and to foods that cause reactions in the pulp. As pressure builds on the nerve itself, pain can become extreme.

Without treatment, tooth decay can continue to spread into the tooth root, periodontium, and bone. Here the process slows, but it does not stop. Over months and years the root and socket are slowly destroyed until the tooth is lost. Without a tooth to stimulate it, alveolar bone is resorbed so that adjacent teeth shift and the bite becomes disturbed. Even worse, infections can spread from tooth root abscesses to other parts of the body, including the lungs and the brain; though uncommon, these infections are disastrous.

Tooth decay can begin when the first teeth erupt in infancy; by two years of age about 10 percent of children have at least one cavity. The risk of decay increases over the years. Without prevention, more than 90 percent of adolescents have tooth decay by age 17, affecting an average of 8 teeth per person. By age 35 the average American has lost one "permanent" tooth to decay and has 10 to 17 decayed or filled teeth.

Tooth decay is a chronic disease. Its damage is irreversible; the body cannot heal decayed teeth, though dentists can restore them, halting further damage. Restoration is obviously far better than pain, infection, and tooth loss. But prevention is best of all.

Preventing Tooth Decay. Although tooth decay is as old as mankind, it is very much a disease of modern culture. Cavities were uncommon before the industrial revolution and are still quite rare in "primitive" societies, until they become "civilized" — hooked on sugary refined foods. Tooth decay *can* be prevented, saving us all enormous amounts of discomfort, time, and expense. And we don't have to return to the primitive world to achieve these benefits; in fact, tooth decay in America has been reduced by about 50 percent over the past 20 years. Excellent progress, but still short of complete prevention, which *is* a realistic goal.

You can prevent tooth decay in three ways: by strengthening your enamel, by fighting oral bacteria, and by improving your nutrition and oral hygiene.

Fluoride. The best way to strengthen enamel is to increase its fluoride content. When fluoride is incorporated into the structure of enamel, it provides great resistance to demineralization caused by bacteria and acid, thus preventing the first steps in tooth decay. Because enamel is formed between birth and age 14 years, childhood is the crucial time for fluoride supplementation.

The benefits of fluoride were first recognized about 50 years ago when dentists noticed that children growing up in communities with naturally fluoridated water had many fewer cavities than children raised in towns with low-fluoride water. Because most water supplies in the United States are fluoride-deficient, fluoride has been added to drinking water since 1945, when Grand Rapids, Michigan, Newburgh, New York, and Brantford, Ontario, led the way. Careful studies in these three communities proved that fluoride supplementation reduces cavities by 50 to 65 percent. These impressive results have been confirmed in more than 150 scientific studies conducted in all parts of the world.

Despite these overwhelmingly favorable results, the fluoridation of drinking water has generated enormous emotional reaction and intense public debate. The controversy was rekindled in early 1990 by headlines proclaiming that fluoride supplementation had been found to produce cancer in rats. In fact bone cancers were found in just four male rats that had been fed fluoride in a concentration 79 times higher than the amount found in drinking water. Moreover, many media reports failed to note that the study involved more than 1,000 animals who remained cancer-free; neither female rats nor mice of either sex developed tumors despite being fed equally high doses of fluoride. And a newer study published in the *Journal of the National Cancer Institute* failed to find *any* evidence of cancer in rats fed more than twice as much fluoride for two years.

Animal studies can be very helpful to screen for the safety of food and water additives. In the case of fluoride, the animal experiments that are best scientifically do *not* confirm a risk of cancer even in extraordinarily high doses. More important, fluoride has been studied in humans for over 50 years. More than 150 studies have been performed and over 35,000 scientific papers have been published. The evidence is incontrovertible: in the doses added to drinking water, fluoride is both effective and *safe.*

Fluoride does not cause cancer in man. In high doses it can cause other side effects, including mottling of teeth and, at very high doses, damage to bones. But to get enough fluoride from drinking water to discolor your teeth or weaken your bones, you'd have to drink about 260 gallons of water per day. In fact, people who drink fluoridated water have stronger bones, less osteoporosis, and fewer fractures than those who don't.

The fluoride controversy is a good example of what can happen when emotion and zeal replace scientific objectivity. Don't let the headlines frighten you; read the whole story and you'll find that the fluoride in your drinking water is safe. Chapter 24 provides some guidelines to help you evaluate medical information appearing in the popular media.

If you are among the 30 percent of Americans who do not drink water containing the recommended one part fluoride per million (1 ppm), you should consider fluoride supplements. The American Dental Association

Table 14-1. Daily Fluoride Supplement for Children

	Age		
Fluoride in your water	birth–2 years	2–3 years	3–13 years
Less than 0.3 ppm	0.25 mg	0.5 mg	1 mg
0.3 to 0.7 ppm	none	0.25 mg	0.5 mg
More than 0.7 ppm	none	none	none

and the American Academy of Pediatrics recommend that you provide fluoride drops or tablets for your children. To calculate the proper dose, first check out your water supply (chapter 22 will tell you how). Then use table 14-1 to find out what's best for your children.

You can also get fluoride in your toothpaste and in mouth rinses. Fluoridated toothpaste makes sense for all children and adults — which is a good thing, since 90 percent of the toothpaste sold in this country is fluoridated. Fluoride mouth rinses are less necessary if you have fluoride in your water, in supplements, or in toothpaste. If you use fluoridated toothpastes or mouth rinses, be sure not to swallow them; they can contain over 1,000 times more fluoride than drinking water, so you could get too much of a good thing. Finally, fluoride can also be applied professionally by your dentist or hygienist; these yearly treatments make most sense for children who are not protected by fluoridated water and for children with active cavity formation.

Fluoride strengthens teeth by increasing their mineral content, helping enamel to resist the harmful effects of bacteria and acid. Fluoride works best on smooth tooth surfaces, but the pits and fissures that are present on every tooth's surface can still provide a fertile ground for cavity formation. Fortunately, there is now a way to protect these tooth surfaces, using professionally applied occlusal sealants.

Sealants. Sealants are thin plastic coatings that can be placed on tooth surfaces without damaging the enamel. Sealants create a mechanical barrier that protects enamel from food debris, bacteria, and acids. They work best on precisely the areas that need protection the most — on pits and fissures. Sealants can reduce cavities by 50 to 100 percent. They should be applied on permanent molars as soon as the pit and fissure surfaces erupt from the gums in children, usually between the ages of four and eight. When properly applied, sealants should last for five or six years; they should be replaced when they're lost, at least until age 25.

Oral hygiene. A fine film of bacteria, called plaque, covers all tooth surfaces from infancy onward. Brushing your teeth removes many bacteria, but they begin to reaccumulate within minutes. In a matter of hours salivary proteins, residual material from food and water, and bacteria form a sticky coating on all tooth surfaces. Dietary sugar fuels the fire, promoting bacterial growth and acid production. Acids eat away enamel, eventually producing tooth decay. In addition, bacterial products injure the gums, leading to gingivitis and periodontitis as well as bad breath. Without preventive action the plaque will begin to accumulate calcium and to harden, eventually producing a tough coating called calculus or tartar. Tartar is great for the bacteria, which continue to multiply deep within the film. And unlike plaque, which can be brushed away, tartar is so tough that you'll need a dentist or hygienist to scale it off.

You can prevent all this.

First, brush your teeth thoroughly at least twice a day. Toothbrushes with soft bristles and rounded contours are easiest on your gums, but the main consideration in picking a toothbrush is to find the one that feels best in your hand and fits best in your mouth. Many brushing techniques have been advocated. To the best of my knowledge, no technique is superior; just be sure you brush all surfaces. You can check your technique by using a disclosing solution to reveal otherwise invisible plaque after you've brushed.

Despite enormous amounts of hype, no toothpaste has been proven superior to the others. Pick the one you like best so you'll use it. Fluoride should be included in the formula, and if you tend to form lots of tartar, look for "anti-tartar" products that contain pyrophosphates. Remember, though, that some toothpastes may be excessively abrasive.

Dental flossing is every bit as important as toothbrushing. In fact, flossing is the key to preventing periodontal disease. Infamous as the most common cause of tooth loss in adults, periodontal disease can actually start in youth. Because of this, flossing should begin in childhood and continue throughout life. Floss at least once a day, spending two to five minutes so that you can maneuver the floss between and around all your teeth. Experiment with waxed and unwaxed floss and with dental tape until you find the preparation that suits you best. Flavored floss is great if it helps motivate you to floss your teeth daily. As with so many aspects of prevention, diligence and technique are more important than flavor and color.

Mouthwash is a big-ticket item for Madison Avenue and the media. The claims that bombard us daily are so extravagant that it's tempting to dismiss them all, to equate mouthwash with hogwash. But antibacterial mouthwashes can reduce oral bacteria, at least in the short run. Listerine was the first brand approved by the American Dental Association; less expensive generic equivalents have subsequently been approved and more are being studied, so you should look for an ADA acceptance seal on your favorite brand. Be on the lookout, too, for new studies evaluating the safety of the alcohol in mouthwash. A preliminary report by Dr. Deborah Winn suggests that regular use of mouthwash containing more than 25 percent alcohol may increase the risk of oral cancer. It's a disquieting possibility, but the data are still tentative. Above all, put mouthwash in perspective: rinsing with an antibacterial mouthwash twice a day may be helpful, but it's no substitute for brushing and flossing.

The peculiarly American fascination with high-tech devices does not stop with oral hygiene, nor does our preoccupation with the quick fix. You can choose among a great variety of water-powered cleansing devices, and you can pay up to $100 for an electric toothbrush. In my view these gadgets are the stationary bicycles of oral hygiene — great if you use them properly and regularly, but useless if they are allowed to collect dust on your bathroom shelf. If you have special problems, your dentist may prescribe a specific device for you. Otherwise, the choice is yours. If high-tech gadgets motivate you to take good care of your teeth, go ahead and use them. But you can do just as well with an old-fashioned toothbrush and a roll of dental floss. Buying high-tech tools won't help unless you use them. After all, dental health, not guilt, is your goal. As usual, successful prevention depends not on good intentions but on good habits.

Preventive Dental Care. Your dentist and dental hygienist can help prevent tooth decay in three ways: by applying occlusal sealants, by applying fluoride if your water supply is not high in fluoride, and by professionally cleaning and scaling your teeth. The first two apply principally to children; in regard to cleaning, there is little scientific evidence that it will add appreciably to excellent home care, but widespread clinical experience supports the tradition of professional prophylactic treatments at regular intervals.

Your dentist can also detect early disease of your teeth and gums. Common sense insists that it's a worthwhile goal, but unfortunately there are no scientific data to tell us how best to go about it. A clinical exam once or twice a year seems reasonable. Dentists also perform routine screening x rays, but they are more controversial. True, x rays can detect cavities before they are visible clinically, but they also expose you to small doses of radiation. Dental health professionals have been unable to agree on what x-ray schedule is best, so individual judgment is required. For children with no cavities, bitewing films every one to two years should suffice; adults with healthy teeth should not need bitewing x rays more often than every one to three years. If active cavities are present, it's reasonable to cut the intervals between x rays in half — but only until cavity formation has ceased. Needless to say, if you have symptoms of dental or periodontal disease, you may need additional films. But even if you're hurting, bitewing or periapical views of the problem areas seem wiser than whole-mouth x rays. When it comes to x rays, I'm not asking you to second-guess your dentist — but I am suggesting that you discuss the question before the films are taken.

How often should you see your dentist? Because there have not been any comparative trials of routine dental care at various intervals, I can't give you an authoritative answer to this simple but important question. But I see no reason to quarrel with clinical tradition. If you have a healthy mouth and a healthy body, a checkup and cleaning every 6 to 12 months seems reasonable. Certain medical conditions also call for dental checkups at least every 6 months; included on this list are abnormal heart valves, insufficient saliva production, and head and neck cancer that has been treated with radiation. Tobacco abuse and heavy drinking are two more reasons for frequent dental visits.

Nutrition and Dental Health. The final element in dental prevention is your diet. I'm sorry to be the bearer of bad tidings about tasty tidbits, but the news should not be a surprise; way back in 1738 Jonathan Swift observed that "sweet things are bad for the teeth," and he was right.

The bacteria on your teeth and gums love sweets every bit as much as you do. They gobble up carbohydrates and metabolize them into acids. Refined sugars are the worst offenders; after you've eaten sweets, your teeth may be coated with acid for up to an hour. You won't feel the acid, but 60 minutes gives it plenty of time to eat at the minerals in your dental enamel.

Sugary foods will increase your risk of tooth decay. Sugar in drinks is neutralized and carried away by saliva relatively quickly, but the phosphoric acid in soda can etch enamel, exposing it to sugar. The sugar in solids lingers on, benefiting your bacteria at the expense of your teeth. Candy is the leading offender, but even "healthy" sweets such as dried fruits will expose your teeth to harmful sugar for long periods of time. In fact, no less an authority than Aristotle observed that eating figs caused rotten teeth in ancient Greece.

You don't have to forsake all sweets to protect your teeth, but you should reduce the amount of sugar you eat; on average, Americans consume 25 percent of their calories in the form of sugar — which is why dentists drive luxury cars. You should also reduce the amount of time that sugary residues remain in your mouth; even if you can't resist that sweet, you can rinse or brush the sugar away shortly afterward.

Fillings. Fluoride, sealants, oral hygiene, good nutrition, and dental care should prevent almost all cavities. Nearly every filling, then, represents a failure of prevention. But do fillings represent more than lost opportunities? Can they actually present a hazard to health?

All that glitters is not silver. The ordinary "silver" amalgam fillings that glint in more than 100 million American mouths are only 35 percent silver. Tin and copper account for 15 percent. Zinc is present in trace amounts. The other 50 percent is mercury, the source of mercurial debate about the safety of amalgam restorations.

The dangers of mercury toxicity have been known since the days of Lewis Carroll's Mad Hatter. In the United States mercury has been banned from felt manufacturing since 1941 and from interior latex paint since 1990. In 1991 the Swedish government prohibited amalgam restorations for pregnant women, but there are no restrictions on amalgam use in American teeth. Should there be?

Mercury that stays put in fillings is entirely safe, but if it's vaporized, it can enter the body. It is true that chewing produces vaporization, and that studies of a few humans have found elevated mercury levels in people with amalgam fillings. It is true, too, that 12 fillings placed in each of six sheep studied in Canada resulted in mercury vaporization. Putting these observations together in December 1990, the TV show "60 Minutes" aired a report titled "Is There Poison in Your Mouth?" The results were predictable, with dental amalgam getting the blame for everything from multiple sclerosis to PMS.

Don't rush out to have your amalgam fillings replaced; instead, chew over a few facts. First, people are not sheep, which spend 15 hours a day chewing on abrasive grains and grasses. Second, even people with extensive amalgam restoration vaporize only 1 to 3 micrograms of mercury per day, less than the 25 micrograms we get daily from food and far less than the 300 to 500 micrograms per day considered safe by the Occupational Safety and Health Administration. Third, careful studies of Swedish patients and American dentists and hygienists have found *no* evidence of disease related to amalgam exposure.

Amalgam has been used in dental fillings for more than 150 years. It's much less expensive than gold, plastic, or ceramic restorations, yet it often outshines the more expensive alternatives in performance. Faced with the mercury debate, the Food and Drug Administration convened a special panel to evaluate amalgam's safety; the unanimous verdict was that the mercury in fillings is safe.

The only element of mystery in the amalgam story is how medical journalism could be allowed to provoke so much unfounded fear. If you have any lingering doubts, ask your doctor to arrange a blood or urine test to measure your mercury levels before you ask your dentist to replace your amalgam restorations.

Periodontal Disease

Periodontal disease is in many ways a mirror image of tooth decay. Cavities begin in the enamel; they are more common in children and are clearly the product of the Westernized life-style. In contrast, periodontal disease begins in the soft tissues that support the tooth itself; it is more common in older people, and it occurs just as frequently in primitive societies as in the industrialized world. Despite these differences, tooth decay and periodontal disease have three important similarities: both are caused by oral bacteria; both can lead to pain, expense, and tooth loss; and both can be prevented by meticulous oral hygiene and good nutrition.

The earliest and mildest form of periodontal disease is *gingivitis*, inflammation of the gums. If gingivitis is allowed to progress, the inflammation will gradually extend to deeper tissues, including the periodontium (see figure 14-1). In time, inflammation spreads from these soft tissues to the alveolar bone of the tooth socket. Next, the bone is absorbed, producing a periodontal pocket of pus. As the tooth socket is damaged, the tooth becomes looser and looser until it falls out.

Periodontal disease is common. At least half of all young adults have gingivitis, and about 90 percent of senior citizens have periodontitis. Gingivitis produces reddened gums that bleed during toothbrushing, and it may also cause bad breath. Because its inflammation is deeper, periodontitis may not be recognized until tooth loosening has occurred. By then, irreversible bone destruction has already taken place. Treatment can still help, but it's time-consuming and expensive. I'm sure you'll agree that the best strategy is to prevent periodontal diseases from getting started in the first place.

Periodontal disease is caused by bacteria that accumulate in the spaces between the teeth and gums. Everyone has bacteria in these gingival crevices, but if plaque is allowed to accumulate here, bacteria gain the upper hand. As they grow, oral bacteria produce enzymes and toxins which injure the gums. Injured tissues invite further bacterial growth, resulting in more toxins, more damage, and more bacterial invasion. Without treatment, this cycle will be interrupted only when the tooth is lost.

Oral hygiene is the key to preventing periodontal disease. The routine is familiar: diligent toothbrushing and flossing are essential, and supplementary antiseptic mouth rinses may help. But it takes dexterity as well as diligence to remove deep plaque — so professional cleaning and scaling once or twice a year is very important as well. Good nutrition, too, is beneficial; the bacteria in gingival crevices like sugar just as much as the bacteria on superficial plaque.

Take care of your mouth; it does require an investment of time and effort, but if you don't make the investment now, you'll be paying your dentist later. Pay now or pay later — the choice is yours. I'll invest in prevention.

Is Dental Care Safe?

Although few people like going to the dentist, most believe they'll leave the office healthier than when they went in. Occasional outbreaks of hepatitis have been traced to dentists over the years, but they've done little to shake public confidence in dental care. In the 1990s, however, a few cases of AIDS have been acquired from faulty dental care; these tragedies have understandably generated a new wave of concern about the safety of dental visits.

Even as I write these words, the Centers for Disease Control are developing standards to protect patients from acquiring infections from their health care providers. Virtually every professional medical and dental association is also at work on the problem. But even before new standards are put into practice, you can protect yourself.

First, understand that the risks of dental and medical treatment are very, very low. Only a handful of infections have been traced to dentists. They are tragedies of the first order. But opportunistic politicians and journalists threaten to fan legitimate concern into hysteria. In fact, all evidence suggests that the risk to health care providers is greater than the risk to patients — and, fortunately, even those risks are very low.

Second, understand that good sterile techniques and appropriate infection-control procedures are the best protection for patient and provider alike.

What does this mean in your dentist's office? You should be sure that the entire staff is taking infection-control precautions. They should wear gloves for all oral exams and treatments, and they should change their gloves every time they leave the room. They should also wear masks and protective eyewear. All equipment must be sterilized before it's reused, and each dental suite should be cleaned between patients. Of importance, too, is the safe disposal of needles and other potentially infected wastes.

Have a look around your dentists' offices, and don't hesitate to ask about their infection-control policies. Most likely you'll find that your dentists are acting as if they don't trust you. But if they're taking precautions against your microbes, you can trust them.

■ Trauma

It makes little sense to brush, floss, and faithfully visit the dentist, only to have your teeth knocked out in an accident. Unfortunately, it's a common scenario — but a preventable one.

More than 50,000 facial injuries are sustained in motor vehicle accidents each year. Many of these accidents can be prevented. But even if an auto accident occurs, simply wearing a seat belt will reduce your risk of facial and dental injuries by 25 percent.

Although exercise is good for health, sports do pose a risk of trauma. Fortunately, sports injuries that threaten life and limb are uncommon; unfortunately, injuries that threaten tooth and jaw are common indeed. Helmets and face masks have prevented many such injuries in hockey and football; they would be just as useful for biking and skateboarding, but it's frustratingly difficult to convince many young people that protective equipment is important. Even more neglected is the mouth guard, a simple device that would prevent many teeth from being knocked out of alignment, cracked, or lost during sports. Think it over; a mouth guard could be your most valuable bit of equipment for biking, basketball, skating, and especially for contact sports.

■ Dry Mouth

Nearly everyone experiences a dry mouth from time to time. In most cases, though, that sticky, uncomfortable feeling is nothing more than a temporary nuisance caused by breathing dry air, dehydration, stress, or too much talking. But some people are troubled by prolonged dry mouth; in fact, more than 40 percent of senior citizens report that their mouths *usually* feel dry. In addition to discomfort, prolonged dryness can lead to medical complications.

The mouth is lubricated by six major and many minor salivary glands. The flow of saliva is stimulated by the thought, smell, sight, or taste of food, as well as by chewing and swallowing. Although the salivary glands are quite small, their productivity is prodigious; normal people secrete more than *one quart* of saliva each day.

Saliva is 99 percent water; the remaining 1 percent contains various chemicals, including digestive enzymes. Saliva is essential for many reasons. It moistens and lubricates food, facilitating swallowing. It begins the digestion of carbohydrates, and it dissolves chemicals in foods so they'll register with our taste buds. Last but not least, saliva cleanses the teeth and mouth, fighting tooth decay and periodontal disease.

What makes the mouth go dry? The most common causes are readily preventable: dry air and dehydration. The treatment is obvious: moisten dry air with a humidifier, and wet your whistle by drinking lots of fluids. Mouth breathing and excessive talking are equally simple causes of Sahara tongue, but these habits are harder to correct.

Another common cause of dry mouth is medication. Culprits include many drugs that doctors prescribe to treat high blood pressure, psychological disorders, and diarrhea. In many cases alternate drugs are available, so you should ask your doctor to consider switching medications if you are troubled by this side effect. Remember, too, that over-the-counter remedies such as antihistamines and decongestants can also reduce saliva flow, making your mouth unpleasantly dry.

Whereas all these causes of dry mouth can be prevented or corrected, other causes may be permanent. More than 1 million Americans have a disorder of the salivary glands that produces persistent dryness; women are most often affected by this problem, called Sjogren's syndrome, which can also cause dry eyes. Other causes of chronic dry mouth include diabetes, underactive thyroid glands, salivary gland infections, and previous radiation therapy.

Even if you can't remedy the underlying problem, you can take steps to prevent dry mouth from causing complications affecting your swallowing, speech, and dental health. Sour and spicy foods will get the most moisture from your salivary glands. Chewing gum and sucking hard candy will also help, but be sure to choose sugarless varieties. Foods to be avoided include salty items that can irritate oral tissues. Alcohol and tobacco are also on the list of irritants. You can use mineral oil, glycerine, or commercial saliva substitutes to lubricate your mouth. The simplest lubricant of all is water; drink small sips as often as possible, particularly while you're eating solid foods that need lubrication. Finally, if you don't have enough saliva to cleanse your teeth normally, you should redouble your attention to oral hygiene.

■ Temperomandibular Joint Syndrome

The name of this common problem is such a mouthful that the simple act of pronouncing it might injure your jaw. Don't worry. Like most dentists and doctors, you can simply call it TMJ syndrome. Although TMJ syndrome is caused by overuse of the jaw, the problem stems not from talking or even chewing but from clenching.

A surprising number of people clench their jaws and grind their teeth. The number is surprising because they deny the habit, not because of shame or sham but because they do it unconsciously, during deep sleep.

Clenching and grinding puts pressure on the TM joint, which functions as the hinge of the upper and lower jaws. When the symptom is jaw pain, the diagnosis is simple. But the pain of TMJ syndrome can be referred to the ears, teeth, neck or head, so it may be mistaken for much more serious problems ranging from arthritis of the neck to sinus conditions to brain disorders.

The puzzle of TMJ pain is usually solved by a roommate or spouse who diagnoses nocturnal jaw clenching. Although the habit is hard to break, mild TMJ pain can often be treated successfully with measures as simple as warm compresses and aspirin. In difficult cases, jaw manipulations and prescription medications may be necessary. For true prevention, however, see your dentist. Using a simple protective bite guard at night can prevent both the pain of temperomandibular joint syndrome and the difficult chore of mastering its name.

■ Oral Cancer

Dry mouth is a nuisance. TMJ syndrome is a pain in the neck. Oral cancer is a killer.

More than 30,000 cases of oral cancer were diagnosed in the United States in 1989. Despite surgery and radiotherapy, nearly one third of oral cancer patients die from the disease, placing oral cancer tenth on the list of cancer killers. The grim statistics are all the sadder in view of the fact that oral cancer shares with lung cancer the frustrating distinction of being the most preventable form of cancer.

The leading cause of oral cancer is tobacco abuse, which contributes to 90 percent of all cases. Alcohol abuse is a close second, playing a role in 75 percent of oral cancers. Simple arithmetic demonstrates that both problems are present in most oral cancer patients, possibly because alcohol dries out oral tissues, increasing their vulnerability to the cancer-causing chemicals in tobacco. Other less common causal factors include radiation, occupational exposure to nickel or wood dust, certain viral infections, and possibly some nutritional deficiencies.

Nearly all cases of oral cancer can be prevented by avoiding tobacco use and alcohol abuse. But oral cancer also raises a unique issue in tobacco abuse, since smokeless tobacco is a major risk to the gums, cheeks, tongue, and mouth.

Smokeless tobacco was widely used throughout the United States in the nineteenth century. Its decline in the early twentieth century can be attributed to influences both good and evil, to antispitting campaigns on the one hand and to mass production of cigarettes on the other. Unfortunately, chewing tobacco and snuff are mounting a worrisome comeback in recent years. Twelve million Americans now use one or the other, with half admitting to regular use. Most users are men; alarmingly, 25 percent are teenagers. Although many social factors contribute to this pattern of usage, role models may bear some of the responsibility, since nearly 40 percent of professional baseball players use smokeless tobacco.

Another factor that contributes to the resurgence of smokeless tobacco is ignorance. Although many people believe that it can be used safely, nothing could be further from the truth. Even without smoke, these forms of tobacco fire many health problems, including a fiftyfold increase in the risk of oral cancer, gingivitis and periodontal disease, receding gums, and nicotine addiction. In fact, nicotine levels are as high in smokeless tobacco users as they are in smokers.

The primary prevention of oral cancer is simple but highly effective: avoid tobacco use in all forms, and avoid excessive alcohol use. But secondary prevention is also a realistic goal, being much easier for oral cancer than for almost any other malignancy except skin cancer. The key is to detect oral cancers when they are just starting, before they've caused any symptoms much less any metastatic spread. The best hope for secondary prevention is a careful oral exam. Smokers and drinkers should be examined carefully twice each year, once by their doctor and once by their dentist. Suspicious areas should be biopsied so treatment can be initiated promptly. Early treatment is life-saving, but radiotherapy is debilitating and surgery may be disfiguring. It is clear that the best approach is to avoid oral cancer in the first place by snuffing out tobacco use and alcohol abuse.

Scientific research first published in 1990 is raising new hopes for the prevention of oral cancer. Patients who have been treated successfully for one oral cancer still suffer from a very high risk of developing second and third cancers. Doctors at the M. D. Anderson Cancer Center in Houston studied more than 100 such patients, administering high doses of isotretinoin to half. The drug, which is licensed only for the treatment of severe acne, provided dramatic protection against second cancers. Side effects were often troublesome, and more research will be needed to confirm these results and improve the treatment program. But these findings should be of interest even to people who have never had oral cancer because isotretinoin is a derivative of vitamin A. It's too early to recommend vitamin supplements to prevent cancer, but I'm strongly in favor of eating lots of vitamin-rich vegetables and fruits (see chapter 20 for a full discussion of vitamins and cancer).

■ Disorders of the Throat and Larynx

The larynx is a marvelous apparatus designed for two roles, swallowing and speech. The vocal cords are small, filmy membranes that are surrounded by cartilage, including the "Adam's apple." During swallowing, the vocal cords close, thus preventing food from "going down the wrong pipe" into the lungs. During speech, fine puffs of air are exhaled past the open vocal cords; vibrations of the cords produce the fundamental tone, which is then modified by the throat, tongue, lips, and teeth to produce the melodious characteristics of healthy speech.

Disorders of the larynx can interfere with both swallowing and speech. You can prevent many of these problems; you should start, in fact, simply by being sure that these dual functions of the larynx are performed sequentially rather than simultaneously.

It may seem insultingly obvious to exhort you to swallow carefully, but you won't take the subject lightly if you've ever witnessed a "café coronary." Hundreds of people choke to death on food that becomes lodged in the larynx, producing spasms which completely close off the airway. Meat is the leading culprit, but nuts and many other foods can also cause the problem. You will find the guidelines for prevention not in a medical text but in your mother's good advice: cut your food carefully, chew slowly, and swallow soberly. I can add only one element to this folk wisdom: learn the Heimlich maneuver so you can help café coronary victims, including, if necessary, yourself.

Many disorders of speech are also preventable. Hoarseness is most often a temporary problem caused by allergies, viral infections, inhalation of dust or fumes, or excessive dryness. But prolonged hoarseness can be a sign of vocal cord polyps or cancers — both preventable.

Vocal cord polyps are caused by abuse or overuse of the voice, which is why they're variously known as screamer's polyps or singer's polyps. Prevention is easy in theory but may be difficult in practice: don't shout, scream, or even talk or sing too much. Voice rest and speech therapy can be very helpful treatments for vocal cord polyps, but if they don't succeed, surgery may be needed.

Cancer of the larynx is responsible for almost 2 percent of all cancer deaths. Much more common in men than in women, laryngeal cancer is nearly always the result of smoking. As in the case of oral cancer, alcohol abuse is frequently a co-factor. Avoiding tobacco use and alcohol abuse would prevent almost all cases of throat cancer, along with so many other medical problems.

Early detection of laryngeal cancer can be life-saving. Hoarseness is almost always the first symptom. Men who smoke and drink should see an ear, nose, and throat specialist if they are hoarse for two weeks; if you don't smoke or drink, it's safe to wait twice as long before seeing a physician. Best of all, as usual, is primary prevention. Prudent living can save your voice and your life. Make the right choice — and speak up about it to your friends and relatives.

▪ 15 ▪

Skin Disorders

As the most visible part of the human anatomy, the skin generates more comment and concern than any other part of the body. Many people use cosmetics to cover the skin, some undergo surgery to alter it, and a few acquire tattoos to decorate it. Because skin disorders are so apparent, people worry about them disproportionately: parents are alarmed by childhood rashes even though they are rarely serious; adolescents despair over acne although it's temporary; and adults become progressively preoccupied with spots and wrinkles with each passing year. Americans spend millions of dollars on "skin care" products, yet few take really good care of their skin. Narcissism notwithstanding, you should understand your skin and tend to it properly; you'll look better and — even more important — you'll prevent disease.

▪ The Normal Skin

In addition to being the body's most visible organ, the skin is also its largest. An average adult's skin has a surface area of nearly two square yards and a weight of 11 pounds. But sheer size is not the skin's only attribute; although most people think of it as a simple passive covering, the skin is actually a complex, active organ with many important functions.

The skin is divided into three layers (see figure 15-1). The outer layer, or *epidermis,* is unique among human tissues. It's a tough barrier which must be intact to prevent infection, yet it's chiefly composed of dead and dying cells. Ten percent of the epidermal cells are pigment-containing melanocytes, but 90 percent are epithelial cells which undergo rapid cell division. More than 500 million new epithelial cells are formed each day to replace cells that have died. Shortly after each cell is formed, it loses its nucleus, the control center that directs cell division. Already doomed to an early demise, the epithelial cells move toward the skin's outermost surface. As they move outward, the cells lose water, become smaller, and gain keratin, a large protein that is responsible for the skin's sturdy exterior. But just when the epidermal cells achieve their life's goal of toughness and dryness, they reach the skin's surface — and are shed from the body, to be replaced

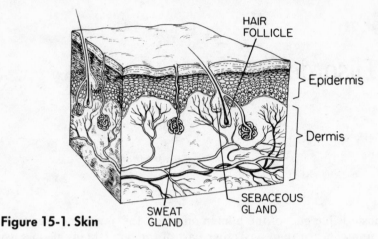

HAIR
FOLLICLE

Epidermis

Dermis

SEBACEOUS
GLAND

SWEAT
GLAND

Figure 15-1. Skin

by a younger cell from below. And you thought only snakes shed their skins!

All of this cell division and shedding requires nutrients and oxygen. The middle layer, or *dermis*, is the skin's support system which fills these needs. It contains the connective tissue that supports the skin, the blood vessels that supply nutrients and remove wastes, the lymph channels that remove fluid, and the nerves that remind you to keep your skin out of harm's way. The dermis also contains the elastic tissue that helps keep the skin firm and smooth.

The deepest layer of the skin is no less complex. It contains specialized structures that actually are part of the skin even though they are usually considered separately. Sweat glands, oil-producing sebaceous glands, and hair follicles populate this third and deepest layer of the skin.

Nature is conservative and economical; when the body's structures are elaborate, there is usually a good reason for the complexity. In the case of the skin, there are actually many good reasons, for the skin has many roles in preventing illness.

The tough, dry outermost layer of skin prevents infection. Microbes cannot penetrate the intact epidermis, but even if they sneak in through a small cut, they find the dry environment inhospitable. With a low water content, however, the skin requires lubrication. The sebaceous glands secrete oils to do the job; not coincidentally, these oils also contain antibacterial chemicals.

The skin keeps the agents of infection out, and it also keeps the fluids of life in. This job seems self-evident, but its importance is illustrated by burn patients who can die because of fluid and protein losses caused by destruction of the skin barrier.

The body's temperature is also regulated by the skin. Sweat glands are responsible for cooling the body. In addition, blood vessels in the dermis will widen when the body is too warm and constrict when it's too cool, dissipating or conserving body heat as needed.

Another role of the skin is to protect the body from injury. The nerves on the dermis fill this role, sounding the alarm if they are exposed to heat, cold, or pain.

The skin is also designed to defend the body's vulnerable internal organs from environmental injury. Many potentially toxic chemicals are unable to penetrate through the skin. In addition, the pigmented melanocytes of the epidermis protect against radiation injury. But these defenses are imperfect: some toxins can penetrate the skin, and ultraviolet radiation is extremely harmful to fair-skinned people.

The skin does a wonderful job in preventing many forms of illness. But it needs your help. With a few simple precautions, you can take proper care of your skin, augmenting its functions. By saving your skin, you can preserve your health.

■ Sunburn

Can something as commonplace and ubiquitous as sunburn be a disease? You can bet on it. Sunlight is your skin's worst enemy.

Sunlight is composed of electromagnetic radiation. Chapter 22 explains all the forms of radiation; for now, though, you should understand that the radiation in sunlight contains energy. The sun's energy warms the world, nurtures its crops, and lights our lives. It also injures the skin.

The harmful element in sunlight is not visible light but ultraviolet radiation. The sun emits three types of ultraviolet radiation. Ultraviolet C is the most potent, but because it's blocked out by the earth's atmosphere, it poses no risk to human health. Ultraviolet B is another matter. It has enough energy to cause disease, and it does penetrate through the atmosphere; as the ozone layer thins out, in fact, more and more ultraviolet B radiation is getting through. The third type of ultraviolet radiation, ultraviolet A, has the longest wavelength. It's the closest to visible light, and it carries much less energy than the other forms of ultraviolet radiation. Because ultraviolet A is not strong enough to cause a sunburn, it was long dismissed as harmless. But ultraviolet A can penetrate deep into the skin, and new evidence suggests that it can be dangerous, with repeated exposures causing cumulative damage to the skin's elastic tissues.

Ultraviolet waves pack a punch; in an attempt to deflect that punch, the melanocytes in the epidermis produce more pigment, putting the tan in suntan. But when ultraviolet rays overwhelm the protective pigment, they cause the tissue injury and inflammation of sunburn. Even worse, ultraviolet B waves contain enough energy to disrupt the structure of DNA, the master material that constitutes our genes. Damage to DNA can have many consequences, including cancer; indeed, sunlight can — and does — cause skin cancer.

Ultraviolet radiation can also do some good for the body, converting vitamin D into its active form in the skin to preserve bone calcium. In fact, if you are very careful to protect yourself from sunlight, you should be equally careful to get extra vitamin D from fortified dairy products (low-fat, please) or from vitamin supplements.

Some sunlight is healthful, but we get far too much. Two forms of human behavior account for our increased exposure to ultraviolet radiation. The first is cultural, our exaltation of the tanned and tawny look. The second is industrial, our use of chlorinated fluorocarbons (CFCs) in refrigerants and aerosols. CFCs leak into the atmosphere, where they deplete the stratospheric ozone layer. For each 1 percent decrease in the ozone layer, the earth receives 2 percent more ultraviolet radiation. So if you warm up in the sun and then use air conditioners and cold drinks to cool off, you are harming your environment as well as your skin.

Sunburn is the most acute and dramatic form of sun injury. Well named, it is quite literally a superficial burn of the epidermis and dermis. Epithelial cells are damaged, so they die and are shed at an abnormally rapid pace, leaving the dermis exposed. Fluid leaks from exposed tissues and accumulates in blisters. Blood vessels in the dermis widen, giving the skin its angry red hue. The dermis is congested and swollen, putting pressure on the nerves, which remind you that a day in the sun wasn't such a good idea after all.

A sunburn hurts. A severe sunburn also produces fever, dehydration, and fatigue. But you'll get over it, won't you? Yes and no. You'll recover, but the risk of skin cancer will linger on. Sunburns are particularly dangerous to children and adolescents; as few as five childhood sunburns will double the lifelong risk of melanoma, the most serious form of skin cancer.

Sunburn is, of course, preventable. My mother used to teach me that the best way to prevent a sunburn was to increase sun exposure gradually each summer. Even without understanding skin biology, Mother was right. Given time, the melanocytes are able to produce their protective pigment. But Mom was also wrong; a "healthy" tan prevents sunburn all right, but it's far from healthy. Ultraviolet damage to DNA is cumulative, so repeated exposure to even small doses will increase your risk of skin cancer and accelerate skin aging. Grandma notwithstanding, my wife and I encourage our kids to cultivate a healthy pallor!

To save your skin, shield it from the sun. You can do this in two ways, one high-tech and the other no-tech.

Sunscreens are the high-tech way to protect your skin. They come in two varieties, physical sunscreens and chemical sunscreens.

Physical sunscreens reflect away all ultraviolet rays, providing excellent protection for the skin. That's the good news. The bad news is that they are greasy and messy; in addition, they rub off easily. Zinc oxide and titanium dioxide are the active ingredients in various physical sunscreen preparations. They are most practical for use on localized areas with intense sun exposure, preventing the red-nosed lifeguard syndrome.

Chemical sunscreens don't reflect away the sun's energy; instead, they absorb ultraviolet rays, capturing the energy in their molecules instead of your skin's. Three groups of chemicals can be used to absorb ultraviolet B radiation: PABA, cinnamates, and benzophenes. Each group contains many compounds that can be used in sunscreens. Most sunscreens contain a combination of chemicals; knowing the exact ingredients is important only if you become allergic to them, in which case you should switch to a sunscreen containing a different class of chemicals. Many sunscreens also contain moisturizers, which can help keep skin healthy, and cosmetic ingredients, which are a matter of personal preference. Various vehicles are available, so sunscreens are marketed as lotions, gels, creams, or ointments; here, too, the choice is entirely yours.

You don't have to be a chemist to compare sunscreens; the manufacturers have done it for you. All sunscreens are rated in two different ways. The SPF, or sun protective factor, rating tells you how effectively the product absorbs ultraviolet B waves. The higher the SPF, the greater the protection. Sunscreens come with SPFs as low as 2 and as high as 50. Most doctors recommend SPF 15; higher numbers provide little extra protection, but they may be helpful for people who are particularly sensitive to the sun.

The second rating system grades the durability of sunscreens, scoring their ability to resist removal from the skin by perspiration or water. *Water-resistant* sunscreens remain on the skin after two 20-minute immersions in water, whereas *waterproof* preparations have passed the sterner test of four 20-minute immersions.

Although these two rating systems are very helpful, a third is needed. As of 1991 there was no system to rate protection against ultraviolet A radiation. Although there is heated debate about the effects of ultraviolet A, most dermatologists agree that it can be harmful and that it should be blocked. Many manufacturers assert that their products' ingredients provide "broad-spectrum" protection against both ultraviolet A and B, but only one ingredient, Parsol 1789, has thus far been FDA-approved for protection against ultraviolet A. As new testing standards are developed, we can expect additional chemicals to win approval, and to find that approval reflected on sunscreen labels. Until then, use the SPF as your guide, but look for Parsol 1789 if you need full protection because of a fair complexion or intense sun exposure.

Choosing a sunscreen can be complex, but using it properly is simple — and essential. Use your sunscreen early and often. For the best protection, apply it liberally to all sun-exposed areas 15 to 30 minutes before you go into the sun. It will take about an ounce to cover your body well. Even if you are using a waterproof preparation, it's prudent to reapply the sunscreen after swimming or after an hour of heavy perspiration. Sunscreens are not recommended for infants younger than six months of age; SPFs above 15 should probably not be used by young children.

Sunscreens are safe; the only known complications are skin allergies, which are infrequent and usually mild. Sunscreens are effective; it is estimated that they would reduce the rate of skin cancers by more than 75 percent if used properly. But they are not a panacea. In my opinion you should take additional precautions against ultraviolet exposure.

Use your sunscreen, and use it properly, but don't let it give you a false sense of security. Back up your high-tech prevention with the "no-tech" method: reduce your exposure to sunlight. Remember that only mad dogs and Englishmen go out in the noonday sun; avoid sun exposure between 10 A.M. and 2 P.M., when the rays are strongest. Beware of reflective surfaces: sand, snow, ice, and concrete can reflect 10 to 50 percent of the sun's energy back at you. Wear a hat and protective clothing. And be very sure to redouble your efforts to protect your children from the sun, since they are at greatest risk of melanoma from exposure.

Can tanning salons give you a safe suntan? I'm sorry to say the answer is no. Avoid even tanning machines that purport to supply only "safe" ultraviolet A waves. There is just no such thing as a safe tan.

■ Skin Cancer

Skin cancers are the most common of all human malignancies. Fortunately, the majority of them originate from epithelial cells; these basal cell and squamous cell cancers are much less dangerous than deadly malignant melanomas that originate from pigmented melanocytes.

About 600,000 cases of basal cell and squamous cell cancer are diagnosed in the United States each year. The most common forms of human cancer, they are also the most treatable; virtually all cases can be easily cured if detected early. Advanced cases can be disfiguring, however, and neglected cases can slowly spread, eventually killing about 2,000 people annually.

Malignant melanomas are much less common, affecting 32,000 people each year. Melanomas can also be cured if they are detected early. Unlike basal cell and squamous cell cancers, however, melanomas have the capacity to spread to the lymph nodes, the lungs, the liver, and other tissues; once this happens, treatment is very difficult, and 6,500 people die from melanomas each year.

It is alarming to note that skin cancers are becoming much more common. Fifty years ago the risk of developing a melanoma was only one in 1,500, but now your lifetime risk is one in 120, a twelvefold increase. Melanomas have increased more rapidly in the past decade than any other form of cancer — and all the evidence points to a continuation of this dangerous trend. Squamous cell and basal cell cancers are increasing as well, at a rate of about 5 percent per year. To make matters worse, the major increase is occurring in young and middle-aged people, formerly at very low risk.

We are in the midst of an epidemic of skin cancer — an epidemic that can be prevented.

The major cause of all forms of skin cancer is sun exposure. Primary prevention depends on reducing the primary cause; use sunscreens, and limit your exposure to sunlight. Skin cancer is also an ideal candidate for secondary prevention. Basal cell and squamous cell cancers enlarge very slowly, and even melanomas grow slowly enough so that early detection can lead to cure. The trick is to detect skin cancers early, before they cause symptoms. Fortunately, screening is simple, requiring no more than a look at the skin — and a trained eye.

Suspect any skin lesion that is enlarging, particularly if it changes in color or bleeds. Sores or ulcers that don't heal are also worrisome. Don't count on pain to warn you that you have skin cancer; most cancers are entirely painless, so you'll have to rely strictly on the visual appearance of the lesions.

Melanomas can be tricky to spot because they can be confused with ordinary benign skin moles. Any pigmented spot that enlarges or bleeds should be promptly examined by a physician. You can also use four additional criteria to tell you whether a lesion should be checked medically: (a) *a*symmetry: most melanomas are irregular in shape, whereas most moles are symmetrical and regular; (b) *b*order: most melanomas have irregular borders that are scalloped, notched, or blurry and indistinct, whereas moles are usually sharply defined by a smooth, regular border; (c) *c*olor: melanomas tend to be multicolored, with varying hues ranging from black to brown to red or even white or blue, whereas moles may be light or dark, but they are usually of a single, uniform hue; (d) *d*iameter: melanomas are usually larger than 6 millimeters at the time of diagnosis. Moles, too, can be large; but lesions smaller than the size of a pencil eraser are more likely to be benign.

You can remember these four criteria by their first initials, *a b c d.* But they will help you only if you use them by examining your own skin at regular intervals.

The American Cancer Society recommends monthly self-examination. Although sun-exposed areas are at greatest risk, you should really check your entire body. To do so, you'll have to undress and inspect yourself in good lighting in front of a full-length mirror. First face the mirror and examine the front of your body. Next, turn to the right, then the left to check both of your sides. To examine your back, turn your back to the mirror and hold a smaller hand mirror in front of you. The hand mirror can also be used to check the backs of your legs and the soles of your feet, while you are sitting in a chair. For completeness, have a look between your fingers and toes. Once you get into a routine, you can accomplish the entire exam in just a few minutes. It can be even quicker if you enlist the help of a spouse or friend.

Report any suspicious lesions to your doctor. You should also be sure your doctor examines your skin during your regular checkups. Finally, you might wish to have a dermatologist examine your skin if you have added melanoma risk factors such as intense sun exposure (particularly in childhood), a family history of melanoma, fair, heavily freckled skin, or previous skin disease.

■ Dry Skin

One of the unique properties of the skin is the low water content of its outermost layer. Indeed, this lack of moisture creates an environment hostile to bacteria, thus helping to prevent skin infection. But things can go too far; excessively dry skin is itchy and unsightly, and it may be a precursor to more serious skin disorders.

Water is *not* the remedy for dry skin. In fact, water can cause dry skin. The problem is not lack of water but lack of the oils that lubricate normal skin. Washing with water can actually remove these oils, exacerbating the problem. In addition, many soaps remove lubricating oils from the skin. Dry skin is also caused by cold, dry winter air. The skin's number one enemy, sunlight, can further contribute to drying.

Dry skin cracks and flakes. It itches. It can develop deep, painful fissures. These can also lead to infections, which may be very serious. The reason is that bacteria that are normally excluded from the deep layers of the skin can creep in through the cracks and fissures in dry skin. Scratching can nudge the bacteria along.

You don't have to give up bathing to prevent dry skin. Simply put the oils back. Use soaps that contain oils — they really make a difference. Bath oil is also very helpful. And if these measures are not enough, apply emollient lotions to your skin after you wash and before you go to bed. Finally, a home humidifier in winter and protection from the sun in summer will help keep your skin well lubricated and healthy.

■ Skin Infections

Dry skin can lead to skin infections; so can wet skin.

Before you accuse me of sounding like a politician, let me explain. Dry skin leads to infection because without enough oil the skin becomes fissured, providing a portal of entry for bacteria. But excessive water causes another type of damage as the superficial layer of the skin becomes macerated or soggy. Waterlogged skin loses its ability to fight off certain bacteria. Even more striking is the way macerated skin nurtures the growth of fungi, leading to "athlete's foot," "jock itch," and "ringworm."

Because these fungal infections are always confined to the outer layers of skin, the epidermis, they are not at all serious. But they are itchy, uncomfortable, and unsightly. They can also damage the skin enough to invite bacteria in, setting the stage for deeper, much more serious infections; athlete's foot, with its cracked, fissured skin, is particularly notorious.

You can treat superficial fungal infections yourself with nonprescription ointments, sprays, creams, gels, or powders; many brands are available. Don't let all the hype confuse you. It's the antifungal medication that does the job, not the slick package or reassuring TV ad. The most effective medications contain one of three antifungals: clotrimazole, miconazole, or tolnaftate. If you start self-treatment early, using one of these medications as directed by the package label, your itching should improve in a day or so, and your rash should clear up in a week or two; if not, check with your doctor to see if your diagnosis was right.

Best of all, take the simple steps that will prevent these infections. Dry your skin thoroughly after you wash or swim; talcum powder can help. If you are prone to athlete's foot, be particularly careful to keep your feet dry. Wear cotton socks in summer and wool in winter to help wick perspiration away; a synthetic fiber, polypropylene, is even better. Avoid nylon socks because they trap moisture. Select well-ventilated shoes for sports and for daily activities; if your feet sweat heavily, invest in a second pair of athletic shoes so you'll always be able to start out with a dry pair.

■ Acne

My daughters would be furious if I let you in on the foolproof way to prevent acne, since I never disclosed the secret method to them. I won't disclose it to you, either — not because of fear of filial wrath, but because there is no secret.

Acne is caused by excessive activity of the sebaceous glands in the deepest layer of the skin. Quiescent until puberty, these glands begin producing an oily substance, sebum, in adolescence; in both boys and girls sebum production is triggered by tiny amounts of testosterone, the male hormone. Because it is viscous and sticky, sebum tends to plug the ducts leading from the glands that produce it, giving rise to the characteristic pustules of acne. Infection with skin bacteria that are ordinarily harmless may add to the inflammation.

Acne often runs in families. But much as acne sufferers might like to trade in their parents, that's not the way to prevent acne. The best way is the simplest: ordinary soap and water, used at least twice a day to remove excessive skin oil and bacteria. An antiseborrheic shampoo will do the same for your scalp. Oily creams and cosmetics should be avoided, but water-based make-up is acceptable.

Teenagers dedicate themselves to an extraordinary array of dietary restrictions to prevent acne. There is no scientific evidence that any nutritional intervention will be effective.

Unfortunately, there is no way entirely to prevent acne. If acne develops despite simple hygienic preventive measures, a variety of abrasives and astringents is available for self-treatment. These can cause skin irritation, however, and they should not be overused. Nor should patients or their families attempt to remove lesions by squeezing or picking them.

Many prescription medications are available for the treatment of acne. All can help, but none is infallible, and, like all medications, they may produce side effects. Let your doctor try to help if simple prevention and self-treatment programs fail to control acne.

My best advice may be the hardest to follow: be patient. Acne resolves with time; it's one of the *good* things about aging.

■ Skin Allergies

You may not realize at first blush that many skin rashes are caused by allergies. Medications are often responsible, but foods can also trigger allergic rashes. These skin reactions frequently resemble viral infections; even stress can cause hives, which may mimic other rashes. Despite their diverse causes, these rashes often look the same because in each case the skin is reacting to a stimulus elsewhere in the body. As a result, systemic allergies produce a red, itchy rash that appears simultaneously on many parts of the body.

The skin, however, can also display allergic reactions to chemicals placed directly on its surface. Since contact is required, this problem, called contact dermatitis, is confined strictly to the parts of the body that are touched by the offending substance. The rash of contact dermatitis is also red and itchy, but weepy blisters appear in more severe cases.

The treatment of allergic rashes is simple: stay away from the culpable chemical, and the problem will resolve. The same tactic will prevent recurrences. The trick is to determine what substance is to blame. In some cases your doctor can use patch tests to fix responsibility. More often, you'll have to do the detective work in a trial-and-error fashion. Remember that the very soaps, lotions, ointments, and cosmetics that you may be using to help your skin can be the cause of allergic reaction. Metals, too, can be the surprise culprits; just ask my daughter, who insists on silver or gold because of an "allergy" to the nickel in costume jewelry.

■ Toxic Chemicals

The skin provides a barrier that keeps many chemicals out of the body. Some chemicals, though, injure the skin by causing allergies, inflammation, or irritation. Still others can penetrate right through the skin, traveling in the blood to produce mischief elsewhere in the body.

The best way to prevent toxins from damaging your skin is to keep chemicals off your skin; gloves and protective clothing can provide crucial help. If toxic chemicals do contaminate your skin, remove them as rapidly as possible. Remember that without prevention, the problem could be more than skin deep, since various chemicals can penetrate through skin. (This is why medicated skin patches can be used for estrogen replacement, motion sickness, high blood pressure, and angina.)

The most serious chemical exposures are inadvertent, but the most common ones are entirely voluntary, to say the least. All cosmetics and skin lotions contain chemicals. Most are completely harmless, but some can cause irritation and allergies. Remember that the chemicals in cosmetics are not subjected to the same safety standards as the chemicals in drugs or food additives. In fact, with the exception of a few additives and coloring agents, the Food and Drug Administration allows cosmetic manufacturers to use any chemicals they choose, without prior safety testing. Moreover, manufacturers can label their products "doctor tested," "nonirritating," or "nonallergenic" without submitting any medical data to the FDA. It's free enterprise at work. Remember, though, that you are free to change brands if your "skin care" product produces adverse reactions. Even better: take good care of your skin, keeping it healthy and youthful so you'll be less tempted to cover it up.

■ Aging Skin

American culture is preoccupied with youth. Because the skin often reveals the most visible evidence of aging, it's the recipient of some $10 billion worth of ointments and lotions that are sold each year to restore youth, or at least the appearance of youth. There is little evidence that these potions do any good. In fact, there is no way to turn back the clock. But there are ways to prevent many of the skin changes associated with aging.

Many factors conspire to make the skin look old. The chief factor is a loss of elastic tissue from the skin's middle layer, the dermis; when elastic tissue declines, the skin becomes flaccid and wrinkled. The skin surface also changes, taking on a tough, leathery appearance. The pigmented cells deep in the epidermis contribute their share to the much-lamented look of maturity; increased melanocyte activity produces brownish "age spots."

Changes in the body's tissues are, of course, irreversible consequences of aging. Just look at any 70-year-old. Now look again: all of our subject's skin is 70 years old, but the skin of the face, neck, arms, and hands looks 15 or 20 years older than the skin of the trunk and thighs, which is of the same vintage.

You don't have to be an Einstein to realize that the theory of relativity does not explain these differences. Clocks tick at the same pace for the back as for the face. The difference is not age but exposure.

Many environmental factors damage the skin, making exposed areas look old. Wind, heat, and chemical toxins all damage elastic tissue, toughen the skin surface, and stimulate melanocytes to produce blotchy pigments. A 1991 study by dermatologists at the University of Utah provides clear evidence that another toxin causes premature skin wrinkling and aging: cigarette smoking. Wrinkled skin, of course, is not the main reason to abjure tobacco, but it joins the many other problems that should bring a furrow to your brow whenever you see a cigarette. Still, even among all these hazards the most potent stimulus to the skin's "aging" is exposure to ultraviolet rays — to sunlight. Ultraviolet B is the main culprit, but even the less potent ultraviolet A rays can contribute to premature skin aging, since they penetrate deep into the skin's elastic tissue layer.

Aging cannot be reversed, but it may be possible to modify some of the changes of photo-aging, to make sun-aged skin look younger. A 1988 study from the University of Michigan evaluated the effects of tretinoin cream (Retin-A) on the skin of healthy adult volunteers. All subjects applied the medication to one side of the face and to one arm, while applying an inert placebo cream to the other side. Neither the patients nor their doctors knew which side was getting the real thing. But after 16 weeks they could tell the difference; nightly tretinoin applications reduced fine wrinkling and increased skin smoothness and pinkness. A 1991 study of tretinoin treatment reported similar results for fine wrinkles, and a 1992 study found that "liver spots," pigmented areas that also result from years of ultraviolet damage, also respond to tretinoin cream.

I wish I had a nickel for each patient who has called me to request a prescription for tretinoin, but I'm glad my nickel didn't depend on writing a prescription. Should you call your doctor? Not yet. The three studies involved only 339 patients, and the improvements, though real, were mild. The only reported side effect was skin irritation, but we should have the benefit of long-term observations of many patients before prescribing a potentially powerful drug for cosmetic purposes. These reservations apply even more strongly to growth hormone, another great hope because of a 1990 study which showed that injections of the hormone can make skin thicker and more elastic. Finally, although estrogen replacement therapy is frequently prescribed for postmenopausal women who'd like "young skin," this is the *least* valid reason to take hormones.

I'm slow to use my prescription pad to right wrinkled skin, but even without offering medication I can offer some hope for ultraviolet injury masquerading as aging. The body has mechanisms to repair damaged DNA. By protecting yourself from the sun, you can forestall further harm — and you'll give your normal repair mechanisms a chance to heal some of the damage.

As usual, the very best approach is primary prevention. The healthful life-style recommended throughout these pages will keep your internal organs vigorous and youthful over the years. Protection from sunlight will keep your skin looking as young as you feel. Life-style changes will be most effective if they are started early in life. Simple advice, but unfortunately, like youth itself, it's often wasted on the young.

■ 16 ■
Infectious Diseases

It may comfort you to learn that no person is ever truly alone. But that sense of comfort may dissipate rapidly when you realize that our constant companions are myriads of microbes. We are indeed surrounded by a bustling world of bacteria. They're everywhere: in air, water, and soil, on all animals, and on all surfaces of the human body itself.

Don't let your comfort turn to alarm. Most micro-organisms are entirely harmless, and some are actually helpful, crowding out more dangerous bugs. And even the most dangerous of organisms can be prevented from causing harm. Good general health is your best defense, but specific evasive tactics will also help.

■ Patterns of Infection

Although microbes evolved long before humanity arose 40,000 years ago, infectious diseases didn't become major killers until perhaps 10,000 years ago, when the agricultural era began. With the rise of farming, people began to store food and water for future use instead of consuming it immediately. They also began to live in larger communities, typically cheek by jowl with domesticated animals. Microbes began to spread from animals to people and from person to person; contaminated food and water provided reservoirs of infection; poor sanitation and hygiene opened the door to many infections; and nutritional deficiencies weakened the body's general health and its immune mechanisms.

As people began to migrate, they took bacteria and viruses with them. The great contagious plagues of the Middle Ages resulted when new organisms ravaged peoples who had never had a chance to build up immunity to such "foreign" bugs.

The modern era of infectious diseases coincides with the modern era of human life. The industrial revolution packed people together in large cities. Crowding, poor sanitation, and contaminated food and water produced epidemics of pneumonia, tuberculosis, intestinal infections, and many other infectious diseases. It's no wonder, then, that in 1900 the leading killers in America were pneumonia, influenza, and tuberculosis.

Fortunately, medical science has learned to fight back. Vaccines and antibiotics have been the major tools for infection control. Some advances have been spectacular: smallpox, an ancient scourge of humanity, has been eliminated from the face of the earth; polio, diphtheria, tetanus, and whooping cough have become rarities in America today; pneumonia and tuberculosis can be cured with powerful new antibiotics.

All this progress calls for congratulations — but not complacency. Far from it. When antibiotics were introduced in the 1940s, many doctors expected infections to dwindle or even disappear. True, pneumonia and influenza have dropped from their lofty position as our number one killers. But they are still in sixth place. In fact, only cardiovascular disease and cancer claim more American lives than infections, which collectively account for about 200,000 deaths annually. In all, infections account for more than 42 million days of hospitalization and 2 billion days of disability in our country each year, at a total cost of more than $20 billion. And in less fortunate areas of the world, infections remain the major causes of death; worldwide there are 5 million deaths from pneumonia, 5 million from diarrhea, 3 million from tuberculosis, and 1 million each from malaria, measles, and hepatitis — *every year.*

You and I can do little to solve the world's infectious disease problems. Nutrition, sanitation, housing, and immunization are the key remedies; antibiotics, though important, are actually less crucial than these fundamentals. But we can do a lot to prevent infections in modern America. And we had best attend to it. Despite all our wealth and progress, old infections persist, affecting especially our most vulnerable citizens, the very young, the very old, and the very poor. Even more disturbing is the appearance of entirely new infectious diseases such as Legionnaires' disease, toxic shock syndrome, Lyme disease, and especially AIDS. No diseases illustrate more clearly the simple principle that prevention is the best medicine.

■ The Microbial World

Infections are unique among the diseases of humanity, being caused exclusively by external agents, or micro-organisms. Although all infections are caused by microbes, these biological agents come in many different forms, causing diseases as diverse as the sniffles and AIDS.

Viruses are the smallest and simplest of microbes, yet they're the most difficult to diagnose and treat. Viruses are so primitive they cannot even live on their own. Composed simply of a tiny amount of genetic code core (DNA or RNA) and a protein coat, these minuscule particles don't have the enzymes necessary for their own metabolism and reproduction. To survive they must invade living cells, using the host cells' metabolic apparatus for their own purposes. Unfortunately, those purposes often include damage to the very cells that have been so hospitable.

Viruses are far too small to be seen with ordinary microscopes. They cannot be cultured using the usual techniques of a diagnostic microbiology lab. Needless to say, these limitations pose problems for your doctors, who must diagnose viral infections on the basis of clinical criteria or specialized lab tests.

Viruses also pose special problems for you because they can *never* be treated with ordinary antibiotics. I wish I had a nickel for each time I've explained this to a patient phoning in to ask for penicillin to treat a cold or flu.

Despite these problems, we are making progress in the control of viral infections. The greatest progress has been in prevention: smallpox, rabies, influenza, hepatitis B, measles, mumps, German measles, and polio are examples of viral infections that can be prevented by vaccines. Chicken pox will soon join this list. And there is even some progress in treating a few viruses: influenza, herpes, and AIDS can now be treated with special medications, though none can be cured by them.

Bacteria are much larger and more independent than viruses, having all the equipment they need to grow and reproduce on their own. But being bigger and stronger does not necessarily mean that bacteria are more harmful than viruses. In fact, many bacteria are quite harmless, though others are potentially lethal. Even the most hazardous bacteria, however, can be diagnosed more rapidly than can viruses, since bacteria can be seen with a microscope and grown in the lab. Also reassuring is the fact that antibiotics can be used to treat almost all bacteria; each bug, however, requires its own type of drug, so a precise diagnosis of bacterial infections is essential for therapy to be most effective.

Most of the harmless microbes that normally reside on the healthy human body are bacteria. But most of the dangerous microbes that cause pneumonia, sinus infections, urinary and genital tract infections, skin infections, bone infections, and joint infections are also bacteria. Prevention, then, involves the challenge of keeping the bad guys away without disturbing the good guys that can actually contribute to health. Avoiding exposure is, of course, the best preventive tactic, but vaccines and antibiotics can also help protect against certain bacteria.

Fungi and *parasites* are even larger and more sophisticated than bacteria. Often considered rare and exotic by patients and doctors alike, fungi and parasites are more likely to cause human disease in tropical and underdeveloped areas than in the United States. Still, they are major causes of human suffering and death around the world. And as the globe shrinks in the jet age, we should all learn how to prevent the major parasitic infections that may cross our far-flung paths.

■ How the Body Fights Infection

We live in a sea of microbes. It's no surprise, then, that infectious diseases are common. More surprising, perhaps, is the fact that we're not ill with infections all the time.

You don't have to read Louis Pasteur to understand why we are not overwhelmed by microbes. True, the greatest microbiologist had a lot to say on the subject. But nearly 300 years earlier the greatest poet, Shakespeare, explained it in a single sentence: the body is "a Fortress built by Nature for herself against Infection."

The human body possesses many lines of defense against infection. The first defenses are simple barriers that keep bacteria from invading our most vulnerable tissues; examples include an intact skin, an active cough reflex, and normal amounts of stomach acid. But even if microbes sneak past these mechanical defenses, they run up against a sophisticated network of antibodies that can neutralize them and white blood cells that can gobble them up.

The best way to keep your defenses strong is to keep your general health good. Chapter 11 details the body's immune system and its proper care and feeding.

There are only three basic tactics to prevent infections: avoiding exposure, taking certain antibiotics, and receiving immunization. Still, there are many variations on these themes. Let's explore some of the specifics.

■ Immunization

Immunity is the key to natural resistance to infection. As you encounter microbe after microbe during the course of daily life, you'll build up protective antibodies and white blood cells that prevent many serious infections.

Understanding this principle, doctors can now help things along by giving you vaccines to produce immunity even before you encounter potentially dangerous micro-organisms. Credit for the first human vaccination belongs to Edward Jenner, who injected cowpox virus into a child in 1796, preventing smallpox. Jenner's approach was crude, but it worked. The basic strategy of vaccination has changed but little in the subsequent 200 years, but our techniques have improved enormously. As a result, immunization is perhaps the most effective tool in all of preventive medicine.

Childhood Immunizations

Pediatricians have been diligent practitioners of preventive medicine, far outshining all other primary care practitioners. Their leadership is most evident in immunizations: about 75 percent of American children receive all their recommended immunizations. For adults, unfortunately, the ratio is reversed, with only about 25 percent fully protected, but it's a shameful failure of prevention in our wealthy country that protection does not approach 100 percent in all age groups.

A simple immunization schedule should be followed for all healthy children:

Age	Immunizations
2 months	Diphtheria-Tetanus-Pertussus (DTP)
	Oral polio vaccine (OPV)
	Hemophilus influenzae B (Hib)
	Hepatitis B (Hep B)

4 months	DTP, OPV, Hib, Hep B
6 months	DTP, Hib, Hep B
15 months	DTP, OPV, Hib
	Measles-Mumps-Rubella (MMR)
6 years	DTP, MMR
16 years	adult-type tetanus–diphtheria (Td)

The results of childhood immunizations have been spectacular. In the United States, for example, the annual incidence of polio has fallen from 20,000 cases to about 20; rubella (German measles) from 60,000 to 300; diphtheria from 350,000 to 30. Most dramatic of all is the total disappearance of smallpox, not only in America but throughout the entire world — which is why the oldest of vaccines is no longer in use. And all this progress has been achieved at modest expense with few side effects.

Despite the fine record of childhood immunizations, however, we should be doing even better. Measles is a case in point. An effective vaccine reduced this serious childhood infection from more than 500,000 cases in 1963 to fewer than 1,500 cases in 1983. Many authorities predicted that measles would be eradicated from the United States before the year 2000. They were wrong. Since the 1980s measles has been making a comeback, rising to about 30,000 cases (with nearly 100 deaths) in 1990. The vaccine is as good as ever, and the measles virus has not gotten any tougher. What's gone wrong? We are simply not getting the vaccine to the children who need it. As in so many aspects of prevention, the solution to the measles dilemma lies not in fancy new technology but in simple measures, in just doing the basic things we know will be effective.

Adult Immunizations

If you've paid your dues in childhood and have received your full complement of shots, you'll need relatively few vaccinations in adulthood.

The only immunization recommended for every adult is *tetanus-diphtheria*. You should get a booster every 10 years to keep up your defenses against these potentially lethal diseases. The side effects are minimal, amounting to a sore arm for a day or so, perhaps accompanied by a transient low-grade fever. But the gains are enormous; not only will you be protected, but you won't have to run to an emergency ward for a tetanus shot every time you get a cut or a puncture wound. If your immunity is not up to date, however, don't neglect to get a shot if you are injured; deep wounds may even call for rapid (though temporary) protection with tetanus immune globulin as well as immunization with the vaccine itself.

Although tetanus-diphtheria is the only immunization recommended for all adults, other adult immunizations are extremely beneficial for individuals who are at particular risk for infections.

To cope with the resurgence in *measles*, the traditional single measles immunization was replaced with a two-shot series beginning in 1990. Most adults, however, got only one measles shot in childhood. Hence, measles boosters are now recommended for college students, health care workers, residents of areas with measles outbreaks, and international travelers. Measles boosters have almost no side effects. They can be administered alone or as part of a combined measles-mumps-rubella vaccine; women who get the combined product, however, should be sure to avoid pregnancy for three months. And people who were born before 1957 don't need any measles shots, since it's likely that they had natural measles in childhood, gaining lifelong immunity.

Rubella (German measles) immunizations should also be considered for some young adults. Unlike measles, German measles is a very mild disease, except for unborn infants whose mothers are infected during pregnancy. I'm glad to report that the devastating malformations of congenital rubella have been nearly eliminated in the United States. But we can't rest on our laurels. Ten to 20 percent of young women are not protected against German measles. Unless a blood test proves immunity, every woman of child-bearing age who did not get a childhood rubella shot should be immunized. Rubella shots may produce some joint pain, but this discomfort is temporary while the protection is permanent. Although there is no evidence that the vaccine can harm a fetus, all women should be sure to avoid pregnancy for three months after this immunization.

Mumps vaccinations should also be considered for people born after 1956 unless they received a vaccination on or after their first birthday or have had physician-diagnosed mumps. Whereas rubella vaccinations are particularly important for young women, mumps vaccinations are especially recommended for nonimmune men, since mumps can produce very painful inflammation of the testicles in adolescents and adults.

Despite shortcomings, immunization for tetanus, diphtheria, measles, mumps, and rubella have dramatically reduced these five diseases in the United States. Unfortunately, the same is not true for *hepatitis B*. An effective vaccine has been available since 1982, but the incidence of hepatitis continues to *increase* annually. To improve this dismal record, scientists need to develop an even better vaccine and pharmaceutical manufacturers need to bring down its cost. But progress does not have to await these developments. The current vaccines are safe and effective. True, they are costly, but they're much less expensive than a case of hepatitis.

Hepatitis B vaccine is recommended for all people living in countries with high infection rates. In the United States hepatitis B vaccine is currently recommended for health care workers who come in contact with blood and body fluids, kidney dialysis patients, intravenous drug users, male homosexuals, sexual and household contacts of hepatitis patients, and residents of certain institutions. Unfortunately, we have not succeeded in persuading vulnerable adults to accept the three-shot series. As a result, hepatitis B was added to the list of recommended childhood immunizations in 1991. The infection is rare in American children, but the program is designed to make sure that the next generation of adults will be protected; chapter 7 explains these recommendations in detail.

It may surprise you to learn that *polio* immunizations are not recommended routinely for American adults, even for those who were not immunized in childhood. Polio vaccine isn't needed precisely because it's so effective; the disease has become so rare in the United States that routine adult immunization is not required. But if you're planning travel to underdeveloped areas where polio still occurs, you should be sure that you are protected. Adults who never received the vaccine in childhood should be immunized with a series of polio shots using the inactivated vaccine before departure. Previously immunized adults, however, may receive a single booster dose of the oral polio vaccine prior to travel.

Travel is the only reason for Americans of any age to receive vaccines against *yellow fever, typhoid*, or *cholera* — all diseases that are vanishingly rare in our country. You can learn more about preventing these illnesses while you are abroad in the next section of this chapter.

Another immunization with a rather narrow target group is the *meningococcal* vaccine. This product does help protect against a bacterium that causes meningitis and blood infections in children and young adults. But since these dreadful infections are uncommon, the meningococcal vaccine is recommended only in domestic outbreaks and for travel to countries with substantial infection rates.

Just the reverse is true for the two final adult immunizations: widespread use *is* recommended. Unfortunately, these recommendations are not being followed.

Influenza and *pneumococcal pneumonia* are both very common throughout the United States. They are particularly severe in older adults and in patients with heart disease, lung disease, and other chronic illnesses ranging from sickle cell anemia to diabetes to kidney failure. Influenza and pneumonia vaccinations are recommended for all people over 65 and for patients of any age whose illnesses make them particularly vulnerable to either infection. Chapter 5 provides the details for these recommendations; unfortunately, they're ignored by nearly 75 percent of the people who should be heeding them.

It has been frustratingly difficult to persuade many adults — and their doctors — to comply with immunization recommendations. But one group of people will almost always do what's good for them: travelers are generally happy to roll up their sleeves so they won't get sick away from home.

■ Travel-Related Health Problems

It is, in fact, a small world.

Infections that originate right in the neighborhood may be hard to cope with; infections from exotic places can be even more difficult. The hazards of imported germs have long been recognized. As far back as 1470 the Venetians instituted a policy of quarantine to control plague brought in by travelers. Panicky proposals to contain AIDS notwithstanding, we've come a long way in infection control since the Middle Ages. Our major concern, in fact, has shifted from the prevention of imported diseases to the protection of Americans who travel abroad. And since 20 million of us venture overseas annually, travel-related health problems are an important issue, particularly for the 5 million Americans who visit underdeveloped countries each year.

Still, only about 50 percent of Americans who travel abroad receive proper medical preparation. Be sure you're among the half who don't take a vacation from prevention.

General Precautions

After you've visited your travel agent, consider a visit to your doctor. Most people planning trips to industrialized areas don't need extra checkups, but older people and those with chronic medical problems should be sure they're fit to travel before they depart. And everybody planning prolonged or arduous trips or travel to underdeveloped or tropical areas should have medical evaluations prior to departure. Schedule your visit at least six weeks before your trip so you'll have ample time for immunizations.

The most important aspect of a pretravel checkup is a general health evaluation. If you have medical problems, you should obtain a medical summary including copies of relevant test results and electrocardiograms. If you take medications or use medical devices, request a letter from your doctor to facilitate your passage through customs and security checks. Be sure you have enough medication for your entire trip, and bring along a clear list of trade and generic names and dosage schedules just in case you need refills. Your list should also include all your allergies and dietary requirements. If you'll be spending more than a week or two in an underdeveloped area, ask your physician about a tuberculosis skin test during your preparatory checkup. Needless to say, it's also the time to discuss immunizations and prophylactic medications.

Even if you don't anticipate health problems, you should check with your insurance company to be sure you'll be covered abroad. And if you have chronic problems or will be in remote areas, obtain a list of trustworthy health care facilities in case emergencies occur.

Some health-related problems may develop even before you've arrived at your destination. Air travel will expose you to reduced oxygen levels and barometric pressures (for details on prevention, see chapters 5 on sinusitis and 22 on mountain sickness). To prevent blood clots from forming in your veins during prolonged sitting, pump your leg muscles several times an hour and walk up and down the aisle every hour or two; if you've had venous disease in the past, consider wearing elastic stockings or taking low-dose aspirin. If you're prone to motion sickness during land, sea, or air travel, obtain a preventive pill or patch from your doctor, and use it before you get sick. Last but not least, you may want to spend a few days gradually altering your sleeping and eating timetables to lessen the effects of jet lag, particularly if you'll be flying across more than two time zones from west to east.

Your Medical Kit

If you'll be traveling to urban centers, you won't need more than a credit card or some local currency to get what you need. But if you'll be in remote areas, consider packing a small medical kit with a few basic supplies:

Band-Aids, Ace bandages, moleskin for blisters
Disinfectants, such as Betadine
Sunscreen, insect repellent, antifungal powder
Aspirin, ibuprofen, or acetaminophen
Diarrhea remedies (Imodium, Pepto-Bismol)
Antihistamines, decongestants, motion sickness preparations
Prescription medications for malaria or diarrhea

Immunizations

Although travelers are most concerned about exotic illnesses, it's crucial to begin with the basics. Be sure your *tetanus-diphtheria* booster is up to date, and get a *flu* shot or *pneumonia* vaccine if you need one. Similarly, check to see if you need boosters for childhood immunizations such as measles and polio.

Only two immunizations are legally required for travel, and only certain countries require proof of immunity before they'll let you in. *Yellow fever* is common in equatorial Africa and in areas of South America. A very effective vaccine is available, but it's administered only by designated medical travel facilities.

Cholera vaccine is required for entry to certain countries. It's a good idea for travelers who'll be in areas where cholera is still common. Though not required for travel, *typhoid* vaccinations should be considered for journeys to tropical and underdeveloped areas. *Hepatitis A* may also be acquired from contaminated food or water in tropical and underdeveloped areas. If you'll be off the beaten path or if you'll be in typical tropical tourist accommodations for more than three months, you should be immunized. Excellent immunity is conferred by gamma globulin, but you'll need a repeat shot every six months. Remember, though, to complete your other immunizations *before* you get gamma globulin.

Tropical Travel: General Precautions

A few simple precautions will go a long way toward keeping you healthy in the tropics. Here are ten important tips:

1. Beware of the sun and the heat. Use a sunscreen, and follow the precautions cited in chapter 15 to keep your skin healthy. To prevent heat-related illnesses, give yourself time to acclimatize, stay well hydrated, and avoid excessive exertion.

2. Avoid all untreated water, including ice cubes. Drink bottled water, and use it to brush your teeth. If high-quality water is not available in sealed bottles, you can treat tap water by boiling it for ten minutes, by adding one iodine tablet per quart at least 30 minutes before you drink the

water, or by using special filters. Bottled carbonated beverages, coffee, and tea are safe. Avoid milk and other dairy products unless you are sure they've been pasteurized.

3. Eat only fruits that you can peel or slice yourself. Avoid fresh vegetables unless you can be sure that they've been thoroughly washed with bottled or treated water.

4. Avoid uncooked or undercooked meats, fish, and shellfish. Whenever possible, select well-cooked foods that are served hot. Breads and canned foods are generally safe.

5. Minimize your risk of insect bites. Be particularly careful to protect yourself from mosquitoes between dusk and dawn, when most malaria transmission occurs. Important protective measures include the use of screening and nets and light-colored clothing that covers most of the body. Use insect repellents; products containing DEET are best against mosquitoes, ticks, fleas, and flies. Protection lasts for several hours, but it's shortened by swimming and heavy perspiration. Permethrum may be sprayed on clothing for additional protection; a single application will protect against ticks and mosquitoes for up to a week, even if the garments have been washed.

6. Do not swim in fresh water if schistosomiasis is present. Chlorinated water in swimming pools is safe. Never swim alone; be especially cautious with ocean swimming, exercising the precautions outlined in chapter 17.

7. Be a defensive driver and a prudent pedestrian. Poor roads, inadequate night-time illumination, unfamiliar or haphazard traffic regulations, and aggressive driving habits make motor vehicle accidents a major hazard for travelers in many tropical areas.

8. Avoid contact with animals, both wild and domestic. If you are bitten, wash the wound thoroughly with copious amounts of soap and water, apply a disinfectant, and seek medical attention, including rabies prophylaxis, as soon as possible.

9. Be absolutely certain to protect yourself against sexually transmitted diseases.

10. Avoid over-the-counter medications. Be judicious about seeking local medical care, avoiding injections unless they are absolutely essential.

Traveler's Diarrhea

Call it *turista*, Montezuma's revenge, or the Aztec two-step. By any name, traveler's diarrhea is no joke, affecting 30 to 50 percent of North Americans who visit tropical and developing countries. Although the cramps and diarrhea usually resolve without treatment, three to five days of discomfort is inconvenient at best, debilitating at worst.

Traveler's diarrhea can be prevented. Because the bacteria that cause it often contaminate food and water, dietary precautions are your best defense. Tropical tips 2, 3, and 4 are the key ways to keep your trip galloping along without detouring into the trots. But even the most careful traveler can sometimes get *turista;* one of my most humiliating personal experiences was a case that developed while I was jogging in Guatemala (perhaps

I should add another tip: never wear white shorts while jogging in the jungle).

Although pills should never replace prudence for the prevention of diarrhea, medications can be a useful supplementary tactic. Medications can be used before diarrhea occurs or to shorten its duration and prevent dehydration after it has hit you.

The simplest preventive medication is bismuth subsalicylate — Pepto-Bismol. Two tablets four times a day can cut your risk of traveler's diarrhea by up to 60 percent. Unless you are allergic to salicylates, such as aspirin, you have little to lose from trying this program.

Antibiotics can also be taken preventively. But these medications can produce side effects, including allergic reactions and sun sensitivity. So except for special cases, such as patients who lack stomach acid, I generally prescribe antibiotics for early self-treatment rather than for prevention. A variety of antibiotics are effective for *turista;* the list includes doxycyline, trimethoprim, trimethoprim-sulfamethoxazole, and ciprofloxacin. All require a prescription, so check with your doctor before you depart.

You can also use nonprescription remedies to reduce the symptoms of diarrhea. Loperamide (Imodium) is effective; take two tablets (4 mg) at first, then one pill (2 mg) after each loose bowel movement up to a maximum of eight pills in 24 hours. Be cautious with your use of loperamide; like other medications that slow bowel contractions, it can actually prolong infections and may even increase the likelihood of certain complications of severe colitis.

Fluid replacement is extremely important. You can make your own solutions to replace the chemicals lost in watery diarrhea. For the first glass mix eight ounces of fruit juice, one-half teaspoon of honey or corn syrup, and a pinch of salt. For the second, dissolve one-quarter teaspoon of baking soda in eight ounces of boiled or carbonated water. Drink alternately from each glass until your thirst is quenched. You may supplement these solutions with carbonated beverages, boiled, bottled, or treated water, or tea made with safe water. Avoid solid foods and dairy products until you've recovered.

In most cases you can prevent or treat traveler's diarrhea on your own. But medical attention is mandatory if you develop a high fever, bloody diarrhea, or unusually prolonged or copious diarrhea. Just the prospect of these complications should persuade you that prevention is, as usual, the best medicine.

Malaria

Traveler's diarrhea is a major nuisance, but malaria is a medical menace.

Malaria is caused by protozoa, tiny parasites that infect red blood cells. Typical symptoms include high fever, shaking, chills, headache, and profound weakness. The most serious form of malaria can be lethal; another variety can cause relapse months or even years after the infection was first acquired in the tropics.

No longer present in the continental United States, malaria is still widespread in tropical and subtropical areas around the world, including parts of Mexico, Haiti, Central and South America, Africa, the Middle East, Turkey, the Indian subcontinent, China, Southeast Asia, the Malay archipelago, and Oceania. Because even brief exposures can result in malaria, all travelers to malarious regions should take preventive medications.

The parasites that cause malaria are transmitted exclusively by the bite of infected mosquitoes. The first step in prevention, then, is to sidestep infected insects (see tropical tip 5).

But malaria is so serious that you cannot rely on insect repellents and fly swatter; preventive medications are necessary. For decades the mainstay of prophylaxis was chloroquine. Unfortunately, many of the most dangerous malaria parasites are now chloroquine-resistant. Fortunately, doctors have again pulled ahead in the constant struggle between the critters that cause infection and the chemicals that kill them. A new medication called mefloquine can now be used to prevent chloroquine-resistant malaria. Mefloquine is easy to use: simply take one tablet a week, beginning one week before you depart and continuing until four weeks after your last potential malaria exposure. You'll need to get a prescription for mefloquine; you should also check to see if the parasites have again begun to outsmart the scientists, in which case you may need alternative medications.

After Your Trip

If you've remained well while abroad, you won't need a medical checkup on your return. The one exception is a tuberculosis skin test, which is a good idea for people who have spent substantial time in underdeveloped areas. In addition, some authorities in tropical medicine recommend routine stool exams for parasites.

Just the reverse is true if you have felt ill during or after your trip: a medical evaluation can prevent complications. Be sure to provide a detailed travel history, and do your best to pick a doctor who knows the territory.

Further Information for the Traveler

Tropical medicine is a highly specialized field. Fortunately, many medical centers now offer travel clinics and tropical medicine referrals; they are often the best resources for preventive information and immunizations, as well as for treatment of exotic travel-related illnesses. In addition, the U.S. Public Health Service offers a telephone information service for travelers. Using a touch-tone phone, call the Centers for Disease Control in Atlanta at (404) 332-4555; the line is open 24 hours a day, but it's a toll call, so have your itinerary — and a pen and paper — ready before you call. You may also want to have a fax number at the ready, since the traveler's information line will offer you the option of receiving a faxed reply that includes a world malaria map. For more detailed information you can purchase the World Health Organization's "International Travel and Health, Vaccination Requirements and Health Advice" by calling (518) 436-9686.

■ AIDS

You don't need me to tell you that AIDS is the most serious preventable disease in the world today. But you may need me to remind you that although AIDS is not yet curable, it *is* preventable — *completely* preventable. Prevention is, in fact, quite simple. Still, it's so important that we must specify in detail the ways to prevent AIDS.

The AIDS Epidemic

First recognized in 1981, AIDS is a new disease. Because it is spread from person to person, AIDS has acquired a momentum of its own; it's the only major killer that's increasing in prevalence each year.

In the first 10 years of AIDS, an estimated 1 million Americans were infected with Human Immunodeficiency Virus (HIV), the cause of AIDS. Approximately one of every 100 adult males and one of every 600 adult females in the United States are infected. More than 160,000 people have developed full-fledged AIDS. Nearly two thirds of these patients are already dead; experts estimate that the death toll will triple by the end of 1993, surpassing 300,000. Tragically, three quarters of all AIDS victims are under 45. As the infection spreads, it has taken an increasing toll of the urban poor and of minority groups.

When compared with the staggering burden of suffering and death, the economic consequences of AIDS may at first seem unimportant. Still, we are spending more than $2 billion annually to care for patients with AIDS, to say nothing of the billions consumed by indirect costs and lost productivity. As the infection spreads, its economic impact is also skyrocketing. In many urban areas entire health care systems and social service networks are on the brink of being overwhelmed by AIDS.

In other parts of the world the situation is even worse. The World Health Organization estimates that in the first decade of AIDS, 10 million people were infected with HIV. The death toll has been enormous, and is increasing rapidly.

The Cause of AIDS

AIDS is caused by the Human Immunodeficiency Virus (HIV). Despite all the harm it creates, HIV is a very fragile virus; it can survive only in blood or body fluids, and it is rapidly destroyed by heat, drying, and disinfectants such as bleach.

To cause disease, HIV must first enter the blood. There is no evidence that it can enter through healthy skin, through the stomach and intestines, or through the lungs. But the virus can enter the body through the mucous membranes such as the tissues that line the genital tract and mouth, particularly if cuts, tears, or ulcers are present. It can also enter through cuts in the skin and by contaminated injections and transfusions.

Once in the blood, HIV multiplies and is carried to many tissues, including the brain and nervous system. But the most severe damage occurs in the blood itself; HIV preferentially infects and destroys the very white blood cells that boost the body's immune system. As these so-called CD4+ lymphocytes disappear from the blood, the body's ability to fight infections and tumors declines progressively. The result: a bewildering array of infections caused by bacteria, parasites, fungi, and viruses, as well as a series of sarcomas, lymphomas, and other malignancies. Although most of these infections and tumors can be treated, they recur inexorably, eventually killing every patient with AIDS.

The Course of Infection

Every patient with AIDS is infected with HIV, but not all people with HIV infection have AIDS.

Like many infections, HIV usually causes no symptoms when it is first acquired. In fact, the sensitive blood tests that detect the virus may remain negative for as long as six to 12 weeks after infection. Even after the blood tests are positive, most HIV-infected patients look and feel perfectly well for months to years. Unfortunately, HIV-infected people can spread the virus through their blood and body fluids during this asymptomatic period.

As time goes on, an increasing percentage of HIV-infected people develop symptoms of disease. The first sign may be a milder illness called AIDS-related complex, or ARC. Patients with ARC develop fatigue, swollen glands, fever and sweats, diarrhea, weight loss, and white plaques in the mouth caused by a fungus infection. Virtually all patients with ARC go on to develop one of the severe infections or tumors that define AIDS. And in many patients AIDS itself is the first symptom of HIV infection. An otherwise rare form of pneumonia (pneumocystis carinii, or PCP) or an unusual malignancy (Kaposi's sarcoma, or KS) is frequently the first manifestation of AIDS.

We don't know exactly what percentage of HIV-infected people go on to develop AIDS. It is clear that the percentage increases with each year of infection; about 5 percent develop AIDS each year, so that half of all HIV-infected people are sick within 10 years of infection. And once AIDS occurs, it progresses inexorably, causing death within two to three years in almost all cases.

How HIV Is Transmitted

AIDS is a truly fearsome disease. But your fear of HIV will be put in proper perspective once you understand that the virus is actually rather difficult to catch.

HIV can be transmitted *only* through infected blood and body fluids. As a result, there are only three ways to get AIDS: through sexual contact with an infected person, through injection of contaminated material, and through transmission from an infected mother to her newborn infant.

Sexual transmission is most likely in male homosexuals and bisexuals. But it is clear that HIV *can* be transmitted through strictly heterosexual encounters, including both genital and anal intercourse. The frequency of HIV transmission during oral-genital sex is less clear, but this mode of transmission has been documented and must be considered a risk.

The risk of sexual transmission of HIV increases with increasing numbers of sexual encounters and partners. Transmission is also facilitated by the presence of genital ulcers and other sexually transmitted diseases. Even in the absence of these risk factors, however, any sexual contact that involves the exchange of body fluids can spread the virus if either partner is infected. The only entirely "safe" sex is monogamous sex between HIV-negative individuals.

Needle transmission of HIV has changed greatly during the first decade of the AIDS epidemic. In the early years, between 1978 and 1985, transfusions of contaminated blood products accounted for many cases of AIDS, particularly in patients with hemophilia. But now that we've learned what causes AIDS, transfusions are very safe: all donors are screened for risk factors; all blood is tested for HIV; and all clotting factors for hemophiliacs are heat-treated to kill the virus. In the United States the risk of acquiring HIV from blood is now less than one per 60,000 transfusions.

Another way of transmitting HIV is through accidental needle sticks. Only medical personnel caring for HIV-infected patients are at risk; this route of spread has been rare but mandates special precautions for all health care workers.

HIV transmission from infected health care personnel to their patients is even less common. In fact, only a handful of cases have been documented. The key to preventing HIV transmission between health care providers and patients is universal precautions. Health care providers should wear gowns, gloves, masks, and protective eye wear while performing invasive procedures. All equipment and devices that enter a patient's body should be sterilized completely before use. All needles and sharp devices should be stored, handled, and disposed of with special care. Equipment and devices that touch but do not penetrate a patient's mucous membranes should be sterilized or disinfected before use; devices that touch intact skin should be cleansed before use. All specimens of blood and body fluids should be handled with precautions. Even without body fluid contact, health care providers should always wash their hands between patient contacts.

Although health care is safe, there has been tragically little progress in controlling the major way in which HIV spreads through needles: intravenous drug abuse. Drug abuse is the most rapidly increasing cause of AIDS in the United States, and drug users who develop HIV infection have a shorter life expectancy than do other HIV-infected people.

The third and final way in which HIV can be transmitted is from infected mothers to their newborn infants. Spread of the virus may occur during pregnancy, during birth, or during breast-feeding. In all, about half of all babies born to HIV-positive mothers will develop the infection. Surely no form of this terrible disease is sadder than pediatric AIDS.

How HIV Is Not Spread

Most of the early panic about AIDS was fueled by ignorance. But even now that we've learned what causes AIDS, many misconceptions persist. Unfortunately, these misconceptions can interfere with humane interactions with

HIV-infected people; they can also distract us from the preventive precautions that really do matter.

You *cannot* catch AIDS from talking with, eating with, or touching infected people. HIV is not spread through the air, even by coughing or sneezing. The virus cannot be transmitted in swimming pools. HIV is not spread by food, water, drinking fountains, or eating utensils. It is never transmitted from clothing, bedding, doorknobs, telephones, or toilet seats. Although HIV can sometimes be found in the saliva of infected people, there has never been a proven example of its spread by kissing. HIV is not transmitted by mosquitoes or other insects. AIDS cannot be spread through normal interactions at school or at work; household and family transmission depends entirely on sexual contact or pregnancy. Nobody can acquire HIV by donating blood.

Primary Prevention of HIV Infection

Despite its dangers, HIV is actually a rather difficult virus to catch. Because its spread is restricted to sexual transmission, needle transmission, and infected pregnancies, effective prevention requires intervention in only those three areas. In fact, I summarize prevention for my patients with two simple injunctions: you'll never get AIDS if you keep your pants up and your sleeves down.

The theory is simple, but practice has proved difficult. You should know the details.

Preventing Sexual Transmission. There are only two ways to prevent absolutely the sexual transmission of HIV: celibacy and monogamous sex with a noninfected partner. Neither method has proved popular. Realistic prevention, then, depends on adherence to sexual practices that if not entirely "safe" are surely "safer."

The risk of contracting HIV infection can be reduced by avoiding multiple sex partners. In contrast, risk is increased by sexual intercourse with male homosexuals and bisexuals, prostitutes, intravenous drug users, and with the sexual partners of such high-risk individuals.

The risk of contracting HIV infection can be reduced by avoiding sexual practices that traumatize tissues or produce bleeding. Anal intercourse is one such practice; the receptive partner is at particular risk.

The risk of contracting HIV infection can be reduced by avoiding the exchange of body fluids during sex. This is best accomplished by the use of condoms. To avoid the spread of AIDS, condoms should be worn during all vaginal, anal, and oral intercourse; the *only* exception is monogamous sex between HIV-negative individuals.

To prevent infection, condoms must be used properly. Use only latex condoms labeled "to prevent disease." Store condoms in a cool, dry place out of direct sunlight. Never use condoms that are torn, brittle, sticky, or discolored. Never reuse condoms. If a condom breaks during intercourse, sex should be immediately interrupted until the condom has been replaced.

Condoms should be put on before any sexual contact occurs. They should be unrolled completely on the erect penis, covering it entirely but leaving a small space at the tip to collect semen; some brands have reservoir tips to serve this function. Remove air pockets by pressing air down toward the base.

Spermicides that contain nonoxynol-9 confer extra protection because nonoxynol-9 inactivates HIV as well as many of the other agents that cause sexually transmitted diseases. Some condoms are manufactured with spermicidal lubricants, but vaginal application of the spermicide will provide additional protection. Water-based lubricants such as surgical jellies are safe for condoms. Never use oil-based lubricants that can damage condoms, such as petroleum jelly, mineral oil, cold cream, hand lotions, baby oil, and vegetable oil.

After ejaculation, the penis should be withdrawn while it is still erect. To prevent spillage, the condom should be held at its base during withdrawal. It should then be gently removed, wrapped in tissue, and discarded in the trash. Afterwards, wash the genitals with soap and water.

Preventing Needle Transmission. The rules for preventing needle transmissions of HIV are even simpler than the rules for preventing sexual transmission. In fact, there is only one rule, and it has *no* exception: don't use intravenous drugs. Unfortunately, drug use remains a critical problem in the United States. One of its most tragic consequences is the transmission of AIDS, not only to other drug users but to their sexual partners and their babies as well.

The prevention and treatment of drug abuse is an extremely complex problem. No definitive solutions are in sight. But until real answers are available, we should do what we can — and that includes interrupting the transmission of HIV between drug users. Needle transmission of HIV can be prevented by using sterile or bleach-treated needles and by never sharing needles. I can understand the qualms about providing needles, or even directions for "safe" needle use, to drug abusers. Still, the threat of AIDS is so great that I believe a needle policy is not only necessary but long overdue. Sterile, single-user needles will do more than protect drug users; they will also reduce the transmission of AIDS to sexual partners of drug users and to newborn infants.

Other Precautions. Because of the limited ways in which HIV can be transmitted, sexual and needle precautions are the mainstays of prevention, and few other precautions are necessary. Because they can be contaminated with blood or saliva, razors and toothbrushes should not be shared. Accidents involving potentially infected body fluids should be carefully cleaned up using bleach freshly diluted with 10 parts of water to one part of bleach.

Secondary Prevention of AIDS

The primary prevention of HIV transmission involves the highly emotional issues of sex education, condom availability and use, and needle exchange programs. But the secondary prevention of AIDS is no less controversial, including the ethically difficult questions of testing, notification, and confidentiality, which pit privacy and individual rights against prevention and community responsibility.

The secondary prevention of AIDS depends on testing to detect early, clinically silent HIV infection. Accurate, rapid, reliable blood tests can now accomplish such screening. The most widely used test is an ELISA assay, which is about 99 percent accurate. Few medical tests score better than 99 percent, but few diseases are more frightening than AIDS. To reduce further the chances of false positive results, medical labs should always repeat positive ELISA tests, and then confirm the results with a different test such as the Western blot assay. Both of these tests measure the body's antibody response to HIV; both can be negative in early infection. High-risk individuals, then, should not take a negative test as absolute proof that they are free of the virus, but should consider repeat testing in three months. Research tests, including viral cultures, can be helpful in special circumstances. And testing should always be accompanied by counseling to help interpret and cope with the results.

Testing for HIV infection is only half the secondary prevention problem, and it's the easier half at that. Far trickier is the question of whom to test.

We are not at the stage where everyone should be tested for HIV — not yet, at least. But high-risk individuals should be tested. HIV testing should be encouraged for gay and bisexual men, intravenous drug abusers, individuals who have had multiple sexual partners (especially prostitutes), patients with other sexually transmitted diseases, and people who have been sexual partners of any of these high-risk individuals. Testing is also reasonable for patients who received transfusions of blood or blood products between 1978 and 1985. Long-term residents of areas with a high prevalence of HIV infection (central Africa and Haiti are examples) should also be offered testing. Health care workers who perform invasive procedures should be tested. Above all, women who belong to high-risk groups should be encouraged to accept testing before or during pregnancy so the question of fetal risk can be addressed. In all cases informed consent should be obtained before HIV testing is performed, confidentiality should be assured, and counseling should be available.

Why test for early HIV infection? There are two reasons. First, people who test positive may derive important health benefits from this information. Early treatment with antiviral drugs may delay the transition from asymptomatic HIV infection to ARC or AIDS. In addition, prophylactic immunizations and antimicrobial therapy may avert some of the terrible infections that complicate AIDS, including pneumocystis pneumonia and tuberculosis.

The second benefit of HIV testing extends beyond the individual to the community. The spread of HIV can be controlled by altering sexual behavior and needle use. Partners who are at risk should be notified, within the limits of preserving individual privacy. Similarly, health care providers should be informed about patients who are HIV-positive. Finally, women who are pregnant or who may become pregnant should be encouraged to consider the implications of a positive test in formulating their plans.

The Control of AIDS

AIDS is the most serious infectious disease in the world today. It is also one of the most preventable.

Medical science has learned an enormous amount about AIDS, but much more research is needed. The most pressing needs, of course, are for drugs that are more effective against HIV and for a vaccine that will prevent infection. Despite great technical difficulties in both areas, I am confident that these research efforts will succeed. To increase the likelihood of success, however, the body politic must devote additional resources to the struggle against AIDS; in this area, at least, it's surely time to escalate from a skirmish to an all-out war against AIDS.

Even with enhanced commitments, scientific efforts to control HIV infection will take time. But when it comes to AIDS, time is already too short. There is more we must do right now.

HIV is the cause of AIDS. But there is another, equally important cause. It's the same thing that causes so many other preventable diseases: human behavior. Even though we can't yet control HIV, we should be able to influence self-destructive behavior. The spread of HIV can be slowed, if not halted. But control of infection will require control of high-risk sexual behavior and of needle sharing. In my view massive public education campaigns are an absolute necessity. And information must be accompanied by practical help, including sex counseling, condom availability, drug abuse prevention and treatment, and needle programs.

I realize that some of these proposals are politically controversial. To still that controversy, I'd like to invite politicians (and voters), educators, and religious leaders to visit the nearest hospital and its AIDS clinic.

We've neglected the basics in preventing many diseases, including AIDS. I fear that it's been easy to put AIDS out of mind by considering it as "their" problem, as a disease affecting mainly gays and drug users. This mental game may be easy, but it's morally wrong. It's also short-sighted. "Their" problem is our problem as fellow humans, as taxpayers, and as members of a community increasingly threatened by the general spread of HIV.

■ Other Sexually Transmitted Diseases

Although none can rival HIV, many other microbes can be transmitted sexually. They are rarely lethal, but they can cause substantial suffering. They can all be prevented, using the same tactics that can prevent AIDS: safer sexual practices, including condoms and spermicidal jellies, case finding and notification, and testing. Fortunately, an additional tactic is available for most of these diseases, since curative therapy is available for all but herpes.

Syphilis

Caused by a special type of bacterium called a spirochete, syphilis produces genital ulcers and can also spread far beyond the genital tract to damage the nervous system and the heart. The spirochete can also cross the placenta; as a result, the infection can spread from pregnant women to their unborn infants.

Like other sexually transmitted diseases, syphilis is most common in people between the ages of 15 and 30. Because the spirochete is readily killed by penicillin, the incidence of syphilis in the United States began to decline in the 1940s, falling eventually to an all-time low of 7,000 cases in 1957. Although the spirochete remains exquisitely sensitive to penicillin, changing sexual practices have produced a resurgence of the disease; at present more than 50,000 cases occur in the United States annually. Especially tragic is the surge in syphilis among newborns, who may suffer permanent disabilities or death from the infection. As recently as 1986, for example, there were only 57 cases of newborn syphilis in New York City, but in 1988 more than 1,000 cases were recognized.

Syphilis is completely preventable. As with other sexually transmitted diseases, prevention involves safer sex (including the use of condoms and spermicides), and case finding and notification. In addition, syphilis can be detected with a simple blood test and can be cured by antibiotics, making it an ideal target for secondary prevention.

Gonorrhea

Each year at least 2 million Americans become infected with the bacteria that cause gonorrhea; most are adolescents and young adults. In men, gonorrhea causes a penile discharge and painful urination. In addition to experiencing pain and discharge, women with gonorrhea can develop pelvic inflammatory disease, which causes fever, severe lower abdominal pain, and a substantial risk of permanent infertility. Blood, joint, and skin infections may occur. Both men and women can also have clinically silent gonorrhea; they continue to feel well, but they can spread the bacteria to their sexual partners.

Although most gonococcal bacteria have become partially or completely resistant to penicillin, extremely effective alternative antibiotics are available. Prevention is complicated by the lack of a blood test to detect latent infection. Still, gonorrhea could be controlled with safer sexual practices, case finding, diagnosis by culture methods, and curative antibiotic therapy. It's a real shame that we've made so little progress against this ancient disease.

Chlamydia

Chlamydia is the sleeper among sexually transmitted diseases. Its name is difficult to pronounce (kla-*mid*-ea), and it is difficult to diagnose with blood tests or cultures. But chlamydia is also a difficult problem for sexually active people, infecting 3 to 4 million Americans annually.

In men, the special type of bacterium that causes this infection produces a penile discharge and painful urination. Mild inflammation and discharge from the cervix is the most common symptom in women, but they may also develop pelvic inflammatory disease and permanent infertility. Pregnant women can also pass the infection to their newborn infants, who can develop eye infections or pneumonia.

Special laboratory tests can be used to detect chlamydia in specimens obtained from the penis or cervix. More important, the infection can be cured by antibiotics. Most important of all, it can be prevented by safer sexual practices, case finding, and treatment of contacts.

Genital Herpes

About 500,000 Americans become infected with the genital herpes virus each year. This number may seem relatively small in comparison with the 6 million infected annually by gonorrhea and chlamydia. But the herpes virus persists in infected individuals and may relapse without additional sexual exposure. As a result, more than 20 million Americans are currently infected with the virus, and each is potentially able to spread herpes to sexual partners.

The herpes virus produces painful genital ulcers, which may be accompanied by fever and swollen lymph glands in the groin area. Pregnant women who are infected can pass the virus to their newborn infants, sometimes with devastating consequences. A new antiviral medication, acyclovir, can control the symptoms of herpes, but it will not eliminate the virus from nerve tissues; as a result, relapses may occur after the medication is discontinued.

Even though genital herpes cannot be cured, it can be prevented by safer sexual practices, including the use of condoms and spermicides.

■ Lyme Disease

Lyme disease is an example of a "new" infection that's not really new. Although it was not officially diagnosed and named until a cluster of cases occurred in Lyme, Connecticut, in 1975, manifestations of the disease were first recognized in Europe nearly 100 years ago. Still, Lyme disease appears to be on the increase, with nearly 8,000 cases reported in the United States annually. The disease has been recognized in at least 46 states, but most American cases have occurred in just three regions: wooded areas of New York, Connecticut, Massachusetts, and other coastal New England and mid-Atlantic states; Wisconsin and Minnesota; and wooded coastal areas of California and Oregon. It also occurs throughout Europe and Australia. Most cases occur between May and August.

Lyme disease is caused by a spirochete. But this specialized bacterium does not naturally infect humans. Instead, it is an infection of animals such as deer and mice. The spirochete is transmitted to humans by tiny deer ticks that become infected when they feed on animals harboring the spirochete.

In 75 percent of cases the earliest symptom of Lyme disease is a rash that's notable for its large size and circular shape, with a red rim on the outside and normal skin toward the middle. The rash fades within several weeks, but some patients go on to develop arthritis, neurological abnormalities, or heart problems. Antibiotics are effective; most patients recover fully, but some can have chronic arthritis or permanent neurological abnormalities.

You can prevent Lyme disease by preventing tick bites. Your doctor can help you avoid the potentially serious consequences of the infection by treating it with antibiotics in its early stages.

Simple measures will go a long way toward preventing tick bites. The ticks that carry Lyme disease favor woods and grasses; if you venture into the woods in spring or summer, you should always wear protective clothing, including shoes and long pants. Use insect repellents, especially in high-risk areas of the country, apply them to your skin, and repeat the application every few hours if you're sweating heavily. Most chemical insect repellents contain DEET, but their DEET concentrations vary from 7 to 100 percent; a 30 percent solution seems about right; higher concentrations are no more effective, and they can produce side effects, especially in children. For extra protection you can spray your clothing with insect repellents that contain permethrin.

Because tick bites are painless, you may not know that the insects have defied your chemical barriers and clothing to reach your skin. To detect ticks, you should inspect yourself carefully when you undress, remembering that these ticks are not much larger than sesame seeds. Don't panic if you spot a tick; even in high-prevalence areas, most ticks are not carriers of the Lyme spirochete. Of course you have no way of telling if a tick is infected. But since it takes many hours for ticks to transmit their infection to people, you can prevent Lyme disease even after you've been bitten by simply removing the tick. Don't squash the insect onto your skin; instead, use a tweezers to grasp the tick as close as possible to its mouth, and then remove it with a slow, steady pull.

There is no Lyme vaccine for humans, but a vaccine for dogs was marketed in 1990; it may help protect dog owners from acquiring the infection from their pets.

See your doctor if you develop symptoms that may reflect Lyme disease. A blood test can often help confirm the diagnosis, and antibiotic treatment (doxycyline or amoxacillin for early disease, ceftriaxone for late disease) can kill the spirochete, preventing complications of the infection.

■ Pneumonia, Influenza, and Tuberculosis

No longer the leading killers in America that they were 100 years ago, these infections are still sixth on the list of fatal diseases. Like nine of the ten leading causes of death, pneumonia, influenza, and tuberculosis can often be prevented; chapter 5 tells you how.

■ Food poisoning

Food poisoning is a major problem in underdeveloped areas where sanitation is poor, but it's also a common, and preventable, cause of discomfort and disease in all Western cultures.

What Is Food Poisoning?

Food poisoning comes in two varieties.

In the first, bacteria contaminate food, where they multiply and produce toxins. The illness that results when the food is eaten is caused not by the bacteria themselves but by the toxins they leave behind in the food. The most common forms of food poisoning, caused by staph or clostridia bacteria, belong in this toxin-induced category. The symptoms are vomiting and diarrhea starting abruptly 6 to 12 hours after the contaminated meal. Needless to say, it's a very uncomfortable problem, but there is never any fever or intestinal bleeding, and the symptoms resolve fully in just 6 to 24 hours. Another form of toxin-induced food poisoning, botulism, is much more serious, but it's now rare in the United States.

In the second form of food poisoning, the microbes that contaminate food establish actual infections in the human intestinal tract. Because the bacteria have to multiply in the gastrointestinal tract, the symptoms can be delayed for a day or two, and they usually begin more gradually than do toxin-induced symptoms. But it takes longer for the body to rid itself of bacteria, so symptoms are more prolonged, sometimes lasting for a week or more. And since there is an actual infection, fever is often present along with cramps and diarrhea, which can contain mucus and blood in more severe cases.

Traveler's diarrhea is one example of the second type of bacterial food poisoning. Home-grown bacteria that are common causes of diarrhea include campylobacter, salmonella, shigella, and yersinia. In underdeveloped areas typhoid and cholera are much more serious intestinal infections transmitted by contaminated food and water.

Several species of viruses are also capable of causing gastrointestinal infections; typically milder than bacterial infections, they produce less fever and rarely cause bleeding. In the underdeveloped world many parasites cause intestinal infections. But you don't need a passport to acquire a parasite; if you have a child in a day care center or if you drink from a clear mountain stream that has been contaminated by beavers, you may already have spent some time cleaning up after a common parasite, giardia.

In all, dozens of bacteria, viruses, and parasites can cause food poisoning. You can learn to prevent them in less time than it would take to learn their names.

Preventing Food Poisoning

Although you don't have to pray for protection against food poisoning, the first step in prevention has been elevated to a lofty status next to godliness: it's cleanliness. Good sanitation that absolutely protects water from contamination by sewage is the first requirement. If you have a public water supply, the bacterial count of your water will be monitored for you; but if you have your own well, you'll have to arrange testing yourself. And to prevent household spread of intestinal infections, handwashing after using the toilet and before cooking and eating is a simple but effective hygienic measure.

The second requirement for preventing food poisoning is proper food preparation. Carefully wash fresh fruits and vegetables, thoroughly cook all meats, fish, and poultry, and diligently refrigerate all cooked foods.

Although these rules are entirely simple, they are broken with distressing frequency. A particular problem is posed by poultry and eggs, since nearly *one third* of all raw poultry is contaminated by salmonella or campylobacter. No wonder there are an estimated 4 million cases of food poisoning due to these bacteria in the United States each year! But they can be prevented. To prevent bacterial multiplication, always defrost frozen poultry in a refrigerator or microwave instead of at room temperature, and never leave fresh or defrosted birds at room temperature for longer than 30 minutes. Cook poultry and eggs above 160 degrees, and refrigerate them at 40 degrees or less. (Yes, it's goodbye to the soft-boiled three-minute egg.) Never use eggs that have cracked shells or are outdated. Be particularly careful to follow these same precautions for leftovers, which should always be finished up within four or five days. Pay extra attention to summer picnics, which are classic occasions for food poisoning; tradition notwithstanding, a modern cooler will serve you much better than a pretty wicker basket.

Although poultry and eggs are the leading sources of bacterial food poisoning, no food is risk-free unless it is handled properly. For example, shellfish from contaminated waters may harbor hepatitis A; chopped meat is a favorite breeding ground for clostridia; cheese may be contaminated by listeria; and staph loves custards and mayonnaise-based salads. All in all, bacteria are less finicky than many people. The moral: prepare, store, and serve all foods as if they were potentially contaminated; the extra protection really takes very little extra work.

Last but not least, rely on your common sense to protect your intestinal tract. If your food looks, smells, or tastes as if it might be spoiled, change your menu. A last-minute dash to the market is better than an all-night journey to the bathroom.

■ The Control of Infectious Disease

Human genetics change very slowly. As a result, human diseases have changed slowly as well, at least until the industrial revolution produced the rapid technological and life-style alterations that have introduced so many new illnesses to humanity. But microbial genetics change very rapidly. As a result, we are confronted with a constant array of new infectious diseases caused by apparently new or different organisms. For example, I spend many hours teaching medical students and doctors about Legionnaires' disease, Lyme disease, toxic shock syndrome, and AIDS — all of which were unknown when I was in medical school just twenty-five years ago.

Fortunately, medical science has been quick to deal with these new infections. Although each burst on the scene as a mysterious threat, all were rapidly understood and — with the important exception of AIDS — controlled.

The contest between microbiologists and microbes will continue unabated. But although you should be grateful for modern medical science, you should not depend entirely on doctors and drugs to protect you from infections, either new or old. Microbes can cause infections only after they gain access to the body, and most cause disease only if the body is first weakened. Prevention, then, depends on the basics: a prudent life-style that keeps the bugs away while maintaining the good general health that will keep them at bay.

∎ 17 ∎

Accidents and Occupational Disorders

I am constantly surprised that most people, even those who take aggressive action to prevent bodily illness, have a fatalistic view of bodily injury. "It's just an accident," they say, "and accidents will happen."

Accidents will happen — if we let them.

It's true that accidents are chance events, random, unpredictable, and unforeseeable. But most injuries are *not* caused by true accidents. Instead, physical trauma results from circumstances that place the victim at risk, from behavior that makes the accident an event that's just been waiting to happen. In fact, many injuries are predictable — and preventable.

Of course, not *all* accidents can be prevented, any more than *all* heart disease or cancers can be avoided. But a little planning and prudence can go a long way toward protecting you and your family from accidental injury at home, on the roads, outdoors, and at work.

The notion that accidents can be prevented may surprise you, but it's hardly new. An early expert in human nature, if not prevention, put it nicely: "Out of this nettle, danger, we pluck this flower, safety" (Shakespeare, *Henry IV*, part 1).

∎ Accidents in America

It's no accident that I've devoted a whole chapter to injury prevention: accidents are the fourth leading cause of death in the United States, and they are the leading killer of Americans between 1 and 44 years of age. Each year about 100,000 Americans die from injuries sustained in accidents; that amounts to 11 deaths per hour. Because so many victims of fatal accidents are young, accidents result in a greater loss of years of working life than heart disease, cancer, and stroke *combined*.

Approximately 50 percent of all fatal injuries result from motor vehicle accidents. Falls are in second place, accounting for 13 percent of deaths. Other leading killers include drowning (7 percent), fire (6 percent), poisoning (4 percent), suffocation (4 percent), and firearm accidents (2 percent). We don't hear much about these deaths, but we do encounter lots of publicity about air travel fatalities, even though they account for just over 1 percent of the total.

Accidental deaths are just the tip of the injury iceberg. Sixty-eight million accidents severe enough to restrict activity or require medical care occur in the United States each year. Nearly 9 million of these accidents are serious enough to cause disability, amounting to about 1,000 per hour. The economic impact of these injuries is enormous; the costs of direct medical care and lost productivity approach 1 percent of the gross national product.

Each and every one of us is at risk of accidental injury or death, but some of us are at higher risk than others. Young children, adolescents and young adults, and elderly people are most vulnerable. Men are at higher risk than women. People working in construction and agriculture are more likely to be injured than are people in other occupations. And the poor are more likely to suffer death or disability from accidents than are the affluent.

Preventing accidents is not an easy matter, but it can be done. Alcohol and other intoxicating agents account for 50 percent of all deaths from motor vehicle accidents, drownings, and shootings, and for 40 percent of deaths from fires. Cigarette smoking is responsible for 25 percent of fatal fires. Unsafe driving practices, neglect of seat belts and child restraints, poor product design, improper storage of chemicals, inadequate lighting, and unsafe working conditions are among the many preventable causes of injuries.

The National Academy of Science tells us that "injury is probably the most under-recognized major public health problem facing the nation today." "Injury" derives from the Latin word for "not right." It's not.

Motor Vehicle Accidents

Like other twentieth-century technological marvels, the automobile has brought us great efficiency, convenience, and pleasure — at a price. By substituting horsepower for leg power, motor vehicles have deprived people of much-needed physical exercise. By producing noxious gases as by-products of internal combustion, automobiles threaten to send us from the freeway to the hospital. By propelling us at enormous speeds, they can subject the human body to much more physical force than it can withstand. Above all, motor vehicles, like other modern technologies, function at the behest of people; human behavior determines whether they will serve us faithfully or injure us fatally.

Nearly 50,000 Americans are killed in motor vehicle accidents each year, and another 2 million sustain disabling injuries. You can avoid becoming a statistic by following a few simple guidelines.

Don't drink before driving. About half of all fatally injured drivers have blood alcohol concentrations above .10 percent, the legal limit in most states. In my view the only entirely safe blood alcohol level for drivers is 0. But even if you follow the "not a drop" rule yourself, you can still be victimized by a drunk driver. There is an urgent need for improved public education, appropriate controls on alcohol sales, and enhanced law enforcement. We also need to find some way to dissociate commercial messages that glorify fast cars and cold beer during the same time-out. And we need action to control other intoxicating drugs, which contribute to more than 10 percent of all serious motor vehicle accidents.

Wear seat belts. The proper use of lap and shoulder restraints can reduce serious injuries and deaths by about 50 percent. Some newer autos are equipped with automatic motorized shoulder belts and manual lap belts. Don't forget to buckle your lap belt; without it you can "submarine" under your shoulder harness during an accident, sustaining needless injury.

Although 37 states have mandatory seat belt laws, only 49 percent of Americans wear seat belts. My patients explain their neglect with many creative excuses ("They don't fit"; "I'm too fat"; "Not comfortable"; "I'll be trapped"; "Takes too long"; "Why should I listen to the government?"). There is *no* valid reason for not wearing seat belts. *Always* buckle up when you are in a moving automobile, whether you're sitting in the front or the rear.

I don't know how many illnesses I've prevented with other advice, but I do know that over the years four patients have phoned me to report that simple seat belt instructions have saved their lives. Seat belts could save your life, too.

Use child restraints. All 50 states require them, with good reason. Unrestrained children are 10 times more likely to die in auto crashes than are children who are properly protected by safety seats. Highway accidents kill as many children as cancer and congenital malformations combined; all childhood deaths are tragic, but these traumatic deaths are doubly sad because they are preventable.

Make safety an important criterion when you buy your next car. Air bags are of proven benefit. Unfortunately, many such safety features are expensive options. But the choice is yours: antilock brakes or turbochargers. Investigate crash-worthiness as well as style. And take good care of your car so it will be safe to drive.

Drive carefully and defensively. Obey traffic laws. The 55-miles-per-hour speed limit was instituted to conserve gasoline (a good idea for a healthful environment as well as a healthy economy), but it also contributed to a 29 percent decline in death by auto. The return to 65 miles per hour in some states has already increased fatalities. Slower is safer.

Don't drive if you are sleepy, sick, or taking medications that may impair your alertness or judgment. If you have serious medical problems, discuss the possible risks of driving with your doctor. Elderly people with imperfect vision, impaired hearing, or slowed reactions should be particularly careful to match their itineraries to their abilities.

Take a safe driving course, particularly if you are an older driver. Experience is a great asset for older drivers, but slowed reflexes can increase their risk of accidents. The American Association of Retired Persons (1901 K Street, N.W., Washington, DC 20049) offers an inexpensive eight-hour "55 Alive" safe driving course for drivers over 50. The National Safety Council (44 North Michigan Avenue, Chicago, IL 60611) offers a defensive driving course that is open to drivers of all ages.

Always wear a safety helmet while riding a motorcycle. Better yet, don't ride a motorcycle.

These guidelines are, I know, obvious to the point of being tedious. Obvious or not, they are neglected with alarming regularity. In this respect, too, motor vehicle accidents are like other preventable illnesses: the simple, obvious measures provide the best protection.

Airplane Accidents

Unless you are a pilot, mechanic, or air traffic controller, there is little you can do to prevent plane crashes. As a voter, however, you can work to be sure the Federal Aviation Administration has the regulations and resources it needs to prevent accidents. Air travel is safe, but it could — and should — be even safer.

Even if you can't prevent air accidents, you can be a safety-conscious passenger. Wear your seat belt and join the campaign for child restraints. Pay attention to the safety information provided before take-off, read the emergency instructions placed in your seat pocket, and familiarize yourself with the plane's safety equipment and emergency exits. Because smoke can interfere with visibility after a crash, it's a good idea to count the number of rows between your seat and the nearest emergency exit.

Recreational Accidents

Swimming and Boating. Drowning claims an average of 6,500 lives each year. Toddlers between the ages of one and three are at greatest risk; they could be protected by installing a securely latched four-foot fence around back-yard pools and by providing adult supervision.

Alcohol is responsible for nearly half of the 1,200 adult boating-related deaths each year; other intoxicants contribute to an additional 10 percent. Sobriety is the key to prevention. Also important are good swimming skills and effective flotation devices for all boaters. Swimmers, too, should exercise simple safety precautions. They must be wary of ocean waves, currents, and undertows. They should never swim alone, even in the "safe" confines of a pool. Very cold water is another potential hazard; body heat is lost 25 times more rapidly in water than in air, so hypothermia, muscle rigidity, and ultimately drowning can result from cold water immersion. Preexisting injuries and illness can also sap strength and endurance; never swim if you have a serious illness or injury, or if you're tired out even before you work out.

Diving is responsible for more than 500 crippling brain and spinal cord injuries each year, mostly caused by diving into shallow water or empty pools; they could be prevented by one simple rule: look before you leap.

Bicycling. Half of all Americans ride bikes. Never having recovered fully from the athletic deprivations of an urban childhood, I belong to the other half. Still, I'm all for biking; it's an excellent form of aerobic exercise and a nonpolluting form of transportation.

That's the good news. The bad news is that bicycle accidents are the most numerous of all recreational injuries, accounting for more than 550,000 emergency ward visits each year. Many bike injuries are minor lacerations and bruises (minor unless you are the patient), but they also include fractures, internal injuries, and 1,000 deaths per year.

Just 12 simple guidelines will reduce substantially your risk of suffering a serious biking injury. The first three guidelines: wear a helmet, wear a helmet, wear a helmet. Helmets reduce serious head injuries by 80 percent; be sure you have a high-quality helmet that's been approved by objective organizations such as the Snell Foundation.

The other nine guidelines are also important. Because 95 percent of biking fatalities involve collisions with motor vehicles, *avoid traffic* when you can, and *obey traffic laws* and safety regulations to the letter when you can't avoid riding in traffic. Wear bright-colored clothing and consider mounting a flag on your bike to *increase your visibility.* Always *use reflectors and lights* at night. *Ride defensively,* assuming the worst of drivers. *Avoid dangerous surfaces* — surfaces that are muddy, sandy, icy, excessively bumpy, or covered with wet leaves. *Stay in control* of your bike at all times, avoiding excessive speed and dangerously sharp turns. *Beware of dogs.* Finally, like the automobile drivers who are your greatest worry, you should *avoid alcohol and drugs* before you hit the road.

Horseback Riding. Thirty million Americans ride, and they suffer serious injuries at a higher rate (one per 350 riding hours) than even motorcyclists (one per 7,000 riding hours). Most are caused by falls. Since riders can travel at 30 miles per hour eight feet above the ground, it's not surprising that head injuries are the greatest worry. Yet only 20 percent of riders wear helmets. For prevention, get protection; strap on your helmet before you gallop off into the sunset.

Falls

Falls pose a major public health problem in America. When young people fall there is usually a reason, good or not; they fall off a bike or a horse, out of a tree, or off their skis. But when older people fall, it is often difficult to identify a predisposing cause. One of every three senior citizens will fall during the course of a year; in all the elderly account for 74 percent of the 13,000 deaths caused by falls annually.

Falls by children can be reduced by using appropriate safety equipment, including crib and bed railings and stair and window guards. Preventing falls among the elderly is more difficult but no less important. Effective prevention involves identifying potential problems in two areas: in the elderly themselves, and in their personal environment.

Impaired vision, weak muscles, and poor coordination can all contribute to falls by the elderly. The best prevention involves maintaining good general health, screening for correctable visual problems, and maintaining regular physical activity to promote strength, endurance, and coordination. Measures to prevent osteoporosis (see chapter 8) will also diminish the risk of injury when falls occur. Good footwear is important. Medications that may impair alertness or judgment should be minimized or avoided; so, too, should medications that may lower the blood pressure excessively. It's up to doctors to use extra care when prescribing sedatives and tranquilizers to older people; it's up to each person to use alcohol prudently if at all.

Because 60 percent of falls by the elderly occur at home, a secure home environment is mandatory. Things that can help include good lighting (including night lights); nonslip flooring; sturdy hand rails on stairways; sensibly arranged, stable furniture (especially high, firm chairs); and nonslip tubs and showers. Stray objects, electrical cords, and torn rugs are particularly hazardous. And many elderly people have benefited from the security of a personal emergency response system to bring help quickly if they fall (or fall ill) at home. Outside, buckled pavement and surfaces that are slippery or icy constitute the greatest threat to keeping our senior citizens upright.

Violence

Whereas most injuries are unintentional, some are not. Violence produces a peculiarly, though not exclusively, American form of death. Homicide has climbed to eleventh place among the leading causes of death. Although no age, race, or sex is immune, young males, especially blacks, are at highest risk. A 1991 U.S. Senate Judiciary Committee report characterized our country as "the most violent and self-destructive on earth." With 25,700 murders in 1991, it's hard to dispute this sorry conclusion.

Violence also accounts for many nonfatal injuries. In 1991 alone more than 2.6 million Americans were raped, robbed, or assaulted — an all-time high. Every *hour* more than 250 Americans fall victim to violent crimes. A large number of these result from domestic violence, which is particularly likely to harm women and children. Several studies have shown that 22 to 35 percent of women who seek care in hospital emergency wards are suffering from physical or mental symptoms caused by battering. All too often, I'm sorry to say, doctors treat the symptomatic injuries without addressing the underlying cause.

Firearms also play an important role in unintentional injuries and deaths. About 70 percent occur at home; many of the remainder are hunting accidents. Most often young males are the victims. It's a serious problem, causing 1,700 deaths in the United States each year. Many lives could be saved by storing firearms in locked cabinets and by keeping them unloaded. Education and abstinence from alcohol could help protect hunters. But in view of the many injuries caused by intentional and accidental firearm use, I believe that gun control legislation is a medical necessity.

Fires

With more than 6,000 deaths from fire annually, America stands shamefully first in fire fatalities, with three times the death rate of Europe, Australia, and Japan. Don't blame our firefighters; we have more firefighters, and they have better equipment and shorter response times, than in other countries. Don't blame our trauma centers; we are well equipped and all too experienced in treating burn victims. Don't blame our home construction methods or fire codes, though both could use improvement. To explain our sorry leadership in fire fatalities, don't look for a scapegoat at all — instead, just look in a mirror.

A few surprisingly simple changes in equipment and behavior could prevent many burns and fire fatalities; you should not get burned even once.

Faulty heating devices are the leading cause of residential fires; kerosene space heaters are particularly risky. Smoking causes about 25 percent of residential fires; fire prevention officials have long advocated the development of self-extinguishing cigarettes and matches to combat this problem. Lacking these products, they advocate safer smoking practices — for example, don't smoke in bed. I have a much better system: don't smoke at all!

The third leading cause of fire fatalities is alcohol; a study from Maryland revealed that the majority of fire victims were intoxicated at the time of death.

Do you still wonder why so many Americans die in fires?

Be sure that your family is well protected from fire. A few simple measures will help:

- If you use an electric space heater, be sure it has been approved by a nationally recognized testing lab. Keep it on the floor when it's in use, being sure that it's at least three feet away from flammable fabrics and that it's turned off when you leave the room.
- Keep your burners and ovens clean. Never leave pot holders on the stove. Don't store things over the stove where someone could be burned reaching for them. Don't wear loose-fitting sleeves when you're cooking. Heat cooking oil slowly, and keep your pot handles turned in to prevent pots from being knocked off the stove. Most important of all, never leave cooking unattended.
- Keep your chimney clean, and always use a metal screen for your fireplace.
- Store matches in cool areas out of the reach of children.
- Have your furnace inspected and serviced regularly. Never store inflammable materials near the furnace. Use only approved containers to store gasoline, paint, and other combustibles.

Have a smoke detector on each level of your house; at least one should be near every bedroom so you'll hear an alarm at night. Smoke detectors come in two varieties, photoelectric and ionizing: both act by sensing smoke particles rather than heat or flames, and both are very sensitive. Test your smoke detector monthly, and change batteries at least once a year. When you change its battery, vacuum the detector to clean the sensing chamber. Never paint over a smoke detector. Consider replacing old units with new ones every ten years or so.

Have at least one fire extinguisher on every level of your home. Multipurpose dry chemical extinguishers (labeled Class A, B, and C) are best because they are effective against electrical fires and burning solvents as well as ordinary fires. Be sure that your extinguishers are fresh and functional, and that everyone in your family knows how to locate and use them.

Prepare your family to escape from fire. Be sure you have a safe exit route from each floor of your house, and run through a fire drill at regular intervals.

Most fire departments have excellent information on fire prevention: many will visit your home to inspect it for fire hazards and to give you firsthand advice on fire control. It's a resource you should utilize. Just one hot tip may prevent your dreams — and your health — from going up in smoke.

Household Hazards

There's no place like home, even when it comes to accidents. As a place where you're likely to be injured, your castle is second only to your car.

Electrical Hazards. In addition to causing 166,000 residential fires, electrical hazards are responsible for many other shocking injuries, including 300 electrocutions annually.

Extension cords are a major problem. Best used only temporarily, they should never be overloaded, wrapped around furniture, nailed to baseboards, or passed under rugs. Always use heavy-duty cords for high-wattage appliances such as heaters, toasters, computers, and power tools, and always plug them into grounded (three-pronged) outlets.

Repair or replace any appliance that is electrically malfunctioning. Even frayed cords on lamps should be replaced. Never use light bulbs with higher wattage ratings than your lamp is designed to accommodate. Don't overload electrical outlets. If you blow a fuse, find out why; never use a fuse with a higher amp rating than its circuit was designed to accommodate.

Use appliances properly. Always use grounded outlets for three-pronged plugs. Unplug hair dryers, irons, and space heaters when they are not in use. Try not to leave home while the washer, dryer, or dishwasher is on. Never, ever use electrical appliances while you are standing on a damp floor or using the bathtub or shower.

Protect your children. Teach them the fundamentals of electrical safety at an early age — and, just to be safe, keep appliances out of their reach and place covers over your electrical outlets.

Call an electrician if you notice warning signs such as repeatedly blown fuses or tripped circuit breakers, sparks, fires, or heat from electrical outlets or switch boxes, abnormal odors, or flickering lights. Correcting electrical hazards to prevent fires and shocks is a bright idea.

Scalding. There are many ways you can get into hot water around the house: scalding is among the more serious household hazards.

Every year 112,000 Americans require emergency treatment for scaldings, half caused by tap water. These incidents could all be prevented simply by setting household water heaters to 120 degrees F. Many are now set as high as 150 degrees F, a waste of energy as well as a health hazard. The moral: get a liquid-crystal thermometer, test your hot water at the tap, and adjust your water heater's thermostat.

Many other household scaldings could be prevented by better product design; wide-bottomed pots and kettles, improved coffee makers, and childproof stove switches are among the modifications that would help.

If prevention fails, you should know what to do until medical care is available. You can reduce the depth of a scald burn with a simple first aid measure: cold water.

Carbon Monoxide. Because it's odorless, colorless, and tasteless, carbon monoxide gas may be difficult to detect before it has done its poisonous work. Early symptoms include headache, dizziness, and loss of mental clarity. Later, shortness of breath and weakness appear. The final symptoms are coma, brain damage, and death.

Carbon monoxide is a natural by-product of combustion. To prevent dangerous concentrations of carbon monoxide from building up, be sure that your gas, oil, coal, or wood heating system is well maintained and is working properly. Of great importance, too, is adequate ventilation of your home. Signs of trouble include stale, smelly, or excessively humid air or soot coming from a heating system or fireplace. If you spot these problems, open the windows and call your heating company — from another room.

And while you're thinking about carbon monoxide, be sure that your car's exhaust system and body are in good shape so that exhaust gases won't seep into the vehicle.

Hazardous Products. The safety of home, indeed. Many of the wonderful technological advances that make the contemporary American home such a nifty place can also produce major injuries. In addition to electrical hazards, excessively hot water, and faulty heating systems, we must also consider the potential dangers of the very products that keep our homes sweet, our gardens green, and our cars humming.

Household cleaners, paints and solvents, pesticides and fertilizers, and automotive products can all be hazardous. Look for "Warning," "Danger," "Caution," or "Poison" on all labels — and follow safety directions to the letter. Leave all hazardous products in their original containers with their warning labels and directives in plain view. And before you use a hazardous product, be sure you know what to do in case of an accidental exposure.

Use hazardous products only in well-ventilated areas. Work outdoors when you can, avoiding windy days; open windows when you must stay indoors. Keep children and pets away from work areas. Take breaks frequently, especially if you feel dizzy, nauseated, or unduly tired. Don't eat, drink, or smoke when you are using dangerous products. Better still, don't smoke at all.

Follow directions carefully. Never mix products unless specifically directed to do so. When necessary, wear appropriate safety equipment such as gloves and protective clothing to safeguard your skin, goggles to protect your eyes, and a mask to protect your lungs. If a spill occurs, clean it up promptly. Wash or shower thoroughly after you've finished using hazardous products.

Use only as much of a hazardous product as you need to do the job. Clean up promptly. Store all potentially dangerous products carefully, out of reach of children and animals. Lids and caps should be tightly sealed and child-proof. Containers should be kept dry. Flammable and volatile materials should be kept in cool, well-ventilated areas far removed from sparks, flames, heat, and sources of emission; store gasoline only in approved containers.

Dispose of hazardous products according to directions so that you will protect your environment as well as your health.

To cut down on your worries about hazardous products, use them as little as possible. Instead, conserve, recycle, and experiment with alternative and natural products that are safer for people and the environment we share.

Child Safety

Surely the most vulnerable among us, children are entirely dependent on family and society for food, shelter, nurturing, and health. Accidents and injuries are particularly threatening to those who are too young to know better. It's up to adult caretakers to prevent childhood accidents.

Childhood poisonings have decreased by 75 percent since child-resistant caps were put on medications and household chemicals. But these containers will protect your children only if you use them properly; keep medications and hazardous products in their original packaging, and always fasten containers securely. Remember, too, that child-resistant is not child-proof. Keep medications and chemicals out of your children's reach, preferably in securely latched cabinets. But since some children seem able to thwart all reasonable precautions, every home with young children should have a bottle of syrup of ipecac to induce vomiting in case of poison ingestion — and the number of a poison control center's hotline.

Lead poisoning is a particularly insidious childhood hazard that can result from lead in old house paint, drinking water, auto emissions, dust, and soil; chapters 4, 11, and 22 discuss these problems in detail.

Choking kills about 150 American children every year. The culprits are usually small round objects, including parts of toys, small balls, undersized infant pacifiers, and balloons that are underinflated or empty. Foods, too, can lodge in a child's small windpipe; peanuts, popcorn, hard candies, grapes, and pieces of hot dog are the leading hazards. The Consumer Product Safety Commission has done a good job in improving the design of products for children, but parents must be vigilant as well. Parents should also learn the Heimlich maneuver (CPR and first aid courses teach this simple technique) so they can save their children should choking occur.

Strangulation and suffocation are two more hazards unique to childhood. Strangulation can be caused by hanging from clothing or high-chair straps, or by wedging the head between crib slats or under the mattress. Suffocation can be caused by plastic bags and sheeting, plastic playpen sides, polystyrene-filled cushions, and even by adult mattresses and water beds if infants are allowed to sleep on them face down. Older children may suffocate if they become trapped while playing in refrigerators or other appliances. Improved product design and warning labels are helping to control these hazards, but parental responsibility remains the key to prevention.

Each year more than 1 million American children under four require emergency treatment for injuries suffered at home. Accident prevention, like other good health habits, should begin in childhood. Starting at the earliest possible age, teach your children how to avoid injuries. Teach them, too, the importance of good nutrition, regular exercise, the avoidance of smoking and substance abuse, and other essential health habits. And remember that the very best way to teach is by example.

■ Occupational Disorders

Throughout our history as a species humans have worked. And throughout human history injury and illness have been unintended by-products of that work. Modern industrial society, however, depends on work of unprecedented complexity, often involving huge machines with great power to injure and tiny chemical compounds with great power to cause illness. There are two obvious ways to prevent all these problems: inherit, or win the lottery. But if you have to work, some basic principles of prevention can help keep you healthy on the job.

Occupational health problems include about 10 million injuries, 350,000 illnesses, and 50,000 to 70,000 deaths annually. The National Institute for Occupational Safety and Health has compiled a list of the ten leading work-related health problems.

1. Lung disease (asthma, inflammation, chronic lung disease, cancer)
2. Musculoskeletal injuries
3. Cancers (skin, bladder, liver, nose, lining of the lung, and leukemia)
4. Severe traumatic injuries (amputations, lacerations, fractures, eye loss or damage)
5. Cardiovascular disease (heart attacks, high blood pressure)
6. Reproductive disorders (infertility, miscarriage, malformations)
7. Nervous system disorders
8. Noise-induced hearing loss
9. Skin disorders (burns, infections, allergies)
10. Psychological disorders (stress, depression, alcohol and drug dependency)

Preventing occupational disorders requires three levels of action: governmental, industrial, and individual. The first got a tremendous boost from the Occupational Safety and Health Act of 1970. Still, much more progress is needed. Corporate America devotes less than 2 percent of its revenues to employee safety and health programs, and only 2 percent of all workers have access to industrial health services. American medicine is not much further along than American industry: although more than 115 million of our citizens work, only 1,000 physicians in this country are board-certified in occupational medicine.

When it comes to preventing occupational disorders, then, you can't rely entirely on your government, your boss, or your doctor. They can all help, but as in so many areas of prevention, the final responsibility is yours.

Accidents

Of the 10 million injuries suffered on the job each year, 3 million are serious enough to require emergency medical care, 2 million are disabling, and 10,000 are fatal. Motor vehicle crashes are the most common causes of fatal industrial accidents, accounting for one third of the total. Among the remainder, falls, industrial equipment injuries, being struck by falling objects, electrocutions, and burns are most common. Although all workers are at risk, the highest injury rates are in agriculture, mining, manufacturing, construction, and transportation.

Work-related accidents occur at a rate more than two times higher than at home or in public places. A full 40 percent of them are preventable. Optimal working conditions (good lighting, safe machinery) are important. So, too, are safety-oriented regulations and standards (reasonable productivity quotas, appropriately timed work shifts and breaks). Training and education can also help prevent many employee injuries. Last but not least, don't overlook the importance of simple personal precautions (carefulness and courtesy, sobriety). A safe working environment, safe equipment, and safe workers can prevent many work-related injuries.

Occupational Illnesses

"How much sickness, death, and misery are produced by the present state of many factories, warehouses, workshops and workrooms?" The question was posed by Florence Nightingale in 1859. Despite all that has happened since, it's a question that still needs to be asked today.

In contrast to industrial accidents, which are sudden and obvious, most industrial illnesses are slow and insidious. Sometimes a single toxic exposure can cause illness years later. More often, repeated exposures cause cumulative damage that becomes evident only after months or years.

With tens of thousands of chemicals in daily use, it's impossible to catalogue all the hazards faced by American workers. Unfortunately, in fact, the toxic potential of many compounds has not even been investigated. But every worker should be alert for certain major exposures:

Oils and coolants
Pesticides and fumigants
Solvents (benzene, trichloroethylene)
Gases (ammonia, carbon monoxide, chlorine)
Mineral dusts (asbestos, silica, coal, talc, fiberglass)
Metal dusts and fumes (lead, mercury, arsenic)
Physical hazards (radiation, heat, cold, noise)

If you work with any of these potential hazards, be sure your health is being protected. Safe working conditions, exacting safety regulations, proper equipment, good training, and appropriate emergency procedures are crucial. Because most exposures occur through inhalation, good ventilation, hoods over hazardous work areas, and protective masks are essential. Skin contact is the second leading type of exposure; always wear gloves and protective clothing. Finally, companies that use toxins should monitor vulnerable employees for exposure *before* illness occurs; using radiation badges and monitoring blood lead levels are examples of secondary prevention in the workplace.

It's very common to change jobs several times in the course of a career. Keep a record of the exposures you may have experienced in each of your positions. Remember, too, that you don't have to be an employee to suffer from potentially harmful industrial exposures. For example, household members can be exposed to dust brought home on the worker's clothing. In addition, everyone living near an industrial site should be aware of potential toxic exposures.

A great range of preventable disorders can occur in the workplace. Table 17-1 summarizes some of them.

Occupational health is complex, and prevention is multifaceted. You can get lots of information and help from the National Institute for Occupational Safety and Health (1600 Clifton Road, N.E., Atlanta, GA 30333; 1-800-356-4674).

Repetitive Motion Disorders

It's possible that many people experience mild episodes of it. It's probable that some are seriously afflicted by it. It's doubtful that many people suffer major consequences from it.

It is the latest worry in the American workplace: the repetitive motion or cumulative trauma disorder.

In 1717 the father of occupational medicine, Bernardino Ramzinni, wrote that "violent and irregular motions and unnatural positions" can produce injury. The latest controversy in occupational medicine hinges on a new question: Can gentle, regular, natural motions cause injury if they are repeated often enough?

The question is simple — but the answer is not.

The repetitive motion disorder has generated great concern among workers and great debate among physicians. Highly emotional publicity has fueled widespread worry that's sometimes tinged with panic. The medical jury has not yet returned its verdict; still, we know enough to be confident that even if concern is warranted, alarm and hysteria are not.

For decades both workers and their physicians have believed that repetitive use produces musculoskeletal injuries, particularly involving the back, neck, arms, and hands. But it's been surprisingly difficult to confirm this belief by objective medical study. In fact, it is now quite clear that repetitive use does *not* cause osteoarthritis, the common form of joint damage that had previously been attributed to "wear and tear."

Table 17-1. Selected Occupational Disorders

Disorder	Occupation/Industry	Cause
Malignancies		
nasal lining	woodworkers	hardwood dust
	radium workers	radium
	nickel smelters	nickel
lungs	construction and maintenance workers handling asbestos, automobile brake repairmen, certain industrial workers	asbestos
	coke oven workers	coke oven emissions
	uranium and fluorospar miners	radon
	smelters	nickel, arsenic, chromates
	chemists	bis-chloromethyl-ether
bone	radium workers	radium
scrotum	lathe operators, metal workers	mineral oils
	coke oven workers, petroleum refiners	soots and tars
kidney	coke oven workers	coke oven emissions
bladder	rubber and dye workers	benzidine, napthylamine, auramine, 4-nitrophenyl
leukemias	radiologists, rubber industry workers	ionizing radiation
Anemias	whitewashing and leather industry	copper sulfate
	electrolytic processes, smelting	arsine
	plastics industry	trimellitic anhydride
	explosives manufacturing	TNT
	radiologists, radium workers	ionizing radiation
	pesticide production	phosphorus, arsenic
	pigment production, pharmaceuticals	arsenic
Infections		
tuberculosis	medical personnel	bacteria
plague, anthrax, rabies	farmers, ranchers, veterinarians	bacteria, viruses
hepatitis	medical personnel, day care workers, staff of chronic care facilities	viruses

▶

Table 17-1. (continued)

Disorder	Occupation/Industry	Cause
Nervous system disorders		
encephalitis	battery, smelter, and foundry workers	lead
Parkinson's disease	welders, manganese processing workers, battery makers	manganese
nerve inflammation	pesticides, pigments, pharmaceuticals	arsenic
	furniture refinishers, degreasers	hexane
	plastics and rayon industries	methylbutylketone, solvents
	battery, smelter, and foundry workers	lead
	dentists, chloralkali plants, battery makers	mercury
	plastics and paper manufacturing	acrylamide
	bakers, blacksmiths, glass blowers	infrared radiation
	fumigators	naphthalene
Lung disorders		
asthma	jewelry and metal workers	platinum
	paint and adhesive workers	isocyanates
	bakers	flour
	woodworkers	wood dust
	foam and latex makers	formaldehyde
lung inflammation or scarring	coal miners	coal dust
	asbestos exposures	asbestos
	quarrymen, sandblasters, miners, ceramics industry	silica
	talc processors	talc
	cathode ray manufacturers	beryllium
	silo fillers, arc welders	nitrogen oxides
	paper, refrigeration, oil industries	sulfur dioxide
	plastics industry	trimellitic anhydride

Table 17-1. (continued)

Disorder	Occupation/Industry	Cause
Hepatitis	dry cleaners, plastics industry, solvent users	carbon tetrachloride, chloroform, trichlorethylene
	explosives and dye industries	phosphorus, TNT
	fumigators, fire extinguisher makers	ethylene dibromide
Kidney failure	battery makers, plumbers, solderers	lead
	electrolytic processes, smelting	arsine
	antifreeze manufacturing	ethylene glycol
	dentists, jewelers, battery makers	mercury
	fire extinguisher makers	carbon tetrachloride
Male infertility	formulators and applicators	dibromochloropropane
Skin inflammation	many occupations	many irritants (solvents, oils, acids, alkalis)

Source: Adapted from P. T. Landrigan and D. B. Baker, "The Recognition and Control of Occupational Diseases," Journal of the American Medical Association 266 (August 1991), 676.

Other studies, however, have suggested that certain occupations may indeed injure the hands and wrists. Vibrating hand-held power tools such as jackhammers appear to cause hand dysfunction, including painful spasms of the blood vessels (Raynaud's phenomenon). Even occupations that are less traumatic may cause hand problems; assembly-line work, meat cutting, grinding, and other mechanically stressful jobs have been blamed for the carpal tunnel syndrome, a thickening of wrist ligaments that produces hand pain by putting pressure on a major nerve as it passes across the wrist. But while some authorities accept the validity of these studies, others do not.

If strenuous industrial occupations spark controversy, clerical work starts wars. And the quintessential American work of the 1990s, computer data entry at video display terminals, is at the heart of the debate. Many thousands of workers have experienced hand, wrist, and arm complaints that have sometimes been severe enough to produce disability or induce surgical therapy. Despite the real misfortunes of individual patients, however, it is far from clear that repetitive use is actually responsible for these problems. In fact, a 1990 Dutch study published in the *American Journal of Epidemiology* found *no* link between repetitive keyboard use and the carpal tunnel syndrome.

Repetitive use can surely cause discomfort and pain. A 1985 Michigan study found that more than 25 percent of workers experienced at least one bout of arm and hand pain during a two-year period. This study, in fact, is the major document cited by proponents of the repetitive trauma concept. But a close look at the investigation itself is instructive; it documents an association between work and wrist pain but *not* between work and objective tissue injury, including carpal tunnel syndrome.

These distinctions may appear to be meaningless hair-splitting. Indeed, pain is pain. But we need to know whether or not these pains reflect actual tissue damage. In 1979 the average workers' compensation claim for wrist injuries cost $618 for medical payments and $1,026 for indemnity compensation. Since then, costs have soared — and so have complaints. In 1989 the U.S. Department of Labor received 147,000 complaints of repetitive motion disorders, a 22 percent increase over the previous year. At present, repetitive motion complaints account for more than half the workplace disorders reported to the Bureau of Labor Statistics. With all this pain, disability, medical and surgical therapy, and expense, we need to sort out the complex biomechanical, psychosocial, and economic factors that contribute to the repetitive motion syndrome.

But until we have more answers, we should encourage simple measures that may minimize musculoskeletal complaints. Work stations should be designed to provide comfort and support, and to allow a natural body position. Padded chairs and good posture seem important. Good lighting, a reasonable work pace, and regular breaks should help reduce muscle tension and stress, particularly if breaks are used for stretching and moving instead of more sitting and staring.

The video display terminal is neither a technological heaven nor an operator's hell. It is an important tool which must be used properly. If employers' expectations for the computer age have been exaggerated, so too have workers' fears. For example, despite years of worry and volumes of strident claims, a 1991 study in the *New England Journal of Medicine* demonstrated that VDT use is *not* linked to miscarriages (see chapter 22 on low-frequency radiation). When used correctly, the VDT can produce important commercial and technical benefits without causing illness. But, as in all areas of occupational health, the worker's comfort, satisfaction, and protection are crucial to both productivity and health.

It won't do you much good to eat a low-fat, high-fiber diet, exercise regularly, get your immunizations, and floss your teeth if you are killed or crippled by an accident, poisoned by a toxic chemical, or injured at work. Together we can help make safety a priority for government and industry. Individually we can do the little things that will go a long way toward preventing accidents and occupational disorders.

▪ 18 ▪

Substance Abuse:
Tobacco, Alcohol, and Drugs

Late one night a member of the Boston Celtics struck two local university students with his van. The news media reported that the driver was intoxicated; the two young women he struck died. At teaching rounds early the next morning I discussed the case of a 34-year-old woman with a life-threatening heart valve infection caused by intravenous cocaine abuse. Returning to my office, I examined two patients with severe emphysema, two with coronary artery disease, and one with lung cancer; all had been heavy cigarette smokers. Then, during my hospital consultation rounds, I evaluated a 23-year-old man who has been in a coma for 17 days because he fell down a flight of stairs while drunk.

All in a day's work.

All tragic, unnecessary, and preventable.

Substance abuse is a major cause of suffering, disability, and death in the United States today. It takes many forms, from the perfectly legal abuse of tobacco products and alcohol to the entirely illicit use of cocaine, heroin, and amphetamines. Although smoking, drinking, and using drugs may seem to be completely unrelated problems, they actually share many key features. In each case voluntary use of a chemical agent can lead to physical and psychological dependency on that chemical — addiction. And in each case continued use of the addicting substance is self-destructive behavior that often leads to dreadful medical, psychological, and social consequences. Today, and every day, 1,100 Americans will die from tobacco abuse, 300 from alcohol abuse, and 20 from drug abuse.

Substance abuse is a multifaceted problem of enormous complexity. Its root causes vary, including genetic factors, psychological issues, social pressures, and economic problems. The successful prevention and treatment of substance abuse must involve progress in all these areas. It should be a top priority for our society. Despite their prime importance, the socioeconomic aspects of substance abuse are beyond the scope of this book (and its author). But we should attend to the medical aspects of substance abuse, and to interventions that may allow vulnerable individuals to recognize substance problems early, to take corrective action, and to prevent disaster.

■ Tobacco Abuse

It may surprise you to find tobacco in a chapter on substance abuse, much less in first place. Smoking is, after all, perfectly legal and extremely widespread. But don't let legal and social norms fool you: tobacco use is substance abuse. The U.S. Surgeon General, the American Psychiatric Association, and the National Institute on Drug Abuse have all found that nicotine is an addicting substance. In fact, animal studies have demonstrated that nicotine is just as addicting as cocaine and heroin. And because smoking is so widespread, cigarettes kill more Americans in *one week* than cocaine and heroin together in *one year*. Are you still surprised that smoking heads this chapter?

The health consequences of tobacco abuse are unimaginably disastrous. *Smoking accounts for one sixth of all deaths in the United States each year.* Claiming 434,175 lives in 1988, smoking is clearly our leading preventable cause of death. The average smoker will die more than six years earlier than the average nonsmoker. During their shortened life span, smokers will also suffer much more discomfort, disease, and disability than nonsmokers.

The economic impact of smoking is also disastrous. The average smoker will incur a lifetime cost of more than $20,000 in medical bills and lost wages — more than $2 for each pack of cigarettes smoked. Tobacco abuse costs our society more than $200 billion each year, costing each *non*smoker more than $220 annually.

Tobacco use is nearly as old as human agriculture, beginning about 5,000 years ago. First cultivated in the New World, tobacco was perhaps the first American export — a tragically successful export that spread rapidly throughout the world. But the health consequences of tobacco remained relatively modest until the mid-nineteenth century, when cigarettes began to replace snuff, pipes, and cigars. In the early twentieth century, new techniques of cigarette manufacturing and marketing fueled an explosive increase in cigarette smoking; for the first time, large numbers of women became addicted to tobacco. Patterns of tobacco use also changed, with inhalation the rule rather than the exception. The net result: the "brown plague," a true modern epidemic.

The dangers of tobacco have been obvious at least since the U.S. Surgeon General's 1964 report on smoking and health. Individuals, private institutions, and government agencies have begun to fight back. In 1965 more than 40 percent of all adults smoked cigarettes; at present just under 30 percent smoke. But 53 million adult Americans still smoke cigarettes, and 1 million teenagers take up the habit each year. In addition to the young, smoking disproportionately affects the poor and members of minority groups. Women, too, have lagged in smoking cessation.

We must do better — much better. Our goal, in fact, should be nothing less than a smokeless society.

Why Is Tobacco So Dangerous?

Tobacco smoke contains more than 4,700 chemicals, at least 43 of which are proven carcinogens. The chemicals in smoke are rapidly absorbed from the lungs, traveling in the blood to all of the body's tissues. It's easy to see why cigarettes account for 30 percent of all cancer deaths and 30 percent of all heart disease deaths in the United States.

Nicotine, the best known of these toxins, is a powerful central nervous system stimulant. Inhaled nicotine hits the brain in less than six seconds — twice as fast as mainlined heroin. The average smoker takes more than 50,000 hits of nicotine each year. In addition to its addicting properties, nicotine is also a circulatory stimulant, causing sharp increases in blood pressure and heart rate. Found only in tobacco, nicotine is actually a potent poison; 60 milligrams of nicotine taken in a single dose will kill the average adult by paralyzing breathing, making nicotine as potent as cyanide.

Nicotine is bad enough, but it is only one of the many toxins in tobacco smoke. Like nicotine, many of these chemicals are natural ingredients of the tobacco leaf itself. Others are by-products of combustion; carbon monoxide is particularly worrisome because it impairs the oxygen-carrying capacity of blood, stressing the heart, circulation, and lungs. Astonishingly, many other chemicals are actually added to cigarettes by the manufacturers to "improve" the taste, aroma, and combustion properties.

Some improvements! Here is a partial list of the major toxic components of cigarette smoke:

nicotine	carbon monoxide
catechols	acetaldehyde
n'-nitrosonor-nicotine	nitrogen oxides
phenol	hydrogen cyanide
polynuclear aromatic hydrocarbons	acrolein
beta-naphthylamine	ammonia
nickel	formaldehyde
cadmium	urethan
arsenic	hydrazine
polonium-210	nitrosamines

It's enough to make you sick.

Low-nicotine, low-tar cigarettes are being promoted intensively. Are they safe? Absolutely not. In actual fact, smokers of "low-yield" cigarettes get just as much nicotine into their systems as do smokers of ordinary cigarettes, to say nothing of carbon monoxide and hundreds of other chemicals. After reviewing all the evidence, the British Health Education Council said it all: smoking low-nicotine, low-tar cigarettes is "like jumping from the 36th floor instead of the 39th."

There is no such thing as a safe cigarette. But is there a safe "dose" of cigarettes? The answer is no. It's true that the heaviest smokers suffer the deadliest consequences of smoking. But because damage from tobacco smoke is cumulative, even light smokers are likely to suffer from their habit.

Table 18-1. Health Consequences of Tobacco Abuse

Body system or function	Tobacco-related disorders
Heart	Coronary artery disease, including heart attacks and angina Abnormal heart rhythms Rapid pulse Sudden cardiac death
Circulation	Narrowing and blockage of arteries Aneurysms of the aorta Blood clots in veins (in conjunction with birth control pills)
Nervous system	Strokes Hemorrhages
Lungs	Cancer of the lungs Cancer of the lung lining (in conjunction with asbestos) Chronic bronchitis Emphysema Asthma and allergies Infections (sinusitis, bronchitis, pneumonia)
Intestinal and digestive	Gastritis and ulcers Cancer of the esophagus, stomach, pancreas
Musculoskeletal	Osteoporosis and fractures
Reproductive	Cancer of the cervix Tubal pregnancies Miscarriages Premature deliveries Low-birth-weight babies Sudden infant death syndrome Male impotence Cancer of the prostate
Kidney and urinary	Cancer of the kidney, bladder
Blood	Decreased oxygen delivery Elevated red and white blood cell counts Malignancies: leukemia, multiple myeloma
Metabolic	Decreased HDL (good) cholesterol Altered metabolism of various medications Central obesity (increased waist-to-hip ratio)
Head and neck	Cancer of the mouth, tongue, larynx (voice box) Tooth loss Periodontal disease

Table 18-1. (continued)

Body system or function	Tobacco-related disorders
Skin	Premature facial wrinkling
Trauma	Burns, smoke inhalation, and death from fire
Psychological	Depression
	Addiction

Women who average just four cigarettes a day, for example, will double their risk of suffering a heart attack.

The only safe cigarette is the one that remains unsmoked.

Other types of tobacco use are not as spectacularly suicidal as cigarettes, but they are still extremely dangerous. The similarity between pipes, cigars, and cigarettes makes it obvious that these forms of smoking are all hazardous. Unfortunately, however, the dangers of smokeless tobacco are often underestimated; a leading cause of oral cancer, snuff and chewing tobacco are used by 10 million Americans.

Health Consequences of Tobacco Abuse

By now you should know that tobacco causes major diseases of virtually all human organ systems. Still, it may be useful to summarize these problems in tabular form (see table 18-1).

It's a fearsome list. While some smoking-related problems are relatively mild, most are highly lethal. And in most cases smoking produces an enormous increase in risk. For example, smoking accounts for 92 percent of all deaths from mouth cancer, 90 percent of deaths from lung cancer, 80 percent of deaths from laryngeal cancer, 78 percent of deaths from esophageal cancer, 48 percent of deaths from kidney cancer, 29 percent of deaths from pancreatic cancer, and 17 percent of deaths from stomach cancer. Smoking causes 115,000 deaths from heart disease each year, about one third of the national total. Every year 57,000 Americans die from chronic obstructive lung disease and 27,500 die from strokes simply because they smoked. And maternal smoking is responsible for 18 percent of low-birth-weight babies, premature deliveries, infant respiratory distress syndrome, and sudden infant deaths.

Passive Smoking

Every cigarette has two ends. One transports smoke into the mouth, throat, and lungs of the voluntary smoker. The other emits smoke into the environment, transforming bystanders into involuntary smokers. To make matters worse, sidestream (secondhand) smoke is actually dirtier than mainstream smoke.

Three out of every four Americans are involuntarily exposed to tobacco smoke. Nonsmokers living in the same household as smokers are at particular risk; elevated blood levels of nicotine and carbon dioxide are usually present, and headache, cough, and eye and nose irritation are common. Passive smoking lowers the HDL (good) cholesterol levels of nonsmokers. As little as 20 minutes in a smoky room can alter the platelet function of passive smokers. Passive exposure to smoke at work also impairs the lung function of nonsmokers.

Nasal irritation, abnormal blood tests, and diminished lung function are troublesome, but passive smoking does far more, none of it good. Children are especially vulnerable. Nonsmoking women who are exposed to passive smoking during pregnancy have an increased risk of fetal loss. The children of smokers are three to four times more likely to develop serious respiratory infections than the children of nonsmokers. These children, too, score lower on standardized intelligence tests than do the children of nonsmokers. Even worse, leukemias, lymphomas, and brain cancers are more common in the children of smokers.

Adults are also harmed by passive smoking. The risk of lung cancer is doubled in adults exposed repeatedly to household smoking. Passive smoking also contributes to heart disease; the spouses of smokers suffer 30 percent more heart attacks than the spouses of nonsmokers.

The Environmental Protection Agency reports that passive smoking causes 3,700 deaths from lung cancer, 10,000 deaths from other cancers, and 37,000 deaths from heart attacks in the United States each year. That means that for every eight smokers who are killed by their habit, one *non-smoker* is killed by secondhand smoke.

Cigarette smoking is the leading preventable cause of death in the United States.

Passive smoking is the third leading killer, ranking just behind alcohol abuse.

Each person is responsible for his or her own health. It's up to each smoker to quit, with as much medical and community help as needed. But when it comes to passive smoking, the responsibility for preventing illness is communitywide.

There ought to be a law. Fortunately, in many communities there is.

Smoking Cessation: Benefits

The best time to quit smoking is before you start. The second best time is now.

It's never too late to stop smoking; even if you've smoked for years, your health will improve once you've kicked the habit. And the benefits are substantial: a 45-year-old smoker who quits can expect to gain five years of life expectancy; a 65-year-old who quits smoking will gain three and one third years of life.

Smoking cessation reduces the risk of cancer. Men who smoke are 22 times more likely to die from lung cancer than nonsmokers; within just 10 years of quitting, however, lung cancer risk declines by about 70 percent. Smoking cessation also dramatically reduces the risk of mouth and throat cancer, pancreatic cancer, and bladder cancer.

Smoking cessation reduces the risk of heart disease. Smokers have double the nonsmoker's risk of fatal heart attacks; in just one smoke-free year this excess risk is cut in half, and after 15 years the risk for former smokers is exactly the same as for people who have never smoked.

Smoking cessation reduces the risk of stroke. Smokers are twice as likely to die from strokes as nonsmokers, but after just five years the risk for former smokers is back to normal.

Smoking cessation improves lung function, helping to prevent pneumonia and influenza and slowing the progression of emphysema. Blood vessels, too, benefit from quitting; the risk of arterial blockages and aortic aneurysms declines substantially in smokers who give up cigarettes. Smokers who have stomach ulcers will experience faster healing if they quit. And pregnant women who quit smoking will have safer pregnancies and healthier babies, even if they delay quitting until the thirtieth week of pregnancy.

The long-term health benefits of smoking may be hard to keep in mind, but there are also immediate personal rewards. Quitting is the best cure for irritation of the eyes, nose, and throat, to say nothing of the smoker's cough. Smoking cessation improves energy, exercise capacity, and "wind." Food tastes and smells better. And people who quit look and smell better to nonsmokers, who are, after all, in the majority.

Finally, smoking cessation is a financial bonanza, saving a one-pack-per-day smoker $730 a year. Reduced medical expenses and sick time will add to the instant rebate.

Is there any reason *not* to quit? No indeed.

Many smokers disagree with me, citing weight control as a reason to delay quitting. It's not a good reason. In fact, the weight gain that results from quitting is modest, averaging only five pounds, and even this modest gain can be minimized by instituting a weight-control program while giving up cigarettes.

Smoking Cessation: Tips and Techniques

If smoking cessation were easy, cigarette sales would plummet; more than 80 percent of adult American smokers say they would like to quit. Nicotine is addicting, and smoking cessation is difficult. As a former smoker I understand those difficulties. But difficult is not impossible: 43 million Americans have stopped smoking. If you smoke, you should do whatever it takes to join us.

Most people who kick the habit do so on their own. Some succeed by gradually cutting down, but most find the abrupt "cold turkey" method best. Here are a few tips that may help your cold turkey fly:

- Reinforce your motivation. Make a list of all the bad things about smoking and all the good things about quitting.
- Pick a date and stick to it. Make it a big day such as a birthday or anniversary. Or join millions in the American Cancer Society's Great American Smokeout each November. In general, it's best to avoid holidays that involve parties in smoke-filled rooms.

- Try to persuade all the smokers in your household or office to join you in quitting.
- Just before your quitting day, have your teeth cleaned, your clothing cleaned, and your house cleaned. Throw out your ashtrays and matches or lighters along with your cigarettes.
- Start an exercise and nutrition program.
- Stock up on sugarless gum, low-calorie candies, and other cigarette substitutes. Spicy flavors such as cinnamon may be particularly helpful.
- Try to avoid situations that trigger your smoking, particularly at first. You won't have to forsake coffee, alcohol, big meals, or parties forever, but you should attempt to spend as much time as possible in smoke-free situations during the first days and weeks.
- Reward yourself. Buy a piggy bank or open a special bank account. Deposit every dollar you save on cigarettes and buy yourself a special gift with the money that accumulates.
- Think positively. You *can* quit. When a "friend" offers you a cigarette, don't explain you are trying to quit. Instead respond simply, "No thanks, I don't smoke." When you feel tempted to smoke, recite or read your motivation list. Think of all the weak-willed people you know who have quit; if you don't know any, think of me.
- Find other ways to relieve tension. Deep-breathing exercises and meditation (see chapter 19) can help. Exercise is also very helpful. Mental exercises that take your mind off your craving are useful. Find ways to keep your hands busy — knitting, doodling, solving puzzles, and manipulating pencils or "worry beads" are all much better than smoking. Allow yourself low-calorie snacks to keep your mouth busy as well.
- Take one day at a time. Don't kid yourself into thinking that you can smoke "just one." As with any other addicting substance, one dose of nicotine is enough to reestablish your habit. Don't allow yourself one puff — not even after months or years of success.
- Don't give up if you fail on your first attempt to quit — or, for that matter, if you don't make it on your second or third try either. Most successful quitters need several serious attempts finally to kick the habit. If you find yourself smoking again, try to figure out what went wrong so you can avoid similar problems the next time around.

If you can't quit on your own, you can get help. Your doctor may decide to prescribe a nicotine skin patch or nicotine-containing chewing gum to get you over the physical withdrawal symptoms that testify to the fact that smoking *is* an addiction. Because smoking cessation is so very important, I've even prescribed mild tranquilizers to help control stress. Hypnosis is another treatment that can be very useful.

Many hospitals, civic groups, and religious organizations offer smoking cessation clinics and groups; employers, too, are increasingly active in helping with smoking cessation. You can also consider one of the many commercial smoking cessation groups listed in the Yellow Pages, or you can contact the American Cancer Society, the American Lung Association, or the National Cancer Institute for helpful information on quitting (see chapter 24 for addresses).

Smoking and Society

Smoking cessation is difficult because nicotine is an addicting substance. But it's difficult, too, because the smoking habit is reinforced by the tobacco industry, by elements of the mass media, and even by some government policies.

Despite all that we know about smoking and health, more than 623 billion cigarettes are sold in the United States annually — over 3,000 per adult. It's no wonder, then, that the tobacco industry remains one of the most lucrative in America, generating nearly $7 billion in annual profits. Some of these revenues, it's true, go to farmers, workers, merchants, and shareholders. But the industry also invested $3.27 billion in cigarette advertising and promotion in 1988, a 27 percent increase over the previous record expenditure a year earlier. Tobacco ads on television and radio have been banned since 1971, but the industry is still getting its pitch across.

One of the results of this advertising muscle is that the media may be reluctant to bite the hand that feeds them. Magazines, in particular, derive nearly 6 percent of their advertising revenues from tobacco manufacturers. It's no coincidence that studies have shown that they tend to underreport news about the adverse health effects of smoking.

Tobacco advertising and promotion efforts are targeted increasingly at minority groups, women, and young people. Not surprisingly, smoking is especially prevalent in these groups. Although 46 states and the District of Columbia have laws restricting the sale of tobacco to minors, about 3,000 teenagers take up the smoking habit each day, providing ready replacements for the 1,100 adults killed daily by cigarettes.

Laws notwithstanding, more than 90 percent of all smokers report that they became addicted before age 21. Unless we change, more than 5 million of today's children will eventually be killed by cigarettes.

Another distressing aspect of the commercial might of the tobacco industry is the export trade. More than 30 percent of our tobacco crop is sold overseas. America is the world's leading tobacco exporter, selling 216,583 tons of tobacco abroad in 1986. Although many federal agencies are leading the fight against smoking in America, our trade representatives are working to *expand* foreign tobacco sales. In 1990 American manufacturers exported 160 billion cigarettes, a record number. And overseas, as at home, the most vulnerable are targeted selectively, so that cigarette sales are rising fastest in developing countries. Worldwide tobacco use has increased by almost 75 percent since the 1964 U.S. Surgeon General's report on smoking and health. At present more than 1 billion people smoke, consuming more than 5 trillion cigarettes annually. The toll is astounding: smoking is responsible for 2.5 million excess or premature deaths annually; world-wide, nearly 5 percent of all human deaths are caused by smoking.

Former U.S. Surgeon General C. Everett Koop, a courageous leader of the fight against smoking, has pointed out that "at a time when we are pleading with foreign governments to stop the export of cocaine, it is the height of hypocrisy for the United States to export tobacco." Hypocrisy indeed, but hardly an accident. After all, a tobacco leaf is carved into the U.S. House of Representatives speaker's rostrum, symbolizing our nation's 200-year-old obeisance to tobacco.

Despite all our efforts, both public and private, tobacco use remains a terrible problem in the United States and around the world. It's a complex problem, too, involving legitimate concerns ranging from free speech to the balance of trade. I am neither a constitutional scholar nor an economist, and I won't pretend to have the answers to these difficult questions. But I am a doctor, and I believe that we must somehow find a way to put health first.

We need to prevent cigarette promotions from convincing our young people that smoking enhances vigor, sophistication, and sex appeal. We need a way to enforce existing laws prohibiting tobacco sales to minors. We need a way to educate the public about the hazards of smoking and the addicting properties of nicotine. We need to develop better techniques for smoking cessation. We need a way to shift excess health insurance premiums and tax burdens from nonsmokers to smokers and to the tobacco industry itself. We need better ways to protect people from passive smoking and environmental pollution.

In 1988 the Canadian government raised cigarette taxes, mandated stern health warnings on cigarette packages, and banned tobacco advertising and promotion. As the price of a pack of cigarettes rose to U.S. $5.50, cigarette sales fell 20 percent in less than two years. In all, 40 percent of Canadian smokers have quit; because of their greater sensitivity to price, half of all teenage smokers have kicked the habit. Our tobacco problems may be more complex, but they are no less solvable. The U.S. Public Health Service has adopted the goal of a smokeless society by the year 2000. It may not be attainable, but it is a worthy call to action which we should all heed.

■ Alcohol Abuse

Two of every three American adults consume alcohol, making it the most widely used drug in the United States. As a nation we consume 5.8 billion gallons of beer, 585 million gallons of wine, and 395 million gallons of distilled spirits every year. As individuals we drink an average of 318 beers, 179 drinks of hard liquor, and 77 glasses of wine annually. This means that the average American over 14 consumes more than two and a half gallons of pure alcohol per year. By any measure, that's a lot.

For most people who drink, alcohol is a well-tolerated drug, providing personal enjoyment and social benefits. In general, alcohol use of up to two drinks a day is considered safe; several studies, in fact, have suggested that one to two drinks a day may actually reduce the risk of coronary artery disease. Although I don't choose to drink, I use the two-a-day rule to advise patients that low-level alcohol use is safe. But as with all rules, there are exceptions: to avoid fetal damage, pregnant women should not drink at all; to avoid accidents, nobody should drink before driving or operating hazardous machinery; to avoid complications, patients who have serious illnesses should check with their doctors before drinking, as should people who require medications. Women should consider the possibility that even low doses of alcohol may increase their risk of breast cancer. And nobody who has had an alcohol-related problem should drink at all.

With these important exceptions, drinking the equivalent of up to two drinks a day is safe. But although a little alcohol is safe, drinking more, even a little more, can be very dangerous.

Alcohol is an addicting drug, and alcohol addiction is widespread. In 1989 10.5 million American adults exhibited symptoms of alcoholism, and another 7.2 million abused alcohol without experiencing symptoms.

Alcohol is a dangerous drug. Men who average more than two drinks a day are twice as likely to die before age 65 as are men who don't drink at all; for women alcohol use triples the risk of premature death. Alcohol is associated with nearly 10 percent of *all* deaths in this country, killing 105,095 people in 1987. Accidents and liver disease head the list of alcohol-related killers.

Alcohol is a drug that is abused by people of all ages. Like tobacco abuse, alcohol abuse often begins in youth. More than half of all seventh- to twelfth-graders drink, as do 80 percent of college students. Many drink heavily; 30 percent of American college students have five or more drinks in a row at least once within any two-week period. True, not many teenagers die from alcoholic liver disease, but 7,000 15-to-24-year-olds die each year in alcohol-related automobile accidents. Nor is the problem improving; whereas teenage drug abuse is beginning to diminish, youthful alcohol abuse is as rampant as ever.

Alcohol is an expensive drug. In 1987 alcohol abuse cost our country $116 billion in lost productivity, medical care expenses, and property damage — even more than the cost of cardiovascular disease. In effect, each of us pays a hidden "alcohol tax" of $300 per year, yet the treasury recaptures only $50 per capita in annual alcohol excise tax revenues.

Despite the pervasive medical, psychological, and social problems they cause, alcohol and alcoholism are sadly neglected in medical education and research. In the political arena, too, these depressing problems are often brushed aside; it seems easier to have a drink and forget our problems than to face our problems and forgo the drink.

Health Consequences of Alcohol Abuse

Like tobacco, alcohol can damage almost all the body's major organ systems. Each chapter of this book details the diseases caused by alcohol; needless to say, all of these problems are entirely preventable. So that you

Table 18-2. Health Effects of Alcohol Abuse

Body system or function	Alcohol-related disorders
Heart	Rapid or irregular heart action Weakened heart muscle function Heart failure Increasing angina
Circulation	High blood pressure
Nervous system	Stroke due to brain hemorrhage Confusion and dementia Seizures Acute intoxication Withdrawal symptoms including hallucinations and DTs Brain degeneration Peripheral nerve damage
Intestinal and digestive	Inflammation of the esophagus and stomach Ulcers Bleeding Inflammation of the pancreas Hemorrhoids Cancer of the esophagus and stomach
Liver	Fatty liver Alcoholic hepatitis Cirrhosis
Musculoskeletal	Osteoporosis Muscle weakness Fractures due to trauma
Breast and reproductive	Fetal damage including mental retardation and growth retardation Fetal alcohol syndrome Breast cancer in women Breast enlargement in men Male impotence

won't have to reread the whole book to review the effects of alcohol, I'll summarize them in table 18-2.

What Is Alcohol Abuse?

Alcohol use, in modest amounts, is safe. Alcohol abuse, however, is hazardous. What's the difference?

Although there is no absolute line between alcohol use and abuse, they can be differentiated in two ways: on the basis of the volume of alcohol consumed and on the basis of the pattern of consumption and its consequences.

Table 18-2. (continued)

Body system or function	Alcohol-related disorders
Kidney	Excessive urination
Blood and immune system	Anemia
	Low white blood cell counts
	Low platelet counts
	Abnormal bleeding
	Impaired immune function
Metabolic	High blood triglycerides
	Low blood sugar levels
	Low blood protein levels
	Low blood magnesium and phosphorus levels
	Malnutrition
	Acidosis
	Altered metabolism of various medications
Head and neck	Cancer of the mouth and larynx
Skin	Itching
	Rosacea and other abnormalities
Infections	Increased susceptibility to many infections
Trauma	Motor vehicle accidents
	Falls
	Fires
	Drownings
	Violence
	Other accidents
Psychological	Addiction
	Depression
	Anxiety
	Antisocial behavior
	Impaired work performance
	Impaired family interactions

Beverages vary in their alcohol content. In order to quantify alcohol consumption, doctors and nutritionists define one drink as containing 15 grams of alcohol, the amount found in 12 ounces of beer, five ounces of wine, or one and a half ounces of 80-proof distilled spirits.

Based on these standards, people who average less than three drinks per week can be considered light drinkers, people averaging less than two drinks per day are moderate drinkers, people averaging two to four drinks per day are heavy drinkers, and people averaging more than four drinks per day are very heavy drinkers. One of every 11 American adults is a heavy or very heavy drinker — and is therefore at risk of serious medical and personal consequences.

Almost all alcohol abusers are in the heavy or very heavy drinking categories. Surprisingly, though, some people can drink heavily without suffering adverse consequences. As a result alcohol abuse must be defined further.

Problem drinking is a pattern of alcohol use that results in disturbances of health, work, or social interactions. Early signs of problem drinking may include medical symptoms such as loss of appetite, morning nausea and vomiting, diarrhea, facial flushing, headaches, impotence, tremulousness, acid stomach, weight loss, and abdominal pain. Psychosocial symptoms may include episodes of intoxication at least once a month, use of alcohol during most recreational activities, skipping meals, blackouts, recurrent lateness or absenteeism from work, use of alcohol to relieve stress or depression, insomnia or nightmares, and the inability to cut down on alcohol use. Frequent accidents or incidents caused by driving "under the influence" may be the first signs of problem drinking. Often, relatives or friends are the first to notice the problem, which is denied by the drinker despite an escalating array of warnings.

Alcohol abuse is a serious type of problem drinking characterized by heavy drinking on a daily basis, heavy drinking on most weekends, or binges of heavy daily drinking interspersed with periods of sobriety. Alcohol abusers are likely to suffer major medical or psychosocial consequences of alcohol.

Alcoholism is the most dangerous pattern of problem drinking — so dangerous, in fact, that it reduces life expectancy by an average of 12 years. The key feature of alcoholism is physical or psychosocial dependence on the drug — addiction. Alcoholics face a double bind: continued use of the drug produces ever greater medical, psychosocial, and financial woes, yet interrupting alcohol intake causes withdrawal symptoms that may include tremors ("the shakes"), hallucinations ("the frights"), seizures ("rum fits"), and delirium tremens (DTs, or "the horrors"). Still, most alcoholics manage to withdraw periodically from the drug, only to take up drinking again. For most, alcoholism is a chronic disorder with a progressive downhill course.

Problem drinking, alcohol abuse, and alcoholism are not confined to Skid Row. They are not restricted to any ethnic group, nor are they exclusively male problems. Far from being "someone else's" problem, alcohol abuse may be surprisingly close to home. In fact, it's likely to be very near at hand: 18 million Americans are affected by some form of problem drinking.

Are You a Problem Drinker?

The first step in controlling any medical problem is to diagnose it. Recognizing alcohol abuse, though, can be surprisingly difficult for physicians, since many of its early medical and psychosocial symptoms are nonspecific. The problem is compounded by the fact that most patients who abuse alcohol deny the problem to themselves so they never report it to their physicians.

For years I confined my screening efforts simply to asking my patients how many drinks they consumed each day. I learned my lesson, however, when a "two-a-day" man finally revealed after five or six years of annual queries that *each* of his drinks contained *eight* ounces of gin. One man's drink is another man's bottle! Now I screen my patients by asking four questions:

1. Have you ever tried to cut down on your drinking?
2. Have you ever been annoyed by criticism of your drinking?
3. Have you ever felt guilty about your drinking?
4. Have you ever had a morning "eye opener"?

You can ask yourself these simple questions. One "yes" does not mean that you are an alcoholic. But even one positive response does mean that you should give your drinking some serious thought.

To think further about your drinking, take the simple ten-question test below.

Answer each question, then add up your score; a score of four suggests problem drinking, and five suggests alcoholism.

	Point Scores	
1. Do you feel you are a normal drinker?	Yes (0)	No (2)
2. Do friends or relatives think you are a normal drinker?	Yes (0)	No (2)
3. Have you ever attended a meeting of Alcoholics Anonymous (AA)?	Yes (5)	No (0)
4. Have you ever lost friends or girlfriends or boyfriends because of drinking?	Yes (2)	No (0)
5. Have you ever gotten into trouble at work because of drinking?	Yes (2)	No (0)
6. Have you ever neglected your obligations, your family, or your work for two or more days in a row because you were drinking?	Yes (2)	No (0)
7. Have you ever had delirium tremens or severe shaking, heard voices, or seen things that were not there after heavy drinking?	Yes (2)	No (0)
8. Have you ever gone to anyone for help about your drinking?	Yes (5)	No (0)
9. Have you ever been in a hospital because of drinking?	Yes (5)	No (0)
10. Have you ever been arrested for drunk driving or driving after drinking?	Yes (2)	No (0)

Source: A. D. Pokorny, B. A. Miller, and H. B. Kaplan, "The Brief MAST: A Shortened Version of the Michigan Alcoholism Screening Test," American Journal of Psychiatry, *129: 342 (1972). Copyright © 1972 American Psychiatric Association.*

If you have reason to be concerned that your alcohol use is becoming alcohol abuse, don't ignore the problem. Early action can help control problem drinking, preventing its potentially disastrous consequences. And plenty of help is available.

Controlling Alcohol Abuse

Understanding the causes of alcohol abuse would greatly facilitate its control; unfortunately, the causes of most problem drinking remain obscure.

Problem drinking does tend to cluster in families, reflecting either a genetic cause or learned behavior. Several studies have investigated children born to alcoholic families who were separated from their families early in life. The offspring of alcoholics do have a much higher-than-normal rate of alcoholism even if they were raised in nonalcoholic households. In some cases, then, there is a genetic predisposition to alcohol abuse. Unfortunately, we don't yet know how to identify the responsible gene, much less how to modify its influence.

Even though heredity can play a role in alcohol abuse, it does not explain the entire picture. Many children of alcoholics never drink at all, and many problem drinkers have no alcoholic relatives. Psychosocial factors are clearly implicated in the origins of alcohol abuse. But those factors are also hard to pin down. There is no single "alcoholic personality"; in some cases of alcoholism, even detailed psychiatric investigations fail to reveal the causal factors.

Because there are many types of alcohol abuse, there are also many treatments. And because the causes of alcohol abuse are still largely unknown, no single preventive program or treatment plan is uniformly successful. Still, most successful programs incorporate two major goals: to reduce or preferably eliminate the use of alcohol, and to replace it with interpersonal interactions that provide support and self-esteem.

In early or mild cases of alcohol abuse, the problem drinker may be able to achieve the first goal on his or her own. But people who are alcohol-dependent generally need medical help for detoxification ("drying out"). Detoxification programs are available in all parts of the country; some are out-patient plans, but many require hospital stays of one to four weeks.

Withdrawing from alcohol is only half the problem. Staying sober is the other. In some early or mild cases of alcohol abuse, the drinker can build a support network to replace alcohol without professional help. In most cases, however, intensive assistance is necessary. Many types of help are available from psychologists, physicians, social workers, community groups, employee assistance programs, religious organizations, and self-help associations. Each problem drinker must find the program — or programs — that suit him or her best. In my practice I've found the most successful organization to be Alcoholics Anonymous (AA).

AA is a wonderful resource for problem drinkers. We might not need it so often, though, if we took steps to change the role that alcohol plays in our society.

Alcohol and Society

Throughout recorded history alcoholic beverages have been part of human society. In its very earliest use alcohol may have been a helpful food preservative, but since the dawn of civilization alcoholic beverages have flourished for their cultural roles rather than their nutritional or medicinal merits. Since antiquity, too, the hazards of alcohol have been obvious: "Inflaming wine, pernicious to mankind, / unnerves the limbs, / and dulls the noble mind" (Homer, the *Iliad*, 850 B.C.).

Although the process of distillation was known to the ancients, for centuries most alcohol was consumed as fermented wine or beer. The industrial revolution, however, changed the pattern of alcohol use as it did so many traditional aspects of human life. Distilled spirits became widely available at low prices, unleashing what became known in England as the "gin epidemic." Attempts to control this modern epidemic have been uniformly unsuccessful; America's futile experiment with Prohibition in the 1930s and the Soviet Union's failed attempt to restrict vodka sales in the 1980s bear witness to the age-old resilience of the alcohol habit.

In contemporary America, however, alcohol's place in society has become institutionalized. Images of alcohol use are everywhere: college newspapers devote 13 times more space to beer ads than to ads for books and soft drinks combined; just three beer companies spend more than $50 million annually sponsoring automobile racing; alcohol use is portrayed 10½ times in an average hour of prime-time television.

Each and every year manufacturers spend more than $1.5 billion to advertise and promote alcoholic beverages. Unlike drugs and tobacco, which are unsafe in any amount, alcohol is both socially acceptable and medically safe in modest doses. But alcohol is very *un*safe in moderate to heavy doses. Yet this message is swamped by ubiquitous images of fast cars and cold beer, sophisticated women and expensive wine, successful men and tall drinks.

To protect American health, we need to find ways to restore alcohol use to its appropriate place in the social order. Without sacrificing free speech, we need ways to balance glamorous images of alcohol with graphic representations of the disastrous medical and social consequences of alcohol abuse. Without sacrificing personal freedom, we need ways to place realistic limitations on the availability of alcoholic beverages. Without stifling economic incentives, we need ways to increase the price of alcoholic beverages, which fell in real cost by 20 to 48 percent between 1960 and 1980.

Each year more American lives are lost to alcohol than were lost in the entire Vietnam war. Acting as citizens, as health care providers, and as the body politic, we must find a way to prevent this carnage.

■ Drug Abuse

Tobacco and alcohol abuse pose very difficult problems for our society; drug abuse presents challenges of enormous complexity.

All medications can be misused and abused, but substances that are addicting create a self-perpetuating cycle of abuse that greatly complicates preventive efforts. Society has placed few restrictions on tobacco and alcohol availability, and the limitations that are in place are enforced only erratically. In contrast, many laws have attempted to control the use of illicit drugs; but despite $7 billion spent on enforcement in 1990 alone, the drug problem remains critical.

Patterns of Abuse

Drugs of abuse fall into three categories. *Legal over-the-counter drugs* include tobacco and alcohol as well as aerosols (spray paint and so on) and solvents (glue, lighter fluid). *Legal prescription drugs* include stimulants, sedatives and tranquilizers, and narcotics and other painkillers. *Illicit street drugs* include marijuana, cocaine, crack cocaine, heroin, and hallucinogens, among many others. Although all can create medical, psychological, and social havoc, our present discussion of drug abuse will focus on illicit drugs and on prescription drugs used illicitly.

Drugs of abuse can be used for five purposes: to alter mood, to alter perception, to increase energy levels, to produce drowsiness or sleep, or to control pain. But the factors that motivate drug abuse vary enormously from individual to individual, ranging from legitimate medical use gone astray, to social experimentation, underlying psychotic illnesses, or desperately self-destructive cultural norms.

Although alcohol can be used socially without being abused, all nonmedical uses of the other substances are abusive. Still, the patterns of abuse vary widely. *Experimental abusers* try drugs briefly and intermittently, usually motivated by peer pressure, easy availability, and curiosity. *Periodic ("recreational") abusers* turn to drugs with more regularity, often in response to stereotyped social situations. *Habitual abusers ("addicts")* consume drugs on a regular, recurrent basis dictated by internal needs rather than social circumstances.

Of these patterns only one is truly stable: addiction is notable for its terrible durability. Unfortunately, experimental abuse often becomes periodic and periodic abuse habitual — which is why all substance use is substance abuse.

The Burden of Drug Abuse

Because of its illicit nature drug abuse is secretive, and statistics are tentative at best. Still, a 1990 National Institute of Mental Health study of 20,291 persons concluded that 6.1 percent of Americans abuse drugs other than alcohol and tobacco. More than half of all drug abuse is tied to a serious underlying mental disorder.

More than 10 million Americans smoke marijuana on a regular basis; most are teenagers and young adults. Two to 3 million Americans sniff, smoke, or inject cocaine or crack on a regular basis; still in widespread use throughout all social strata, cocaine is beginning to concentrate in the inner city. Heroin, injected habitually by 500,000 people and periodically by up to 2 million others, is found principally in impoverished urban centers.

Consequences of Drug Abuse

Like alcohol abuse, drug abuse has disastrous medical, psychological, and social effects. Unlike alcohol, which is socially sanctioned, drugs are illicit, thus adding criminality and violence to the already formidable hazards of abuse. In New York City, for example, two out of every three men who are arrested test positive for cocaine.

Even the most benign of the drugs of abuse, marijuana, can be dangerous. Impaired judgment, alertness, and perception make accidents and trauma the chief hazards of its use. Respiratory tract irritation is another common complication of marijuana smoking. Because the smoke contains cancer-causing chemicals and tars, long-term marijuana use may eventually produce even more serious medical consequences.

Despite those very real dangers, marijuana is so much less hazardous than the other drugs of abuse that it belongs in a class of its own. Recognizing this, many communities impose much milder sanctions on its use. And doctors are now finding beneficial uses for marijuana, including the treatment of glaucoma and the prevention of nausea caused by cancer chemotherapy treatments.

The other drugs of abuse are much more destructive.

Intravenous drug abuse is a major cause of our terrible AIDS epidemic. Shared needles spread the virus from person to person; sexual partners of drug abusers may be infected as well. There are about 1 million intravenous drug abusers in America; up to half are already infected with the AIDS virus. Hepatitis, syphilis, tetanus, pneumonia, tuberculosis, and heart infections are among the other infectious complications of drug abuse.

The cardiovascular system, too, bears a major burden of drug abuse; complications include abnormal heart rhythms, heart attacks, and sudden death. Drug overdoses can also kill by paralyzing breathing. Nervous system problems include seizures and strokes, especially strokes caused by brain hemorrhages.

A particularly tragic consequence of drug abuse during pregnancy is fetal damage which can produce stillbirths, prematurity, malformations, newborn syphilis, and pediatric AIDS. Infants born to drug abusers may actually be addicted at birth, giving rise to severe withdrawal symptoms in the first days of life. It is now becoming apparent that long-term behavioral problems and intellectual deficiencies are often the childhood legacy of maternal drug abuse.

The psychosocial consequences of drug abuse are no less devastating. Addiction, depression, lethargy, irregular sleep patterns, paranoia, psychosis, and violence are among the many personal hazards of drug abuse. Some psychological problems abate with abstinence, but others are permanent.

Drug abuse is directly responsible for 5,000 to 10,000 deaths in our country each year. Many others die from indirect consequences of drug abuse; included in this number are one quarter of all AIDS victims.

This tremendous burden of suffering, disability, and death carries a crushing financial cost as well. Drug abuse costs the U.S. economy well over $60 billion annually.

The Control of Drug Abuse

I suspect that many of my readers use alcohol from time to time. A few may still be smokers. But my guess is that drug abuse is rare among those of you who have read through 18 chapters of this book. If I'm right, very few of you will need the details of drug detoxification and rehabilitation programs. But all of us need to know at least two facts about these treatments: they do work, but they are often unavailable to the people who need them most.

Even if few of us abuse drugs, we must all approach the drug problem as if it were our problem. Indeed it is: at least 6 million Americans have serious drug problems, and many others are harmed indirectly by the medical, economic, and criminal complications of drug abuse.

Although I hope none of you is ever even tempted to experiment with drugs, I hope all of you will think about these problems. Each of us must be alert for drug problems in our relatives, friends, co-workers, and — above all — our children. All of us must help vulnerable people get the professional treatment they need for prevention, control, and rehabilitation. Like most alcohol abusers, but unlike many smokers, nearly all drug abusers need professional help to conquer their problems.

Although doctors can't resolve our drug crisis, the vantage point of preventive medicine is, I believe, relevant. It's too late for the primary prevention of drug abuse in America — the illness is already here. It's also too late for secondary prevention — the symptoms are already very evident. But there is still time to prevent further complications, to practice tertiary prevention — if we start now.

We need better drug laws and improved law enforcement. But seven of every ten drug-control dollars are already spent on interdiction and punishment, with success that is limited at best. We have an acute need for vastly expanded drug treatment facilities. We are in desperate need of a massive campaign to halt the spread of AIDS in drug users. Needed, too, are effective educational programs to prevent drug abuse from getting started in the first place.

America is, I'm sorry to say, the drug capital of the world; with only 2 percent of the world's population, we consume 60 percent of its illicit drugs. To control substance abuse we need to make structural changes in our society; to improve family stability, housing, economic opportunities, and education; to redress the ills that breed drug abuse. A tall order indeed, but the health of our nation depends on our commitment, collective effort, and success.

■ T H R E E ■

A Comprehensive Program for Health Enhancement

▪ 19 ▪
Psychological Health

Even my most devoted reader will, I suspect, experience at least a tiny sensation of relief after completing Part Two of *Staying Well*. I hope you're eager to begin Part Three; still, I'll ask you to pause for just a moment and turn back to chapter 1 and its list of the ten leading causes of death in the United States. Only the eighth, suicide, is primarily a mental disorder. Even one of ten may be enough to convince you that psychological factors are important to health, but it's only the tip of the iceberg. Psychological factors also contribute to the leading cause of death, heart disease. Insofar as stress raises blood pressure, mental influences contribute to the third and tenth causes of death, stroke and atherosclerosis. And although the evidence is much less complete, many authorities speculate that emotional factors may even contribute to cancer, our number two killer, by weakening the body's immune system.

Psychological factors can contribute directly to the causes of many diseases, but they are even more influential indirectly. Personal experiences, educational influences, and emotional states determine human behavior — and behavior (diet, exercise, smoking, alcohol and substance abuse) is a key determinant of *all* ten leading causes of death.

A nine-year study by Drs. Lisa Beckman and Leonard Syme evaluated nearly 7,000 adults in Alameda County, California. This investigation identified one factor that increased the risk of dying during the study period by 2.8 in women and 2.3 in men. This crucial risk factor is not smoking, nor is it drinking, sloth, or nutritional neglect. Instead, the risk factor is social isolation; people with the fewest social ties had the greatest risk of dying from heart disease, circulatory ailments, and even cancer.

Research is just beginning to elucidate the many ways in which mind and body interact. But even now it is obvious that psychological factors help establish the balance between illness and health, tipping the scales in one direction or the other. In addition to health, mental factors contribute to the fullness and pleasure of life.

■ Mind and Body

More than 2,300 years ago the great Greek physician Hippocrates recognized that a sound mind and a sound body are equally important determinants of human health and well-being. Plato, too, understood that "the right education must tune the strings of the body and mind to perfect spiritual harmony." But in our modern world, alas, mind and body are often out of tune. Restoring their harmony could help put civilization back into Western civilization; it would also help enhance health and prevent disease.

Mental and physical functions are equally important for health because they are not two separate entities; instead, they are two aspects of a single human being.

Some links between mind and body are obvious. We all know "physical" illness can affect mental function. When we're sick, we often feel depressed and logy. For decades doctors assumed this was simply a psychological reaction to the loss of physical health, but new research suggests the link is even more intimate. Infections, allergies, inflammatory conditions, and even certain tumors cause the body's white blood cells to release excessive amounts of a small but powerful chemical called interleukin-1, or IL-1. If it is injected into animals, it promptly puts them to sleep. In humans IL-1 passes from white cells into the blood, which carries it to the brain. It's no wonder, then, that we experience impaired concentration, depression, and even somnolence when we have infections and other illnesses.

In contrast, physical well-being is typically associated with relaxation and optimism. Like the low spirits that accompany illness, the high spirits of health may have a chemical basis. Exercise, for example, causes the body to produce a family of chemicals called *endorphins*. Endorphins act on the brain to reduce pain and elevate mood. The good mood you experience when you are well does not depend strictly on the absence of doctors' bills; fitness and good health actually stimulate "happy" molecules.

Physical illness causes mental depression; fitness and health contribute to psychological well-being. But the interaction between body and mind is a two-way street: emotional factors can also produce chemical, hormonal, and neurological alterations that affect bodily function.

Psychic arousal causes immediate physical arousal. The heart pumps faster, the blood vessels narrow, the blood pressure rises, and even the pupils widen. In contrast, mental relaxation can slow the body's motor down. Meditation, biofeedback, and other relaxation techniques can actually slow the heart, reduce blood levels of stress hormones, and improve the circulation. Stress and depression can also affect the blood cells and proteins of the body's immune system. The brand-new scientific discipline of psychoneuroimmunology is studying the interactions between the mind, the nervous system, and the immune apparatus. At this early stage we can say only that these interactions are numerous but subtle and complex. Still, it is possible that they affect the body's resistance to infections, tumors, and other illnesses.

W. B. Yeats, arguably our century's greatest poet, asks, "How can we know the dancer from the dance?" Like a ballet, mind and body are inseparable steps in the endlessly fascinating and varied choreography of humanity.

■ Psychosomatic Illnesses

All too often in today's world the mind and the body fall out of step. The result: problems that range from mental dis-ease to physical disease.

In some cases people who are physically healthy interpret emotional distress as physical illness. Unaware of depression or stress, they complain instead of headaches, chest pain, breathing difficulties, or abdominal discomfort. Almost everyone will experience such "functional" symptoms from time to time, and virtually everyone will worry occasionally about illness. But when these symptoms recur or persist despite good health, they suggest a "hypochondriac" personality style. Doctors often refer to patients whose physical complaints are caused by mental distress as the "worried well," but I think it's more appropriate to characterize them as "worried sick." In fact, although these patients may not have diseased hearts or intestines, their chest or abdominal pains are just as "real" and important as the sickest patient's pain. Indeed, these symptoms can be disabling. The physician must, of course, be sure that these symptoms do not have an organic basis. The next task, which is no easier, is to help put a worried mind back in step with a healthy body.

The Mind and the Heart

There is no doubt that mental factors can do more than produce physical *symptoms;* they can also contribute to actual physical *disease.* Consider the nation's number one killer, coronary heart disease.

Heart disease, of course, has many causes; chapter 2 reviews the role of high cholesterol levels, high blood pressure, smoking, physical inactivity, gender, and heredity. But the list of risk factors also includes psychological elements. Emotional disturbances are the most controversial of the cardiac risk factors, and they are probably less potent than the others. Even so, I'm convinced that in some patients heartfelt emotions contribute importantly to angina and heart attacks.

The link between personality and the heart was clarified in 1959 by Drs. Meyer Friedman and Ray Rosenman, who found that people with a particular personality profile were unusually susceptible to heart attacks. They coined the term *Type A personality* to describe the emotional characteristics that *triple* the risk of heart attacks. Type A people are tense and driven. They will work long hours and accomplish a great deal, but they tend to be competitive, demanding, and perfectionistic. When faced with frustration or delay, Type A's are prone to outbursts of anger and hostility. Their "short fuses" are expressed not only in their tempers but in their body language: Type A people have taut facial expressions, rapid or irregular breathing, and staccato speech. They walk quickly, with short, choppy strides, and they are fidgety and restless when sitting down. Always rushing from task to task, Type A people are the most extreme example of the hurry sickness that affects so many people living in the fast lane of modern industrial society.

That's the bad news. The good news is that Type A behavior can be modified by special counseling. In fact, studies by Dr. Friedman and his colleagues have shown that psychological interventions can reduce a Type A heart patient's risk of a second heart attack by as much as 50 percent.

Not all cardiologists and psychiatrists agree that the Type A personality is a key cardiac risk factor. Some authorities have implicated social isolation and free-floating hostility in men and anxiety in women as the major emotional risk factors. Other research identifies pessimism as a cardiac risk factor, and a 1992 study found that living alone increases the probability that heart patients will die of their disease. Despite these disagreements, most experts agree that mental factors can predispose to heart attacks. And that's my message: psychological factors *can* lead to physical illness.

Mental Contributions to Bodily Disease

Many organ systems can be affected by psychosomatic illnesses. Neurological symptoms, including migraines, tension headaches, neck pain, and tremors, are often triggered by stress. In the respiratory system asthma or hyperventilation may be precipitated by emotions. Worry and stress are also traditionally implicated in some cases of gastritis, peptic ulcer disease, diarrhea, and irritable bowel syndrome. Although the causes of low back pain are often mysterious, mental stress seems to contribute to the muscle tension that plagues so many patients. In the reproductive system emotional factors are clearly of major significance in many women with menstrual irregularities and in many men with impotence. Although the kidneys are not directly affected by emotions, the bladder may be — resulting in either urinary frequency or incomplete emptying.

The immune system, too, can be affected by depression and stress, but the clinical consequences of these changes are not yet known. Among the endocrine and metabolic disorders, thyroid overactivity can sometimes be triggered by stress, and the eating disorders are prime examples of psychological disorders that lead to physical illness. Even the skin can display the link between mind and body; in fact, hives, itching, and skin rashes are often highly visible reminders that emotions affect bodily function. And when it comes to accidents and substance abuse, the psyche is obviously the key to the behavioral determinants of health and illness.

I've selected these examples to emphasize my theme: when it comes to your health, your mind *does* matter. To prevent illness, you should attend to your emotional health. Not surprisingly, your efforts will be rewarded by greater personal happiness as well as by enhanced health.

■ Psychological Disorders in America

Emotional disorders, ranging from temporary psychological disturbances to major mental illnesses, rank among the most common health problems in our country.

Because they're sometimes subtle — and always personal — it's hard to be sure just how many people are affected by these problems. Still, the National Institute of Mental Health estimates that in any six-month period, 18.7 percent of adults suffer from psychological illnesses. Anxiety disorders head the list (8.3 percent), with alcoholism and drug abuse (6.4 percent) and depression (6 percent) close behind. Schizophrenia, antisocial personality disorders, and major thought disorders are much less common, each affecting about 1 percent of the populace. Add them up and you'll see that at least 30 million Americans have major psychological problems at any given time. And in addition to causing suffering, disability, and even death, mental illness is expensive, consuming more than 7 percent of all health care dollars.

■ Stress and Anxiety

Stress is as old as humanity. Inevitable in the course of everyone's life, stress is not simply a necessary evil. Instead, some types of stress are actually *desirable;* stimulation and challenge are the names we give to the "good" forms of stress that add spice to life, promoting optimal function of individuals and societies. But if some stress is good, excessive stress can be very bad indeed, contributing significantly to human discomfort and disease.

Like it or not, we live in an era of excessive stress, an age of anxiety. Far from conquering humanity's three age-old enemies, modern industrial society actually faces intensified versions of each: modern technology and nuclear capabilities have added a frightening new face to war; political turmoil has compounded the horror of famine; and AIDS threatens us with a contagion of unrivaled destructiveness. Even the nurturing aspects of nature have become sources of stress, as humanity continues to deplete and pollute the environment.

Global stress is bad enough, but for most people it serves principally as a backdrop for the smaller stresses of daily life which are felt much more intensely because they are so much closer. The workplace is competitive and uncertain. Financial stresses are all but universal. Daily life is harried and hurried, paced by fast cars and slow traffic, fast tempos and loud noises, fast food and nutritional short-cuts.

At the same time, many of humanity's traditional coping mechanisms have lost their power. Recreation is far from creative, depending instead on the passive persuasions of the mass media. Too often, exercise is an oddity. Worst of all, family life is itself stressful rather than supportive, as interpersonal social networks progressively loosen.

American physicians write more than 100 million prescriptions for tranquilizers each year. I myself write some of them, and these medications can be helpful. But you can find much better long-term solutions to stress and anxiety. Excessive stress and its internal counterpart, anxiety, are not necessary parts of life in today's world. Stress can be identified, and it can be controlled.

What Is Stress?

Although many people think of stress in strictly psychological terms, it's actually a complex physiologic state involving the nervous system, hormones, and blood chemicals as well as the mind. Stress is a very primitive, basic human response to threat.

Many physiologists and psychologists have contributed to our understanding of stress, but the work of two pioneering scientists stands out. First, in the early part of this century Dr. Walter B. Cannon of Harvard pointed out that the stress reaction is a primitive series of reflexes that mobilizes the body's defenses against external threats. Mental alertness is heightened as soon as the alarm sounds. Almost immediately the sympathetic nervous system is activated. The heart pumps faster and harder, so it can deliver more oxygen to the body's tissues. Blood pressure rises. Blood vessels in the digestive organs and skin narrow, shifting blood to the skeletal muscles, which need it most. Deprived of some of its circulation, the skin becomes cool and clammy and hair shafts become erect. The lungs, too, are activated; breathing speeds up and bronchial tubes widen, enabling the body to take in more oxygen and expel more carbon dioxide. The adrenal glands also go into action, pumping large amounts of adrenaline and cortisone into the blood stream. Blood sugar levels rise, providing an instant source of energy for the metabolism to use in an emergency. In addition, the blood's clotting mechanisms are activated, preparing for possible injury. Muscles become taut and ready to spring into action. Even the eyes prepare for maximum effort by widening their pupils to admit more light.

The net effect of the stress response is that the body is shifted into overdrive, ready to respond to a crisis. Cannon aptly called this the "flight-or-fight" response. It's an ancient, automatic adaptation as old as humankind itself. Indeed, the flight-or-fight response is entirely appropriate when the threat is physical and external, when it's a rumbling landslide or a roaring saber-toothed tiger. But human genetics have changed little, while the world around us has changed enormously. As a result, the primitive stress response has remained intact and is activated in its original form even when the threats are mental rather than physical. The racing heart, high blood pressure, rapid breathing, and tight muscles that served us so well in the forest serve us poorly in the corporate boardroom, the college classroom, or the hospital emergency room.

The second major contributor to our understanding of stress was Dr. Hans Selye of Montreal, an endocrinologist. His experiments of the 1950s showed that the stress reaction is divided into three stages. First is the stage of alarm, the initial phase of arousal that triggers the entire stress reaction. Next comes the stage of heightened function, in which the body is prepared to resist threats, to cope with crisis. But the stage of resistance is followed by a third and final stage, that of exhaustion. The stress reaction inevitably takes its toll, depleting the body's coping mechanisms. When stress is severe or prolonged, the first two stages of heightened function invariably culminate in a third phase of impaired function.

Stress has many faces. It can be an appropriate response to physical challenges ranging from athletic competition to sudden emergencies, a sign that we are stimulated or "turned on" for an important meeting, a big exam, or a challenging creative task. But even "good" stress will leave us exhausted if it's too intense or too prolonged. Even worse is "bad" stress, an inappropriate, maladaptive mobilization of primitive mechanisms. Excessive and inappropriate stress can do more than just cause exhaustion; it can also cause illness.

Stress and Anxiety

Stress is the body's response to an external threat; anxiety is the response to an internal stimulus. Stress may be appropriate and helpful or inappropriate and harmful; anxiety is always maladaptive and it's often harmful. If stress is flight or fight, anxiety is fright.

Like it or not, anxiety is an inevitable consequence of modern life. We all experience it sometimes, but we may not always recognize its symptoms. Apart from the absence of an obvious threat, anxiety mimics stress. Mental symptoms range from worry to irritability or hostility to sensations of dread, foreboding, or panic. Muscles are tense, resulting in fidgetiness, taut facial expressions, headaches, or neck and back pain. The mouth is dry, sometimes producing the sensation of a lump in the throat which makes swallowing difficult. Clenched jaw muscles can produce jaw pain and headaches. The skin can be pale, sweaty, and clammy. Intestinal symptoms range from "butterflies" to heartburn, cramps, or diarrhea. A pounding pulse is common, as is chest tightness. Rapid breathing is also typical, and may sometimes be accompanied by sighing or by a recurrent cough. In extreme cases hyperventilation can lead to tingling of the face and fingers, muscle cramps, light-headedness, and even fainting.

Anxiety sounds pretty bad, and it can feel even worse. Fortunately, most bouts of anxiety are brief and mild; stage fright is a good example. Stage fright resolves when the curtain opens; minor anxiety spells also resolve, either spontaneously or as a result of improved circumstances, mental distractions, or physical exercise. But when anxiety is prolonged or severe, it represents a more serious problem requiring more intense interventions.

Anxiety Disorders

Anxiety disorders are common, affecting more than 8 percent of American adults. These disorders come in many forms.

Situational anxiety affects most people at one time or another. It may, for example, strike you when you visit your doctor's office, or it may hit me when I open the first reviews of this book. In most cases situational anxiety will resolve on its own when the stressful circumstances resolve.

Generalized anxiety disorder is more serious because it lasts for months or even years, unpredictably waxing and waning in severity. Patients with chronic anxiety often regard their tension as "normal"; their friends and relatives may also simply accept them as "uptight" people with "short fuses." Indeed, the chronic anxiety disorder can be so persistent that it becomes a basic life-style. Still, it is a disorder and it can be treated.

Panic attacks are episodes of severe anxiety characterized by intense apprehension and major physical symptoms, including a pounding heart, rapid breathing, light-headedness, headaches, and chest tightness. Unlike chronic anxiety disorders, which often go unrecognized, panic attacks are impossible to overlook. Patients suffering from panic attacks know they are ill, and they often come to the emergency ward for help. But they typically seek medical treatment instead of psychiatric help because they are convinced that their problems are "physical" rather than "mental."

Burnout feels like exhaustion, but it's the result of excessive stress. Everyone who works hard, mentally or physically, will feel tired or stale from time to time. But burnout is more than fatigue, and it takes more than a weekend away to restore enthusiasm.

Phobias are disabling symptoms of anxiety. Patients with burnout struggle with stress until they can struggle no more; patients with phobias attempt to cope by avoiding situations that trigger anxiety. Fear of flying is one example; when mild it's a common, easily conquered form of situational anxiety, but when it's severe it can be a phobia intense enough to keep its sufferers grounded. Even more disabling is agoraphobia — a fear of public places, public transportation, and people in groups.

Post-traumatic stress disorder may be expressed in many ways, including generalized anxiety, panic attacks, violence, substance abuse, or sleep disturbances. It can result from any severe stress, but the cataclysm of war is its most frequent cause.

Recognizing Stress and Anxiety

All people experience stress; indeed, the world would be dull and dreary without some stress. Most people learn to cope with it, to resolve conflicts whenever possible, and to adapt to the stresses that won't just go away.

Many times, however, stress becomes internalized, leading to anxiety. Temporary anxiety is as universal as stress — unpleasant, but no big deal. But when anxiety is recurrent, severe, or chronic, it *is* a big deal, affecting health as well as happiness.

To find out if you have a problem with anxiety or stress, ask yourself the 18 questions below. Add up your score. Totals above 61 suggest severe anxiety; scores between 46 and 60 suggest moderate anxiety; those between 31 and 45 suggest mild anxiety; and those below 30 do not indicate anxiety.

	Almost never	Some- times	Often	Almost always
1. I am "calm, cool, and collected."	4	3	2	1
2. I feel that problems are pil- ing up so that I cannot over- come them.	1	2	3	4
3. I feel my heart racing or pounding without exercising.	1	2	3	4
4. Some unimportant thought runs through my mind and bothers me.	1	2	3	4
5. I feel secure and at ease.	4	3	2	1
6. I feel I am dizzy, light- headed, or faint.	1	2	3	4
7. I wish I could be as happy as others seem to be.	1	2	3	4
8. I feel joyful and confident.	4	3	2	1
9. I feel worried and tense.	1	2	3	4
10. I am afraid of people and things.	1	2	3	4
11. I have stomach pains or indigestion.	1	2	3	4
12. I am inclined to take things hard.	1	2	3	4
13. I sleep poorly or have nightmares.	1	2	3	4
14. I enjoy sitting quietly.	4	3	2	1
15. I feel rushed or hurried.	1	2	3	4
16. I get headaches or neck pains.	1	2	3	4
17. I get flushed or sweaty with- out exercising or I get hives.	1	2	3	4
18. I am eager for new chal- lenges and tasks.	4	3	2	1

Source: C. D. Spielberger, Manual for the State-Trait Anxiety Inventory. *Consulting Psychologists Press, Palo Alto, California.*

Don't let a high score on this self-assessment test add to your anxiety. Instead, double-check your results by asking a close relative or friend if your responses are accurate. If your results are confirmed, take action by exploring the coping techniques discussed at the end of this chapter. It may take time, it may take effort, and it may take help — but you can learn to cope with stress, thus preventing its harmful consequences.

■ Grief and Depression

Every life has its ups and down. Challenge and stimulation spark the "ups," but "up" can become "uptight" when stress and anxiety are excessive. Rest and relaxation provide the "downs," but this too can become excessive, resulting in boredom or apathy. Much more troublesome are down periods that are severe or persistent; far from being normal, they represent clinical depression.

Depression rivals anxiety for its frequency, its seriousness, and its protean physical and psychological manifestations. We are living not only in an age of anxiety but also in decades of depression. More than 25 percent of patients with medical illnesses are depressed, no surprise in view of the unity of mind and body. But even without medical problems, more than 8 percent of all Americans will develop a major depressive episode at some time during the course of their lifetime; minor depressions occur in up to 30 percent. Depression is twice as likely to affect women as men.

Depressive illnesses always cause suffering, and they can cause long-term disability and even death. Depression is also very expensive, costing Americans more than $16 billion each year in direct and indirect expenses.

What Is Depression?

Stress and anxiety represent an excessive or maladaptive response to a threat, which may be real or imagined. Depression represents an excessive or maladaptive response to a loss, which may be real or imagined. The prototype of anxiety is fear, of depression grief.

Like anxiety, depression involves the whole person, including both mind and body. Like anxiety, depression ranges from mild to major. Like anxiety, it involves symptoms that may be psychological or physical. And like anxiety, depression is often unrecognized by patients, relatives, and doctors.

The emotional symptoms of depression can be understood as an exaggeration of the blue or "down" moods that we all experience in reaction to disappointment or loss. But clinical depression goes further. Its sufferers lack self-esteem. They feel hopeless, helpless, and worthless. Pessimism is universal and guilt common. Loss of interest in the world around them leads depressed people to become isolated, withdrawing from professional and social contacts. Depression impairs the ability to concentrate and focus. Patients complain of memory loss, and their productive thoughts are often replaced by recurrent ruminations about physical symptoms, illness, and death. Despite all this self-preoccupation, self-neglect is the rule. Whereas passivity and withdrawal usually predominate, anxiety and agitation can be features of some depressive illness.

Physical symptoms are also part of most clinical depressions, and in severe cases they can predominate. Loss of energy is typical, often leading to slow movements, slow speech, and striking inactivity. Loss of appetite is just as common; despite physical inactivity, weight loss can be severe.

Sexual dysfunction, extreme fatigue, constipation, backache, and other bodily complaints may be more worrisome to the patient than the mood disturbance itself. Sleep is usually abnormal; in most cases insomnia and early morning wakefulness occur, but excessive sleep can also be a symptom of depression.

What Causes Depression?

Despite its frequency and severity, depression remains a medical mystery. In some cases it's caused by specific medical disorders, by medications, or by alcohol. Any loss of health, in fact, can cause depression.

But in most cases of clinical depression physicians cannot identify an underlying medical illness. Sometimes a traumatic life experience, typically a major loss or separation, accounts for the lack of self-esteem that is central to depression. But clinical depression often occurs without obvious psychological trauma. Heredity seems a likely culprit in families plagued by depression in generation after generation. Neurochemical abnormalities must be responsible for many, if not most, cases of depression, but research has not yet pinpointed these disturbances.

Loss and Grief

Although it's not actually a form of depression, bereavement demonstrates many features of true clinical depression. Indeed, the distinction between sadness and depression can blur, and normal grieving can merge into clinical depression.

About 8 million Americans experience the death of a family member every year. Although the loss of a loved one always occasions grief and sorrow, the death of a child or a spouse is particularly traumatic. Indeed, in addition to experiencing grief, the surviving spouses themselves exhibit an increased incidence of illness and death during their first year of bereavement.

Normal bereavement first produces shock and disbelief, then loneliness and longing for the lost person, and then despair and social disorganization often tinged with guilt. The normal mourning process proceeds through these stages over the course of three to six months, and then enters the final stage of recovery and social reorganization, which can occupy another three to six months. About half of all mourners become clinically depressed at some point during the year following the death of a loved one. Sixteen percent remain depressed for more than a year, thus crossing the line between normal grief and clinical depression. The weakening of family ties, social networks, and traditional mourning rituals in our modern, mobile society surely contributes to these pathological grief reactions.

Types of Depression

Reactive depression is an emotional reaction that follows a loss. The loss of a marriage, a friendship, or a job are examples. Although reactive depressions can be distressing, they are self-limited; in time the pain of loss recedes and self-esteem returns.

Anniversary reactions are resurgences of depression that occur on the anniversary of a loss; these low spells are usually relatively mild and brief.

Chronic depression is characterized by pessimism, self-doubt, and unhappiness, but it does not include the physical symptoms of major depressions. Chronic depression can be so prolonged that it's perceived as a sign of a gloomy personality rather than a psychological disorder.

Major depression is just what it sounds like, an intense phase of despair accompanied by major physical symptoms such as extreme fatigue, loss of appetite, or sleep disturbances. Suicidal thoughts may be prominent. Medical help is necessary to treat major depressions.

Manic-depressive illness is a puzzling disorder in which periods of depression are punctuated by bursts of excessive energy or euphoria. During their manic phases patients are lively, talkative, and hyperactive, but they display inappropriate judgment, grandiose ideas, and insomnia. Often familial, the manic-depressive disorder also requires specialized medical treatment.

Seasonal affective disorder — SAD indeed — is a form of depression just now gaining recognition by the medical community. A cyclic disorder, seasonal depression appears in the late fall and resolves in the late spring. Unlike the other depressive illnesses, it's usually accompanied by increased appetite, weight gain, and sleepiness. Seasonal depression appears to be caused by an abnormal sensitivity to the lack of daylight. In fact, enlightened psychiatrists are now using phototherapy to treat these patients.

Suicide

Claiming 30,000 American lives each year, suicide is our eighth leading cause of death. Many suicides are preventable.

Suicide often occurs in the context of depression, panic attacks, alcohol and drug abuse, or major medical or mental illness. Because adolescents are particularly vulnerable, they should be taught to recognize signs of depression in themselves and in their peers. Early recognition and skilled intervention may help.

Not all suicides can be prevented. In fact, ethicists, jurists, and physicians are now starting to ask if all suicides *should* be prevented. It's a vexing question, but many thoughtful people have come to believe that suicide may be a morally and legally appropriate choice for certain individuals suffering from terminal illnesses. But since they're irreversible, such choices must always depend on a clear and measured appraisal of all the facts and alternatives. Depression and anxiety prevent dispassionate decision making and are never acceptable as the basis for a decision to terminate life. At present, nearly all suicides in America result from mental illness.

Recognizing Depression

Depression has many forms, and it may even be masked or disguised. To find out if you have a tendency toward depression, ask yourself the

20 questions below. A total score below 30 is reassuring; scores between
31 and 45 suggest mild depression; those between 46 and 60 indicate
moderate depression; and those above 61 raise the possibility of severe
depression.

Like the anxiety self-assessment test, these questions are intended to
provide a guideline, not a diagnosis. If your self-test suggests depression,
be sure to look into the possibility — and to take steps to correct the
situation.

	Almost never	Some-times	Often	Almost always
1. I feel blue or sad.	1	2	3	4
2. I feel confident and hopeful about the future.	4	3	2	1
3. I feel like a failure.	1	2	3	4
4. I don't enjoy things the way I used to.	1	2	3	4
5. I feel guilty.	1	2	3	4
6. I have a feeling that something bad may happen.	1	2	3	4
7. I am pleased with myself.	4	3	2	1
8. I blame myself for everything that goes wrong.	1	2	3	4
9. I have crying spells.	1	2	3	4
10. I get irritated or annoyed.	1	2	3	4
11. I am interested in people and enjoy being with them.	4	3	2	1
12. I am unsure of myself and try to avoid decisions.	1	2	3	4
13. I feel that I look attractive and healthy.	4	3	2	1
14. I sleep poorly and am tired in the morning.	1	2	3	4
15. I am energetic and eager to take on new tasks.	4	3	2	1
16. My appetite is not as good as it used to be.	1	2	3	4
17. I am as interested in sex as I used to be.	4	3	2	1
18. I am concerned about my stomach and my bowels.	1	2	3	4
19. I feel healthy.	4	3	2	1
20. I have trouble doing my work.	1	2	3	4

Source: A. T. Beck et al., "An Inventory for Measuring Depression," Archives of General Psychiatry 4, pp. 561–65 (1961).

■ Psychological Health: Coping Strategies

Everyone experiences stress, frustration, and disappointment. To stay healthy, each person needs to establish a repertoire of coping mechanisms. Here are some fundamentals that can help.

Identify Your Sources of Stress

Often this is the easy part: an illness, the death of a loved one, a financial crisis, a job change, a family conflict or other major stress is easy to spot. But subtle stress can be just as harmful as overt stress. Think about patterns of stress to identify the situations that produce mental discomfort. Many times it's simply overload — too many things to do, too little time to do them. Ambiguous situations are also stressful; problems develop if you don't know what role you're expected to fill in professional or social situations. Loss of control over the outcome of a situation can be even more stressful than the lack of information. Last but not least, the lack of personal support and positive feedback greatly compounds any stressful situation.

Self-knowledge is the key to avoiding stress. If you know yourself, you'll be able to anticipate stressful situations before they occur, allowing you to plan ways to minimize these pressures.

Express Yourself

Self-expression can be every bit as important as self-understanding. Don't try to deny your feelings or to hold them in. Suppressed feelings take a toll; suppressed anger, for example, increases the risk of heart disease. Pent-up feelings may erupt when you least want them to, placing stress on other people and adding to your own problems.

The best way to express your feelings is to talk them out with a friend, a relative, or a counselor. Sometimes just talking to yourself will help. If you do talk things over with yourself, remember to tell yourself to look on the bright side; emphasize the positive, and look for the kernel of humor that is invariably hidden in even the most stressful situation.

Another good way to express feelings is to write them down. Try a letter; even if you don't mail it, you may gain a lot from simply organizing your thoughts and expressing your feelings.

Structure Your Life-Style to Reduce Stress

Establish realistic goals and expectations, avoiding extremes when you set your sights. If you expect too little of yourself, you'll run the risk of boredom, guilt, and a loss of self-esteem that can lead to depression. But if you take on too much, you'll run the risk of overload, stress, and anxiety. Know your abilities, and use them to the fullest. Know your limits also, and live within them.

Be flexible. Even the best plans may go awry; to avoid stress, learn to cope with the unexpected. Leave some room in your schedule so you can adjust to circumstances, thus avoiding overload.

Pace yourself. Give yourself enough time to accomplish your goals. Alternate stressful tasks with more relaxing ones. Take breaks, allowing yourself reasonable amounts of down time. If you are able to control your work schedule, you may want to book an appointment with a nonexistent visitor so you'll have 15 minutes to yourself; use the time to catch up with work, to meditate, to get a little exercise, to read, or just to stare into space. Take vacations, three-day weekends, or the occasional long lunch hour whenever you can. At home, take the phone off the hook and enjoy a little peace and quiet. Allow yourself the luxury of doing nothing at all once in a while.

Seek variety, both at work and at play. A routine can be reassuring and comfortable, but variety will keep you stimulated, fresh, and enthusiastic. Consider new horizons at work, and experiment with new forms of recreation and relaxation.

Establish priorities. No person can do it all. By omitting or deferring your less important tasks, you'll be able to focus your energies on your key goals. By attempting less, you may well accomplish more — with considerably less stress.

Make People Your Top Priority

Interpersonal interactions can be the greatest source of stress or the firmest source of support.

The great philosopher Jean-Paul Sartre once wrote that hell is other people. Indeed, few things can raise your blood pressure faster than conflicts with hostile or demanding people. Learn to handle them. Listen carefully, trying to understand what's behind their anger. Instead of fighting fire with fire, acknowledge hostility and try to defuse it ("You sound angry; how can I help?"). Stay calm, but don't always retreat. Instead, learn to assert yourself to protect your own rights and interests.

Remember the other side of the coin: friends are good medicine. Cultivate relationships with friends (and even with relatives!). Invest thought, effort, and time to build the social networks that will help you get through crisis and stress. Remember that social isolation is a major risk factor for heart disease; don't let yourself drift away from your community.

Don't Depend on Alcohol or Drugs

You can run but you can't hide. Substance abuse is escapism, but it won't enable you to escape your problems. Instead, both your psychological and your medical problems will be multiplied many times over by attempts at self-medication with alcohol or drugs. Nicotine is no better; don't turn to tobacco for relief of stress; only your health will go up in smoke. Even caffeine may add to feelings of stress by speeding up your heart and your mind.

Exercise

Physical exercise is as good for your mind as it is for your body.

Exercise improves mood, dissipates stress, and fights depression. By promoting physical health, exercise will increase your energy and vigor. As your body improves, your self-image is bound to improve. Learning to control your body will also add to your sense of mastery and self-confidence.

In addition, exercise and sports provide many opportunities to make friends and build networks. Getting into shape is hard work at first, but once you're fit, exercise is fun. "All men," wrote Aquinas, "need leisure"; exercise is indeed a wonderful form of recreation.

Neurochemical mechanisms also help explain how exercise affects the psyche. Endurance exercise increases the body's supply of endorphins, which fight pain and elevate mood. You may not get a "runner's high" when you work out, but you can expect to feel relaxed, optimistic, and happy after vigorous exercise.

The best way to attain these benefits is through aerobic exercise. Chapter 21 will help you construct the fitness program that's best for you.

Sleep

Physical exertion is beneficial for both mind and body; its polar opposite, sleep, is also important for both aspects of health.

Sleep gives the body a break from physical exercise, and it affords the mind a respite from mental work. But sleep is more than just rest. In fact, normal sleep is divided into recurrent cycles of rest and activation. In the down phases, called non-R.E.M. sleep, the metabolism, the heartbeat, and the respiration are all slowed down, and the brain's nerve cells are inactive. In R.E.M. (rapid eye movement) sleep, however, the pulse and respiratory rate rise, though the muscles are relaxed. More important, the brain is active. Brain wave recordings during R.E.M. sleep resemble patterns seen during wakefulness; dreaming occurs during this phase of the sleep cycle. Both types of sleep are important. They alternate continually during normal sleep, with a single cycle taking about 90 minutes.

There is no ideal amount of sleep. Healthy people average seven to nine hours per night, but the amount of sleep that people need varies widely. In general, sleep requirements are greatest in children and young adults; they level off in adulthood, then diminish in advanced age.

Allow yourself to get enough sleep, no matter how busy you are. Sleep deprivation is self-defeating; it will reduce your efficiency and impair your ability to cope with stress. Experiment with different schedules to find what works for you. Some people can cut back on sleep when they are under pressure, but others need more sleep to function well. You may even want to experiment with napping; a 10- to 20-minute midday nap has been found to improve the performance of airline pilots, and it may suit you. In contrast, long siestas are likely to keep you up at night, thus doing more harm than good.

You'll know your sleep pattern is right if you awaken alert and refreshed. But a good night's sleep can be hard to come by. All of us experience insomnia from time to time, but 15 to 20 percent of us have recurrent or persistent insomnia.

Insomnia has many causes. *Psychological factors* are responsible about half the time, with anxiety disorders and clinical depression heading the list. *Medical problems* account for another 10 percent of sleep disturbances; breathing problems such as sleep apnea (see chapter 5), heart disease, and urinary tract disorders are the chief culprits. *Drugs and chemicals* explain another 10 percent; both stimulants (caffeine, nicotine, decongestants, asthma treatments) and sedatives (alcohol and other drugs) can interfere with normal sleep. In a third of all insomnia sufferers, however, the true cause remains obscure.

If you have insomnia, consider first the possibility of psychological, medical, or chemical causes. If none is present, try these simple measures to improve your sleep:

- Establish a regular schedule, going to bed and getting up at nearly the same time each day. Avoid daytime naps.
- Be sure your bed is comfortable, and reserve it for sleeping. Use your chair for reading or watching television, restricting your bed for sleep and other horizontal activities.
- Be sure your bedroom is quiet and dark. It should also be well ventilated and kept at a constant, comfortable temperature.
- Get plenty of exercise during the day.
- Eat properly. Avoid caffeine and alcohol, especially late in the day. Try to avoid all beverages after dinner if you find yourself getting up at night to urinate. If you enjoy a bedtime snack, keep it bland and light.
- Above all, don't worry about sleep. Watching the clock never helps. Try not to lie in bed reviewing your problems or plans; instead, think of something relaxing and pleasant. If you can't manage to relax in bed, don't lie there thrashing about; get up, do something different — and then try again.

Chronic insomnia is very frustrating. If you can't correct it with these simple measures, consider meditation and progressive muscle relaxation techniques. Or get help; sleep clinics are now available in many medical centers, and your personal physician may have some ideas. But don't just ask for sleeping pills; they can be useful for brief periods, but they can have side effects, and they cannot be expected to provide long-range solutions for insomnia.

Meditate

Meditation illustrates the unity of mind and body. Modern studies of Indian yoga masters have shown that meditation can actually slow the heart rate, lower blood pressure, reduce the oxygen consumption and breathing rate, lower blood adrenaline levels, and change the skin temperature.

Although meditation is an ancient technique of Eastern religions, you don't have to become a convert or a pilgrim to put it to work for you. In fact, the leading American proponent of meditation is not an Indian spiritualist but a Harvard physician, Dr. Herbert Benson. Dr. Benson's studies have demonstrated that meditation is easy to learn, and that it can be used successfully to reduce stress and treat hypertension.

Dr. Benson's relaxation technique involves four elements:

1. Select a time and place that will be free of distractions and interruption. A semidarkened room is often best; it should be quiet and private.
2. Get comfortable. Find a body position that will allow your body to relax so that physical signals of discomfort will not intrude on your mental processes.
3. Achieve a relaxed, passive mental attitude. Close your eyes to block out visual stimuli. Try to let your mind go blank, blocking out thoughts and worries.
4. Concentrate on a mental device. Most people use a mantra, a simple word or syllable that is repeated over and over again in a rhythmic, chantlike fashion. You can repeat your mantra silently or say it aloud. It's the act of repetition that counts, not the content of the phrase; even the word "one" will do nicely. Some meditators prefer to stare at a fixed object instead of repeating a mantra. In either case, the goal is to focus your attention on a neutral object, thus blocking out ordinary thoughts and sensations.

Muscle Relaxation and Deep-Breathing Techniques

In meditation, mental relaxation is used to regulate bodily as well as psychological functions. In progressive muscle relaxation and deep breathing, physical relaxation is used to achieve mental calm.

The technique of progressive muscle relaxation is easier to master than meditation. Like meditation, muscle relaxation is best performed in a quiet, secluded place. You should be comfortably seated or stretched out on a firm mattress or mat. Until you learn the routine, have a friend recite the directions or listen to them on a tape, which you can prerecord yourself.

Progressive muscle relaxation focuses sequentially on each major muscle group. Each muscle is tightened. The contraction is maintained for 20 seconds and then slowly released. As the muscle relaxes, concentrate on the release of tension and the sensation of relaxation. Start with your facial muscles, then work down your body.

Forehead	Wrinkle your forehead and arch your eyebrows. Hold, then relax.
Eyes	Close your eyes tightly. Hold, then relax.
Nose	Wrinkle your nose and flare your nostrils. Hold, then relax.
Tongue	Push your tongue firmly against the roof of your mouth. Hold, then relax.
Face	Grimace. Hold, then relax.
Jaws	Clench your jaws tightly. Hold, then relax.
Neck	Tense your neck by pulling your chin down to your chest. Hold, then relax.

Back	Arch your back. Hold, then relax.
Chest	Breathe in as deeply as you can. Hold, then relax.
Stomach	Tense your stomach muscles. Hold, then relax.
Buttocks and thighs	Tense your buttocks muscles. Hold, then relax.
Arms	Tense your biceps. Hold, then relax.
Forearms and hands	Tense your arms and clench your fists. Hold, then relax.
Calves	Press your feet down. Hold, then relax.
Ankles and feet	Pull your toes up. Hold, then relax.

The entire routine should take 12 to 15 minutes. Practice it twice daily, expecting to master the technique and experience some relief of stress in about two weeks.

Deep breathing is even easier and less time-consuming. Best of all, you can sneak breathing exercises in to any part of your day, using the technique to dispel stress as it occurs:

1. Breathe in slowly and deeply, pushing your stomach out so that your diaphragm is put to maximum use.
2. Hold your breath briefly.
3. Exhale slowly, thinking "relax."
4. Repeat the entire sequence five to ten times over, concentrating on breathing deeply and on inhaling and exhaling slowly.

You can use deep breathing whenever you need it most. If you find it helpful, plan to repeat the sequence five times a day — even on good days.

Get Help If You Need It

Self-help techniques can go a long way toward controlling stress and depression. But sometimes they are not enough. If you are still troubled despite your best efforts, get skilled help.

That help can come in many forms. Support groups can provide the guidance and information you may not be able to get on your own; Alcoholics Anonymous is an outstanding example. Take a course in stress control or attend a stress management clinic; they can help you learn stress control techniques, and many clinics also offer biofeedback devices that allow you to monitor muscle tension, heart rate, blood pressure, or skin temperature as you learn to relax.

Counseling is also a good way to attain psychological health. A broad range of professionals can help; psychiatrists, psychologists, social workers, psychiatric nurses, mental health workers, pastoral counselors, and group therapists are all available. Techniques vary, but the basic goal is to work through problems and conflicts by talking them out, gaining insight, and learning to use these insights to control emotions, make choices, and establish healthy relationships. Sometimes just a few sessions will be remarkably helpful, but in other cases more intense therapy is needed.

Psychiatrists and other physicians can also prescribe medications to treat psychological problems. Ideally these drugs are temporary aids that are used to help establish a long-term program for recovery and mental health. Drug therapy has improved rapidly during the past few years; medications are particularly beneficial for the serious psychological disorders that seem to have a neurochemical basis.

Build a Balanced Life

Just as moderation is the key to physical health, balance is the key to psychological health. Balance work and play, exercise and rest, discipline and indulgence. Balance independence and interdependence, solitude and companionship. Balance thought and fantasy, effort and relaxation, routine and spontaneity. Balance your needs with those of your family and your community. Balance your mind and your body to keep both healthy and fit.

■ 20 ■
Nutritional Health

Nutrition is central to health. Good nutrition is one of the most important tools for disease prevention; bad nutrition is a major cause of many serious illnesses.

It sounds simple. But even though everyone agrees that nutrition is important, the details of what's good and what's bad seem to be embroiled in endless controversy. In part these controversies derive from legitimate scientific uncertainties. To an even greater extent, however, the confusion depends on deeply ingrained eating habits and cultural traditions. Economic pressures generated by industrial giants in agriculture, food processing, and marketing compound the debate and make change difficult to achieve.

Fortunately, nutritional science is now pointing the way toward healthful eating. Interestingly, the new direction it's pointing is backwards, to the basics of human nutrition.

■ Historical and Genetic Perspectives

It's hard to be sure just what was eaten at the dawn of humanity, 40,000 years ago, but anthropological research provides some provocative clues. Drs. S. Boyd Eaton and Melvin Konner estimate that the Stone Age diet was composed of 65 percent vegetable foods and 35 percent animal foods. Because of the high animal content, the diet was high in protein, deriving one third of its energy from protein. But since wild game meat is very lean, the diet was low in fat at about 20 percent; most of the fat, in fact, was of the unsaturated variety. The remainder of the caloric content, about 45 percent, derived from carbohydrates. Vegetable carbohydrates also contributed about 100 grams of fiber per day — huge quantities by current standards. The primitive diet was high in potassium and calcium but low in sodium; it contained adequate quantities of iron, vitamins, and other micronutrients.

Human genetics have changed but little since the Stone Age; in contrast, the human life-style has changed enormously. Today's diet would be unrecognizable to primitive people, but the changes occurred gradually. Humans learned to cultivate crops and domesticate animals about 10,000 years ago. Grains and cereals became the main vegetable foods, replacing wild fruits, seeds, and nuts. Domesticated animals replaced wild game, and dairy products became a staple. The result: more saturated fat, less fiber, and less dietary diversity.

The agricultural era diet persisted until the industrial revolution of the nineteenth century. With industrialization, human living patterns changed at a startling pace. Mechanization and agricultural technology have kept pace with the astounding population explosion; with the tragic exception of famine zones in the underdeveloped world, the quantity of food is no longer a problem. But the quality of food has been drastically altered, contributing to new diseases of modern life.

Our diet can improve, and these diseases can be prevented.

■ The American Diet

You don't have to be an anthropologist to comprehend the link between our changing diet and our changing diseases; America's recent history proves the point. In just 100 years the American diet has moved from vegetable foods to animal foods, from carbohydrate to fat, from fiber to refined foods, from potassium to sodium. Total caloric consumption has not changed, but obesity has increased dramatically. It's no coincidence that heart disease, high blood pressure, strokes, gallstones, diabetes, bowel diseases, and cancers of the colon and breast have also increased substantially. Our new lifestyle has created new diseases.

What did you eat for lunch? If you're like 20 percent of Americans, you ate at a fast food restaurant. Perhaps you had a cheeseburger with fries and a shake; 200 burgers are sold in the United States every second. Your fast lunch may have tasted good, and the price seemed reasonable. But there is a hidden cost: sound nutrition. In just a few minutes you consumed 1,500 calories, nearly enough for the entire day. You also ate 75 grams of fat and 1,800 milligrams of sodium — more than you should take in all day. You are well on your way to exceeding your daily quota of protein, but you've done little to meet your need for fiber.

Our most affluent and best-educated citizens have made significant dietary improvements, but children and young adults are more easily influenced by America's corporate taste makers and have not yet established wise nutritional patterns. In addition, the poorest among us continue to eat the most fat, animal protein, sugar, and salt, and the least fiber and vegetable protein. And even in the midst of our staggering epidemic of overnutrition, there are many pockets of hunger and malnutrition in our country.

All segments of American society can benefit from improved nutrition. You don't have to eat like a hunter-gatherer to prevent disease; it's not a bad idea, but I'll settle for a good old American diet, circa 1900.

■ Cultural Perspectives

Heavily dependent on social traditions and customs, economics, and agricultural resources, dietary patterns differ greatly from country to country.

Not surprisingly, differences in the world's pantries parallel differences in the world's hospitals.

The famous Seven Countries Study, which tracked more than 12,000 men for ten years, found that men eating the most fat had the highest blood cholesterol levels and the most heart disease. Finland, for example, led the way in both dietary fat and heart disease; the United States was close behind. In Greece, where the average fat consumption is below 30 percent, coronary heart disease is three times less common than in the United States, where fat consumption exceeds 40 percent.

Dietary fat is a leading cause of cancer as well as heart disease. American women eat 1,000 more calories per day than Japanese women, mostly because they eat three times more fat; Americans also have five times more breast cancer. Blacks in Nigeria eat much more fiber than blacks in America, who have ten times more colon cancer. Hindus in India eat largely vegetable protein and are virtually free of colon cancer; Parsis in India eat a Western diet and have Western rates of colon and breast cancer.

The average diet in China derives just 7 percent of its protein from animal sources, the average American diet nearly 70 percent. Americans eat 20 percent *fewer* calories than the Chinese, yet we are 25 percent fatter. The reason: 77 percent of the calories in China come from complex carbohydrates such as rice and other grains; only 45 percent of America's calories come from carbohydrates, half of these from refined sugars. The Chinese eat much more fiber, the Americans, much more fat. As a result, the average blood cholesterol level in China is nearly 100 points lower than it is in America, and heart attacks kill 67 of every 1,000 American men but only 4 of every 1,000 Chinese men. American women have five times more breast cancer and eight times more cervical cancer than Chinese women. American women also have much more osteoporosis even though they eat many more dairy products; our higher protein intake and lower exercise levels may explain this apparent contradiction.

It's no secret that Third World countries envy the Western life-style. Who can blame them? I, for one, wouldn't trade my citizenship for any other in the world. But many aspects of our life-style are detrimental to health: sedentary living, stress, smoking, drinking, and substance abuse are tragically obvious examples. Our diet, too, belongs on the undesirable list, yet it is envied the world over. Immigrants to our shores adopt our diet in short order. As a result, their disease patterns change drastically, rapidly approaching Western prevalence rates. Worldwide differences, then, are based not on genetics but on life-styles.

It is fashionable today for nutritionists to recommend a "Mediterranean" diet, high in pasta and olive oil. I'm all for it. More radical nutritionists advocate an "oriental" diet, rich in fish and rice. I'm even more enthusiastic. But the nutritional ploy I like best of all transcends all geographic restrictions, bypassing even Scarsdale and Hollywood. It's a basic human diet, founded not in cultural traditions but in the history of our species. It's very low in fat and high in fiber, low in animal protein and high in vegetable products, low in sodium and high in potassium, calcium, and vitamins. It may seem drastic, but viewed from the perspectives of human history and cultural diversity, it's really very conservative. It can also be delicious and economical.

I present this dietary plan not as a given but as a goal, not as an absolute but as an alternative. Indeed, my family and I continue to change slowly toward this nutritional goal. With some planning and patience you can also progress in these directions. As you do, you can expect to help prevent disease, to enhance health, and to discover lots of tasty eating.

■ Diet and Health

The links between diet and health are complex, and they often seem controversial. Some of the debates arise because so many people have an economic interest in food. Add family traditions, cultural norms, and personal taste and preference. Stir in a woefully inadequate system of health education. Spice it up with cultural prejudice. Mix in doctors who know shockingly little about nutrition and politicians who judge vegetables by voter appeal rather than vitamin content. Add a dash of sensational journalism, and simmer with the inevitable resistance to change. The result: a recipe for confusion and uncertainty. It's not tasty, and it has not done much to advance the cause of nutritional reform.

Even well-informed, highly motivated people are discouraged by the confusion over diet and health. Indeed, some frustration is inevitable because the rules *do* change as science learns more about nutrition. Shellfish, long taboo because they contain so much cholesterol, are now acceptable because they contain so little fat. Margarine, formerly given a pat because of its low saturated fat content, is now viewed with concern because it has large amounts of trans-fatty acids that can raise blood cholesterol levels. Fish oil is favored, then forgotten. Some authorities claim that salt is not responsible for the ups and downs of blood pressure, while others tell us to shake the habit. Calcium supplements are in, then out, now in, as we struggle to learn how to prevent osteoporosis. Oat bran, too, has gone from panacea to pariah — only to find its way back to respectability as a useful aid to lower blood cholesterol levels.

What's a mother to do? Try to keep up with the latest research, but learn to distinguish between breakthroughs and ballyhoo, facts and fads. Above all, keep the big picture in view: even if we debate the merits of margarine and butter or oat bran and wheat bran, we should not lose sight of the irrefutable facts that dietary fat predisposes toward disease while fiber promotes health.

Table 20-1 presents an outline of the big picture. It may be subject to quibbling, if not debate. I've added asterisks to indicate areas of conflicting data. In addition, some recommendations will change as the science of nutrition advances. But even if some details shift, the major facts are likely to remain secure.

To dispel any lingering doubts about the nutritional program that's best for health, just add up the number of times key items appear in table 20-1.

Table 20-1. Diet and Health

Disease	Dietary factors that contribute to the illness	Dietary factors that help prevent the illness
Coronary artery disease	Saturated fat Cholesterol Salt*	Fiber Fish Alcohol Polyunsaturated fats* Carotene-rich vegetables* Vitamin E*
High blood pressure	Salt Excessive calories Fat* Alcohol	Calcium* Potassium*
Blood clots		Root vegetables*
Varicose veins		Fiber
Stroke	Salt Fat Excessive calories Alcohol	
Lung cancer		Carotene-rich vegetables
Asthma	Preservatives containing sulfites*	
Colon cancer	Fat Meat protein* Excess calories	Fiber Vitamin D* Vitamin C* Carotene-rich vegetables*
Diverticulosis		Fiber
Hemorrhoids		Fiber
Hernias		Fiber
Constipation and irritable bowel		Fiber
Cancer of pancreas		Fiber
Cancer of esophagus	Alcohol	Carotene-rich vegetables
Cancer of stomach	Smoked, dried, and salted foods Nitrates* Alcohol	

▶

Table 20-1. (continued)

Disease	Dietary factors that contribute to the illness	Dietary factors that help prevent the illness
Gastritis and ulcers	Alcohol* Caffeine*	Fiber*
Cirrhosis of the liver	Alcohol	
Gallstones	Fat Excessive calories Ultra-low-calorie diets	Fiber
Osteoporosis	Excessive protein Alcohol	Calcium
Breast cancer	Fat Excessive calories Alcohol	Fiber* Carotene-rich vegetables*
Cancer of uterus	Fat Excessive calories	Carotene-rich vegetables
Prostate cancer	Fat	
Bladder cancer		Carotene-rich vegetables
Impaired kidney function	Excessive protein*	
Kidney stones	Excessive calcium	
Anemia		Iron Vitamin B$_{12}$ Folic acid
Obesity	Excessive calories Fat	Fiber*
Diabetes	Excessive calories	
Cataracts		Carotene-rich vegetables*
Dental cavities	Sugars	
Cancer of mouth and larynx	Alcohol	

*Indicates preliminary or inconclusive data

Fat appears in the bad column nine times, while fiber appears on the good list eleven times. Caloric excess shows up as a cause of disease eight times. Alcohol makes the trouble category ten times, the helpful category only once. Carotene-rich vegetables appear exclusively in the desirable column, where they are found seven times. Remember that animal products tend to be high in fat and calories and that plant foods tend to be high in fiber and vitamins, and you'll be well on your way to nutritional health.

Eat like a hunter-gatherer? Perhaps it's not such a bad idea after all.

■ The Elements of Nutrition

I hope you're convinced that a sound diet can help prevent disease. Still, to improve your own diet you need to know the details. Let's consider first the individual building blocks of good nutrition. In later sections we'll see how these elements come together in foods — and then in a total eating plan that's enjoyable, practical, and healthful.

■ Cholesterol

As the leading topic of dietary conversation, cholesterol is on everyone's lips. Despite all this talk, however, I'm afraid that cholesterol is still too prominent on most folks' menus.

Even people who are concerned about cholesterol are surprised to learn that it's not actually a fat. Instead, cholesterol is a soft, waxy material belonging to an entirely different group of chemicals called *sterols*. Because dietary cholesterol and saturated fat have similar roles in health and disease, the chemical distinction between them may not seem very important. But this technical difference explains how some foods can be free of cholesterol yet high in harmful fats, while other foods are high in cholesterol but low in fat. You should understand just enough chemistry to outwit unscrupulous food manufacturers who trumpet "no cholesterol" in large print while reluctantly disclosing fat content in tiny letters.

Cholesterol is present in all animal tissues; it is an essential part of the membranes that surround all animal cells. In contrast, all vegetable products are entirely cholesterol-free.

Cholesterol is important for your health in two ways. Your *blood* cholesterol levels are major determinants of your risk for coronary artery disease, atherosclerosis, and stroke. Chapter 2 explains the two types of cholesterol in your blood, and describes the ways you can lower your bad, or LDL, cholesterol while raising your good, or HDL, cholesterol.

Cholesterol in *food* is also important for health. It would seem obvious that the more cholesterol you eat, the higher your blood cholesterol level will be. Indeed, this logic holds true — but only to a point. Dietary cholesterol accounts for only one third of blood cholesterol; the other two thirds is manufactured by your own liver. Eating saturated fat stimulates your liver to manufacture more of the harmful type of cholesterol. So to lower your blood cholesterol, it's actually even more important to reduce the saturated fat in your diet than to eliminate cholesterol-rich foods. Now you know why we can give shrimp, high in cholesterol but low in fat, a cautious OK.

Even if dietary cholesterol is not the crucial determinant of blood cholesterol levels, you should keep your cholesterol consumption as low as possible. In fact, most foods that are high in saturated fat are also high in cholesterol, so by restricting your consumption of liver, red meat, whole milk products, butter, eggs, and cheese, you'll make progress on both fronts.

The average American eats about 450 milligrams of cholesterol per day. Because your body makes all the cholesterol it needs, the optimum amount of dietary cholesterol is probably none at all. The American Heart Association tells us to eat no more than 300 milligrams. I'd be even happier if you stayed under 200; my own daily quota averages 130 milligrams.

■ Fats

Cholesterol gets most of the blame for our nutritional excesses; fats deserve it.

Before I proceed to hold fat up to the fire of prevention, I should point out that some fat is essential for health. Fat is a critical component of all human organs and tissues. It is the body's major form of energy storage. In addition, fatty tissue insulates the body and cushions its vital internal organs. Fats are also crucial carriers of vitamins A, D, E, and K, which will not dissolve in water.

We all need fat in our bodies and in our diets. But the typical American eats far more fat than necessary, averaging about one third of a cup of pure fat — the equivalent of 22 pats of butter — per day. About 40 percent of our daily caloric intake comes from fat; the American Heart Association recommends a decrease to 30 percent, but I'd favor a progressive reduction all the way down to 20 percent.

Why reduce dietary fat? There are three major reasons. First, fat is the most calorie-dense of all foods (see table 20-2); as a result, America's high fat intake contributes significantly to America's excessive body fat.

Second, fat contributes to heart disease. But while all fats have the same caloric content, they differ greatly in their impact on blood cholesterol levels and cardiovascular disease. Unfortunately, in addition to eating too much fat, Americans are eating the wrong types of fat. The typical American consumes 11 gallons of ice cream, 261 eggs, and 79 pounds of beef each year. Instead of all this animal fat, we should be eating modest amounts of vegetable fats. Indeed, you can get enough of the essential fatty acid that is indispensable for health from just tiny amounts of vegetable oil.

The third reason to reduce your dietary fat intake is cancer. The risk of colon cancer, uterine cancer, and prostate cancer are increased by excessive fat consumption. As with heart disease, animal fat appears to be the

Table 20-2. Caloric Content of Nutrients

Nutrient	Calories	
Fat	9 calories per gram	252 per ounce
Alcohol	7 calories per gram	196 per ounce
Carbohydrate	4 calories per gram	112 per ounce
Protein	4 calories per gram	112 per ounce

main culprit; a multinational study published in the 1990 *Journal of the National Cancer Institute* reports that the risk of colon cancer doubles with every 10 grams of saturated fat in the daily diet above 10 grams a day.

Obesity, heart disease, and cancer: three good reasons to reduce the fat in your diet — and to substitute unsaturated fats of vegetable origin for saturated fats from animal products.

Good Fats, Bad Fats

Not all fats are created equal; some are more harmful than others. *Saturated* fats are those in which all the carbon atoms have hydrogen atoms attached, while *unsaturated* fats have "empty" carbon atoms with unfilled hydrogen slots. *Monounsaturated* fats have one unfilled slot; *polyunsaturated* fats have two or more.

Even if you can't tell carbon from cookies, you can tell the difference between saturated and unsaturated fats. Saturated fats tend to be solid at room temperature, whereas unsaturated fats are generally liquid at room temperature.

There are two key differences between saturated and unsaturated fats. First, saturated fats generally come from animal sources, whereas unsaturated fats have vegetable origins. Second, saturated fats elevate blood cholesterol levels while unsaturated fats do not; some unsaturated fats, in fact, may even lower cholesterol levels.

It's simple enough — so far. But there are some important exceptions to this lean outline.

Tropical oils are the first exception. Palm oil, palm kernel oil, and coconut oil come from plants and are liquid at room temperature, but they otherwise behave like animal fats: they are saturated, and they raise blood cholesterol levels. As a result, you should treat palm and coconut oils like animal fat: avoid them as much as possible. Unfortunately, tropical oils are used in many commercial baked goods because they are plentiful, inexpensive, and stable. To avoid them you'll have to be a careful label reader. Look beyond the big print that says "100 percent vegetable oil" to see if the fine print lists either of these tropical "animals." Chocolate lovers should beware, too, of cocoa butter, which is also composed principally of saturated fat despite its vegetable origins.

Another exception: partially hydrogenated vegetable oils. In most cases these are polyunsaturated fats which are used in food preparation; to improve their culinary properties, manufacturers add hydrogen atoms to the fatty acids. As a result they become more nearly saturated — hardly an improvement for health. Because they are used in so many commercially prepared foods, it's hard to avoid them entirely. But partially hydrogenated fatty acids pose problems which came to light in a 1990 study of margarine.

The margarine story goes back to the earliest days of "oleo." Manufacturers of this new "artificial" food wanted to do everything they could to duplicate the taste, color, and texture of the "high-price spread," butter. Color and flavor were achieved easily enough, but to solidify margarine and give it the feel of butter, food processors had to hydrogenate the poly-unsaturated vegetable oils which are margarine's main ingredients. But hydrogenation does more than simply make the fatty acids more nearly saturated; in addition, the process changes the configuration of the fats, straightening out their normal comma shape. Chemists call this a shift from the *cis-* to the *trans-* configuration. Food manufacturers call it a bonanza, since the straighter trans-fatty acids can be packed closer together, producing a semisolid fat with a longer shelf life which can still be labeled "unsaturated." Cooks call it an advance, since trans-fatty acids make margarine smooth and raise its melting point. Doctors and nutritionists, however, call it trouble.

A team of Dutch investigators raised the alarm when studying the effects of various fatty acids on blood cholesterol levels. The new observation was that even though they are unsaturated, trans-fatty acids also raised blood LDL cholesterol levels. In fact, LDL cholesterol levels were nearly as high on the trans-fatty acids as on a saturated fat diet. Even worse, the trans-fatty acids also lowered the HDL or "good" blood cholesterol levels, while the saturated fats did not. All in all, this study in the *New England Journal of Medicine* suggests that trans-fatty acids may be even more harmful for blood cholesterol levels than saturated animal fats.

Should we switch from margarine back to butter? No. The total fat and caloric content of butter and its closest imitator, stick margarine, is identical, but butter is much higher in saturated fat and contains 31 milligrams of cholesterol per tablespoon, whereas margarine has little saturated fat and is cholesterol-free. But stick margarine is made up of 25 percent partially hydrogenated trans-fatty acids. You can do better. The softer the margarine, the less it's been hydrogenated, and the lower its content of trans-fatty acids. Tub margarines, for example, average 17 percent trans-fatty acids. "Diet" or "imitation" margarines have even less fat, and liquid margarine is the lowest of all in both saturated and trans-fatty acids.

You don't have to give up margarine, but you should use it intelligently. Choose the least hydrogenated (least solid) preparation that will satisfy your palate — and, as with all fats, use it sparingly. Needless to say, pure liquid vegetable oils that are not even partially hydrogenated are the best of all.

Since the 1990 Dutch study, nutritionists have begun to warn us about stick margarine, and health-conscious consumers have begun to get the message. But many people still overlook the trans-fatty acids present in other partially hydrogenated vegetable oils. These oils are used in many commercially prepared foods, including nondairy creamers, frosting, imitation cheese, candy, hydrogenated peanut butter, and cereals. Baked goods are often very high in trans-fatty acids; for example, a typical pastry or donut contains about six grams, while even a "heart-healthy" bran muffin contains four grams.

The moral: read the fine print and choose products with nonhydrogenated unsaturated vegetable oils whenever possible. Even better: do the cooking yourself, using mono- or polyunsaturated oils.

Nutritional Health

The unsaturated fatty acids also present many choices. Numerous scientific studies have investigated the relative merits of mono- and polyunsaturates, and have compared the effects of various polyunsaturates on blood cholesterol levels. The data are complex and often contradictory; the debates that result are more notable for their heat than their light. In my view the differences among unsaturated fats are less important than their similarities. All are much better for your cholesterol levels than are the saturated or trans-fatty acids, but all should be used in moderation. Until we have additional data, you can let taste, convenience, and price dictate your choice among the unsaturated oils. All things being equal, I'd tend to favor canola oil and olive oil.

Because of their unique properties, another type of unsaturated fatty acid deserves additional thought. Although it is not of plant origin, its beneficial properties may exceed those of polyunsaturated vegetable oils. Too good to be true? No, but it is a fishy story: the unsaturated fatty acids in question are found in fish oil.

The current interest in the medical benefits of fish goes back to the observation that despite a diet that is very high in animal fat, Eskimos get very little heart disease. The reason: the animal fat eaten by Eskimos comes from *marine* animals instead of *land* animals. And a careful investigation of 852 middle-aged Dutch men found that those who ate the equivalent of two fish meals a week enjoyed a 50 percent reduction in heart disease over a 20-year period.

Fish oil contains unique unsaturated fats called omega-3 fatty acids; eicosapentaenoic acid (EPA) is considered the most beneficial of these. Although therapy with fish oil capsules has been a disappointment, the benefits of eating fish have been validated in studies performed in Sweden, America, and Wales. Note also that among the vegetable oils, canola oil is unique because it's also rich in omega-3's, which account for 10 percent of its content.

Table 20-3 compares the properties of various fats and oils.

Facing the Fats: Calculation and Guidelines

At this point you are undoubtedly saturated with facts about fat. Five major principles are all you'll really need to stay healthy — if you apply them properly to your diet. To review:

1. Eat a diet low in fat. Most major health organizations recommend that no more than 30 percent of your daily calories come from fat, but I join other authorities who prefer a target of about 20 percent. If 20 percent seems too restrictive, remember that the Ornish and Pritikin diets have achieved excellent results for heart patients by providing less than 10 percent fat.

2. Avoid saturated fat. No more than one third of your daily fat intake should be in the form of saturated fat.

3. Avoid animal fat. Most of it is saturated, and animal products also contain cholesterol. An exception is fish oil, which is desirable because of its high content of omega-3 polyunsaturates.

Table 20-3. Fats and Oils

	Fatty acid contents (as % total fat)		
	Saturated	Mono-unsaturated	Poly-unsaturated
Animal fats			
Undesirable			
Butter, cream, whole milk	66	4	30
Beef, tallow	52	44	4
Lard (pork fat)	42	45	13
Chicken fat	30	49	21
Desirable			
Fish oil	29	31	40
Vegetable oils			
Undesirable			
Coconut oil	92	6	2
Palm kernel oil	81	11	2
Cocoa butter	63	34	3
Palm oil	51	39	10
Desirable			
Peanut oil	18	48	34
Olive oil	14	77	9
Cottonseed oil	27	19	54
Soybean oil	15	24	61
Corn oil	13	25	62
Sunflower oil	11	20	69
Safflower oil	9	13	78
Canola (rapeseed) oil	6	58	26

Principal source: Nutritive Value of Foods, *U.S. Department of Agriculture*

4. Favor vegetable oils. Most of them are low in saturated fats. Exceptions are coconut oil, palm and palm kernel oils, and cocoa butter, which are high in saturated fat.

5. Favor mono- and polyunsaturates; olive oil and canola oil are particularly desirable. Exceptions are partially hydrogenated vegetable oils; although not technically saturated fats, they contain trans-fatty acids which mimic many of the deleterious effects of saturated fats.

If you're like most people, you eat not fatty acids but fatty foods. To apply even these five simple guidelines to your diet, you'll need to estimate the fat content of your food. You can do this in either of two ways: by calculating the percentage of fat in food or by tallying the total fat content of your diet.

The percentage method may appear to be the easier approach, but appearances are deceiving. Many food manufacturers boast that their products are low in fat because they are 90 or 95 percent fat-free. These numbers imply that only 5 to 10 percent of the food is fat, and that you can eat all you want. It's not necessarily so. Foods are labeled by weight; a food can be *low* in fat by *weight* but *high* in fat by *caloric* content.

"Two-percent" milk is one example. An eight-ounce serving has 5 grams of fat but weighs 250 grams; the fat is indeed 2 percent by weight. But most of the weight of milk is water, which has no calories. The 5 grams of fat in your glass of low-fat milk will contribute 45 calories — almost exactly one third of its total caloric content. "*Two*-percent" milk actually just fits the *30* percent guideline when you calculate its calories rather than its weight.

You can use the percentage method to evaluate the fat content of your diet, but you'll have to do the math yourself:

$$percent\ fat = \frac{900 \times grams\ of\ fat}{total\ calories}$$

We can use whole milk as an example. It contains only 3.3 percent fat by weight. But eight ounces contain 8 grams of fat and 150 calories. Hence:

$$percent\ fat = \frac{900 \times 8}{150} = 48$$

Whole milk may be "97 percent" fat-free, but a whopping 48 percent of its calories come from fat (most of which is saturated fat).

During the course of a day you'll eat some fat-free foods and some high-fat foods. What really matters is not the percentage in each item but your total fat consumption. Hence, I prefer the gram-counting method; it's more informative — and also easier.

First, turn back to chapter 12. Estimate your daily caloric needs from table 12-4. Next, pick your target fat intake, which may be the American Heart Association's 30 percent guideline, my 20 percent target, or something in between. Now check table 20-4 to find what your maximum daily intake of fat should be. The table is easy to use. If you eat 1,800 calories per day and aim for a 25 percent fat intake, for example, your goal is 50 grams of fat per day. To find your maximum intake of saturated fat, simply divide your total fat intake by 3. In our example, one third of your 50-gram daily goal would allow you up to 17 grams of saturated fat per day.

To use either method, of course, you'll need to know the fat content of

Table 20-4. Your Goals for Daily Fat Consumption

Daily calorie intake	Total grams of fat at various target percentages		
	20%	25%	30%
1,200	26	33	40
1,800	40	50	60
2,400	53	66	80
3,000	66	83	100

Table 20-5. The Fat, Cholesterol, and Calories in Foods

Food	Portion size	Choles- terol (mg)	Total calories	Total fat (g)	Satu- rated fat (g)	% Calories from fat
Dairy products						
Whole milk	8 oz	33	150	8	5	48
Low-fat milk (1%)	8 oz	10	102	3	2	23
Buttermilk	8 oz	9	99	2	1	20
Skim milk	8 oz	4	86	trace	trace	5
Yogurt, plain	6 oz	21	105	6	4	47
Low-fat yogurt (plain)	6 oz	3	94	trace	trace	3
Cottage cheese	4 oz	17	117	5	3	39
Low-fat cottage cheese (1%)	4 oz	5	82	1	1	13
Sour cream	1 oz	12	61	6	4	87
Cream cheese	1 oz	31	99	10	6	90
Ricotta cheese (whole milk)	1 oz	58	197	15	9	67
Ricotta cheese (part skim milk)	1 oz	25	156	9	6	52
Cheddar cheese	1 oz	30	114	9	6	74
Parmesan cheese	1 oz	22	129	9	5	59
Swiss cheese	1 oz	26	107	8	5	65
Feta cheese	1 oz	25	75	6	4	72
Egg yolk	1	272	63	6	2	80
Egg white	1	0	16	trace	0	0
Meats (cooked)						
Hot dog (beef)	1	31	158	14	6	82
Bologna (beef)	3 slices	58	312	28	12	82
Salami (beef)	3 slices	65	262	20	9	71
Chuck roast	3½ oz	99	350	26	11	67
Ground beef	3½ oz	87	272	19	7	61
Corned beef	3½ oz	98	251	19	6	68
Rib roast	3½ oz	80	225	12	5	47
T-bone steak	3½ oz	80	214	10	4	44
Liver	3½ oz	389	161	5	2	27
Lamb chop	3½ oz	215	215	9	4	39
Bacon	3½ oz	85	576	50	18	78
Ham	3½ oz	92	178	9	3	46
Veal cutlet	3½ oz	128	271	11	5	37

Table 20-5. (continued)

Food	Portion size	Choles- terol (mg)	Total calories	Total fat (g)	Satu- rated fat (g)	% Calories from fat
Poultry						
Duck	3½ oz	89	201	11	4	50
Chicken (with skin)	3½ oz	91	253	16	4	56
Chicken (without skin)	3½ oz	91	205	10	3	43
Turkey (with skin)	3½ oz	117	182	7	2	35
Turkey (without skin)	3½ oz	112	126	4	1	24
Fish						
Shrimp	3½ oz	195	99	1	trace	10
Lobster	3½ oz	72	98	1	trace	6
Cod	3½ oz	55	105	1	trace	9
Halibut	3½ oz	41	140	3	trace	19
Trout	3½ oz	73	151	4	1	26
Tuna	3½ oz	49	184	6	2	31
Salmon	3½ oz	87	216	11	2	46
Frozen desserts						
Ice cream (premium)	1 cup	88	349	24	15	61
Ice cream (regular)	1 cup	59	269	14	9	48
Sherbet	1 cup	14	270	4	2	13
Frozen yogurt	1 cup	0	216	2	0	8
Frozen yogurt (nonfat)	1 cup	0	175	0	0	0
Nuts and seeds						
Coconut meat	1 oz	0	187	18	16	88
Pecans	1 oz	0	187	18	2	89
Walnuts	1 oz	0	182	18	2	87
Peanuts	1 oz	0	164	14	2	76
Pistachio nuts	1 oz	0	164	14	2	76
Sunflower seeds	1 oz	0	165	14	1	77
Breads						
Whole wheat	1 slice	0	70	1	trace	13
White	1 slice	0	65	1	trace	14
Bagel	1	0	200	2	trace	9
Pita	½ shell	0	165	1	trace	5

▶

Table 20-5. (continued)

Food	Portion size	Choles-terol (mg)	Total calories	Total fat (g)	Satu-rated fat (g)	% Calories from fat
Baked goods						
Croissant	1	13	235	12	4	46
Donut	1	20	210	12	3	51
Bran muffin	1	24	125	6	1	43
English muffin	1	0	140	1	trace	6
Chocolate chip cookies	1	4	46	3	1	54
Oatmeal cookies	1	1	61	3	trace	37
Chocolate brownie	1	14	100	4	2	36
Fig bar	1	5	52	1	trace	17
Cream pie	1 slice	8	455	23	15	46
Apple pie	1 slice	0	405	18	5	40
Chocolate cake	1 slice	37	235	8	4	31
Pound cake	1 slice	64	110	5	3	41
Waffle	1	102	245	13	4	48
Pancake	1	16	60	2	trace	30
Beans and grain products						
Garbanzo beans	1 cup	0	269	4	trace	14
Lima beans	1 cup	0	217	1	trace	3
Kidney beans	1 cup	0	225	1	trace	3
Split peas	1 cup	0	231	1	trace	3
Rice	1 cup	0	225	1	trace	2
Egg noodles	1 cup	50	160	2	1	11
Spaghetti	1 cup	0	155	1	trace	6
Oatmeal	1 cup	0	145	2	trace	15
Corn flakes	1 cup	0	98	trace	trace	0
Granola	1 cup	0	595	33	6	50
Vegetables						
Potato (baked)	1	0	220	trace	trace	0
Broccoli	1 spear	0	50	1	trace	25
Carrot	1	0	30	trace	trace	0
Lettuce	1 wedge	0	20	trace	trace	0
Mushrooms	1 cup	0	20	trace	trace	0
Squash	1 cup	0	35	1	trace	30
Tomato	1	0	25	trace	trace	0
Fruits						
Apple	1	0	80	trace	trace	0
Avocado	1	0	305	30	5	88

Table 20-5. (continued)

Food	Portion size	Choles-terol (mg)	Total calories	Total fat (g)	Satu-rated fat (g)	% Calories from fat
Banana	1	0	105	1	trace	8
Berries	1 cup	0	80	1	trace	11
Dates	10	0	230	trace	trace	0
Melon	¼	0	40	trace	trace	0
Orange	1	0	60	trace	trace	0
Snacks and sweets						
Pizza	1 slice	56	290	9	4	28
Peanut butter	1 tbsp	0	95	8	1	76
Potato chips	1 oz	0	147	10	3	62
Pretzels	1 oz	0	10	trace	trace	0
Popcorn (oil popped)	1 cup	0	55	3	trace	49
Popcorn (air popped)	1 cup	0	30	trace	trace	0
Salted crackers	4	4	50	1	trace	18
Rye crackers	2	0	56	1	trace	16
Chocolate	1 oz	6	145	9	5	56
Gum drops	1 oz	0	100	trace	trace	0
Hard candy	1 oz	0	110	0	0	0
Chocolate pudding	½ cup	15	150	4	2	24
Gelatin	½ cup	0	70	0	0	0
Sauces and dressings						
Mayonnaise	1 tbsp	8	99	11	2	100
Imitation mayonnaise	1 tbsp	4	35	3	1	75
Russian dressing	1 tbsp	0	76	8	1	92
French, Italian (low-cal)	1 tbsp	0	20	1	trace	45
Hollandaise sauce	½ cup	94	353	34	21	87
Barbecue	½ cup	0	94	2	trace	22

Principal source: Nutritive Value of Foods, *U.S. Department of Agriculture*

the foods you eat. Table 20-5 lists the fats in representative foods; you can get more detailed information by ordering the USDA's authoritative publication *Nutritive Value of Foods,* for sale at a modest cost from the Superintendent of Documents, U.S. Government Printing Office, Washington, DC 20402.

If you wish to be precise, tally up the fat in all the food you eat for three consecutive days. But for a general estimate of your diet, simply compare your average fare against the targets in table 20-4; you'll quickly see if you need to improve. Later in this chapter I'll discuss simple ways to turn your new goals into realities.

I hope you understand why it's important to monitor the amount of fat in your diet. It may seem laborious, but you don't have to put a calculator in your hand every time you put a fork in your mouth. Spend a week or two reading labels and checking table 20-5; after just a short time you will have learned the approximate fat content of most of the foods you eat so you won't have to look up most items on your menu.

Monitoring your fat intake is one thing; reducing it is another. Here, too, it will take effort at first. But if you're like most people, your tastes will gradually change, and you'll actually come to prefer low-fat, vegetable-based foods. And if you still crave an occasional high-fat food, there is plenty of room for flexibility (cheating). It will simply be up to you to decide if you want to invest half your day's fat quota in a premium ice cream cone or have a frozen yogurt instead, saving 24 grams of fat for later in the day. Once you have a target fat intake, you'll be in control, able to make the choices that will allow you to eat healthfully *and* enjoyably.

■ Carbohydrates

Bread is the staff of life, and carbohydrates are the stuff of bread.

I hope I've persuaded you to turn the other cheek when you are facing fats. Now you can find out what to eat instead: carbohydrates. As you decrease the fats in your diet, replace them with carbohydrates, increasing your intake from the American average of 45 percent so that 65 or even 70 percent of your calories come from carbohydrates. It sounds good — and it is. But there is one proviso: as you increase your carbohydrate consumption, you should also switch from simple sugars to the complex carbohydrates that are better for health.

What Are Carbohydrates?

All carbohydrates contain just carbon, hydrogen, and oxygen. Simple carbohydrates are sugars, small molecules familiar to you as the sucrose of table sugar and the fructose of fruit sugar. Complex carbohydrates are merely simple sugars joined together into long strands; they are well known to you as starches.

Carbohydrates are found in plants. The only animal source of simple carbohydrates is the lactose in milk; the only animal source of complex carbohydrates is the very small amount of glycogen stored in muscle and liver tissues.

Since all carbohydrates, simple and complex, are converted into glucose before your body uses them, it seems logical that all would have the same impact on health. Logical, yes. Correct, no.

All carbohydrates have the energy value of 4 calories per gram. But sweets, rich in simple sugars, are much more calorie-dense than are starches, rich in complex carbohydrates. Simple carbohydrates contribute significantly to obesity; complex carbohydrates do not.

Sugars are absorbed rapidly into the blood stream; because they must first be digested, starches are absorbed slowly. The rapid absorption of simple carbohydrates raises the blood sugar abruptly, causing the pancreas to pump out large amounts of insulin; complex carbohydrates raise the blood sugar gradually, requiring substantially less insulin for their utilization. Simple sugars should be avoided by diabetics, who lack insulin; complex carbohydrates are recommended as the cornerstone of the diabetic's diet.

Simple sugars not only end up on the hips, but they also linger on the lips — or at least on the teeth. Sweets feed the bacteria that form dental plaque, promoting tooth decay. Complex carbohydrates are safe for your teeth.

Simple sugars are empty calories; sweets contain few nutrients other than sugar itself. In contrast, foods rich in carbohydrates, particularly unrefined carbohydrates, are generally abundantly endowed with other important nutrients.

Simple sugars are not filling. Complex carbohydrates, particularly those present in fruits, vegetables, and whole grains, add bulk and fiber to your diet. The fiber is very important for health and it *is* filling. A piece of candy and an apple, for example, may each have 80 calories, but try eating eight apples!

America's Sweet Tooth

Simple carbohydrates contribute about 25 percent of the calories in the typical American diet. Sugar is everywhere: we start the day with sugared cereals, quench our thirst with soda pop, grab some candy for a quick pickup, and choose sugary morsels for snacks and desserts. It wasn't always that way; in 1900 the average American consumed 75 pounds of sugar in a year, but we've now moved up to 130 pounds annually, and the total continues to rise.

Most of the simple carbohydrates consumed in our country are in the form of refined sugars. But don't mistake "natural" sugars for health foods; the sugar in honey, corn syrup, or molasses has exactly the same effect on your body as the sugar in your candy bar or sugar bowl. Brown sugar is no more healthful than white.

Food manufacturers don't go out of their way to make it easy to recognize sugar in their products. By any name, a simple carbohydrate is just as sugary; here are some of the forms of sugar that appear on food labels:

Sucrose	Maltose	Honey
Glucose	Lactose	Corn syrup
Dextrose	Mannitol	Maple syrup
Fructose	Sorbitol	Molasses

Remember that all of these sugars will affect your body in exactly the same way.

Two artificial sweeteners are in widespread use in the United States. Both saccharine and aspartame have been extensively studied in animals and appear to be safe. Even more important, neither has been proven to cause human disease, despite the use of saccharine since 1879 and of aspartame since 1974. A third sweetener, cyclamate, was withdrawn from the market because it caused bladder cancer in mice, but new data suggest that this observation has no bearing on humans, and the ban is being reconsidered.

Artificial sweeteners appear to be safe, but are they effective? They certainly succeed in making food sweet, but there is *no* evidence that they assist in weight control, which is the principal reason for their use.

At least 90 million Americans consume foods that contain artificial sweeteners. On the one hand, there is no compelling medical reason to discourage their use, though moderation seems prudent, especially for children and pregnant women. On the other hand, there is certainly no reason to encourage their use for weight control.

Above all, artificially sweetened foods and drinks should be used appropriately, as part of an overall program of nutritional health. Sweet nothings, be they bogus or bona fide, should not be allowed to replace the nutritious complex carbohydrates so important for good health.

Complex Carbohydrates: The Simple Facts

Complex carbohydrates — starches — provide only 25 percent of the calories in the average American diet. In many less industrialized societies starches supply more than 75 percent of the calories. We should learn from our neighbors, as well as our past, and aim to triple our complex carbohydrate intake.

It strikes me as ironic that many people in rich countries are reluctant to increase their consumption of complex carbohydrates precisely because many people in poor countries are dependent on them. Starchy foods are plentiful and inexpensive. They have been the staples of the lower economic classes throughout history, and they continue to fill this role in the underdeveloped world today. As people acquire wealth, they turn from their roots, changing from starchy foods to diets high in fat, protein, and refined sugars. Animal products are much more expensive and hence prestigious — but they are much less healthful than vegetables, legumes, fruits, and grains, which are high in starch, fiber, and other nutrients.

Somehow we've got it all backwards. Starchy foods are not considered nutritious — but they are. They are branded as fattening — but they're not. How often have you seen dieters eat their steak but leave their potatoes? How many of them know that a six-ounce potato has only 150 calories and many useful nutrients, while a six-ounce steak has 600 calories and many harmful fats, to say nothing of cholesterol and potentially excessive amounts of protein?

Complex Carbohydrates in Your Diet

Moderation is not my middle name, though I understand why it may seem to be. After pages and pages of "no," "maybe," and "sometimes," after chapters and chapters of "prudence" and "precaution," it is a pleasure to change my tune. When it comes to complex carbohydrates, the watchword is "yes"—go for them!

Starchy foods should be the mainstays of a healthful diet. They should be your main course rather than just side dishes. But even if you eat mainly starchy foods, they need not be boring or burdensome; many varied vegetable products are rich in starch, and many delicious recipes are available to make them as exciting for your palate as they are healthful for your body.

There are many good sources of complex carbohydrates, including:

Breads, cereals, flours
Pasta, noodles
Barley, rice
Legumes (dried peas, beans, and lentils)
Starchy vegetables (potatoes, sweet potatoes, corn, peas, lima beans)

All of these foods will serve you well, and they can be used interchangeably in your diet. But even when you are choosing among them, you should remember a few points.

First, favor unrefined foods such as whole-grain breads, cereals, and pastas; they are all higher in nutrients and fiber then their refined counterparts.

Second, choose your pastas mainly for their taste and texture, but pay some attention to their added ingredients. Whereas whole wheat pastas can provide extra fiber, a plus, egg pastas and noodles have added fat and cholesterol, a minus. Trickiest of all are "high-protein" or "lite" pastas marketed for their extra health benefits. While there is certainly nothing harmful about these products, they are no lower in calories and they miss the point: you are eating pasta to get complex carbohydrates, not protein.

Third, and most important, don't spoil your starchy foods by adding fat to them. Spaghetti is spaghetti, but Alfredo sauce is trouble. Sour cream is the perfect way to ruin the benefits of a baked potato. And when it comes to spoiling potatoes, chips take the prize.

■ Fiber

I don't know who first learned to separate the wheat from the chaff, nor when this landmark event occurred. I do know that the process did not become widespread until the industrial revolution, when milling became mechanized. Since then, refined flour has become the norm in Western societies. Another gold star for human ingenuity. Another setback for human health.

I have no quarrel with either mechanization or milling. I can see nothing wrong with separating grain from husks. But I do object to what occurs next: we should not be discarding the husks. Instead, bran should once again become a normal part of the human diet — along with other sources of dietary fiber.

Because of our preference for refined grains instead of whole grains and for animal products instead of vegetable products, the fiber content of the average American diet has declined by 28 percent in the twentieth century to a paltry 11 grams per day. We should be eating at least three times more fiber. Even if we tripled our dietary fiber, we would still be far below the fiber intake of many less developed societies. Perhaps if we approached their high-fiber, low-fat, vegetable-rich diets, we could also attain their much lower levels of cardiovascular disease, cancer, bowel disease, gallstones, diabetes, and obesity. It's surely worth a try.

What Is Fiber?

Your mother called it *roughage,* and her mother called it *bulk.* Food chemists first called it *crude fiber,* but nutritionists now call it *dietary fiber.* For many people all of these terms conjure up the image of eating bark or rope, things that would truly be rough on your system. Nothing could be further from the truth. Fiber may sound tough, but it's only a special form of complex carbohydrate.

By any name fiber is the structural backbone of plant stems, leaves, and seeds. Unlike other carbohydrates, fiber cannot be digested by human intestinal enzymes; as a result, it remains in the intestinal tract instead of being absorbed into the body. Since fiber is not digested, it has no caloric value; as a result, it was dismissed for years as being unimportant for human health. Since the 1960s, however, many excellent studies have proven that fiber has lots of nutritional value even though it has no caloric value.

Although we all speak of it in the singular, dietary fiber is actually a complex mix of hundreds of plant carbohydrates. Chemists call them gums, pectins, lignins, mucilages, and celluloses. All are large compounds composed of hundreds of sugar molecules linked together into huge branched chains. Even if you can't tell a pectin from a lignin, you should know that there are two major types of dietary fiber, soluble and insoluble.

Insoluble fiber will not dissolve in water. It passes through the intestines unchanged, drawing water into the fecal contents. As a result, the stools become bulkier and are eliminated from the body more rapidly. Insoluble fiber is found in wheat bran, fruits, and vegetables.

Soluble fiber will dissolve in water, but since it can't be absorbed by humans, it remains in the intestinal tract. It swells in water, producing a gel-like texture that makes the intestinal contents bulkier and softer. Soluble fiber delays stomach emptying and sugar absorption, improving blood sugar levels in diabetics. In the stomach this produces a feeling of fullness. In the colon it makes the stools softer and easier to pass. Soluble fiber, which also helps to lower blood cholesterol levels, is found in oat bran, psyllium, legumes, and some fruits and vegetables.

Both forms of fiber are important for health. Only 25 percent of the fiber in the typical American diet is the soluble variety.

Soluble Fiber and Blood Cholesterol: The Oat Bran Saga

The ability of soluble fiber to lower blood cholesterol levels was responsible for the oat bran craze of the 1980s. Between 1984 and 1988 a series of studies on volunteers with high cholesterol levels demonstrated that daily dietary supplementation with 50 to 100 grams of oat bran or with dried beans could lower blood cholesterol levels by up to 23 percent. A 1989 study found that daily administration of 10 grams of psyllium, another soluble fiber, also produced significant reductions in blood cholesterol levels.

Ever eager for a quick fix, the American public began to gobble up everything with an oat on its label. Ever eager for a quick sale, food manufacturers began to add a pinch of oat bran to a bewildering variety of baked goods, from bread to muffins to (it's true) cupcakes.

It was, of course, too good to last. Oats were on a roll only until 1990, when studies from Harvard and Syracuse found that subjects eating oat bran had better cholesterol levels mainly because they substituted oat products for high-fat foods, not because the oat bran itself lowered blood cholesterol. Oats were out.

But the controversy won't go away. In 1991 three studies found that oatmeal, oat bran, and psyllium *do* have a specific ability to lower blood cholesterol levels. A fourth study found that eating 12 prunes a day, which provide about 4 grams of soluble fiber, also lowers cholesterol.

What can we conclude from all this controversy? I'll offer three thoughts. First, it's clear that we still have a lot to learn about the soluble fiber in your diet and the cholesterol in your blood. Science often moves slowly, zig-zagging forward as one study after another adds information about complex problems; chapter 24 will explain how you can evaluate conflicting claims and keep up with developments in prevention.

Second, although there is room for disagreement, I believe the weight of the evidence suggests that soluble fiber *can* help improve cholesterol levels. But don't expect oat bran to be a cholesterol cure. There is no quick fix; instead you'll need a balanced program of nutrition and exercise to improve your cholesterol profile and cardiovascular health.

Third, even though oats, beans, and psyllium are not short cuts to immortality, soluble fiber should be an important part of your diet.

The Fiber in Your Diet

There is no "minimum daily requirement" for dietary fiber. The National Cancer Institute suggests 20 to 30 grams per day. Again shedding my mask of moderation, my rough estimate of the ideal is 30 to 40 grams. As I see it, the more fiber the better — unless, of course, dietary fiber causes discomfort or displaces other valuable nutrients from a balanced diet. Putting my stomach where my mouth is, I average 50 grams of fiber in my daily diet.

How can you get enough fiber? Instead of relying on a single source of fiber, you should eat a variety of fiber-rich foods. Variety will ensure that you get all types of fiber and that you get plenty of other nutrients as well. Variety will also make a high-fiber diet a joy instead of a chore.

Remember that dietary fiber is found only in vegetable products; a single small, juicy strawberry has more fiber than a large, stringy steak. In general, the more refined the product, the lower its fiber content. Apples, for example, have lots of fiber, applesauce only a little, and apple juice none. Although crunchy foods are often fiber-rich, you cannot rely on a food's texture to estimate its fiber content; corn and potatoes are high in fiber, but corn flakes and potato chips are not, even though they are crunchier than their unprocessed counterparts.

When selecting packaged foods for their fiber content, you must read labels carefully. The large print may say "fiber-rich," "highest fiber," or "bran," but the actual fiber content may be rather *low*. Read the small print to find out how many grams of fiber are contained in a serving, and be sure the serving size is specified and realistic. Remember, too, that you should be counting dietary fiber rather than crude fiber toward your 30 gram daily target.

You can find dietary fiber in many foods (see table 20-6). The best sources are whole grain products, vegetables, fruits, and legumes. All are available in your food market. But one form of fiber is found in your drugstore. Long used as an aid to bowel function, psyllium is a natural grain from India that has gained attention recently as a source of soluble fiber that can lower blood cholesterol levels. Psyllium supplements (Metamucil, Fiberall, Perdiem) will add fiber to your diet, but they're expensive, and they won't provide the other nutrients present in whole grain foods. They are safe, even for prolonged use in high doses. If psyllium powder is inadvertently inhaled, however, it may provoke allergic reactions in some sensitive individuals.

Counting Fiber

Eating should be one of life's greatest pleasures rather than an exercise in chemistry and math. Still, fiber is so important that I'll ask you to count the grams of fiber in your diet, at least for a few days. You may find it surprisingly hard to reach 30 grams of fiber per day. Often, a high-fiber breakfast cereal (a really high-fiber cereal, that is) is the best way to reach your goal. And if you still have trouble getting all the fiber you should have from whole foods, dietary supplements of bran or psyllium make good sense.

Can You Get Too Much Fiber?

Yes and no. There is no evidence that very large amounts of dietary fiber cause illness; so-called primitive peoples eat more than 100 grams per day without experiencing any difficulties. I know of no upper limit on the safety of dietary fiber, providing it is part of a well-balanced diet.

But fiber can cause temporary discomfort, including bloating, flatulence, and diarrhea. To minimize these problems, increase your intake gradually. Eat slowly, chewing your food well without swallowing air. Eat a variety of high-fiber foods. If gas becomes a problem, try to determine which foods are responsible so you can switch to other sources of fiber; beans and other legumes are likely culprits. You can also try adding three to eight drops of Beano, a commercial enzyme preparation, to your first bite of high-fiber "gassy" foods.

Although dietary fiber helps reduce the risk of diverticulosis, people who already have this condition are well advised to avoid seeds and nuts, which may cause intestinal irritation. With these exceptions, dietary fiber is a critical element in the treatment of this common ailment.

Table 20-6. Sources of Dietary Fiber

Food	Serving	Fiber content (to nearest gram)	Calories
Grains and flours			
Whole wheat	1 cup (cooked)	10	400
Barley	1 cup (cooked)	8	700
Brown rice	1 cup (cooked)	5	230
Oats	1 cup (cooked)	3	132
White rice	1 cup (cooked)	trace	225
Refined wheat	1 cup (cooked)	trace	420
Baked goods			
Ry Krisp	1 square	5	55
Graham cracker	4 squares	2	120
Bran muffin	1	2	100
Whole wheat bread	1 slice	1	61
Bagel	1	1	145
Pasta			
Spaghetti	½ cup (cooked)	1	155
Legumes			
Baked beans	½ cup (cooked)	9	155
Kidney beans	½ cup (cooked)	7	110
Lima beans	½ cup (cooked)	5	64
Lentils	½ cup (cooked)	4	97
Greens			
Kale	3½ oz	6	50
Spinach	3½ oz	3	22
Romaine lettuce	3½ oz	2	16
Iceberg lettuce	3½ oz	1	13
Vegetables, raw			
Carrot	1 medium	4	30
Tomato	1 medium	2	20
Mushrooms	½ cup	2	10
Celery	½ cup	1	10
Cucumber	½ cup	trace	8
Vegetables, cooked			
Potato (with skin)	1 medium	3	106
Sweet potato	1 medium	3	160
Parsnips	½ cup	3	51
Broccoli	½ cup	2	20
Zucchini	½ cup	2	11
String beans	½ cup	2	16

▶

Table 20-6. (continued)

Food	Serving	Fiber content (to nearest gram)	Calories
Asparagus	½ cup	1	15
Cauliflower	½ cup	1	5
Fresh fruits			
Apple (with skin)	1 medium	4	81
Pear (with skin)	1 medium	4	90
Orange	1 medium	3	62
Banana	1 medium	3	115
Raspberries	½ cup	3	35
Strawberries	½ cup	2	23
Peach (with skin)	1 medium	2	37
Cantaloupe	¼ melon	1	30
Cherries	10	1	49
Grapes	¼ cup	1	50
Plum	1 medium	1	20
Fruits, dried			
Figs	6	19	255
Prunes	6	8	120
Dates	6	4	140
Apricots	6	4	120
Raisins	¼ cup	3	106
Nuts and seeds			
Peanuts	10 nuts	1	105
Almonds	10 nuts	1	79
Popcorn (air popped)	1 cup	1	54
Breakfast cereals			
All-Bran Extra Fiber	1 oz	14	50
Fiber One	1 oz	13	60
All-Bran	1 oz	10	70
100% Bran	1 oz	10	70
Bran Buds	1 oz	10	70
Oat Bran (hot)	1 oz	6	110
Bran Flakes	1 oz	5	90
Corn Bran	1 oz	5	98
Raisin Bran	1 oz	5	110
Cracklin' Oat Bran	1 oz	4	110
Shredded Wheat	1 oz	3	90
Cheerios	1 oz	2	110
Oatmeal	1 cup	2	108
Corn flakes	1 oz	trace	110

Table 20-6. (continued)

Food	Serving	Fiber content (to nearest gram)	Calories
Dietary supplements			
Wheat bran	1 oz	12	n/a
Wheat germ	1 oz	3	62
Psyllium (Metamucil, Perdiem, Fiberall, and others)	1 tsp or 1 wafer	4	varies
Methylcellulose (Citrucel and others)	1 tsp	2	varies

Principal source: Diet, Nutrition, and Cancer Prevention: The Good News, *U.S. Department of Health and Human Services*

Perhaps the best way to prevent fiber from being rough on your system is to drink plenty of fluids. Fiber draws fluid into your feces, which is one of the ways it helps protect your colon from disease. But you have to provide enough fluids to let fiber do its work without depriving your body of the water it needs for its other functions.

■ Protein

Proteins are essential for health. They provide the structural strutwork of our bones and the contractile power of our muscles. They form the enzymes that are vital for all metabolic processes and the antibodies that protect us from infections. Proteins are vital for growth and for the repair of damaged tissues.

Without adequate protein in the diet, all these functions would suffer terribly. But it takes surprisingly little dietary protein to meet the body's needs. An average 150-pound person's body contains only *three pounds* of protein; as little as *two ounces* of pure protein in the daily diet will provide plenty of material to replenish the body's protein stores.

A little protein in the diet is more than just good — it's essential. But protein deficiency is exceedingly rare in the developed world; in fact, the average American diet contains twice the amount of protein it should. And excess protein is more than just wasteful — it may even be harmful.

What Are Proteins?

Proteins are large molecules built from much smaller subunits called amino acids. Each amino acid is composed of carbon, hydrogen, oxygen, and nitrogen; the nitrogen is what makes amino acids and proteins unique, distinguishing them from carbohydrates and fats.

There are hundreds and hundreds of proteins in your body. All are built from just 20 amino acids. Your body's proteins are so numerous and diverse because the amino acids in each are linked in a unique order; the sequence of amino acids determines the structure of each protein and how it functions in your body. If it sounds complex, just think of the alphabet; all the words in this book are made up from just 26 letters linked together in unique sequences.

Like the proteins in your body, the proteins in your diet are composed of chains of amino acids. But the proteins in food are too large to be absorbed from the intestinal tract. Instead, they are digested into individual amino acids that are absorbed into your blood, carried to your liver and tissues, and reassembled into proteins.

Although all proteins are made of amino acids, not all dietary proteins contain each of the 20 amino acids. Your body does not need to get all 20 from your food, since it can actually manufacture 11 of these amino acids. But the other 9 amino acids must be supplied from food; the best way to be sure you'll get enough of all 9 essential amino acids is to eat a variety of foods that contain a balanced mix of proteins.

The Pitfalls of Excess Protein

Can too much of a good thing be harmful? The answer for dietary fat, sugar, and calories is yes; for protein maybe.

Excessive protein consumption may or may not be harmful, but it is certainly wasteful. Ever since ancient times, high-protein diets have been recommended to build muscle strength and power. The Greeks started it all, but today's athletic training tables still groan with steak and eggs, and today's athletes spend millions of dollars on amino acid pills and powders as dietary supplements. They don't work. Extra protein will *not* build muscles; the only way to do that is with exercise. What happens, then, to excess protein? The carbon, oxygen, and hydrogen *are* stored in the body — as fat. The nitrogen is excreted in the urine, where it may be harmful.

Although the proof is not all in, many scientists believe that excess protein contributes to impaired kidney function. Certainly patients with diabetes and those with kidney failure can protect their kidneys by restricting their protein consumption. More experiments will be required to learn if protein restriction protects healthy kidneys as well; until the results are reported, I think it would be prudent for all of us to avoid excess dietary protein.

Perhaps because excessive protein consumption increases urinary nitrogen levels, it can have other adverse effects on the kidneys. High-protein diets increase urine calcium loss; every time dietary protein is doubled, urine calcium levels increase by 50 percent. Two problems may result: kidney stones can be caused by too much calcium in the urine, and osteoporosis can be caused by too little calcium in the bones.

Do you still want to load your menu with high-protein foods? If so, consider this: high levels of dietary protein have been shown to increase the risk of colon cancer. In this case, however, not all high-protein foods are equally guilty. A six-year Harvard study of 88,751 American nurses found that eating large amounts of red meat increased the risk of colon cancer by two and one half times.

Consider also that you fill your plate not with pure protein but with food. Except for egg whites, which are almost all protein, protein-rich foods also contain many other nutrients. In the case of animal protein, these nutrients are often saturated fat and cholesterol; in the case of vegetable protein, these nutrients are often complex carbohydrates and dietary fiber.

Compare the traditional high-protein food, steak, with a neglected source of high-quality protein, beans. A five-ounce steak has 300 calories, while a cup of pinto beans has 265. But the steak comes with 44 grams of protein, 120 milligrams of cholesterol, and 12 grams of fat, much of it saturated. In contrast, the beans contain 15 grams of protein, no cholesterol, and only 1 gram of fat, which is polyunsaturated. The steak has no carbohydrates and no fiber; the beans have 49 grams of complex carbohydrates and 15 grams of fiber. The beans have more potassium and less sodium than the steak; the iron content of the two foods is identical, but your body is more efficient at absorbing iron from animal sources. Add the enormous price differential to your comparison and you'll see that beans are a much better nutritional bargain than steak.

Even a single small portion of steak has enough protein for an entire *day*. Americans are eating too much protein, and it's the wrong kind of protein. Two thirds of the average daily protein intake is of animal origin and only one third comes from vegetable products. The ratio should be reversed. Our reliance on animal protein, however, will be hard to change. American society's overemphasis on high-protein foods, particularly meat and dairy products, reflects long-standing, deep-seated traditions and habits. It also reflects cultural and economic biases against starchy foods; important people, after all, debate meaty issues, and wealthy people live high off the hog.

Excessive animal protein means excessive saturated fat, cholesterol, and calories. Often it also means deficient fiber and complex carbohydrate consumption. This combination of excesses and deficiencies is the link between the Western diet and Western diseases: heart disease, high blood pressure, obesity, diabetes, cancers of the colon, breast, uterus, and prostate, and many bowel diseases.

You don't have to become a vegetarian to prevent these problems (though it wouldn't hurt). But you should gradually switch to a diet that makes vegetables, legumes, fruits, and grains the main dishes, reserving lean meat and low-fat dairy products for side dishes.

If more people bypassed steak, fewer people would need to have operations to bypass clogged coronary arteries and obstructed colons.

Protein Quality

People cannot live on beans alone. While it's a good idea to avoid excess dietary protein, it's also very important to be sure that the protein in your diet contains all the amino acids your body needs.

Animal protein does have the advantage of having the amino acid combinations needed by our animal bodies. For this reason, animal protein has been considered to have the highest biological value or quality. No single vegetable food contains sufficient amounts of all nine essential amino

Table 20-7. Dietary Sources of Protein

Food	Serving size	Protein content (to nearest gram)	Calories	% Calories from protein
Legumes				
Soybeans	1 cup	20	235	34
Garbanzo beans	1 cup	18	270	27
Kidney beans	1 cup	16	230	28
Split peas	1 cup	16	230	28
Lima beans	1 cup	16	260	25
Vegetables				
Potato	1 medium	5	220	9
Broccoli	1 spear	4	40	40
Corn	1 ear	3	85	14
Carrot	1 medium	1	30	13
Tomato	1 medium	1	25	16
Fruits				
Apple	1 medium	trace	80	—
Banana	1 medium	1	105	4
Orange	1 medium	1	60	7
Pear	1 medium	1	100	4
Strawberries	1 cup	1	45	9
Grain products				
Barley	1 cup	16	700	9
Pasta	1 cup	7	190	15
Rice	1 cup	5	230	7
Coffee cake	1 slice	5	230	7
Bran muffin	1 medium	3	125	10
Bread	1 slice	2	65	12
Meat				
Steak	6 oz	51	348	59
Pork	6 oz	48	550	35
Veal	6 oz	46	370	50
Hamburger	6 oz	40	490	33
Poultry				
Chicken	6 oz	27	280	39
Fish				
Tuna (water-packed)	6 oz	60	270	89
Sardines	6 oz	40	350	46
Haddock	6 oz	34	350	39
Dairy products				
Skim milk	1 cup	8	85	38
Whole milk	1 cup	8	150	21

Table 20-7. (continued)

Food	Serving size	Protein content (to nearest gram)	Calories	% Calories from protein
Yogurt (low-fat)	8 oz	12	145	33
Cheddar cheese	1 oz	4	70	23
Cottage cheese	1 cup	28	235	48
Egg	1 medium	6	80	30

Principal source: Nutritive Value of Foods, *U.S. Department of Agriculture*

acids; beans, for example, are low in methionine. But by eating a combination of vegetable foods, you can get all the amino acids you need; rice, for example, is high in methionine.

Good nutrition mandates eating a variety of foods. When it comes to protein, a mix of legumes, grains, and vegetables can provide all the amino acids you need. Supplementing these vegetable proteins with modest amounts of animal protein is not nutritionally necessary, but of course it's perfectly acceptable as part of a balanced diet.

How Much Protein Do You Need?

Although I've asked you to be fairly diligent in counting your dietary fat and fiber, it's not necessary to be so careful in estimating your protein intake. In fact, if you keep your fat consumption low and your fiber intake high, your protein consumption will take care of itself.

If you want a more exact handle on your protein requirements, you can estimate your needs with either of two methods. First, you can aim for a diet that provides about 15 percent of its calories from protein. Use table 12-4 to calculate your daily caloric intake, and divide by 30 to determine your approximate protein need in grams.

An easier method is to aim for .36 grams of protein for each pound of body weight. I'll do the math for you:

Weight in pounds	Daily protein requirements (in grams)
100	36
120	43
140	50 (maximum needed by women*)
160	58
180 and above	63 (maximum needed by men)

To find out if your diet meets — or exceeds — your protein needs, consult table 20-7.

---

* Women who are lactating or pregnant require an extra 30 grams of protein per day; higher amounts may increase the risk of premature delivery.

■ Vitamins

Ever eager for a quick fix, the American public spends more than $2.7 billion annually to purchase vitamin pills. Ever eager for a quick buck, vitamin purveyors push their products to cure arthritis, improve athletic performance, increase energy, fight insomnia, relieve stress, and correct impotence. These claims — and dozens of similar promises — are bogus. Still, emerging scientific evidence is beginning to suggest that higher-than-minimum intakes of certain vitamins may contribute to health. But with a few exceptions, this evidence points to the value of vitamins in foods, not in pills.

What Are Vitamins?

Vitamins are organic molecules that are required for many of the body's metabolic processes. Because the body cannot manufacture them, vitamins must be consumed for these chemical reactions to proceed normally. All 13 vitamins are essential nutrients, but only tiny amounts are needed to prevent vitamin deficiency diseases.

There are two basic groups of vitamins. The fat-soluble vitamins (A, D, E, and K) are absorbed into the body with dietary fat and are stored in the body's fatty tissues. Healthy people can store enough fat-soluble vitamins to last for months. But the capacity to store fat-soluble vitamins is a double-edged sword; you can get along without them for weeks or months, but if you take excessive amounts, you can gradually build up toxic levels, especially of vitamins A and D.

The water-soluble vitamins (the B vitamins and vitamin C) are not stored by the body to any appreciable degree. Extra doses of these vitamins are passed into the urine, so toxic reactions occur only if very large amounts are ingested. Because there is no body depot for water-soluble vitamins, you must consume them frequently (if not daily) to ward off deficiencies. Since these vitamins dissolve in water, excessive processing and cooking can remove them from food. Because only tiny amounts are required, however, a well-balanced diet will always provide plenty of these nutrients.

Vitamins and Health

It's hardly news that vitamins prevent disease. The great nutritional investigations of the early twentieth century established a list of diseases that could be prevented by vitamins: night blindness (vitamin A), beriberi (vitamin B_1), pellagra (B_3), various types of anemia (vitamins B_6 and B_{12} and folic acid), scurvy (vitamin C), rickets (vitamin D), and bleeding disorders (vitamin K). These pioneering experiments also established the minimal daily requirements for vitamins which are, with minor modification, still in use today.

Our current interest in vitamins, however, goes far beyond the deficiency diseases. It now appears that certain vitamin-rich foods can help prevent several types of cancer. Although the evidence is still preliminary, vitamins may also have a role in reducing the risk of cardiovascular disease, cataracts, and possibly certain birth defects.

Cancer and Vitamins

Dietary factors have been causally implicated in up to 30 percent of all human cancers. Many of these cancers (colon, breast, uterus, and prostate) are related to excessive dietary fat and animal protein, excessive caloric intake, and deficient dietary fiber. Salt-cured, pickled, and smoked foods contribute to cancer of the stomach and esophagus. Charcoal broiling, too, can produce carcinogenic chemicals in foods. But in addition to these well-established links between diet and cancer, vitamins play an important role.

We don't know exactly how vitamin-rich foods help prevent cancer, any more than we know what causes cancer. But one theory seems promising.

Many of the body's chemical reactions result in the formation of potentially toxic compounds called *free radicals* and *reactive oxygen molecules*. While all healthy people produce free radicals, their production is further stimulated by exposure to tobacco smoke, solvents, pesticides, and various pollutants, all of which cause cancer. It's not certain that free radicals actually cause cancer, but it is clear that they can attach to cell membranes, alter proteins, and attack the genetic material of cells — DNA. In combination, these events could transform a healthy cell into a cancer cell capable of growing rapidly and invading healthy tissues.

Although the vitamins that protect against cancer are structurally distinct, they have an important property in common: they are antioxidants. Vitamin A and its precursors, vitamin C, and vitamin E can all trap free radicals and reactive oxygen molecules, protecting tissues and — if the theory is right — preventing certain forms of cancer. The evidence is best for vitamin A.

Vitamin A is actually a family of related compounds. Vegetable foods are rich in a precursor of vitamin A called beta carotene. In animal tissues, including the human body, beta carotene is converted into vitamin A. In addition, fruits and vegetables contain many related carotenoid compounds which cannot be converted into vitamin A.

At least 16 studies performed in population groups around the world demonstrate that eating foods rich in beta carotene cuts the risk of developing lung cancer in half. It doesn't take much beta carotene to achieve maximum protection; one carrot a day will provide all you need.

Studies of cancer of the colon, rectum, and bladder also find that foods rich in beta carotene have a protective effect. Only two studies have evaluated beta carotene–rich foods and female reproductive cancer, but both demonstrate protection. The evidence for breast and prostate cancer is mixed, with some studies showing protection but others finding no benefit.

A study of more than 1,200 elderly Massachusetts residents found that people eating the smallest amounts of green and yellow vegetables had three times more cancer deaths than did people eating the largest amounts.

Compounds in the vitamin A family are also being used experimentally to prevent second cancers in patients who have been treated successfully for their initial malignancies. A study using high doses of isotretinoin, a synthetic analog of vitamin A, found protection in patients with head and neck cancers, but a study of beta carotene found no benefit in patients with skin cancer.

Spurred by these findings, many studies of beta carotene supplements are in progress. But until we have the results, the best evidence suggests that beta carotene–rich *foods* are protective, but none of it proves that beta carotene itself is the protective element.

Dark green and yellow-orange vegetables and fruits are the richest sources of beta carotene (see table 20-8). Needless to say, all these foods contain many other nutrients plus fiber; any combination of these constituents could explain the protective effects of vegetable-rich diets.

Vitamin C. More than 50 studies have shown that people with the highest intake of vitamin C–rich foods have the lowest risk of cancer. The evidence for protection is best for cancers of the esophagus, stomach, colon, and cervix. While these results are not as convincing as the beta carotene studies, it seems prudent to include foods with lots of vitamin C in your diet; many fruits (including citrus fruits) and vegetables (including cruciferous vegetables) are excellent sources of vitamin C.

Vitamin E is another good antioxidant and free radical scavenger. But its possible role in cancer prevention is still undefined. Studies of vitamin E are difficult because of its many chemical forms and its presence in so many foods, and because of technical problems in measuring vitamin E levels in blood specimens.

Vitamin D is not an antioxidant, but a 1989 study of 25,000 subjects in Maryland found that people with the highest levels of vitamin D in their blood had the lowest risk of colon cancer. Women living in sunny climes appear to have less breast cancer than women who get less sunlight, presumably because sun increases vitamin D levels. We're a long way from prescribing vitamin D to prevent cancer, but we may be close enough to encourage a glass of vitamin-fortified milk (low-fat, please) each day.

Cardiovascular Disease

Doctors are now starting to ask if antioxidants may help prevent cardiovascular disease. Ongoing laboratory research suggests that free radicals in the blood may alter cholesterol molecules, making them even more likely to clog arteries. If free radicals make bad (LDL) cholesterol even worse, vitamins may be able to help, but the evidence is very preliminary. Several studies have reported that people with low blood levels of vitamin C have higher blood pressure readings and more blood vessel disease than people with normal levels. A 1991 study of 6,000 Scotsmen also linked low vitamin C levels to angina, but concluded that this association might be spurious since smoking, which is known to lower vitamin C levels, seemed to be the cause of excess heart disease in patients with low vitamin C levels. The study did find, however, that low vitamin E levels increased the risk of angina by more than two and a half times. Even more recently, preliminary reports of an ongoing study of 87,244 American nurses noted that women taking more than 100 milligrams of vitamin E daily had 36 percent fewer

Table 20-8. Antioxidant Vitamins in Selected Foods

Food	Serving size	Vitamin A (international units)	Vitamin C (mg)	Calories
Cruciferous vegetables				
Cabbage	1 cup	90	33	15
Cauliflower	1 cup	20	72	25
Broccoli	1 spear	2,540	113	50
Brussels sprouts	1 cup	1,110	96	60
Vegetables				
Asparagus	4 spears	2	16	15
Beets	1 cup	20	9	55
Beet greens	1 cup	7,340	36	40
Carrot	1 medium	20,250	7	30
Corn	1 ear	170	5	85
Kale	1 cup	8,260	33	50
Parsley	10 sprigs	520	9	5
Green pepper	1 medium	390	95	20
Potato	1 medium	0	26	220
Pumpkin	1 cup	2,650	12	50
Spinach	1 cup	3,690	15	10
Squash, summer	1 cup	520	10	35
Squash, winter	1 cup	7,290	20	80
Sweet potato	1 medium	24,880	28	115
Tomato	1 medium	1,390	22	25
Turnips	1 cup	7,920	39	30
Turnip greens	1 cup	13,080	36	30
Fruits and juices				
Apple	1 medium	70	8	80
Apricot	3 medium	2,770	11	50
Banana	1 medium	90	10	105
Cantaloupe	½ melon	8,610	113	95
Cherries	10	150	5	50
Grapefruit	one half	10	41	40
Grapes	10 grapes	40	5	35
Lemon juice	1 cup	50	112	60
Lime juice	1 cup	20	72	65
Orange	1 medium	270	70	60
Orange juice	1 cup	190	97	110
Peach	1 medium	470	6	35
Pear	1 medium	30	7	100
Strawberries	1 cup	40	84	45

Principal source: Nutritive Value of Foods, *U.S. Department of Agriculture*

heart attacks and 23 percent fewer strokes than women who were getting less than 30 milligrams each day.

Vitamin A levels did not correlate with heart disease in the Scottish investigation. But an American study of 333 male physicians with angina found that the administration of 50 milligrams of beta carotene every day reduced the occurrence of heart disease and stroke by about 50 percent. The nurses' study, too, found that 15 to 20 milligrams of beta carotene per day was helpful, cutting the risk of heart attacks by 22 percent and of stroke by 40 percent.

The average American consumes less than 2 milligrams of beta carotene per day. To get 25 milligrams per day, the average amount given in the Physicians' Health Study, you'd have to eat two cups of cooked carrots, a cup of sweet potatoes, a cup of canned pumpkin, or two cantaloupes every day. Because the trial did not investigate lower doses of beta carotene, it's not known if very high doses are really needed to produce cardiac protection. And since the study is small and preliminary, it will have to be confirmed before we can be sure that it's valid. With all these reservations I can't justify prescribing beta carotene for my patients with angina, but I certainly don't discourage them from taking it.

Cataracts

The hope that antioxidants may help prevent cataracts is also based on preliminary evidence. A 1991 Tufts University study of 112 subjects found that people who ate the smallest amount of fruits and vegetables were six times more likely to develop cataracts than the subjects who ate the most vitamin-rich foods. Another 1991 Boston study of 1,380 people found that diets low in vitamins increased cataract risk, and that supplementary vitamin pills appeared to decrease risk by 37 percent.

Infections

Vitamin C has been widely promoted as a way to prevent infections, including the common cold. A number of distinguished scientists are among the leading proponents of vitamin C. But doctors have subjected these claims to careful study and have found that vitamin C has no ability to prevent infections. Despite this data, however, many people swear by vitamin C. Medical science seems unable to snuff out folk remedies for the sniffles — in part, I confess, because we don't have anything better to offer.

Vitamin A supplements have been shown to protect children in India from severe complications of measles. Most of these subjects, however, were nutritionally deficient. Fortunately, we have a much better approach in our country: measles vaccine.

Should You Take Vitamin Supplements?

I wish I had a nickel, or even just a penny, for each time I've been asked this question. I've given it a lot of thought and study, and I've asked the question of many experts. After all this preparation I'm ready to give you my answer: it's a resounding maybe.

It's true — I'm hedging. But if you let me explain, my answer may be more helpful than it seems.

If you're healthy, you don't need to take vitamin supplements to prevent deficiency diseases. This is true even for people on the average American diet; faulty though it is, a typical Western diet provides an abundance of vitamins. Although their diets are usually very healthful, strict vegetarians should take B_{12} supplements because this vitamin is found only in animal products. People with chronic medical illnesses, including liver disease, kidney disease, and intestinal ailments that interfere with the absorption of nutrients, should take vitamins. I also prescribe vitamins for pregnant and lactating women, for many elderly people who may have erratic dietary patterns, for patients with eating disorders, and for those with wasting or debilitating diseases.

But we are beginning to hope that vitamins may do more than prevent deficiency disease. Should healthy people take vitamins to reduce their risk of cancer, heart disease, or cataracts?

With the exception of one small study of beta carotene and heart disease, a preliminary study of vitamin E and heart disease, and a large study of multivitamins and cataracts, all the data that demonstrate protection attribute these benefits to *foods,* not vitamin supplements. Indeed, protection may depend on chemical forms of vitamins that are present in foods but not in pills, on combinations of nutrients, or on food constituents that are still undiscovered. There is, in fact, precedent for the possibility that foods may succeed where supplements fail; for example, eating fish protects against heart disease, but taking fish oil capsules does not.

My best advice, then, is to eat a healthful diet rich in unrefined whole foods, including deep green and yellow vegetables and fruits, cruciferous vegetables, citrus and other fruits, whole grains, and legumes. If you are able to achieve nutritional health, you should not need supplementary vitamins. But if you are unable to eat properly, supplementary vitamins make sense.

Granting that vitamin pills are a poor second to a healthful diet, is there any reason *not* to take them? Aside from considerations of cost and convenience, I can think of no compelling argument against vitamin supplements. The choice is yours; work hard to achieve an ideal diet, but feel free to supplement vitamin-rich foods with vitamin pills if they make you feel more secure.

If you choose to take vitamins, you should consider a few tips:

1. Vitamins should never be a substitute for good nutrition: they can never replace missed meals. Vitamins cannot provide the carbohydrates and fiber you need for health. Nor can they substitute for other preventive practices; it makes no sense to take vitamin A to prevent lung cancer or vitamin C to prevent heart disease if you smoke.

2. Vitamin pills vary enormously in price. In general, you should pick the least expensive supplement that meets your requirements. Look for a reliable manufacturer. Select products that are fully labeled as to contents, doses, expiration dates, and conformity with United States Pharmacopeia

standards. Remember that natural vitamins are no better than synthetic vitamins.

3. Pick an appropriate dosage, avoiding "megavitamins." Remember that high doses of vitamins can be toxic. Vitamins A and D are fat soluble, so even modest overdoses may gradually accumulate in your body, eventually reaching toxic levels. Vitamins C and B_6 (pyridoxine) and niacin are water soluble and will not build up; still, very high doses can have harmful side effects.

Since we don't know if supplementary vitamins are really helpful, it's impossible to recommend an optimal dose. Multivitamins contain 100 to 800 percent of RDAs, which seems quite reasonable. If antioxidants attract you, daily doses of 25 milligrams of beta carotene (equivalent to about 20,000 international units of vitamin A), 500 milligrams of vitamin C, and 400 IU of vitamin E are the best guestimates I can provide.

Should you take vitamins? I've gone a long way to confess that unless you have certain medical or nutritional problems that require vitamins, I can't give you a definitive answer. Nor am I embarrassed to confess this uncertainty. We simply need more medical studies to find scientifically valid answers. Dr. James Lind began these studies some 250 years ago; with our modern investigative techniques, we should be getting the answers any year now.

At present, one third of all Americans take nutritional supplements on a regular basis. This has not prevented the nutritional health in our country from being terrible. New studies may define new roles for vitamin pills, but supplements will never supplant the vital, if neglected, role of good nutrition.

I don't take vitamin pills.

A Glossary of Vitamins

We all have a lot to learn about vitamins. Still, you may want to review the facts that are currently available.

- **Vitamin A**
  Roles: Night vision, healthy skin
  Antioxidant that may reduce cancer risk
  Sources: Deep green and yellow-orange vegetables
  Fortified dairy products and cereals, meats
  *Recommended Daily Allowance:** 5,000 international units (IU)/day, or
  1,000 retinol equivalents (RE)/day
  Overdoses: Brain swelling, eye disorders, skin damage at doses above
  20,000 IU per day

---

*Recommended Daily Allowances are the U.S. RDAs established by the Food and Drug Administration. U.S. RDAs are based on the RDAs of the National Academy of Science. The U.S. RDA is a single value for each vitamin that should ensure adequate intake for almost all healthy people; the National Academy RDAs can vary according to age, sex, pregnancy, and other factors.

- **Vitamin B₁** (thiamine)
  Roles: Carbohydrate metabolism; prevents beriberi
  Sources: Whole and fortified grains; legumes, nuts, poultry, meat
  Recommended Daily Allowance: 15 milligrams per day

- **Vitamin B₂** (riboflavin)
  Roles: Release of energy from foods, healthy skin
  Sources: Fortified grains, dairy products, meat
  Recommended Daily Allowance: 1.7 milligrams per day

- **Niacin** (vitamin B₃)
  Roles: Release of energy from foods
      Prevents pellagra
      High doses can be used to improve blood cholesterol
  Sources: Fortified grain products, peanuts, fish, poultry, meat
  Recommended Daily Allowance: 20 milligrams per day
  Overdoses: Headaches, flushing and itching, liver damage, high blood
      sugar, gout

- **Vitamin B₆** (pyridoxine)
  Roles: Nervous system function, red blood cell formation
  Sources: Whole grains, soybeans, peanuts, bananas, vegetables, poul-
      try, meat
  Recommended Daily Allowance: 2 milligrams per day
  Overdoses: Nerve damage

- **Vitamin B₁₂** (cobalamine)
  Roles: Red blood cell formulation, nervous system function
      Prevents pernicious anemia
  Sources: Found only in animal products, including poultry, fish, dairy
      products, meat
  Recommended Daily Allowance: 6 micrograms per day

- **Folic acid**
  Roles: Formation of red blood cells
  Sources: Legumes, grains, fruits, vegetables, poultry, meat
  Recommended Daily Allowance: 200 micrograms per day

- **Vitamin C** (ascorbic acid)
  Roles: Healthy connective tissue and blood vessels, wound healing, pre-
      vents scurvy
      Antioxidant that may reduce cancer risk
  Sources: Citrus fruits, many other fruits, vegetables
  Recommended Daily Allowance: 60 milligrams per day
  Overdoses: Diarrhea, kidney stones

- **Vitamin D**
  Roles: Healthy bones, calcium metabolism
  Sources: Fortified dairy products, fish, egg yolk, liver
  Recommended Daily Allowance: 400 IU per day
  Overdoses: Elevated calcium levels

- **Vitamin E**
  Roles: Antioxidant that may reduce cancer risk
    Prevents cell membrane damage
  Sources: Leafy green vegetables, vegetable oils, wheat germ, marga-
    rine, butter, liver
  Recommended Daily Allowance: 10 milligrams per day

- **Vitamin K**
  Roles: Blood clotting
  Sources: Leafy green and cruciferous vegetables
    Intestinal bacteria
  Recommended Daily Allowance: 80 milligrams per day

- **Pantothenic acid**
  Roles: Functions in metabolism
  Sources: Whole grains, cruciferous vegetables, meat, egg yolks
  Recommended Daily Allowance: 4 to 7 milligrams per day

- **Biotin**
  Roles: Metabolism
  Sources: Many foods
  Recommended Daily Allowance: 30 to 100 micrograms per day

■ Minerals

As you begin to plan for a healthful balance of minerals in your diet, be prepared to confront a hard fact: the excellent nutritional program that reduces your need for vitamin pills may actually increase your need for mineral supplements.

Your diet should contain at least 15 mineral compounds. For most, only small amounts are needed; a good diet will provide plenty of these trace elements. But even the best of diets may not satisfy the iron requirements of menstruating women or the calcium requirements of postmenopausal women. Most American diets would be low in fluoride if fluorides were not added to the water. Although potassium supplements are required only by patients taking diuretic medications, many healthy people might benefit from extra servings of potassium-rich foods. In contrast, most Americans get far too much sodium in their diets.

Minding your minerals can help you stay well.

Salt

Salt is a very simple compound, composed of only two elements: sodium and chloride. But if salt is simple for chemists, it is nonetheless complex and controversial for doctors and nutritionists.

Salt is a vital constituent of all the body's fluids, including blood. Salt is so vital, in fact, that the body contains an elaborate series of regulatory mechanisms to ensure that the blood's salt concentration will be just right. When the body's salt supply threatens to get low, the kidneys can recapture nearly all the salt in the urine. In times of need, the skin's sweat glands can also conserve salt almost completely. Although it may seem paradoxical, the human body has acknowledged its dependence on salt by evolving systems that allow it to function beautifully with only tiny amounts of dietary salt.

As is so often the case, unfortunately, human behavior has not adapted as wisely as human biology. For primitive humans, salt was a scarcity. When it was available, salt was not added to food but was used for barter. Even today many primitive peoples living in Africa, in the Amazon rain forest, and on isolated Pacific islands eat virtually no salt; not coincidentally, they also have virtually no high blood pressure, vascular disease, or strokes.

Because it was rare, salt became valuable. Because it was valuable, salt became sought after. People learned to harvest salt from evaporated sea water and to mine it from the depths of the earth. For centuries, however, salt was too expensive for the diet of ordinary people. But with industrialization, salt became plentiful. The rich retained their monopoly on gold and silver, while the populace indulged their pent-up lust for salt by making it a dietary staple. By reverse alchemy, then, salt was transformed from valuable to victual. The consequences have been far from tasty.

Salt, Blood Pressure, and Health. Dietary salt is not the only dietary cause of high blood pressure; obesity, alcohol abuse, and excessive consumption of animal fat have also been linked to high blood pressure, as has deficient consumption of potassium and calcium.

Where does salt rank among these preventable causes of high blood pressure? Some authorities rank excessive dietary salt consumption right at the top, while others downplay its influence. Indeed, many healthy people seem to get away with eating enormous amounts of salt without developing high blood pressure, and some patients with high blood pressure don't appear to get much benefit from dietary salt reduction.

Why is salt so controversial? Studies that have compared non-Western with Western cultures demonstrate that Western diets contain much more salt, and that Western populations have consistently higher blood pressure and much more vascular disease. But comparisons of high- and low-salt diets *within* industrialized societies have been less convincing.

I'm happy to report that three papers published in the 1991 *British Medical Journal* may finally help dissolve the salt dispute. In these papers Drs. M. R. Law, C. D. Frost, and N. J. Wald evaluated studies of diet and blood pressure in 24 communities throughout the world. In all, more than 47,000 people were included. Their conclusions: "The association of blood pressure with sodium intake is substantially larger than is generally appreciated and increases with age and with initial blood pressure."

These findings are important enough to warrant a closer look. Dr. Law and his colleagues found that for each 6 grams of dietary salt (2,400 milligrams of dietary sodium), blood pressure increases by about 10 points. Dietary salt has virtually the same effect in industrialized and underdeveloped countries. Moreover, salt increases blood pressure even more strikingly in people who have high blood pressure and in the elderly; in other words, salt is most harmful to the very people who are most likely to suffer damage from high blood pressure.

In a companion study these same British scientists examined the ability of salt restriction to lower blood pressure readings. The results were encouraging: even a moderate reduction in dietary salt lowers blood pressure substantially in as little as five weeks.

What does this mean for the American diet? The average diet contains more than 10 grams of salt (4,000 milligrams of sodium) per day; simply cutting it in half could reduce the occurrence of strokes by 26 percent and of heart attacks by 15 percent, saving thousands of lives every year. When it comes to salt, we should all shake the habit.

The Salt in Your Diet. How much salt should you include in your diet? It's a simple question with a complex answer.

Unlike other minerals, salt has no minimum daily requirement. People can get along perfectly well on nearly salt-free diets.

People with high blood pressure, heart disease, and certain types of kidney and liver disease should drastically restrict their salt intake. People who are healthy and who have normal blood pressure readings can tolerate much more sodium. But even young, healthy people have no *need* for added salt. It seems to me that all people might benefit in the long run from adopting low-sodium diets. Remember that if you eat high-sodium foods, your blood pressure will tend to rise with age, and that your risk of heart attack and stroke rises as your blood pressure increases, even within the "normal" range.

Decreasing dietary salt is less of a sacrifice than it may at first seem. Only 10 percent of our dietary salt comes from the natural salt content of food; 15 percent comes from the salt shaker on the stove or table, and 75 percent comes from processed food. In addition to salt, these processed foods often contain saturated fats and excess calories while lacking vitamins and fiber. So by going back to basics, we can address many nutritional problems at once.

How much salt should you eat? The less the better. Three grams of salt (1,200 milligrams sodium) per day is more than enough; 1 to 2 grams (400–800 milligrams sodium) would be even better.

Salt and Sodium. Salt and sodium are not synonymous. Salt is composed of both sodium and chloride; in fact, it's only 40 percent sodium. But it's the sodium that counts.

Most of the sodium in the American diet comes from salt. One teaspoon of table salt contains 5 grams of sodium chloride; since it's only 40 percent sodium, that means you get 2,000 milligrams of sodium in every teaspoon. By any measure just one spoonful is more than enough for a whole day!

To restrict the sodium content in your diet you'll need to know where it's coming from. Remember that salt by any name is still 40 percent sodium; sea salt, brine, seasoned salt, onion salt, and garlic salt all contain sodium chloride. Remember, too, that sodium in other compounds is just as likely to raise your blood pressure as sodium chloride. Baking powder, baking soda, and monosodium glutamate (MSG) are examples of high-sodium ingredients.

Read food labels to detect all sodium-containing additives. Don't be misled by the big print proclaiming "unsalted"; it means only that no salt has been added during processing. The designation "reduced sodium" is more useful, telling you that the product has 75 percent less salt than comparable items. Even better, "low sodium" tells you that each serving has less than 140 milligrams of sodium, and "very low sodium" means less than 35 milligrams per serving.

Best of all: count the actual sodium content of your food. Read labels or use table 20-9 to find out how much sodium you are actually eating.

Reducing Your Dietary Sodium. If you follow the healthful diet outlined throughout this chapter, you will probably be enjoying a low-salt diet without ever thinking about sodium. Fresh vegetables, grain products, fruits, fish, and poultry are all naturally low in sodium. But if you are starting with a typical Western diet, salt restriction may seem very difficult at first. By making changes gradually, you can ease the transition. Most people, in fact, actually end up *preferring* low-salt foods.

Here are some grains of advice to help you save grams of salt:

1. Don't add salt at the table or to your cooking. Learn to use other spices to enhance the flavor of foods. Salt substitutes, which usually contain potassium instead of sodium, may be useful.

2. Fast foods, processed and "convenience" foods, condiments, and other "junk" foods are particularly high in salt. Avoid chips, salted nuts, pretzels, salted crackers, and salted popcorn. Pickles, olives, and sauerkraut are all very high in salt. Find substitutes, too, for catsup, prepared mustard, and barbecue sauce.

3. Choose fresh or frozen foods instead of canned foods. Stay clear of canned tomato and vegetable juices. Despite its other virtues, canned fish is also high in salt. Avoid canned soups, bouillon, and dried soup mixes.

4. Although fresh meat is low in sodium, cured and processed meats (hot dogs, sausage, bacon, luncheon meats) are very high in salt. Dairy products, too, are high in sodium.

5. You can't read food labels in restaurants, but you can ask about salt content before you order. Remember that soy and teriyaki sauces are very high in sodium.

Potassium

Potassium is the major mineral in the fluids inside all the body's cells. Like sodium, potassium is vital for proper cellular function, indeed for life itself. Like sodium, potassium is closely regulated by the body's control mechanisms; healthy kidneys can excrete excess potassium when blood levels are high, and they can retain potassium when the body's supplies are low.

Because your body can regulate potassium so carefully, you don't have to count the potassium in your diet. Still, you should give your body enough

Table 20-9. Approximate Sodium Content of Selected Foods

Food	Serving size	Sodium content (mg)
Grain products		
Pasta, rice, or cooked cereal	½ cup	less than 5
Bread	1 slice	110–175
Cake and pastry	1 slice	100–400
Muffins and biscuits	1	170–390
Pancakes (from mix)	1	150
Ready-to-eat cereals	1 ounce	100–360
Vegetables		
Fresh (cooked, without salt)	½ cup	most less than 50
Frozen (without sauce)	½ cup	most less than 70
Frozen (with sauce)	½ cup	140–460
Canned (without sauce)	½ cup	140–500
Legumes		
Dried beans, peas, lentils (cooked without salt)	1 cup	less than 5
Baked beans, canned	1 cup	600–900
Nuts		
Peanuts, cashews, almonds, walnuts, pistachios (fresh or roasted, unsalted)	1 cup	less than 20
Salted nuts	1 cup	600–1,200
Fruits		
Fresh, frozen, canned fruits	½ cup	less than 10
Meat, poultry, fish		
Fresh meat	3 oz	less than 90
Ham	3 oz	1,100
Bacon	2 slices	275
Corned beef	3 oz	800
Chipped beef	3 oz	3,600
Hamburger (fast food restaurant)	3 oz	450
Hot dog	1	700
Bologna, salami	1 slice	235
Poultry		
Fresh poultry	3 oz	less than 90
Turkey roll	3 oz	500
Frozen turkey or chicken dinner	1 dinner	1,000–2,000
Fish		
Fresh fish	3 oz	less than 90
Tuna, canned	3 oz	300
Salmon, canned	3 oz	300–440

Table 20-9. (continued)

Food	Serving size	Sodium content (mg)
Sardines, canned	3 oz	550
Shrimp, canned	3 oz	2,000
Herring, smoked	3 oz	5,200
Dairy products		
Egg	1	60
Egg substitute, frozen	$\frac{1}{4}$ cup	120
Milk	1 cup	120–160
Yogurt	1 cup	120–160
Unsalted butter or margarine	1 tsp	2
Salted butter or margarine	1 tsp	115
Natural cheeses	$\frac{1}{2}$ oz	110–450
Cottage cheese	$\frac{1}{2}$ cup	450
Processed cheese or spread	2 oz	700–900
Juices and soups		
Fruit juice, fresh, frozen, or canned	1 cup	less than 10
Tomato or vegetable juice, canned	1 cup	800
Canned, condensed, and dehydrated soups	1 cup	600–1,200
Condiments and dressings		
Oil and vinegar	1 tbsp	less than 5
Prepared salad dressing	1 tbsp	80–250
Catsup	1 tbsp	150
Meat tenderizer	1 tbsp	1,750
Mustard	1 tbsp	65
Barbecue sauce	1 tbsp	130
Soy sauce	1 tbsp	1,000
Teriyaki sauce	1 tbsp	690
Worcestershire sauce	1 tbsp	69
Tomato sauce	1 cup	1,500
Tomato paste	1 cup	77
Snack and convenience foods		
Pizza	1 slice	500–1,000
TV dinner	10 oz	1,000–2,000
Candy	1 oz	less than 25
Peanut butter	1 tbsp	26
Pickle	2 oz	700
Olives	2	385
Pretzels	1 oz	450
Potato chips	1 oz	250
Crackers, plain	1 cracker	30–60
Crackers, cheese flavored	1 oz	300

▶

Table 20-9. (continued)

Food	Serving size	Sodium content (mg)
Popcorn, air popped	1 oz	1
Popcorn, buttered and salted	1 oz	550
Beverages		
Coffee, tea	1 cup	2
Carbonated beverages	8 oz	less than 40
Wine	4 oz	12
Beer	12 oz	25

Principal source: Nutritive Value of Foods, *U.S. Department of Agriculture*

potassium to work with. Although it's not conclusive, there is some evidence that potassium-rich diets may help lower blood pressure. And, except for patients with kidney failure, there is no harm in consuming even very large amounts of dietary potassium.

There is no minimum daily requirement for potassium, but the Food and Nutrition Board of the National Academy of Sciences suggests a ration of at least 2,000 milligrams per day. Oranges, bananas, and other fresh fruits, raisins, dates, and other dried fruits, fish, and most dairy products are high in potassium. Potatoes and most vegetables are also rich in potassium, but much of it will be lost during cooking if the water is discarded. Have a glance at table 20-10 to be sure you are eating some potassium-rich foods every day.

Calcium

As the major mineral in bones, calcium constitutes nearly 25 percent of the body's weight. Calcium is critical for strong bones and teeth. Calcium is essential for muscle contraction, blood clotting, and the proper function of all cell membranes. An adequate intake of calcium may also help prevent high blood pressure.

Recognizing the importance of dietary calcium, in 1989 the National Academy of Sciences increased the recommended daily allowance of calcium for adults by 20 percent to 1,200 milligrams per day. It's easy to increase the RDA, but it's been difficult to increase dietary calcium; women still average only 565 milligrams per day, while men get 975 milligrams. And if the gap between the recommended and the real were not large enough, many experts suggest that postmenopausal women aim for 1,500 milligrams of calcium per day, nearly *three times* their average intake.

Dairy products are the best dietary source of calcium, but they tend to be high in sodium, saturated fat, and cholesterol; low-fat milk, yogurt, and cottage cheese eliminate the fat problem, but they're still high in salt. Fish, tofu, broccoli, and spinach are also good sources of calcium. Table 20-11 details the calcium content of various foods.

I endorse the recommendations for a daily calcium intake of 1,200 mil-

Table 20-10. Potassium Content of Selected Foods

Food	Serving size	Potassium (mg)
Fruits		
Apricots	1 large	100
Banana	1 large	740
Cantaloupe	¼ melon	250
Dates	1 cup	1,150
Orange	1 medium	270
Peach	1 medium	170
Raisins	1 ounce	210
Vegetables		
Asparagus	4 spears	186
Lima beans	1 cup	740
Beets	1 cup	530
Broccoli	1 spear	491
Carrots	1 medium	233
Mushrooms	1 cup	259
Potato	1 medium	844
Spinach	1 cup	307
Squash, winter	1 cup	896
Tomato	1 medium	255
Dairy products		
Milk	1 cup	370
Yogurt	8 oz	442
Fish, poultry, meat		
Cod	3½ oz	336
Tuna	3½ oz	301
Chicken	3½ oz	200
Hamburger	3½ oz	298
Grain products		
All Bran cereal	1 oz	350

Principal source: Nutritive Value of Foods, *U.S. Department of Agriculture*

ligrams for men and younger women, and 1,500 milligrams for postmeno-pausal women. To get this much calcium from your diet without overdosing on salt, fat, or calories takes a bit of doing. In fact, unless you are a true fan of broccoli and tofu, you may need to consider calcium supplements; chapter 8 discusses them, and chapter 10 reviews the only major complication of calcium excess, kidney stones.

Iron

Iron is an essential component of hemoglobin, the oxygen-carrying pigment of red blood cells; iron deficiency is the most common cause of anemia in the United States.

Table 20-11. Calcium Content of Selected Foods

Food	Serving size	Calcium (mg)
Dairy products		
Milk	1 cup	292
Skim milk	1 cup	302
Yogurt	1 cup	415
Low-fat yogurt	1 cup	452
Cottage cheese	1 cup	138
American cheese	1 oz	174
Swiss cheese	1 oz	272
Feta cheese	1 oz	140
Vegetables		
Broccoli, cooked	1 cup	205
Spinach, cooked	1 cup	245
Fish		
Salmon, canned	3½ oz	237
Sardines, canned	3½ oz	240
Crab	1 cup	140
Oysters	1 cup	111
Other foods		
Tofu (bean curd)		
Firm	1 cup	516
Regular	1 cup	260

Principal source: Nutritive Value of Foods, *U.S. Department of Agriculture*

A small amount of iron is lost every day through the intestinal tract and the skin; a daily dietary intake of 10 milligrams of iron is enough to replace these losses for men. Some long-distance runners lose more iron and may therefore develop "runner's anemia." But the biggest losers are women, who shed about 30 milligrams with each menstrual period; to replace this extra iron, women should take in 15 milligrams of iron daily.

The best dietary source of iron is far from the best of foods: red meat. If you follow a healthful diet low in saturated fat and cholesterol, you won't be getting much iron from meat. Instead, you'll have to rely on deep green vegetables, legumes, and certain fish. You can also get iron from grain products; although they are naturally low in iron, they have been fortified with supplementary iron for the past 50 years. Table 20-12 lists the iron content of various foods.

It looks as if it should be easy to get all the iron you need from cereals, legumes, and vegetables. But there is a catch: the iron in vegetable products is not as well absorbed as the iron in animal products.

Most American men get enough iron. But American women — even meat eaters — average only two thirds of the recommended daily iron in-

Table 20-12. Iron Content of Selected Foods

Food	Serving size	Iron (mg)
Vegetables		
Spinach, cooked	1 cup	2.9
Broccoli, cooked	1 spear	2.1
Peas, frozen	1 cup	2.5
Potato	1 medium	2.7
Legumes and nuts		
Lima beans	1 cup	5.9
Pinto beans	1 cup	5.4
Black beans	1 cup	2.9
Lentils	1 cup	4.2
Peanuts	1 oz	1.0
Grain products		
Bread, baked from fortified flour	1 slice	0.7
Cereals, fortified	1 oz	1.0–4.5
Fish		
Clams	3 oz	5.2
Oysters	3 oz	4.8
Tuna	3 oz	1.6
Poultry		
Chicken	3 oz	1.0
Meat		
Pork	3 oz	3.3
Steak	3 oz	3.0
Ham	3 oz	1.2

Principal source: Nutritive Value of Foods, *U.S. Department of Agriculture*

take. A healthful diet can close the gap. Still, menstruating women may wish to consider iron supplements while they are adjusting to beans and greens. Iron supplements are generally prescribed for women who are pregnant or lactating.

A Glossary of Trace Minerals*

In addition to the four major minerals, at least eleven others should be part of your diet. Fortunately, a balanced diet will provide these in abundance, so you can enjoy your pasta without fretting over your phosphorus. Still, you may encounter a variety of claims for these minerals, so you should be able to separate fact from fiction.

---

*Principal source: *Recommended Daily Allowances,* 10th ed., Food and Nutrition Board, National Academy of Science.

- **Selenium**
  Roles: Antioxidant; may help to prevent cell damage from free radicals, possibly aiding in cancer prevention
  Sources: Fish, shellfish, poultry, garlic, tomatoes, meat, egg yolks
  Recommended Daily Allowance: 55 micrograms for women, 70 micrograms for men

- **Zinc**
  Roles: Normal growth; wound healing, protein synthesis
  Maintains senses of taste and smell
  Sources: Oysters, crabs, poultry, grain products, meat, dairy products
  Recommended Daily Allowance: 12 milligrams for women, 15 milligrams for men

- **Magnesium**
  Roles: Bone formation, protein synthesis, muscle metabolism
  Sources: Whole grains, legumes, leafy green vegetables, seafood, soybeans, nuts, apricots, bananas
  Recommended Daily Allowance: 280 milligrams for women, 350 milligrams for men

- **Manganese**
  Roles: Normal cell function, bone growth
  Sources: Whole grains, fruits, beets, and other vegetables, cocoa, nuts, egg yolks
  Recommended Daily Allowance: 2–5 milligrams (estimated)

- **Molybdenum**
  Roles: Normal cell function
  Sources: Grains, beans, peas, dark green vegetables, meats
  Recommended Daily Allowance: 75–250 micrograms (estimated)

- **Chromium**
  Roles: Normal sugar metabolism
  Sources: Whole grains, legumes, peanuts, brewer's yeast, meat, cheese
  Recommended Daily Allowance: 50–200 micrograms (estimated)

- **Copper**
  Roles: Formation of red blood cells, metabolism
  Sources: Oysters, lobster, crab, cereals, barley, legumes, nuts, organ meats
  Recommended Daily Allowance: 1.5–3 milligrams

- **Fluorine**
  Roles: Bone and tooth formation, prevention of dental cavities, possibly prevention of osteoporosis
  Sources: Naturally or artificially fluoridated water, fish, tea, gelatin; supplements may be needed in areas with low-fluoride water
  Recommended Daily Allowance: 1.5–4.0 milligrams (estimated)

- **Iodine**
  Roles: Thyroid function, cell metabolism
  Sources: Iodized salt, seafood, vegetables
  Recommended Daily Allowance: 150 micrograms

- **Chlorine**
  Roles: Fluid balance (with sodium)
  Sources: Salt, seafood
  Recommended Daily Allowance: Not established

- **Phosphorus**
  Roles: Promotes healthy bones and teeth (with calcium)
    Helps release energy from foods
  Sources: Most foods
  Recommended Daily Allowance: 1,200 milligrams, ages 11–24; 800 milligrams beyond age 24

■ Water

It's colorless, odorless, and tasteless (or it should be!). It's abundant and inexpensive (for now, at least). It's usually taken for granted. But it's no less important than the other elements of nutrition. It's the forgotten nutrient.

Accounting for nearly two thirds of the body's weight, water is as abundant in the human body as it is in nature. Indeed, water is vital for all the body's function. Respecting this importance, the body has devised an elaborate series of control mechanisms to maintain a healthy water balance. If you became dehydrated, your urine and sweat become concentrated to conserve water, and your thirst mechanism encourages you to refill your tank. If you have too much water, your kidneys will rapidly rid you of the excess.

The average adult needs about two quarts of fluid daily; about two thirds is provided by the beverages you drink, while one third is contained in the foods you eat.

Even if you don't have to think about the quantity of the water you drink, you should think about its quality. Healthy water is essential; chapter 22 will explain how to evaluate — and protect — your water supply.

■ Food Safety

Chemicals, chemicals, chemicals. If there is one thing that characterizes modern life, it's our reliance on chemicals. For better or worse, food is no exception. Chemicals are added to soil to fertilize crops. Pesticides are sprayed on food to deter insects and blights. Hormones and antibiotics are injected into animals or added to their food to spur growth or boost milk production. Preservatives are added to food to keep it fresh. Artificial colors are used to enhance appeal, and chemicals are used to tenderize, moisturize, and flavor our food.

All of this is done by design. In addition, both chemicals and microbes can enter our food inadvertently, as a result of pollution, contamination, improper processing, or accidents.

Is our food safe to eat?

Not always.

Food-borne illnesses are as old as food. Throughout history the most common have been infection caused by the contamination of food with bacteria, fungi, or parasites. Even today food poisoning is the leading food safety problem, affecting up to 10 million Americans annually. Most cases are mild, but some are very serious indeed. The solutions: tougher standards for the food industry and much more meticulous food inspections. But don't wait for the government to step up its efforts. You can protect yourself and your family with careful shopping, painstaking personal hygiene, diligent refrigeration (below 40 degrees F) and thorough cooking (to an internal temperature above 160 degrees F; set your oven temperature above 300 degrees F).

If food poisoning is an old worry, pesticides and pollutants are relatively new concerns. They are also much more difficult for the individual consumer to detect, since chemically induced illnesses typically result from cumulative exposures and take years to appear. It's also more difficult for individuals to protect themselves from pesticides and pollutants. Together we can generate political momentum for government action. Individually we can protect ourselves by favoring organically and locally grown produce, by carefully washing or peeling fruits and vegetables, and by selecting our fish wisely.

It's hard enough to wash off pesticides from the outside of produce and to avoid buying fish from polluted waters. It's impossible to remove the chemicals that manufacturers add to foods during processing.

In 1958 the U.S. Congress passed the Food Additives Amendment, and in 1960 it added the Color Additives Amendment to the Federal Food, Drug, and Cosmetic Act. Since then, manufacturers have been obliged to prove that additives are safe before they are legally sanctioned. Among the requirements: no substance can be added to food if it harms test animals even at doses *100 times* higher than the proposed human exposure; and no substance can be added if it causes cancer in laboratory animals at *any* dose.

Some consumer advocates call for even tougher standards. I'm sure there is room for improvement, but the current standards have done a good job of protecting us. In the case of cyclamates, for example, the standards are probably stricter than they need to be (see chapter 10).

A few additives, though, deserve special mention. Nitrites are banned from vegetable products, but they are allowed as preservatives in processed meats. Indeed, they are very effective at preventing botulism and other bacterial contaminations. Nitrites themselves are harmless, but they are converted by the body into nitrosamines, chemicals that are carcinogenic in laboratory animals. I think the government should do more to reduce our exposure to nitrites; they provide another reason (along with saturated fat, cholesterol, and sodium) to avoid processed meats. Still, most of the nitrites that arrive in the human stomach come not from food additives but from the metabolism of nitrates, chemicals found in spinach, lettuce, carrots, beets, and other common — and healthful! — vegetables. And the greatest human exposure to nitrosamines comes not from food or water but from cigarette smoke.

Sulfites are also a concern because they can provoke asthma and other allergic reactions in sensitive individuals. I'm glad that sulfites were banned from fresh fruits and vegetables in 1986, and I'm all for further controls. Still, sulfite sensitivity is rare, even in patients with asthma. In fact, allergic reactions to the *natural* chemicals in foods (especially shellfish, nuts, strawberries, and tomatoes) are much more common than are allergic reactions to chemical additives.

We should all remain vigilant about food additives, but we should view the problem in perspective. After all, the tens of thousands of *natural* chemicals in foods greatly outnumber the chemicals that are added in processing; your morning coffee, for example, contains more than 2,000 chemicals. In fact, some natural chemicals are much more likely to cause disease than chemical additives; saturated fat and cholesterol head my list of "natural toxins."

Consider, too, that the great majority of food additives are not exotic chemicals but common ingredients: spices, corn syrup, baking soda, and salt. In my view sodium and sugar are the additives that deserve the most worry, yet they get the least attention.

Finally, remember that food additives do a lot of good. They include many vitamins and minerals that are beneficial for health. They also include chemicals that help us enjoy food; without additives cakes wouldn't rise, breads would become moldy, and many foods would be labeled with tomorrow's date as an expiration deadline.

Food additives are a $10 billion-a-year industry. For all that money we get convenience, improved textures and flavors, useful vitamin and mineral supplements, and protection against spoilage and infection. We also get much more sodium and sugar than we need, as well as a variety of chemicals that seem safe but could be harmful to some individuals. It's a mixed picture: some additives are beneficial, others harmful. On balance, though, they do more good than harm; by reading labels carefully and doing your best to reduce your intake of sodium and nitrites, you can enjoy the benefits of additives while minimizing their risks.

Much the same is true of pesticides and fertilizers; by increasing crop yields, they have produced enormous gains for humankind. We must redouble our efforts to test these chemicals, to ban potentially harmful ones, to minimize the use of even the safest of them, to set tougher safety standards, to improve the inspection of domestic and imported foods, and to seek even better ways to improve agricultural productivity. But in the meantime it seems quite clear that even the imperfect chemicals we use today have done much more good than harm. Indeed, your risk of getting cancer from contaminated fruits and vegetables is much much lower than your risk of getting cancer because you don't eat these fiber- and vitamin-rich foods.

Is our food safe to eat? From the point of view of chemical additives and pesticide residues the answer is yes. True, food could be even safer; but the greatest health risks come not from exotic additives but from natural fats and cholesterol and from sodium, a chemical additive used so widely that we often mistakenly assume that it, too, is natural.

It will take time to improve the regulations that govern chemical additives, pesticides, and fertilizers. But you don't have to wait to find a few simple ways to protect your family from unwanted chemicals. Take a moment to consider the ways you cook food, the ways you store it, and the ways you serve it.

Microwave cooking has been a real boon because of its speed and convenience. It has been an asset for nutrition, too, because it allows foods to be cooked with less fat and because vegetables steamed in microwave ovens retain their nutrients exceedingly well. Microwaves can even be used to make grilling safer; open-flame cooking is less apt to produce nitro-pyrenes and other cancer-causing chemicals if meat is microwaved for several minutes before it is grilled.

When microwave ovens were first introduced, there was understandable concern about radiation exposure. Fortunately, these concerns have proved to be unfounded; strict regulations have limited radiation leakage to less than 5 milliwatts per square centimeter two inches from the oven door. Recently, however, new concerns have been raised about the safety of microwave cooking. Only time will tell if these concerns are justified; until then, a few simple precautions will eliminate any potential risks.

The concern relates not to radiation but to cooking temperatures, and it doesn't implicate food as much as food packaging. At very high temperatures chemicals in plastics and in plasticized paper and cardboard can undergo changes that may render them carcinogenic. To prevent these chemicals from entering your food during microwave cooking, simply transfer your food to glass containers before cooking. And if you use plastic wrap to cover your food while it is being cooked, be sure that the wrap doesn't actually touch the food.

Conventional cooking also requires some attention to cookware. Cast-iron skillets can shed some iron into food, which is actually a good thing since iron is an essential nutrient that may be in short supply if you follow a healthful diet that's low in red meat. Don't rely on iron cookware to make up dietary deficiencies, however, since the iron leached from skillets is not in a form that is absorbed efficiently.

More modern cookware is more problematic. Small amounts of aluminum can leach from pans into food. This has caused worry because some patients with Alzheimer's disease have excessive levels of aluminum in their brain. But the aluminum-Alzheimer's connection is highly speculative at best, and the amount of aluminum that enters food from pots and pans is very low — less than the amount of aluminum in foods naturally, and much, much less than the amount in buffered aspirin and certain antacids. As far as I'm concerned, if you enjoy cooking with aluminum pots, go right ahead. But if you buy a new aluminum pot, it seems prudent to wash it thoroughly and then to boil some water in it before you use it for cooking.

Copper cookware is another matter. If these luxurious and lovely pots are lined with steel or nickel, they are perfectly safe. But if they are all copper, excessive amounts of this mineral can contaminate your food. If you have an all-copper pot, retire it to your kitchen wall and buy a new pot with a safe lining.

Nonstick pans lack the elegance of copper, but they also avoid its problems. Teflon surfaces seem to be perfectly safe even if they are scratched or chipped. In fact, they are a health asset because they allow you to cook with less fat.

Ceramic cookware, by contrast, can be hazardous. The problem is the lead used in ceramic glaze; if the glazing is not done properly, substantial amounts of lead can leach from ceramic containers into food. You can't tell if ceramic ware is safe just by looking at it. Your choices: buy a simple kit to test for lead, or use nonceramic cookware and containers.

Lead is one of the most pervasive and serious environmental toxins. Until 1979 lead was often present in the solder used to seal metal food cans; lead has been removed from almost all domestic cans, but may still be present in some imported cans. If you eat large amounts of canned food, you may want to buy a home lead testing kit to check the cans for yourself. Lead is also present in the foil capsules used to cover the corks of wine bottles. Lead levels in wine often exceed the levels considered safe for drinking water; imported wines are more likely to have high lead levels than domestic wines. The FDA has not yet established standards to regulate the lead in wine; until regulations are available, avoid wine from bottles with leaky corks, and wipe the bottle's rim with a damp towel before you pour the wine. Cork liners are not the only source of lead in beverages; fine crystal glassware, too, contains lead. With prolonged exposure, lead can leach into alcoholic beverages from crystal. Your crystal goblets are safe for wine and brandy, but your crystal decanters should not be used to store alcoholic beverages.

Food safety is an important concern. To prevent problems, think of the chemicals placed in soil, sprayed on produce, and added to foods. Think of the microbes that can contaminate food. Think, too, of cookware and food containers. But above all, think about the food itself. Your greatest risk from food is from overexposure to harmful constituents (saturated fat, cholesterol, sodium) and from underexposure to vital nutrients (fiber, vitamins, minerals, complex carbohydrates).

Nutritious food is safe food.

■ Creating a Balanced Diet

To create a balanced diet you need to learn new ways of thinking about food. Most of us were raised in an era when milk, eggs, cheese, and meat were thought to be health foods, while grains, potatoes, beans, and starchy vegetables were dismissed as fattening. We now know, of course, that just the reverse is true. It seems like a radical change, and it can be confusing. But the scientific data that support this new way of thinking are extremely impressive. Moreover, this seemingly new approach to food is not really new at all but represents a return to the basic human diet that served our species so well for thousands of years.

To enjoy a balanced diet you need to learn new ways to prepare food. Dr. William Castelli estimates that the typical American family subsists on just ten recipes. If yours are like the average recipes, you'll need ten new ones. Even better: don't stop at ten. Instead of dreading your new diet, explore the many pleasures of healthful eating. Experiment with a wide array of good foods and good recipes. Many cookbooks specialize in low-fat, high-carbohydrate recipes that are healthful and delicious; my current favorite is *Jane Brody's Good Food Gourmet,* but you should test several to find the approach you like best. If you become an enthusiast, invest in a food processor and a microwave; both appliances will save time and improve the nutritional value of your food, especially for vegetable-based dishes.

To achieve a balanced diet, change slowly. By the time you are 40, you will have eaten about 40,000 meals, to say nothing of all those snacks. Don't expect yourself to change overnight. Instead, plan to improve your diet slowly but steadily. Target one item per week, and stick to your plan. This week, for example, you might substitute bran muffins for donuts and croissants; later you can substitute English muffins, whole wheat toast, or bagels for the bran muffins. Similarly, you can change gradually from butter to tub margarine, to jam alone, then from whole milk products to low-fat and then nonfat dairy products. Little by little you'll learn to like your new style of eating; far from missing fat and salt, you'll actually prefer healthful foods. One change per week will have you eating well — and liking it — in just a few months.

To benefit from a balanced diet, establish the goals that are right for you. Consider your blood cholesterol levels, blood pressure, blood sugar, and Body Mass Index. Factor in your risk for colon cancer and for cancers of the breast, uterus, and prostate. Include your family health history and your personal health habits in the equation. Remember, too, to consider your personal preferences and pleasures so you can retain the things that mean the most to you. Use all these factors to establish an individualized nutritional plan that will serve your health and your tastes.

To survive a balanced diet, be relaxed about it. You will never find a perfect food. Not everything on your menu needs to have a higher purpose. If you are healthy, your balanced diet will contain plenty of flexibility so that you can "cheat" with a fatty or salty morsel from time to time. Don't worry about every meal, much less every mouthful. Your nutritional peaks and valleys will balance out if your overall plan is sound.

To maintain a balanced diet, understand and accept the broad principles that should govern your nutrition:

- Eat a variety of foods; since no single food is perfect, you need a mix of foods to get all the nutrients you should have.
- Eat fewer animal products and more vegetable products.
- Eat fewer processed and commercially prepared foods and more fresh and homemade foods.
- Eat less fat, especially saturated fat, and less cholesterol.
- Eat more dietary fiber.
- Eat more complex carbohydrates and less sugar.
- Eat protein in moderation.
- Eat less sodium and more potassium and calcium.
- Eat more grain products, especially whole grain products.
- Eat more vegetables, especially those rich in vitamins A and C.
- Eat more fruits, especially those rich in vitamins A and C.
- Eat more legumes.
- Eat more fish.
- Eat chicken and turkey in moderation, always removing the skin.
- Eat little meat, avoiding prime and other fatty cuts, organ meats, and processed meats.
- Eat only low-fat or nonfat dairy products.
- Eat eggs sparingly.
- Use vegetable oils in moderation, favoring olive and canola oils, restricting partially hydrogenated oils (including those in margarine), and avoiding tropical oils and cocoa butter.
- If you choose to use alcohol, do so sparingly.
- Adjust your intake of calories to maintain a desirable body weight; if you need to lose weight, reduce your fat intake and increase your fiber consumption (and your exercise).

If you learn these 20 answers, you won't have to question the percentages, grams, and ounces of each item in your menu. But until your sound nutritional program is under way, use the tables and tips in this chapter to find the hidden fat, salt, and sugar in your foods as well as the sometimes elusive fiber, starch, vitamins, and minerals you need. To be precise, calculate the targets that fit your body and your goals. But if you prefer simple guidelines, aim for my "rule" of 30 plus 40 plus 50 — 30 grams of fiber, 40 grams of fat, and 50 grams of protein daily.

To preserve a balanced diet, work with your family and friends to change together. Far from being alone, you will be among the many thousands of people who are achieving good nutrition. It's not always easy. You'll have to learn new facts and change old habits, to resist the convenience of fast foods and the slogans of the Dairy Council and Beef Board, and to assimilate new styles of eating and new techniques of cooking. But you can succeed.

To evaluate your progress toward a balanced diet, look at your calendar instead of your watch. Your goal is not instant reform but a lifelong pattern of good nutrition. Your rewards will be tangible and multiple. Because grains, legumes, vegetables, and fruits are less expensive than meat and dairy products and processed foods, you'll save money. You'll also gain the pleasures of a varied and interesting diet. Above all, you'll be rewarded with good health and with many more pages on your calendar.

▪ 21 ▪

Exercise, Fitness, and Health

Here's a turnabout: a physician asking his readers to provide a consultation. But the case is easy, and after reading 20 chapters of this book you should do very well. In fact, you may even do a better job than some doctors!

Your "patient" is a 34-year-old man who is entirely free of symptoms. His physical examination is almost as mundane; the only abnormalities are blood pressure which is high at 156/94 and a body weight of 200 pounds, exceeding ideal weight by 15 percent. You inquire further into his background and discover a stressful professional life, tobacco abuse which has been abandoned only recently, and a family history that includes heart disease before age 40 in his father and sudden cardiac death before age 43 in his mother and uncles. No longer quite so bored, you order some lab tests: his blood count, urine, kidney function, and blood sugar are all normal, but his cholesterol is very high, at 292, despite avowed efforts to follow a low-fat diet.

Your diagnosis: atherosclerosis waiting to happen. But your treatment options are fewer than you think; it's 1976, long before the new generation of cholesterol-lowering drugs became available. Your prognosis: trouble ahead.

Because more than 15 years have passed, you can get an instant follow-up. Happily, your prognosis was wrong: the patient has not had a heart attack or stroke. In fact, he feels better than ever. On physical examination he looks less tense. Even more remarkably his weight is now 166, and his blood pressure is normal at 130/84. The lab tests are unchanged except for his cholesterol, which is way down to 220, with an HDL or "good" cholesterol that is extremely high (protective) at 110.

A nice result, to be sure. But modern medicine cannot take the credit for this one. The patient has not been on medication, and his caloric intake is actually higher than ever before. What has occurred?

You take some additional history, finding that you overlooked another coronary risk factor that was present in 1976: sedentary living. More than simply sedentary, the patient was positively inert. But on July 4, 1976, he dusted off his virginal college sneakers and hit the road. A mere .4-mile jog nearly sent him to the emergency ward, but the next day he tried again, then again, and again. By 1977 he was running marathons, and by 1981 he won the New England Athletic Congress 50 Mile Silver Championship, demonstrating a hundredfold increase in physical work capacity in just five years.

This metamorphosis notwithstanding, the patient is not a world-class athlete. He did not slip into a phone booth to strip off his mild-mannered exterior. Far from being a superman, he is really quite an ordinary chap. You guessed it — it's me!

What made Harvey run? Not my knowledge of exercise and health, for like most doctors I knew little about exercise in those dark days. Not my personal physician, for like most doctors I didn't have one of my own. I started to run not because of medical wisdom but because of my wife's common sense — and her firm insistence!

By now most people have heard stories like mine, and many seem to understand the importance of exercise. Unfortunately, the American public does not practice what it preaches. We venerate athletes and spend many hours watching them play — while we sit in a stadium seat or on a living room sofa. Fewer than 15 percent of American adults exercise at optimal levels. Doctors are not much better; according to one survey, only 27 percent of all physicians exercise for even one hour per week, even in California. Perhaps that's why another survey found that only 8 percent of primary care physicians felt they were very successful in helping their patients establish exercise programs.

Exercise is the best-kept secret in preventive medicine.

I didn't learn about fitness in medical school. In fact, exercise itself was my introduction to preventive medicine, changing my way of thinking about health and fitness every bit as much as it changed my body. It can also be your gateway to prevention.

■ Exercise and Fitness

To be fit, you have to be healthy. But being fit is more than just being free of disease. In 1976 I was healthy but far from fit; it took months of slow, steady, repetitive exercise for me to attain fitness. I changed; you can too.

What is fitness?

Physical exertion puts stress on all parts of the human body. But when properly performed, it's *good* stress, and your body will respond in good ways. Your tangible reward is fitness, an *enhanced ability to withstand stress*. When you're fit, you'll be able to withstand physical stress: your body's functions and performance will improve, both in sports and in daily life. When you're fit, you'll be able to withstand mental stress: your self-esteem and satisfaction will improve, both at play and at work. And when you're fit, your ability to withstand the stress of illness will improve: you'll reduce your risk of becoming ill, both when you are young and when you are older.

True fitness involves your whole body, and it can be measured in several ways.

Cardiovascular fitness means that your heart, lungs, and blood vessels are in top condition. It's best measured by your aerobic work capacity, evaluated by monitoring your oxygen uptake while you run on a treadmill or pedal an exercise bike. But even without fancy tests you'll know that you have achieved cardiovascular fitness when you can walk, jog, swim, bike, dance, play tennis, or work in the yard for amazingly long periods of time without getting tired.

Musculoskeletal fitness means that your muscles, ligaments, bones, and joints are in top shape. Most people think of it simply as muscular strength, but there is more to it: your muscles should also have endurance, and your ligaments and joints should be strong and flexible. You'll know you have a fit musculoskeletal system when you can play and work harder and more efficiently than ever without being injured.

Add to these *metabolic fitness*, when your body's chemical constituents are balanced optimally, and *psychological fitness*, when you are able to withstand mental stress without becoming anxious or depressed, and you've attained an enhanced state of happiness, enthusiasm, and energy.

There are no short cuts to true fitness, no pills, potions, or programs that will get you there overnight. There are no secrets of any kind. In fact, regular exercise underlies it all.

■ How Your Body Responds to Exercise

Exercise puts your whole body to work. If your body is not used to exercise, you can injure it by trying to do too much. But if you work yourself into shape gradually, your body will respond in remarkable ways.

Your *heart* pumps about 5 quarts of blood per minute while you're at rest. But when you exercise, your muscles need much more blood. As a result, your heart may have to pump up to 20 quarts per minute during all-out exertion. If you exercise regularly, your heart will be equal to the task. Like other muscles that are properly trained, your heart muscle will become stronger and larger so that it will be able to propel more blood with every beat. It will also become more efficient, requiring less oxygen to do its work. When you're in shape, your resting heart rate will be lower than average because each beat is stronger; for the same reason, your heart won't have to beat as rapidly to keep up with the demands of exercise. All in all, a fit heart can work harder and longer with less strain.

Your *blood vessels and circulation* will also benefit from regular exercise training. Repetitive exercise widens blood vessels and lowers the amount of adrenaline in the circulation. The results: a lower blood pressure and improved blood flow to muscles and other tissues.

Your *lungs* are also put to work by exercise. When you are physically active, your breathing rate increases dramatically, as does the amount of air that you inhale and exhale. When you work out regularly, you'll find that your "wind" will improve. But repetitive exercise training won't actually do much for your lungs themselves. Instead, your improved breathing capacity will depend on improvements in your heart, blood vessels, and muscles.

Your *musculoskeletal* system will improve dramatically with regular exercise. Muscles that are trained with resistance exercises become stronger and larger. Muscles that are trained with aerobic exercises develop an enhanced ability to use oxygen efficiently, leading to much greater endurance. Ligaments and tendons also tend to become stronger with exercise. That's the good news; the bad news is that they also become shorter and tighter. Fortunately, however, stretching exercises can make these tissues more flexible than ever. And regular exercise also increases bone calcium content, making bones stronger and more resistant to fractures.

The *metabolic* effects of regular exercise are every bit as impressive. During exercise your body burns calories up to 20 times faster than it does at rest. If you exercise regularly, your body fat will decrease. Even better, your cholesterol profile will improve. Fitness also enhances the efficiency with which insulin binds to tissues, so blood sugar levels are lower.

Exercise training affects your *blood,* too. If you work out regularly, your blood plasma volume will increase, making your blood "thinner." Your platelets will become less sticky, thus reducing the likelihood of unwanted blood clots. And for extra protection, your body's clot-dissolving mechanisms will also be activated by exercise.

Your *intestinal tract,* too, is influenced by exercise. Bowel contractions are enhanced by physical activity, stimulating eliminations.

The *neurological* and *psychological* effects of exercise are no less important than all these "physical" effects. In fact, the mental side of training has a chemical basis. Exercise increases blood levels of chemicals called *endorphins.* Endorphins, in turn, may account for the improved mood and reduced stress and anxiety that are experienced by many people who exercise regularly.

■ Exercise and Health

Fitness itself should be enough to reward you for maintaining a regular exercise program. But you'll also earn lifelong health benefits from exercise.

Heart disease remains the number one killer in America: heart attacks claim about 500,000 lives each year. Fortunately, the cardiovascular system is also the number one beneficiary of regular exercise. Sedentary people are 1.9 times more likely to suffer heart attacks than are fit people. In our country alone, regular exercise could save more than 200,000 lives annually. Be sure that yours is among them.

High blood pressure affects 58 million Americans, nearly one third of our adult population. Exercise can help; people who are fit are 30 to 50 percent less likely to develop high blood pressure than are sedentary people. And even if you have hypertension, it's not too late to get into shape. Exercise is an excellent way to treat hypertension, reducing blood pressure by an average of 10 to 15 millimeters; in hypertensive patients, however, exercise should be supervised medically.

Stroke ranks third among the causes of death in America, claiming 150,000 lives each year. By fighting atherosclerosis, hypertension, and blood clotting, exercise should protect against strokes. It does; sedentary people are nearly three times more likely to suffer strokes than are fit people.

Colon cancer is distressingly common in the United States, with 150,000 new cases — and 60,000 deaths — each year. Diet is the best way to prevent colon cancer, but exercise can also help; sedentary people are 1.3 to 1.6 times more likely to develop colon cancer than are physically active people.

Osteoporosis afflicts more than 24 million Americans, accounting for 1.3 million fractures annually. Pain, disfigurement, and disability are the obvious consequences, but osteoporosis can also be life-threatening, since elderly women have a 20 percent risk of dying in the first year after a hip fracture. Exercise helps: it increases bone calcium in young athletes, and it will do the same in elderly women. At every age exercise makes bones stronger.

Breast cancer strikes one of every nine American women, and more than 70,000 develop *cancer of the reproductive tract* each year. The role of exercise in preventing these cancers is impressive but sadly neglected. Women who begin to exercise during their early reproductive years can expect to enjoy a 50 percent reduction in their lifetime risk of developing these cancers.

Diabetes and *obesity* are also on the list of major medical problems that can be treated, or even prevented, by regular exercise. About 11 million Americans have diabetes, and 34 million are obese; these numbers should be enough to get all of us to exercise.

Anxiety, depression, and *unhealthful behavior* are even more common. It's harder to quantify the benefits of exercise in these areas, but many studies show that fitness is linked to improved mood, to better performance at work and school, and to more healthful life-styles.

Fitness will improve the quality of your life. Regular exercise will also help prevent disease and disability. Best of all it will actually prolong your life. Even if you don't start exercising until age 40, you will reap enormous benefits from a regular exercise program. If you get into shape and continue exercising for about three hours a week, you can expect to outlive your sedentary peers by about 13 months. That means you'll live two hours longer for each hour you exercise — a good thing to remember the next time you're "too busy to work out."

■ Exercise-induced Illnesses

If prevention were perfect, we'd live like gods, happy, healthy, and immortal. Good as it is, however, prevention is far from perfect. The same is true for exercise; while the net result of exercise is enormously beneficial, adverse effects can sometimes occur. Fortunately, careful planning will enable you to avoid most exercise-induced problems. By learning to listen to your body and to respond to its messages, you can correct most exercise-related problems before they cause any harm.

The health benefits of exercise require long-term adaptations to regular, repetitive exercise. In contrast, most of the undesirable consequences are short-term reactions to single episodes of exercise.

Of greatest concern are the *cardiac complications* of exercise. Every month or two your newspaper will carry a story about someone who died while exercising. Although they're rare, these tragic events get a lot of publicity. Precisely because so many more people die in their sleep, "ordinary" deaths get much less attention than do exercise-related deaths. Don't let the publicity frighten you away from exercise; a large body of scientific evidence proves that exercise will reduce your risk of cardiac death. Still, these well-publicized deaths should remind you to take the simple precautions that will protect your heart when you work out.

Exercise-related heart problems fall into two distinct groups.

When young athletes die during exercise, the most frequent cause is congenital heart disease. Many varieties of heart disease have been implicated, including the excessive thickening of the heart's main pumping chamber which killed college basketball star Hank Gathers, and the abnormal hook-up of the main coronary artery which killed pro basketball great Pete Maravich. It's hard to predict these sudden disasters, and harder still to prevent them. Every athlete should have a competent physical exam, which may sometimes detect worrisome heart murmurs, abnormal heart rhythms, or cardiac enlargement. Athletes with close relatives who died prematurely, especially during exercise, should be considered for an additional test called an echocardiogram. Above all, athletes of any age must be taught to seek medical attention if they faint during exercise, or if they develop chest pain, weakness, undue shortness of breath, or erratic heartbeats. They should also learn to avoid exercise when they have fever and flu-like symptoms, since an inflammation of the heart called myocarditis may result from strenuous exercise during certain viral infections.

When middle-aged and older people die during exercise, the cause is usually undiagnosed coronary artery disease. Perhaps the best-known example is Jim Fixx, who died while jogging in 1984 at age 52. Many similar deaths are preventable. People who are at risk of heart disease should have detailed evaluations before they exercise: Fixx, a former three-pack-a-day smoker whose father died from a heart attack at age 43, never had such an evaluation. Even more important, be alert for symptoms. Most often warning symptoms occur in advance of the cardiac catastrophe: Fixx never reported his "indigestion" to his doctor. Last, but not least, exercise properly so that you will train your heart without straining it. I'll discuss guidelines for safe exercise later in this chapter.

Is exercise dangerous? For people who exercise right, the risks are very low. At Dr. Kenneth Cooper's famed Institute for Aerobics Research, for example, no deaths have occurred in more than 375,000 hours of exercise, including more than 1.2 million miles of walking and jogging. Even in unsupervised settings the risk is low; Dr. Paul Thompson studied runners in Rhode Island, finding one death per 396,000 hours of jogging.

The greatest risks occur in "weekend athletes" — people who engage in strenuous exertion when they are not in shape. Studying the residents of Seattle, Washington, Dr. David Siscovick found that sedentary people who exercise strenuously have a substantial risk of sudden death during exertion, exceeding their risk at rest by 56 times. People who exercise regularly, though, are at much lower risk. In fact, Dr. Siscovick found that regular exercise actually *reduces* the risk of sudden death by 60 percent. The moral: get into shape gradually, and stay in shape by exercising regularly.

Perhaps the best evidence that exercise is safe comes from the most vulnerable people of all — heart patients. Exercise training can be used for rehabilitation and prevention even after heart attacks and bypass surgery. And even in those high-risk patients, fatalities are limited to one for every 783,979 hours of exercise. Far from risking heart damage, these patients benefit greatly from regular exercise, reducing their risk of heart attacks and cardiac death by 25 percent. Of course, heart patients require detailed evaluations and medical supervision to exercise. If you are healthy, it will be much easier for you to exercise safely; still, you will benefit from guidelines similar to those we have developed for our heart patients at the Harvard Cardiovascular Center.

These guidelines will also help prevent the less serious side effects of exercise that are discussed later in this chapter. But the most important guideline of all is the simplest: listen to your body. Even if its messages include relatively common problems such as muscular aches or relatively uncommon problems such as exercise-induced asthma, heartburn, diarrhea, and urinary abnormalities, you don't have to give up on exercise. Instead, check a fitness book or see a sports medicine expert to find out how you can overcome the difficulty.

■ Exercise and the Cycle of Life

Exercise is a natural function of the human body. As our species evolved, the human heart, lungs, and muscles developed an enormous capacity to perform physical work. Indeed, survival depended on daily exertion: up until the time of the industrial revolution, for example, 30 percent of all the energy used by the factories and farms in America was supplied by human labor. The figure now is well under 1 percent. What has changed? Not the human body; it is still engineered to work best when it's worked hardest. But the human mind evolved to solve problems, and one of its signal achievements is the invention of machines that do our work for us. It's been a great boon for civilization, but a real bane for health.

To recapture their potential for fitness and health, people must turn back the exercise clock. Strenuous physical activity is as old as human-kind; it's the sedentary life-style of industrialized Western societies that's new. But we don't have to toil in the fields to become fit; instead we can use the leisure time given to us by tractors to play. Recreational exercise can refresh the mind as it invigorates the body.

The best time to start is in childhood. Even in contemporary America children are naturally physically active — for a while. Unfortunately, it doesn't take long for the video culture to turn an active child into a sedentary one. According to the 1990 National Children and Youth Fitness survey, only 36 percent of America's children exercise appropriately. Is it any wonder that only 32 percent of our children can pass a simple test of muscular strength, flexibility, and cardiovascular endurance? Or that American children were fatter in 1990 than they were in 1980? Even more alarming, a Michigan survey of elementary school students found that 98 percent had one or more risk factors for developing coronary artery disease, including high cholesterol levels in 41 percent and high blood pressure in 28 percent.

The seeds of sedentary living are sown in childhood and harvested in adulthood. If our kids are sedentary, our adults are positively slothful; in our society people exercise less with every passing year.

Far from being kids' stuff, exercise is important for all age groups. It may even affect the pace of the aging process itself.

Suppose we take a perfectly healthy 30-year-old and measure maximum oxygen uptake, cardiac function, blood pressure, body fat, cholesterol, blood sugar, muscle mass, and bone density. Next we put our subject to bed rest for three weeks, then repeat all the measurements. What do we have? All the measurements tell us our subject is now about 45 years old. Fortunately, this instant seniority is reversible; with a few weeks of modest exercise the subject is back to age 30. And if the exercise program is sustained for several months, all the measurements will improve still further; the aerobic work capacity, for example, may actually *double* with three or four months of regular exercise.

You don't have to be an exercise physiologist to understand these results. Helen Hayes put it succinctly when she said "Resting is rusting," and nearly 300 years earlier John Gay explained that "exercise thy lasting youth defends." Many of the physiological changes attributed to aging are not actually caused by *age* itself but by *disuse* and *disease*. Regular exercise prevents disuse; as part of a balanced program of prevention, it helps prevent disease. The next result: a physiologically younger body at every age.

The capacities demonstrated by senior athletes can be truly extraordinary. Albert Gordon moved up from a lifetime of middle-distance running to conquer the London marathon — at age 80. Kenneth Beer didn't take up tennis until age 30 — and 57 years later he was still winning national Super Seniors singles championships. John Fleck entered the 50-, 100-, and 400-meter freestyle swimming races and the 400-meter race walk at the 1991 Senior Olympics — at age 99. Herman Johannsen learned cross-country skiing in his native Norway at age 2; he brought the sport with him when he immigrated to Canada, exercising daily until his death in 1987 at age 111.

The achievements of older athletes are impressive, but individual cases don't prove that exercise itself is actually responsible for these triumphs over time. During the past few years, however, doctors at the University of Toronto, Tufts University, and the Johns Hopkins Medical School have performed carefully controlled physiological studies of senior athletes and of senior citizens who have remained physically active even without competitive sports. The results: 75- and 80-year-olds with the cardiac capacities, metabolic measurements, muscle strength, and bone densities of 50- or 60-year-olds.

It's never too late to start; many studies have shown that even elderly people benefit from exercise. I don't know who had the courage to fund the 1990 Boston study of weight training in nursing home residents, but the results were revealing: nine people between the ages of 87 and 96 completed a two-month program of weight lifting, demonstrating impressive gains in muscular strength.

Exercise is not the fountain of youth, and it cannot actually turn back the clock. But it can help preserve youthful capacities even as it extends life. The ancient wisdom of Hippocrates explains why regular exercise is so very important at all stages in the cycle of life: "That which is used develops; that which is not used wastes away." And if the Greek physician does not persuade, perhaps the Roman poet Cicero will: "Exercise and temperance will preserve something of our youthful vigor, even into old age."

■ What Type of Exercise Is Best?

Although any type of exercise can be worthwhile, one type stands alone for its health benefits. Aerobic training is the best way to enhance your cardiac function, improve your blood cholesterol and sugar levels, strengthen your bones, and reduce your risk of heart attacks, high blood pressure, strokes, and even certain cancers. Regular aerobic exercise will reduce your body fat so you'll look better. It will improve your muscles' endurance so you'll work better. And it will clear your mind so you'll feel better.

In aerobic training your large muscle groups work in a rhythmic, repetitive fashion for long periods of time. Your heart rate increases and you work up a sweat, but if you're doing it right you won't be winded or uncomfortable. In fact you should find yourself enjoying the brisk walking, jogging, swimming, biking, aerobic dance, or racquet sports that constitute typical aerobic exercise programs.

Aerobics should be the core of your exercise program for fitness and health, but you should supplement it with other forms of exercise.

Flexibility training is essential; without it your muscles will become tight and stiff as they grow stronger, thus increasing your risk of injury. Stretching routines are the key to flexibility; they are also ideal for the warm-up and cool-down periods that should always surround active exercise.

Strength training is desirable; it, too, will help prevent injury and enhance performance, and you'll enjoy the way it improves your muscle tone and appearance. But strength training can raise the blood pressure, stressing the heart and circulation. While that's no problem for healthy young athletes, middle-aged people should plan strength training carefully to be sure it's safe; patients with cardiovascular disease can do modified strength training — *if* they are medically supervised.

Speed training is entirely optional; it will do little for health but is important for optimal athletic performance. Speed training is physically stressful; it is not appropriate for people with medical problems, and even healthy athletes must be careful to avoid injury from speed training.

■ How Much Exercise Is Best?

People exercise for three reasons: for health, for recreation, and for competition. The amount of exercise that's best for you depends very much on your health, your fitness level, and your personal goals. But if getting into shape and maintaining good health are your aims, useful medical guidelines are available.

We can estimate how much exercise is best by evaluating two standards: aerobic fitness, and health and longevity.

Aerobic fitness is easy to quantify on a treadmill or bike by measuring work capacity and oxygen uptake. As little as 20 minutes of endurance exercise three times per week will improve your aerobic fitness. But if you work out longer or harder, you will improve further. Eventually, however, you'll reach a plateau that is dictated by your age, gender, and genetic endowment; no matter how hard I work, for example, I'll never have the aerobic capacity of a champion endurance athlete (darn it!).

For fitness, the first hour of aerobic exercise per week is the most important, but additional gains can be attained from additional training. The same is true of health and longevity.

The landmark 1978 study by Dr. Ralph Paffenbarger and his colleagues at Stanford University and the Harvard School of Public Health provides the best quantitative information. These investigations evaluated 16,936 graduates of Harvard College, comparing their risk of heart attack and death with the amount of exercise they performed every week over the years. Exercise was quantified as the number of calories burned up each week. As little as 500 exercise calories per week produced significant gains. Higher exercise levels produced further protection, up to a maximum of about 2,000 calories per week, which reduced the risk of heart attacks by 26 percent. Beyond that level health and longevity benefits plateau, neither improving nor declining with additional exercise.

How can you translate Dr. Paffenbarger's college alumni results to your daily life? Even without a Harvard degree, 20 miles of jogging or walking, 80 miles of biking, or 4 miles of swimming will consume about 2,000 calories. If you are more comfortable watching the clock, you can estimate that

Table 21-1. The Time It Takes to Burn 2,000 Calories

Activity	Time
Strolling	10 hours
Bowling	8 hours 30 minutes
Golf	8 hours
Raking leaves	7 hours
Doubles tennis	6 hours
Brisk walking	5 hours 30 minutes
Biking (leisurely)	5 hours 30 minutes
Ballet	4 hours 30 minutes
Singles tennis	4 hours 30 minutes
Racquetball, squash	4 hours
Biking (hard)	4 hours
Jogging	4 hours
Downhill skiing	4 hours
Calisthenics, brisk aerobics	3 hours 30 minutes
Running	3 hours
Cross-country skiing	3 hours

it will take about an hour of moderate exercise to burn about 500 calories; three to four hours of moderate to strenuous exercise will consume about 2,000 calories. Compare your exercise schedule with table 21-1 to see how you measure up.

As you get into shape, you may find that you've come to enjoy exercise so much that your goals are shifting from health to encompass also recreation or even competition. If so, you may want to work out longer or harder. Is it safe to exercise at these higher levels?

My favorite answer to this question comes not from an exercise physiologist or cardiovascular epidemiologist but from Mae West, who said, "Too much of a good thing is . . . wonderful." Fortunately, all the medical data agree: you can push your fitness horizons beyond exercise for health. As you do so, however, it will become increasingly necessary to follow the guidelines that help prevent injury.

■ Exercising for Endurance: Your Program for Aerobic Fitness

Aerobic activity is the most important part of your exercise program for fitness and health. But aerobic exercise should not be the first part of your program: instead, it should quite literally be the centerpiece, following a ten-minute warm-up period and preceding a five-minute cool-down period.

Warm-Ups and Cool-Downs

To protect your health, always warm up before, and cool down after, vigorous exercise. Warming up will loosen your muscles, tendons, and ligaments, greatly reducing your risk of strains, sprains, and tendinitis. Cooling down will also protect your muscles and joints by reducing tightness and preventing spasms and cramps. No less important is the protection that these routines will gain for your number one muscle, your heart. Warming up will allow your heart rate to increase gradually, just as cooling down brings it down slowly. The result: less stress on your heart, protecting it from erratic pumping rhythms and other complications.

It's easy to devise good routines for warming up and cooling down. Walking is ideal; simply start at a strolling pace, then slowly speed up before you embark on your brisk aerobic walk or jog. When your aerobic period is over, slow down gradually. Similarly, if you're using a bike, rowing machine, treadmill, or other exercise device, start at a slow pace with low resistance, picking up your pace only very gradually; reverse the process to cool down.

You can improve your warm-ups and cool-downs by adding stretching exercises and calisthenics, which also promote flexibility and strength.

Resist the temptation to skimp on stretching, warm-ups, and cool-down. Don't try to jump-start your muscles and your heart; it won't work any better than trying to start your car in high gear.

Planning for Aerobics

To decide how to exercise, consider three elements: the frequency, duration, and intensity of your exercise.

The *frequency* is the easiest to plan. At first, exercise three times a week or every other day. This plan will give your muscles at least 48 hours to recover from exercise; muscles that are rested are resistant to injury, and they'll be fresh and energetic when it's time to exercise. As you get into shape, you may choose to maintain an alternate-day routine or switch to a daily schedule. If you exercise daily, be sure to alternate hard workouts with easier ones so your muscles can recover adequately.

The *duration* of exercise is also easy to plan. Remember your goal: one hour of aerobics per week is a minimum, and three to four hours is optimal. If you're out of shape, begin with a humble ten minutes three times a week. Lengthen your aerobic sessions gradually, always listening to your body to be sure that your muscles and joints agree with your plan.

The *intensity* of your exercise is the trickiest part of your plan. It is also the most important for safety's sake. Begin your fitness program with easier workouts, progressing to more intense activities only gradually.

There are three ways to gauge the intensity of your exercise: you can look it up in table 21-2, you can evaluate it subjectively, or you can measure your heart rate during exercise. By any method your goal is to exercise in the aerobic range, hard enough to get the benefits of endurance training but gently enough to avoid exhaustion and injury.

Table 21-2 summarizes the intensity of exercises, starting gradually, build up to 5 to 7 calories per minute (300 to 420 per hour). To get your 2,000 calories per week, you can maintain this modest level for five to

Table 21-2. The Intensity of Exercise

Intensity level	Daily activities	Recreational activities
1 calorie per minute	Complete rest	
2 to 2½ calories per minute	Standing Desk work Driving an automobile Typing (electric)	Strolling (1 mile per hour) Playing cards Sewing, knitting
2½ to 4 calories per minute	Auto repair Radio, TV repair Janitorial work Typing (manual) Bartending Riding lawn mower	Level walking (2 miles per hour) Level bicycling (5 miles per hour) Billiards, bowling Shuffleboard Woodworking (light) Driving a powerboat Golf (using a power cart) Canoeing (2½ miles per hour) Horseback (walk) Playing various musical instruments
4 to 5 calories per minute	Bricklaying, plastering Pushing a wheelbarrow (100-lb. load) Machine assembly Driving a tractor-trailer in traffic Welding (moderate load) Cleaning windows Housework Pushing light-power mower	Walking (3 miles per hour) Cycling (6 miles per hour) Horseshoe pitching Volleyball (6-man, non-competitive) Golf (pulling bag cart) Archery Sailing (handling small boat) Fly-fishing (standing with waders) Horseback (sitting while trotting) Badminton (social doubles) Energetically playing various musical instruments
5 to 6 calories per minute	Painting, masonry Paperhanging	Walking (3.5 miles per hour)

►

Table 21-2. (continued)

Intensity level	Daily activities	Recreational activities
5 to 6 calories per minute	Light carpentry Raking leaves Hoeing	Cycling (8 miles per hour) Ping-Pong Golf (carrying clubs) Dancing (fox trot) Badminton (singles) Tennis (doubles) Various calisthenics
6 to 7 calories per minute	Digging in garden Shoveling light earth Average sexual activity	Walking (4 miles per hour) Cycling (10 miles per hour) Canoeing (4 miles per hour) Horseback (posting while trotting) Stream fishing (walking in light current in waders) Ice- or roller-skating (9 miles per hour)
7 to 8 calories per minute	Shoveling (10-lb. load 10 times per minute) Splitting wood Snow shoveling Hand lawn mowing	Walking (5 miles per hour) Cycling (11 miles per hour) Badminton (competitive) Tennis (singles) Square-dancing Downhill skiing (light) Cross-country skiing ($2\frac{1}{2}$ miles per hour in loose snow) Water-skiing
8 to 10 calories per minute	Digging ditches Carrying 80 lbs. Sawing hardwood	Jogging (5 miles per hour) Cycling (12 miles per hour) Horseback (gallop) Downhill skiing (vigorous)

Table 21-2. (continued)

Intensity level	Daily activities	Recreational activities
		Basketball
		Mountain climbing
		Ice hockey
		Canoeing (5 miles per hour)
		Touch football
		Paddleball
10 to 11 calories per minute	Shoveling (14-lb. load 10 times per minute)	Running (5½ miles per hour)
		Cycling (13 miles per hour)
		Cross-country skiing (4 miles per hour in loose snow)
		Squash (social)
		Handball (social)
		Fencing
		Basketball (vigorous)
Above 11 calories per minute	Shoveling (16-lb. load 10 times per minute)	Running 7 miles per hour = 12 calories per minute
		Running 8 miles per hour = 13 calories per minute
		Running 9 miles per hour = 15 calories per minute
		Running 10 miles per hour = 17 calories per minute
		Cross-country skiing (5+ miles per hour in loose snow)
		Handball (competitive)
		Squash (competitive)

Note: These are average levels for a person weighing 150 pounds; people who weigh more will consume more energy at each activity. Excitement or anxiety will also increase the intensity of some of these activities.

Source: Modified from H. B. Simon, "Exercise, Health, and Sports Medicine," in Scientific American Medicine. *E. Rubenstein and D. Federman, eds.,* Scientific American, *New York, 1992.*

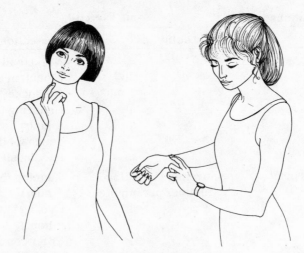

Figure 21-1. Taking carotid and radial pulses

six hours per week — or you can continue to work up to 10 to 12 calories per minute (600 to 720 per hour) so you can get the full benefits of exercise in about three hours each week. Best of all, include both gentle and strenuous exercise; variety will help keep your body fresh and your mind enthusiastic.

The second way to gauge the intensity of your exercise is the simplest, but it's the most subjective. Aim for the "talking pace." You should be working hard enough to work up a sweat, but you should have enough wind to carry on a conversation without gasping for breath. If you're huffing and puffing, slow down and hold a steady pace until it's time to cool down. As you get into shape, you'll be amazed to discover how much your body is able to do without causing breathlessness.

The third way to gauge the intensity of your exercise is the most precise, but it takes a little practice. The first step is to measure your heart rate. In this high-tech world you can buy a variety of pulse meters that will give you an instant digital electronic heart rate readout. If you like gadgets, you may want to invest in one of these transistorized marvels. Or you can measure your heart rate the way doctors and nurses do — with your fingers and your watch.

Figure 21-1 shows you how to take your pulse. Because you'll find it easiest to count your pulse when your heart rate is slow, practice taking your pulse while you're resting quietly. When you are confident that you can feel every beat, practice taking your pulse after exercise. Count every beat for ten seconds and multiply by 6 to find your heart rate.

The next step is to know your maximum heart rate. A stress test is the most accurate way to determine it, but if you are healthy, the low-tech way is good enough: simply subtract your age in years from the number 220.

The third step is to calculate your target heart rate, which ranges from

Table 21-3. Target Heart Rates for Aerobic Exercise

Age	Maximum heart rate	Target range (beats per minute)		10-Second pulse count	
		Low (70% max.)	High (85% max.)	Low	High
20	200	140	170	23	28
25	200	140	170	23	28
30	194	136	165	22	27
35	188	132	160	22	26
40	182	128	155	21	26
45	176	124	150	20	25
50	171	119	145	20	24
55	165	115	140	19	23
60	159	111	135	18	23
65	153	107	130	17	22

70 to 85 percent of your maximum rate. Begin your fitness program at the low end, gradually working up as you get into shape.

I've done the math for you in table 21-3.

Monitoring the intensity, duration, and frequency of your exercise will enable you to write your own exercise prescription using exactly the same principles we rely on to prescribe exercise for patients with heart disease. Once you've learned the simple principles of safe exercise, you can turn to the enjoyable activities that put theory into practice. Experiment to find the ones that suit you best. Even better, learn to combine a variety of sports into a balanced fitness program.

Walking

Can an activity as simple and universal as walking be the basis of a fitness program? Ask Erasmus ("Before supper, walk a little, after supper do the same"), Emerson ("You will never break down in a speech when you have walked 12 miles"), or Dickens ("Walk and be happy, walk and be healthy"). Or if theologians, philosophers, and writers are not your chosen authorities, ask exercise physiologists. They all agree: the answer is yes.

Walking has many advantages. The technique is entirely natural, requiring no special skill or ability. The equipment, too, is minimal: you'll need only a first-rate pair of walking shoes and clothing appropriate for the climate. You can walk year round, wearing a T-shirt and shorts in summer, a light nylon athletic suit in fall and spring, and a heavier suit (Gore-Tex is ideal), gloves, and hat in winter. Add layers as the temperature falls; zippered jackets are best because they allow you to adjust easily to the heat you generate during vigorous exercise. Walk outdoors to enjoy nature or indoors to escape from inclement weather. Walk alone or with a friend.

Walk for transportation, for recreation, for health and fitness, or for competition.

Walking has an important medical advantage: because one foot is on the ground at all times, walking is a low-impact activity, easy on muscles, joints, and tendons.

Are there any drawbacks to walking? I can think of only two. First, it does relatively little for the arms and upper body. Still, by swinging your arms while you walk, you can promote upper-body muscular endurance; carrying light weights (one to five pounds) will do even more, but may also increase the risk of injury. Second, walking is time-consuming. Even brisk walking is less intense than many other aerobic sports, so you'll have to put in more time to get your full exercise benefits. For most people, walking at four miles per hour is a good goal; start with a gentler gait, but make a conscious effort to push your pace as you improve. To achieve maximum fitness, learn the race-walking technique; you can join a walking club or enter competitions to add spice to your walking routine.

Jogging and Running

It's true that you should always walk before you run. But it's also true that you should consider running before you move on to other sports.

Like walking, running is entirely natural. And naturally enough, the two share many advantages. Like walking, running requires little in the way of skill, technique, and equipment. Like walking, running can provide solitude or companionship, indoor exercise or outdoor activity, recreation or competition.

Despite these similarities, running does have a fundamental difference from walking. Whereas walkers have one foot in contact with the ground at all times, runners are entirely airborne for some time during each stride. As pace increases, moving from jogging to running to sprinting, the percentage of the stride that's airborne increases; competitive runners have "flight times" of about 45 percent.

Why run if you can walk for fitness and health? The greater intensity of jogging or running will allow you to achieve your weekly exercise quota faster. And once you're in shape, the extra intensity can be challenging and enjoyable.

The intensity of running provides efficiency and challenge, but it also increases the risk of injury. Unlike walking, running is a high-impact exercise. It's simply a matter of gravity: what goes up must come down. Airborne runners return to earth with each stride, putting a stress equal to eight times body weight on their feet, legs, hips, and neck. In just one mile runners' legs will have to absorb more than *100 tons* of impact force; it's a testament to the wonderful construction of the human body that this can be done with so few problems. But the faster the pace, the greater the impact — and the greater the risk of injury.

Running is more traumatic than walking, but it can be safe. Pay extra attention to warm-ups and stretching. Be sure your shoes are in top condition, and seek out the softest running surfaces you can find. Above all, listen to your body. If your muscles and tendons protest your running, you can take corrective action in plenty of time to avert long-term problems. In most cases you'll be able to resume running, and to continue running for fitness and fun. In fact, although many studies show that a high percentage of runners have injuries from time to time, an excellent 1987 California study of 498 long-distance runners found that they actually had fewer musculoskeletal problems than did age-matched sedentary people.

Running is not for everyone. People who are overweight, very much out of shape, or in the older age groups should certainly start with walking, hiking, or swimming. Arthritis and back pain are two more reasons to pick swimming or walking. But many people find that running is a wonderful way to get their exercise and enjoy it too. The benefits can be little short of amazing; no less an authority than the Old Testament tells us "They shall run and not grow weary" (Isaiah 40:31).

Swimming and Water Exercises

Life on earth evolved from the water. Perhaps it's appropriate, then, that humans return to the water for fitness and health.

In many ways swimming is *the* ideal form of exercise. It builds cardiovascular fitness, and, because it uses the back, upper body, and arms, it builds balanced muscular strength. Swimming also has the unique advantage of enhancing the body's flexibility. Above all, swimming is easy on muscles, joints, and bones; because water is buoyant, it supports 90 percent of the body's weight, greatly reducing the risk of injury.

For all its assets, swimming has four drawbacks.

First, it requires ability. Anyone can learn to swim, but it takes time and effort to learn to swim well. Fortunately, there are excellent aquatic alternatives. Aquadynamics are water exercises that can be performed by non-swimmers; many community pools and YMCAs offer instruction and group classes. Or you can wear a buoyant vest or belt that allows you to stay afloat so you can run in water, getting all the benefits of running without any of the trauma.

The second drawback to swimming is the risk of drowning. It's a small risk, but it must be taken seriously. Chapter 17 discusses the principles of aquatic safety.

The third disadvantage is the hardest to overcome: to swim, you need water. The logistics can be difficult, but this problem, too, can be solved; look for a lake or community pool in summer and a school, YMCA, or health club pool for use during the cool months.

Swimming's final drawback is that it lacks some of the metabolic benefits of weight-bearing exercises; it appears to be less efficient for weight loss, and it may be less effective in retaining calcium in bones. Still, it's excellent for improving cholesterol and blood sugar metabolism as well as for cardiovascular conditioning and muscular endurance — with a very low risk of injury.

Lap swimming is a solitary activity. At first it may seem boring, but the peacefulness can be relaxing and the rhythmic exercise invigorating. Consider getting in the swim of things for fitness, health, and pleasure.

Biking

Requiring only a modicum of skill and coordination, biking can be enjoyed by people of all ages and fitness levels. But unlike walking, running, and swimming, biking requires an additional element — a machine.

Depending on your preferences, the machine is either biking's beauty or its bane. If you are a gadgeteer, you'll love to study the advantages of ten-speed racers, mountain bikes, and all-terrain hybrid models. If you are a tinkerer, you'll love to adjust and tune your machine. But even if your childhood three-speed remains your ideal, you can select a durable and serviceable bicycle and enjoy it for fitness, for recreational touring, and even for transportation.

Biking is good for the heart and circulation, the metabolism, and the leg muscles. As a low-impact form of exercise, it spares muscles and joints from most overuse injuries. But accidents are a major threat. More people are injured while riding than during any other recreational activity; chapter 17 details the prevention of biking accidents, stressing the importance of high-quality helmets and prudent pedaling.

Accidents and traffic, inclement weather, and moderately costly equipment are the only significant drawbacks of biking. You can ride away from these limitations while experiencing the benefits of biking by using a stationary cycle. Whether on the road or in your rec room, biking is a splendid fitness option.

Aerobic Dance

Long familiar as a performing art, a social skill, and a romantic recreation, dance took its proper place as a fitness activity in the 1970s. Dance has two key advantages: it provides a unique brand of camaraderie that can help motivate regular participation, and it conditions all major muscle groups. Because traditional aerobic dance is a high-impact activity, its major drawback is its potential to cause musculoskeletal injury. Dance injuries can be minimized by careful stretching and warm-ups, high-quality aerobic shoes, good instruction, and resilient dance floors. Newer low-impact dance techniques are also very promising.

I'm told that another advantage of dance is its modest requirement for skill. My own attempts to keep up with dance classes lead me to question this assertion. But most people have the grace and coordination I lack, so they can use aerobic dance to attain the fitness I've earned by running, walking, and swimming.

Skating

Ice-skating, roller-skating, and the newest craze, roller-blading, are all excellent endurance activities. They can be used to build aerobic fitness, to condition leg muscles, to have fun, and to compete. They do require equipment that can be expensive, and they demand moderate levels of skill and coordination. Falls and accidents also must be counted among the drawbacks of skating. Still, skating is a low-impact sport that glides nicely into a balanced fitness program.

Cross-Country Skiing

Although downhill skiing is far more popular, cross-country skiing is far superior for fitness. Unlike downhill skiing, cross-country is superb for aerobic training; it also provides excellent muscular conditioning for the arms, back, and trunk as well as the legs. As a low-impact sport, cross-country skiing causes few overuse injuries. Accidents are less common and less serious than they are on the downhill slopes. Cross-country gear is less expensive than downhill equipment; still, it makes walking shoes or swim goggles look like a bargain.

The downside of cross-country skiing, of course, is its absolute dependence on snow. You don't have to drive to a mountain or wait in a lift line to ski cross-country, but you do have to wait for the white stuff. But if your climate features snowy winters, cross-country skiing is a wonderful way to shake the February blahs. You'll find the skiing best on groomed trails, the scenery best on country roads, but the convenience best at the closest golf course. Take a few lessons to learn the relatively easy cross-country technique. Rent equipment to be sure cross-country is for you before you invest in your own gear. It's certainly more complicated than simply heading out your front door to walk or jog, but cross-country skiing can provide a wonderful workout that may even help you look forward to winter.

Needless to say, even the most devoted cross-country skier needs other forms of exercise to stay fit and healthy the year round. A cross-country ski machine can do the trick — and it can also bring all the fitness benefits of the sport to people who would rather never see a snowflake.

Rowing

Like cross-country skiing, rowing is an esoteric sport. It rivals cross-country in its splendid attributes: superior cardiovascular conditioning, balanced muscular development, low impact, and few injuries. But although rowing ranks at the top for fitness, it ranks last for practicality. Rowing requires very expensive equipment, rather special water conditions, and a moderately difficult technique.

Despite these drawbacks, rowing is gaining steadily in popularity. No longer the exclusive domain of elite prep schools and colleges, it's becoming widely available to many people through rowing clubs. If rowing is available to you, consider making it part of your balanced fitness program. Or consider a rowing machine; you won't have the support of other rowers, the pleasures of nature, or the thrill of succeeding in a new sport, but you'll get all the fitness benefits of rowing without its logistical and economic pitfalls.

Table 21-4. How Far You Must Go to Burn 2,000 Calories

Activity	Distance
Swimming	5 miles
Walking	20 miles
Running	20 miles
Cross-country skiing	20 miles
Skating	60 miles
Biking	100 miles

Aerobic Sports and Your Exercise Quota

So many sports, so little time. Many considerations will influence your choice of sports; since all will help keep you healthy, you can let convenience, efficiency, expense, ability, and simple personal preference govern your decision. Best of all, try your hand (and your feet!) at a variety of activities, and build the ones you like best into a balanced exercise program.

You can use tables 21-1 and 21-2 to compare the efficiency and intensity of various exercises. Table 21-4 offers another way to compare aerobic sports.

There is no short cut to fitness. But if you put in your miles on a regular basis, you'll travel all the way to health and longevity.

Competitive Sports

Don't count on competitive sports to get into shape. Instead, use aerobic sports or exercise machines to get into aerobic shape. Add the flexibility drills and supplementary strength work you need. Then use your balanced fitness to enjoy competitive sports; you'll play better and have fewer injuries. And after you've walked your way into shape, you can count your games toward your healthful exercise quota (see tables 21-1 and 21-2).

Table 21-5 compares the pros and cons of selected competitive and recreational sports to help you decide how they can best fill your needs for fitness and enjoyment.

■ Home Exercise Machines

Although most Americans are sedentary, many are caught up in the idea of fitness. Running, tennis, and aerobic dance have taken turns as the leading exercise fads. Exercise machines are the current trend-setters; in 1990 Americans spent more than $1.8 billion on home exercise equipment, a threefold increase over the 1980 expenditure.

Exercise machines offer many advantages. Because they can be installed in the home, they are extremely convenient. They're excellent for aerobic fitness and muscular conditioning. Little skill is required to use exercise machines, but a few minutes of instruction will help ensure that they are used properly. When used correctly, they'll cause very few injuries. Finally, exercise machines can be adapted to every fitness level, from low-intensity exercise to training for competition.

Each machine is available in many models. In general, the low-end varieties tend to be flimsy and hard to adjust precisely. But many modestly to moderately priced machines are sturdy and efficient. At the high end are sleek devices with bells, whistles, and computers to record caloric consumption, speed, and mileage; these gadgets are not necessary for fitness, but they can help provide feedback and motivation.

Despite their many advantages, exercise machines have a drawback; often, they gather dust. Good intentions motivate people to buy exercise machines. Unfortunately, it soon becomes clear that it takes more than intentions to achieve fitness. Machines won't make you fit; only your muscles, your sweat, and your time will.

Nothing illustrates the gap between plans and practice as well as the stationary bicycle. A leading manufacturer of exercise bikes conducted a survey of its customers, expecting to document the durability of its product. Indeed, their bikes rarely broke down — in no small part because the average total lifetime use per machine was just 87 miles! Needless to say, the survey results never made it to Madison Avenue. In my own experience with hundreds of patients and friends, exercise bikes have proven again and again to be extremely efficient devices for cardiovascular fitness that feature two pedals, one seat, and no rider.

Exercise machines are great — if you use them. If they appeal to you, try them at a health club or YMCA to decide if their appeal will last, then invest in a sturdy, durable model for your home.

Stationary bikes really don't deserve to be singled out as a cautionary tale; they're used less often than other exercise machines only because they're purchased more often. Indeed, stationary bikes are the workhorses of most fitness programs, including Harvard's Cardiovascular Health Center.

Stationary bikes are reasonably compact and quiet; without the frills, they're economical, too. Injuries are very infrequent; knee discomfort is usually the first signal that you're doing too much.

Look for a sturdy bike with a rigid frame, adjustable handlebars, and a comfortable seat that adjusts easily to fit your anatomy. Pick a bike that pedals smoothly; in general, the bikes with the heaviest flywheels are the smoothest. One-piece pedals with stirrups are best. Above all, look for precise, easy-to-use resistance settings.

If stationary bikes are the old reliables of fitness, *stair climbers* are the newest craze. There is nothing new, of course, about climbing stairs. As a daily activity walking upstairs can contribute significantly to fitness. For years college athletes have run up stadium steps to build endurance. Doctors used stairs for the earliest exercise stress tests. Aerobic dancers have caught on, too, often incorporating step aerobics into their routines.

Stair climbing for fitness caught fire in 1985 with the introduction of the StairMaster. More than 8 million StairMasters are sold each year, mostly to health clubs. And in the past few years many high-quality, affordable machines have been sold for home use.

Stair climbers provide intensity without impact. At maximum levels you can burn up to 50 percent more calories than you can running; few people, however, can achieve this intensity, though many are attracted to stair climbers for a "quick fix." Still, if your expectations are realistic and you spend enough on your climber, you'll build aerobic fitness and you'll condition your leg muscles. Because the impact is low, injuries are few. Since stair climbers are relatively new, however, it will take more time to be sure that repetitive intense climbing is truly easy on the knees.

Stair climbers at health clubs allow you to program varied and challenging workouts. But at a tenth the cost, home climbers can do the job nicely. Look for a machine with large, comfortable pedals, a sturdy frame, and adjustable handrails that fit your height. The step height, too, should be adjustable to match your natural stride. Above all, look for smooth piston action and easy-to-use, precise resistance setups.

Like bikes and stair climbers, *treadmills* can be used for aerobic fitness

Table 21-5. A Comparison of Sports

	Aerobic training efficiency	Muscular conditioning		
		Legs	Back and trunk	Arms
Aerobic activity				
Walking	Moderate	Moderate	Low	Low
Running	High	High	Low	Low
Swimming	High	Moderate	High	High
Biking	High	Moderate	Low	Low
Aerobic dance	High	Moderate	Moderate	Moderate
Cross-country skiing	High	High	Moderate	Moderate
Skating	High	Moderate	Low	Low
Rowing	High	High	High	High
Competitive sports				
Baseball	Low	Low	Low	Low
Basketball	Moderate	Moderate	Low	Low
Bowling	Low	Low	Low	Low
Golf	Low*	Low	Low	Low
Gymnastics	Moderate	High	High	High
Downhill skiing	Low	High	Moderate	Low
Soccer	Moderate	High	Low	Low
Tennis	Moderate	High	Moderate	Moderate

*Moderate if golfers walk the course carrying their clubs

and for endurance conditioning of leg muscles. Like bikes and stair climbers, treadmills come in deluxe, computerized health club models and in utilitarian versions for use at home. Affordable home models, however, tend to be flimsy; unlike club or hospital treadmills, they are not motorized, so they can be hard to adjust precisely. And if you move up to high-intensity exercise on a treadmill, your legs will be subjected to the impact of jogging and running.

Rowing machines and *cross-country ski machines* have an advantage over bikes and stair climbers: they exercise the upper body as well as the legs. Both machines come in lower-priced models that use pistons to provide resistance and in expensive models that use cables and flywheels. Both do the job, but the flywheels can be adjusted more precisely, and have smoother action that mimics the "feel" and motion of rowing or skiing.

■ Exercising for Flexibility

People should not exercise for aerobics alone. Flexibility exercises are also important: they help prevent injuries and bring grace and coordination to

Impact	Injury potential	Accident potential	Requirement for skill	Convenience
Low	Low	Low	Low	High
High	Moderate	Low	Low	High
Low	Low	Moderate	Moderate	Low
Low	Low	High	Low	High
Moderate to low	Moderate to low	Low	Low	Moderate
Low	Low	Moderate	Moderate	Low
Low	Low	High	Moderate	Low (ice) High (roller)
Low	Low	Moderate	Moderate	Low
Low	Moderate	Moderate	High	Moderate
High	High	Moderate	High	Moderate
Low	Low	Low	Moderate	Moderate
Low	Low	Low	High	Moderate
Low	Moderate	Moderate	High	Moderate
Low	Moderate	High	High	Low
Moderate	Moderate	Low	Moderate	Moderate
Moderate	Moderate	Low	High	Moderate

your body at work and at play. Last but not least, stretching exercises will make your body feel good and your mind feel relaxed.

Although some people are naturally more limber than others, all people tend to become stiffer as they grow older. Although it may seem paradoxical, endurance exercise can also impair flexibility because as muscles grow stronger, they become tighter and stiffer. All in all, the older you get and the more you work out, the more you need to stretch. You may never recapture the loose and limber ligaments of youth, but you will improve; like aerobic fitness, flexibility is an acquired trait.

Like any form of exercise, stretching can do more harm than good if it is overdone or done badly. Listen to your body, never stretching to the point of pain. Plan a routine that is suited to your body and your needs. Because most people exercise predominantly with their legs, lower body stretching is a high priority. People who use their arms for work or sports should also stretch their shoulder and neck muscles. Because all people are vulnerable to back sprains and pain, all should exercise to promote back flexibility. Start with a basic stretching routine:

Achilles stretch
Calf stretch
Hamstring stretch
Thigh stretch
Hip stretch
Groin stretch
Leg spread
Williams exercise for the back
Cat's back exercise
Shoulder stretch
Neck stretch

Detailed directions for doing these stretches are available in most fitness books; if you have special needs, consult a physical therapist, qualified trainer, or yoga teacher; an individualized flexibility prescription can be a real asset for fitness.

When should you stretch? Early and often. Stretching can be a great way to limber up at the start of the day and to relax at bedtime. Best of all, incorporate stretching into the warm-up and cool-down routines that should surround every aerobic workout. Flexibility exercises don't take long, but their rewards will stretch on for months and years of musculo-skeletal fitness and health.

■ Exercising for Strength

Until quite recently, most people associated physical fitness with the muscular physique of the weight lifter. At present, fitness is more likely to evoke the lean look of the marathoner or the supple grace of the dancer. These images need not be contradictory; although aerobic fitness and musculoskeletal flexibility are of prime importance to health and prevention, muscular strength is also important. Strong muscles look better, but they also work better; strength training can improve your ability to perform well in sports, to function efficiently in daily life, and to avoid injuries.

There are three ways to exercise for strength: by using your body's own weight in calisthenics, by using dumbbells and barbells, and by using machines such as Nautilus. All are adaptable to the training strategy that is best for health. The trick is simple: reduce resistance and increase repetitions. Instead of lifting a 100-pound weight once, for example, lift a ten-pound weight ten times. You'll build your muscles, but you'll minimize the stress on your circulation.

You'll need to join a health club or YMCA to use Nautilus machines, and you'll need instruction to use them properly. I'm all for it, as long as you don't let strength training become a substitute for aerobic exercise. Some health clubs promote Nautilus circuit training as an alternative to aerobics. But although circuit training's fast-paced, high-repetition, low-resistance routine is good for muscles, it provides only limited benefit to the heart, circulation, and metabolism. Strength training — even using circuit training programs — should be used as a supplement to aerobics, but never as a substitute for endurance exercise.

You can develop very nice strength-training routines at home using calisthenics alone; as you improve, light weights may give you an extra lift. As with all forms of exercise go slowly, listening to your body as you progress. You don't need to push yourself very hard to benefit from strength training; 15 minutes twice a week is a reasonable goal. Here is a basic strength-training routine:

Calisthenics	Weights
Windmills	Lateral raises
Body twists	Curls
Knee-ups	Press
Push-ups	Front and rear raises
Leg raises	
Side leg raises	
Bent-knee sit-ups	

Detailed directions are available in most fitness books; if you have special needs, consult an exercise instructor or sports trainer.

■ Exercising for Speed

Runners call them intervals, swimmers call them sprints, and rowers call them power pieces. By any name, speed training means going all out — not just once, but over and over again.

As you know, I urge you to exercise for endurance and aerobic fitness. I encourage you to exercise for flexibility. And I recommend at least a bit of exercise for strength. But I discourage exercising for speed — unless you are preparing for competitive sports. Still, you can use the principles of interval drills to improve your aerobic training; alternate hard and easy exercise, applying the stress of the more intensive periods only in a controlled, graduated fashion.

■ Exercise-induced injuries

Although the human body is built for vigorous physical activity, it can be injured by exercise. Most often injuries are caused simply by *overuse,* by doing too much too soon. Injuries can also result from *overstress,* from a single false step or excessive motion that damages tissues. *Muscle imbalance* and the *lack of flexibility* also predispose to injuries. *Poor equipment* and *improper technique* are the other major causes of tissue damage. A balanced exercise program should be able to correct all these problems before they cause harm.

You don't need a degree in medicine, nursing, or physical therapy to treat most sports injuries. Instead, seven simple principles — and a lot of common sense — will do the job.

First, recognize the injury. It sounds simple, and it is. But an amazing number of athletes deny their symptoms, ignoring mild pain, swelling, discoloration, or dysfunction until the problem has become undeniably, and unnecessarily, large.

Second, identify the cause so you can correct it. If it's overuse, reduce your exercise schedule. If it's faulty technique, get some instruction. If it's poor equipment, treat yourself to new gear. If it's muscle imbalance, strengthen your weak muscles. If it's inflexibility, stretch.

Third, use RICE to treat acute soft tissue injuries. Don't be confused: I'm not hauling you back to the chapter on nutrition, but I am advocating a four-point program that contains more than a grain of truth. You can prevent many problems by instituting the RICE program as soon as you've identified an injury:

- Rest: Stop using the injured structure, and don't resume until it's better.
- Ice: An ice pack is the best way to reduce inflammation in its early stages. Apply an ice pack to the injured area for 15 minutes, and repeat ice treatments four times a day for the first 48 hours.
- Compression: A simple elastic bandage can provide lots of protection and support. Wrap it tightly enough to provide support, but be sure it's not so snug that it impairs your circulation.
- Elevation: Let gravity help prevent inflammation. Prop up your injured leg or arm so that tissue fluids will drain away instead of adding to the swelling, pressure, and discomfort.

Fourth, consider taking aspirin or ibuprofen to treat inflammation or pain. You must be cautious with all forms of self-treatment; be doubly cautious with medications, even ones you can buy without a prescription. Read the warnings and precautions on the drug labels, and follow them to the letter.

Fifth, begin rehabilitation. As you begin to feel better, switch from four-a-day ice treatments to four-a-day heat treatments, using a heating pad or hot water bottle for 15 minutes. Follow each heat treatment with gentle range-of-motion movements. As you improve, resume daily activities. Finally, you can return to exercise — but do so cautiously and gradually. Even when you're back to full activity, it can help to apply heat before exercise and ice afterwards.

Sixth, be prepared to get help. In most cases you can take care of your own injuries. But if your problem is unusual, serious, or stubborn, consult a doctor, physical therapist, or sports trainer. If your usual health care providers are not knowledgeable about exercise, find ones who are; sports medicine clinics are available in most communities, providing excellent multidisciplinary care for exercise-induced injuries.

Last, work toward a balanced program that will provide all the benefits of exercise while reducing the risk of recurrent injury. Nearly 300 years ago John Dryden explained that exercise itself can be the key to the rehabilitation and prevention of sports injuries: "The wise, for cure, on exercise depend. God never meant his work for man to mend."

■ Creating a Balanced Exercise Program

Exercise is essential for optimal health. But to be able to work out often enough, long enough, and hard enough to reap all the benefits of exercise, you'll have to avoid injuries, boredom, and frustration. The key is a balanced exercise program.

Here are 20 tips for creating a program of your own:

1. Make physical activity part of your daily life. Modern mechanization is a great time saver, but it's hardly a health saver. Don't turn away from the twentieth century, but don't fail to seek ways to use your natural muscle power.

Walk whenever you can. Walk for transportation. When distances are too great or your time too short, compromise: get off the bus a stop or two early or hunt for a parking space farther away from your destination. Walk stairs (especially up!) whenever you can; start with a flight or two at a time, then gradually see how far you can get. But as you discover your legs, be sure to remember your feet; comfortable, supportive shoes are just as important on the office stairs as running shoes are on the track.

Look for other excuses to use your body. Carry your own groceries and parcels. Try gardening. Consider an old-fashioned hand mower — or, if you use a power mower, make a commitment to use the time you've saved to work out.

Daily activities will not put you in the aerobic training range. They are not a substitute for a formal exercise program. But every little bit helps. Do as much as you can; you'll enjoy your new sense of independence, and you'll save time that was wasted waiting for an elevator, bus, or parking space.

2. Get a physical examination before you start a serious fitness program. Although it sounds formidable, this evaluation is really very simple; it amounts to little more than a thorough checkup, with particular attention to your cardiovascular system, joints, and muscles. The only extra test that should be considered is an exercise stress test. The American Heart Association recommends stress tests prior to vigorous exercise programs for all people over 40. It's an appealing idea, since its goal is to detect hidden heart disease during controlled exercise in the hospital so it won't crop up unexpectedly in the gym. Unfortunately, the stress test is not all it's made out to be.

Chapter 2 details the pros and cons of stress testing. Expense and inconvenience are among the negatives, but they would be easily outweighed if stress tests prevented cardiac problems during exercise. Can stress tests do this? Not very well. A 1991 study by Dr. David Siscovick and his colleagues evaluated pre-exercise stress testing in 3,617 men between ages 35 and 59. All subjects were free of known cardiovascular disease, but all had high cholesterol levels, making them prime candidates for hidden coronary heart disease. Still, *annual* exercise testing predicted only 18 percent of the cardiac problems that developed during the study period, which averaged seven years. Even though stress testing was not useful, exercise itself was quite safe in these high-risk men, with only 2 percent developing exertion-induced heart problems during the seven years of exercise.

Before Dr. Siscovick's results were published, I recommended routine pre-exercise stress tests for men over 50 and women over 60, even if they were perfectly healthy. Now I'm doubtful that routine stress tests are useful in healthy people of any age. Despite the recommendations of the Heart Associates, many doctors agree: only 17 percent of physicians who run marathons have had stress tests done on themselves.

Stress testing remains mandatory before people with suspected heart disease begin vigorous exercise programs. But for healthy people, the general guidelines cited in chapter 2 seem best.

3. Make exercise a priority. True, time is a precious commodity — but so is health. Don't count on *finding* the time for exercise; make the time. President Bush makes time to run, walk, lift weights, use a stair climber, pitch horseshoes, and play tennis and "aerobic golf." True, he doesn't swim for fitness. But Mrs. Bush spends an hour a day in the White House pool. If the president and his wife can make the time to exercise, so can you.

4. Choose the exercises that are right for you. There are many ways to get an aerobic workout. Don't take up jogging simply because your neighbor runs. Instead, pick the activity best suited to your body and to your personal preference, skills, and athletic experience. Take convenience, cost, and social considerations into account. You are much more likely to stick with a program if it's handy, affordable, and enjoyable. Remember to

include exercises for flexibility in your program, and consider some strength training as well. Never stint on warm-ups or cool-downs.

5. Set realistic goals. Health is your first priority, but recreational and even competitive goals are also worthwhile. But in each sphere your aspirations must match your fitness level and skills.

6. Make progress slowly but steadily. Shakespeare said it best in *Romeo and Juliet:* "Too swift arrive as tardy as too slow." Fitness takes time to develop; if you try to do too much too soon, you'll find yourself back at the starting line. But with patience and persistence, you are likely to find that your "realistic" goals were actually lower than necessary. If so, raise your expectations a notch, again giving yourself enough time to achieve your new targets.

7. Keep a fitness log. Record the type and amount of your exercises and how you feel. If losing weight is among your goals, jot down your weight every week. Your progress may seem slow, but if you look back over your log after a month or two, you'll be amazed to find how far you've come.

8. Exercise regularly. Weekend athletes are the most likely to become weekday patients. One-season athletes are even more vulnerable. Don't try to pack a week's exercise into a single day; there is no substitute for regular exercise.

9. Be flexible. Important as they are, your goals and plans should not become rigid ultimatums. It's okay to slack off if you're very busy, and it's mandatory to cut back if you're injured or ill. Be sure to get back on track when things return to normal, but don't try to make up for lost days by overdoing your exercises.

10. Adjust your activities according to the weather. Heat, humidity, and air pollution are always hard to take, but they can make exercise downright hazardous. Cold temperatures, ice, and snow can be equally difficult. Follow the guidelines in chapter 22 to avoid thermal illnesses during exercise.

11. Aim for variety. If you learn to master a mix of activities, you'll be able to develop balanced fitness. By alternating your exercise routines, you'll reduce your risk of injury — and you'll find it much easier to compensate for changes in the weather and in your schedule. Variety will also prevent you from getting stale, keeping your exercise interesting and enjoyable. Variety is the spice of fitness.

12. Eat and drink appropriately. The nutritional requirements of athletes are no different from the needs of sedentary people, except that athletes need more calories and more water. If your goals include weight loss, don't increase your caloric intake until your weight is where you want it. If you need extra calories to maintain your weight, get them from complex carbohydrates. But don't eat anything at all during the two-hour period prior to vigorous exercise. Remember, however, to drink plenty of fluids before, during, and after exercise, particularly in hot weather.

13. Dress appropriately. Style and sparkle are great, but comfort and convenience should be your first priority. Learn to match your clothing to your climate.

14. Use high-quality equipment. Remember that your shoes are the most important equipment for weight-bearing exercises. Be sure they are well made and well fitting; break them in gradually, but change them before they become well worn.

15. Make safety a high priority. Avoid traffic whenever possible. Walkers and runners should always face traffic, while bikers should ride with the traffic; all should wear bright clothing, including reflectors if it's dark. And all should be extremely defensive on the roads. Be wary, too, of dogs — and, I'm sorry to say, of suspicious-looking people. Always wear a helmet for riding a bike (or a horse) and goggles or safety glasses for racquet sports. Swimming and boating require special precautions. Chapter 17 details many of these safety tips.

16. Exercise with other people. It's true that there is safety in numbers, which is particularly important for female walkers and runners. But companionship is also very helpful for motivation and enjoyment.

17. Get instruction. Often an experienced exercise companion can provide helpful tips to get you over the rough spots. If not, consult an exercise instructor or coach; there are no short cuts to fitness, but there are lots of tricks that can make exercise easier and safer.

18. Learn new sports. The challenge and stimulation of new activities will help motivate you to stay fit. Take lessons to help master new sports.

19. Consider entering competition. Don't aim to become a pro, and don't expect a six-figure contract to endorse athletic shoes. But everyone who finishes a fun run or a road race is a winner. Tennis tournaments, basketball leagues, and swim meets are often stratified by age and ability; if you can find one that's right for you, the challenge and companionship of competition may help motivate you to exercise regularly.

20. Listen to your body. Once you've achieved fitness, its message will be positive; you'll actually feel a *need* to exercise. But even after you become devoted to exercise, you can never afford to overlook your body's distress signals.

Exercise only when you are feeling well. Minor aches in your muscles and joints may call for nothing more than extra stretching and warming up, but more substantial discomfort or illness calls for reduced exercise or rest.

Be particularly alert for any symptoms that may suggest heart problems, including pressure or pain in the chest, neck, jaw, or arms, a rapid or irregular pulse, unexpected breathlessness, undue fatigue, excessive sweating, nausea, and fainting or light-headedness. Listen, too, for warnings from your other internal organs, including your nervous system (headaches), lungs (breathlessness or wheezing), your intestinal tract (heartburn, diarrhea, or bleeding), your reproductive organs (menstrual irregularities), and your urinary tract (bleeding). Fortunately, none of these problems is common, and all can be managed successfully — if you recognize them and report them to your doctor. Musculoskeletal aches and pains related to exercise are much more common but are usually amenable to self-treatment — if you recognize them early and react appropriately.

The personal stereo is almost as much a part of the fitness scene as running shoes and T-shirts. Listen to music, listen to news, listen to exercise tapes. But always listen to the signals from your own body.

In 1873 Edward Stanley, the earl of Derby, wrote, "Those who think they have not time for bodily exercise will sooner or later have to find time for illness." More than a century later exercise remains the best-kept secret in preventive medicine. It's a sorry condition, but one that you can correct. Once you know the secret, you can plan an exercise program that will be safe, effective, and enjoyable. It will take some thought and some time — and it will take lots of work. But your rewards will be a lifetime of fitness, health, and fun.

▪ 22 ▪

The Environment
and Your Health

The human species is a newcomer to the planet Earth. Throughout the 40,000 years of human existence, people have depended on their world for sustenance, shelter, and survival. Nature has provided the air, water, and food required for health. But nature has also threatened health with droughts, floods, fires, earthquakes, and other natural disasters. Now, as 40,000 years ago, human health depends on the environment. In this respect humankind is no different from other living things.

During the past 200 years, however, the environment has come to depend on human activity. Unlike other species, humans have the ability to change nature. For millennia these changes were gradual and subtle. But with industrialization humankind began to exert an enormous impact on the natural world, an impact that is increasing every year.

Human activity has changed the water and land nearly everywhere on the earth's surface; altered, too, is the atmosphere that surrounds the globe. Many of these changes reflect the improved standard of living enjoyed by current generations in affluent societies. Many, however, threaten the health of future generations.

▪ How Humanity Affects the Environment

Environmental abuse occurs when good things are taken out of nature's cycles or when bad things are put in. Both resource depletion and environmental pollution have resulted from two events, the industrial revolution and the population explosion.

The earth's resources are finite. In just one year, however, humanity consumes the amount of energy it took nature 1 million years to produce. In just the past four decades the planet has lost 20 percent of its topsoil. A huge amount of water has been removed from the hydrologic cycle, with a volume equal to all of Lake Huron being lost each year. The earth's forests have shrunk by 2 million square miles, an area larger than all of Europe; tropical rain forests are being destroyed at the rate of one and a half acres per second.

Even as our natural resources are shrinking, they are being asked to support an unprecedented explosion of human numbers. It took 40,000 years for the human population to reach 1 billion but less than another 200 years for the population to reach 5 billion. Nearly 80 percent of all the people who have ever lived have been born in the past 50 years. And the population bomb continues to tick: our planet is being asked to support an additional 88 million people each year.

To sustain increasing numbers of people in the face of declining resources, humans have turned to new means of agriculture, irrigation, and production. The by-products of these new technologies contribute to environmental change, much of which is permanent. In the past 200 years industrial output has increased one hundredfold. In this time the concentration of carbon dioxide in the atmosphere has increased by 25 percent and the concentration of methane by 100 percent. In the past 50 years human endeavors have resulted in an eightfold increase in industrial output, electricity production, and numbers of automobiles. But the costs of productivity include the 6 billion tons of carbon emissions that will be added to the atmosphere from this year's combustion of fossil fuels, to say nothing of the countless tons of solid wastes and chemical toxins that will be deposited in our soil, water, and air.

As we enter the twenty-first century, the developed nations bear most responsibility for industrial pollution while the underdeveloped world contributes most to the population explosion. And all countries share blame for depleting the earth's resources, with wealthier lands consuming the most energy and poorer ones depleting the greater share of the world's forests, grasslands, crop lands, and water.

Environmental problems are global problems.

■ How the Environment Affects Your Health

The environment is not a usual concern of preventive medicine. But I'm asking you to include it in your program of prevention for two reasons. First, many ailments that afflict people today result from environmental exposures. The current epidemic of melanomas and other skin cancers caused by depletion of the stratospheric ozone layer is only one example. Second, the specter of environmental illnesses looms over future generations. We must act now to prevent environmental hazards from causing these epidemics in the technological era ahead.

■ The Role of Preventive Medicine

The concept that humankind's external environment affects its internal environment, or health, is hardly new. The Greek physician Hippocrates wrote, "Whoever wishes to investigate medicine properly should proceed thus: in the first place to consider the seasons of the year . . . then the winds . . . common to all countries, and . . . to each locality." Roman physicians, too, recognized the importance of environmental illnesses; indeed, the naturalist Pliny correctly blamed mercury poisoning for the deaths of many Roman miners.

But as the number and complexity of environmentally induced diseases have increased in the modern world, so too have the challenges facing medicine. Can physicians offer guidance to environmentalists, engineers, economists, and politicians? Not much, perhaps. But preventive medicine *has* learned a lesson that is being overlooked. Most of our environmental efforts are now devoted to secondary prevention, to limiting damage after we've created it. Scrubbers that clean up power plant emissions are an example. Like medications that treat coronary artery disease they are useful and important, but they do not address the root cause of the problem. Instead of taking a Band-Aid approach, we need to address the underlying illness. Medicine calls this primary prevention, and it would benefit the planet's health as it does human health. Instead of merely prescribing drugs to bolster the sick heart, we should be preventing atherosclerosis with diet, exercise, smoking cessation, blood pressure control, and stress reduction. Instead of simply removing industrial pollutants after they're manufactured, the world's leaders, too, should practice primary prevention by promoting energy conservation and finding alternatives to fossil fuels.

■ Your Role in Environmental Health

The environment poses complex global problems, far beyond the reach of any one individual, group, or nation. But solutions must start with each person, acting one at a time. In this chapter we'll explore the ways you can evaluate your own environment and make the changes necessary to prevent illness in yourself and your family. We'll also peek beyond the confines of human health to look briefly at the simple things each of us can do to preserve the world's health.

Although individual actions are necessary, we also need to act together as a community, indeed as a community of nations, to arrive at lasting solutions. To protect individual human health we must collectively protect the environment's health. But even here progress must begin with personal efforts. If you agree that the environment is important for your health today and critical for your children's health tomorrow, you should begin to consider the ways you can exert political pressure to achieve social change.

You can make a difference. If you won't, who will?

■ Toxins

Not even the most dedicated environmentalist would advocate the return to a preindustrial economy to protect the environment. Not even the most health-conscious consumer would advocate the elimination of all chemicals to protect health. How can we tell which environmental factors really cause illness so we can concentrate our corrective efforts where they'll do the most good?

How Are Toxins Identified?

Environmental health hazards can be recognized in three ways. The first clues often come from observations of individual cases: a patient is able to relate an illness to an exposure, and a doctor is alert enough to understand the significance of the association. But causality is hard to establish from just a few cases; indeed, many suspected links don't withstand scientific scrutiny. The second way to establish toxicity is through epidemiology; in large population groups the hazards of toxins become clear because hundreds or thousands of cases can be linked to exposure. Finally, animal experiments can be used to document toxicity. Scientists share the public's concern for animal welfare but understand that careful and humane experiments are sometimes the only way to identify toxins, establish acceptable exposure levels, and discover the remedies that will prevent human illness and save human lives.

What Determines Risk to Human Health?

Even after the toxicity of a substance is proven, however, its potential to cause human disease is far from certain. Risk depends on three factors. The first is *the route of exposure*. Most toxins enter the body through the lungs, the intestinal tract, or the skin.

The second factor is the *intensity of exposure;* the risk of illness depends on the dose of the toxin and the duration of exposure. Although in an ideal world we'd like to avoid all exposures, it's comforting to know that in the real world low doses of many toxins are safe; x rays are an example of a potential toxin that is extremely hazardous in large doses but harmless in small amounts.

The third factor in risk is *individual susceptibility*. Allergies can render a substance extremely dangerous to one person even though it's harmless to others. Underlying diseases can enhance susceptibility; smog, for example, is much more dangerous to patients with emphysema than to people with healthy lungs. Finally, co-factors can affect susceptibility; asbestos is 50 times more dangerous to smokers than to nonsmokers.

Toxins and Your Body: Patterns of Illness

Environmental toxins can cause *disease and dysfunction of the body's organ systems*. Sometimes the damage is immediate, as in the case of carbon monoxide poisoning. In other cases the damage is slow, depending on cumulative exposure; lead poisoning, for example, causes anemia and neurological dysfunction gradually as lead levels build up over months and years. Table 22-1 contains additional examples.

Environmental factors can also cause *cancer*, which always develops slowly. Although we still have much to learn about the way it happens, the basic scenario seems clear. Chemicals or radiation injure a cell's genetic material, DNA. Damaged DNA leads to abnormally rapid cell division. The body contains mechanisms to repair DNA and to detect and kill runaway cells. But if these mechanisms are overwhelmed, the damaged cells con-

Table 22-1. Selected Toxins That Damage Human Organs

Environmental toxins	Organ systems affected
Lead, carbon monoxide, arsenic, mercury, pesticides, organic solvents	brain and nervous system
Sulfur dioxide, nitrogen oxides, ozone, particulates, beryllium, asbestos, radon	respiratory tract
Carbon monoxide, carbon disulfide, cobalt, nitrates	heart and circulation
Carbon tetrachloride, aflatoxins, vinyl chloride, pesticides	liver
Nitrates, lead, fluoride	stomach and intestines
Benzene, lead, cadmium, mercury, pesticides	blood
Lead, cadmium, mercury, chromium, carbon tetrachloride, trichloroethylene, benzidine	kidney and urinary tract
Lead, fluoride	bones
Ultraviolet radiation, heavy metals	skin
Hydrocarbons	fat

tinue to proliferate in an uncontrolled manner, eventually increasing in number to be recognizable clinically as cancer. Table 22-2 lists some environmentally induced cancers.

The third type of environmentally induced illness is *reproductive toxicity*. The damage may occur long before pregnancy if egg or sperm cells are injured. More often, though, the damage occurs during pregnancy since fetal tissues tend to be much more vulnerable than adult organs. Reproductive toxicity can take the form of infertility, spontaneous miscarriage, or the birth of babies who are premature, ill, or deformed. Some reproductive toxins are:

Lead
Carbon monoxide
Methyl mercury
Polychlorinated biphenyls (PCBs)
Trichlorophenoxyacetic acid
Dioxin
Tobacco smoke, alcohol, illicit drugs, many medications

Are You Being Harmed by Environmental Toxins?

With so many potential toxins and such diverse types of toxicity, how can you tell if you are suffering from an environmentally induced illness? First, know if you are being exposed. Chapter 5 reviewed radon and chapter 7 discussed occupational exposures; in the next few pages you'll also learn how to evaluate the safety of your air, water, and food supplies. Second, listen to your body; if you have symptoms, discuss them with your doctor to see if they might be environmentally induced. In some cases simple blood tests can be used to determine if you've been exposed; lead is an example. Third, continue routine medical care and monitoring; if your history suggests particular exposures, your doctor may add special screening tests such as chest x rays and lung function tests for asbestos exposure.

When you think about environmentally induced illnesses, you'll focus chiefly on problems "they" have caused, on toxins, pollutants, and radiation produced by industry, agriculture, and governments on a massive scale. Remember, though, that the most dangerous toxins are not the responsibility of "them" but of "us": tobacco, alcohol, and illicit drugs are by far the toxins that cause the most human disease. Natural chemicals such as saturated fats, cholesterol, and salt are not far behind. Even "good" chemicals such as medications can have side effects that produce illness.

A final bit of advice: strike a balance between awareness and anxiety, between precautions and paranoia. This chapter, of course, stresses the things that can go wrong with our environment. They are important indeed, but most readers can protect themselves through simple precautions. And

Table 22-2. Proven Environmental Causes of Human Cancer

Carcinogen	Cancer site
Aflatoxin	liver
Aromatic amines	bladder
Arsenic	lung, skin
Asbestos	lung
Benzene	leukemia
Chloromethyl ether	lung
Chromium	lung
Ionizing radiation	almost all organs
Mustard gas	lung, larynx, sinuses
Nickel dust	lung, sinuses
Polycyclic hydrocarbons	lung, scrotum, skin
Radon	lung
Tobacco smoke	lung, mouth, larynx and throat, esophagus, pancreas, kidney, bladder
Ultraviolet radiation	skin, eye
Vinyl chloride	liver
Wood dust	sinuses

even though hundreds of chemicals can contribute to human disease, thousands are safe, actually contributing to human well-being. Think about your environment and work to improve it, but don't become unduly preoccupied. There is still plenty of enjoyment and safety in the natural world.

■ Air Pollution

Humankind has always worried about ill winds. Since the industrial revolution, however, a new problem has emerged: sick air. And it's a problem that's getting not better but worse. The air we breathe is in danger of becoming a toxic dump.

The earth's atmosphere is 99.9 percent nitrogen and oxygen. Although these gases have not changed in quantity or quality, the air has deteriorated, and the trace gases that account for only one tenth of 1 percent of the atmosphere are responsible.

Major Sources of Air Pollution

Fossil fuel combustion is the chief source of air pollution; industry accounts for two thirds and the world's 500 million automobiles for the rest.

What goes up must come down. What becomes of emissions that enter the air? Some remain in the atmosphere unchanged, but others are altered chemically by the action of sunlight. Water-soluble pollutants dissolve, returning to earth in rain or snow. Finally, some chemicals return directly to earth, being deposited on dry land and in water — and in human lungs.

Each of the major air pollutants causes unique problems.

Sulfur dioxide is produced by fossil fuel combustion and ore smelting. Sulfur dioxide itself produces few problems, though in very high concentrations it can irritate the respiratory tract. But sulfur dioxide undergoes chemical reactions in the atmosphere which transform it to sulfuric acid, a corrosive substance that dissolves in water and returns to earth as acid rain, acid dew, acid fog, and acid snow.

Nitrogen oxides are produced by fossil fuel combustion, with automobile tailpipes the major source. Other sources are fertilizers, deforestation, and biomass burning. Total emissions have doubled in the past 40 years. Like sulfur dioxide, nitrogen oxides undergo chemical reactions resulting in nitric acid, another component of acid rain. Excess nitrogen in water also stimulates the growth of algae, depleting oxygen and causing fish kills. Finally, nitrogen oxides react with hydrocarbons and sunlight to produce photochemical pollutants — smog. As smog, nitrogen oxides are extremely irritating to the respiratory tract, causing shortness of breath, coughing, irritation of the eyes and nasal passages, and increasing susceptibility to pneumonia.

Carbon dioxide, a greenhouse gas that contributes to global warming, is on the rise because of fossil fuel combustion and deforestation. In tropical and subtropical regions, large forests and grasslands are being burned to create range lands and crop lands; biomass combustion and deforestation increase atmospheric carbon dioxide. In high concentrations carbon dioxide is a central nervous system depressant, but atmospheric levels are very far below these toxic concentrations.

Carbon monoxide results from the incomplete combustion of fossil fuels and biomass burning. It displaces oxygen from the blood; commuters, urban pedestrians, and smokers often have blood carbon monoxide levels in excess of 4 percent. The results can be exercise intolerance, shortness of breath, abnormal cardiac rhythms, and angina.

Methane originates from fossil fuel products, the intestinal tracts of cattle, rice fields, and landfills. One of the greenhouse gases responsible for global warming, methane contributes to stratospheric ozone depletion but has no direct toxic action on the human respiratory tract.

Chlorinated fluorocarbons (CFCs) originate from refrigeration coolants, aerosol sprays, and foams. Though not directly toxic to humans, CFCs impair health indirectly by harming the atmosphere, depleting the stratospheric ozone layer and contributing to the greenhouse effect.

Ozone is a gas with a split personality. In the upper atmosphere, where it belongs, ozone is a good guy, shielding the earth from the sun's harmful ultraviolet rays. But at ground level ozone is produced from the interaction of nitrogen oxides, hydrocarbons, and sunlight. High-voltage electrical equipment and lightning generate some ozone, but fossil fuel combustion is its major source. Ground-level ozone, a major component of smog, is extremely irritating to the respiratory tract. Chronic lung disease, bronchitis, and heart disease can all be exacerbated by ozone. Asthmatics, too, can suffer from its effects; a 1991 study from Toronto found that ozone concentrations considered "safe" by the EPA (.12 parts per million) double the likelihood of allergy-induced asthma attacks. Is it any wonder that hospitalizations for asthma have nearly tripled in the United States since 1970?

Particulates. At last, an area in which we can report progress. Particulates contribute to "gray air" and respiratory tract irritation; soot is carcinogenic. But thanks to the Clean Air Acts of 1970 and 1977, all power plants in the United States are now equipped with electrostatic precipitators or filters that remove up to 99.5 percent of the particulates from smokestack emissions. In the United States particulate emissions declined by 62 percent between 1970 and 1987. Progress has been at least as good in Japan, Canada, and western Europe; unfortunately, eastern Europe and the developing nations lag far behind.

Lead. More progress. Our increasing use of unleaded gasoline has removed lead from the fuel pipe and the air. Nearly 35,000 tons of lead entered the air in 1984, but only 1,000 tons were emitted by American automobiles in 1988, and the amount continues to decline. Still, lead toxicity is a major public health problem in our country — not from air pollution but from paint and industry.

Sick Air and Sick People

Despite real progress with particulates and lead, air pollution remains a major problem. In 1987 alone American industry pumped 2.6 billion pounds of hazardous pollutants into the air, including 235 million pounds of cancer-causing chemicals. The EPA estimates that 150 million people in this country breathe unhealthy air. The American Lung Association reports that 382 counties, home to more than half of all Americans, are currently out of compliance with the EPA's own ozone standards. Los Angeles is the worst offender, averaging 138 days of dangerous ozone levels per year in the late 1980s.

In 1952 more than 4,000 Londoners were killed by the Black Fog, history's worst episode of air pollution. Such a calamity is most unlikely today. Still, the EPA estimates that 2,000 Americans die each year from cancer produced by air pollutants. Many thousands with chronic lung disease also die from pollution-induced respiratory failure, heart failure, and pneumonia. In other parts of the world such as eastern Europe, the problem is even more severe.

Air pollution is a leading cause of human illness today. But unless we change our ways, the worst is yet to come. Health will suffer even more from the long-term impact of air pollution, which includes the effects of stratospheric ozone depletion, global warming, and acid rain.

Controlling Air Pollution: National Priorities

What should be done to make the air healthy again? In the short term, tighter government standards will coerce industry to reduce emissions of sulfur dioxide and nitrogen oxides just as they reduced particulate emissions. The technology is already available: scrubbers can reduce sulfur dioxide from power plants by 95 percent, and selective catalytic reduction can do almost as well for nitrogen oxide. Japan has already upgraded 90 percent of its plants to utilize these techniques, which are admittedly very expensive. The United States lags far behind, but the Clean Air Act of 1990 will help.

Automobile efficiency should also be improved greatly. Engineers assert that the internal combustion engine can be made cleaner. Simply improving gas mileage would help immeasurably. For example, at 18 miles per gallon a single car produces 57.7 tons of carbon dioxide over its lifetime; at 28 miles per gallon only 37 tons would be emitted.

Technological improvements can also help protect the stratospheric ozone layer by replacing CFCs in aerosols and refrigerators. We've done a good job with the former but not the latter, again lagging behind much of the industrialized world.

Clean air will not come cheaply. Antipollution equipment to reduce sulfur dioxide and nitrogen oxides will cost American industry $4 billion annually, but at least as much will be saved by protecting farms, lakes, and forests. Reducing urban pollution and chemical emissions will be even more expensive, and the economic returns are harder to calculate. But air pollution itself is very expensive, costing up to $40 billion annually in health care and lost productivity, to say nothing of illness and death. Cleaning up the air and treating illness are both very costly; it's up to us to decide how to spend our money.

Even though modern technology is largely responsible for air pollution, high-tech Band-Aids will not provide long-term solutions. For that we need nothing less than a change in our value system to reduce our dependence on fossil fuels. It's a worldwide problem, but Americans are the worst offenders; each year we consume more than 1,000 gallons of oil per person, about twice the average for Japan and western Europe. We are in dire need of a national energy policy to prevent further damage to our country's economy, ecology, international security, and health.

Controlling Air Pollution: Personal Contributions

What can any one person do in the face of such overwhelming national and international problems? Plenty. We should all institute our own energy policies. Conservation is best: insulate, turn down the thermostat, purchase efficient lighting, cars, and appliances — and use them prudently.

To protect our environment and our health, we must reduce oil use. Forty-three percent of the oil used in America is consumed by private automobiles. Alternate transportation systems will help. But we need not abandon autos; merely increasing fuel economy from the present 27 miles per gallon to a technically feasible 40 miles per gallon would save 2.8 million barrels of oil each day.

Recycling will also go a long way toward conserving energy, thus reducing air pollution. Tips for recycling will appear later in this chapter.

Last but not least, you should support the development of alternative sources of energy, including solar, hydroelectric, wind, geothermal, biomass, and — if safety standards can be improved substantially — even nuclear power.

Protecting Your Health from Sick Air

It will take time and effort to improve the health of our air. Meanwhile, how can you protect your health from air pollution?

First and foremost, keep your heart and lungs healthy so you'll have enough reserve to cope with unavoidable pollution. Second, minimize your exposure. Add environmental quality to the equation when you choose a place to live and work. Don't exercise in areas of smog and urban pollution. Third, stay tuned for pollution alerts. Your eyes, nose, and lungs will let you know when ground-level ozone is very high, but your newspaper and radio station can give advance warning. You can't flee to the mountains every time air quality deteriorates, but you can stay indoors; I actually "prescribe" air conditioning and indoor refuge for my patients with heart and lung disease during air quality warnings. To be effective, however, this strategy requires clean indoor air.

■ Indoor Air Pollution

Environmental problems are global in impact, and their solutions are international in scope. Nevertheless, all pollution is local, at least initially; indoor air pollution is a case in point.

Almost as if we were anticipating outdoor air pollution, we have shut ourselves into tight urban towers that depend entirely on internal ventilation systems. The good news is that we can shut polluted air out; the bad news is that we can also shut polluted air *in*. All in all, indoor air pollution is currently a greater health hazard than outdoor air pollution. Fortunately, indoor pollution is easier to correct.

The Major Pollutants

The most dangerous form of indoor air pollution is tobacco smoke. Passive smoking is the third leading preventable cause of death in the United States, contributing to lung cancer, emphysema, heart disease, and all the other problems caused by firsthand smoking. The danger is great, but the solution is easy: no smoking. Designated smoking areas and good ventilation are important backup remedies. Public buildings, workplaces, and restaurants have made great strides in reducing indoor smoke exposure; do the same for your own house.

Tobacco smoke is easy to see and smell. But the second most dangerous indoor air pollutant is odorless and invisible. A natural radioactive gas, it is much more of a problem for private homes than for office and apartment buildings. It kills an estimated 16,000 Americans each year, most of whom have never heard of it. But if you've read chapter 5, you know how to test for it and how to eliminate it from your home. It's radon.

Another indoor air pollutant is asbestos. Like radon, asbestos causes cancer; like radon, it is especially dangerous to cigarette smokers. Asbestos has been a terrible problem for shipyard employees and other workers. Until the mid-1970s asbestos was used for insulation in apartment buildings and schools. In the absence of structural damage, asbestos insulation appears safe. Still, if you suspect that your home, workplace, or school is at risk for contamination with asbestos, you can arrange to have it tested; your local EPA office will tell you what to do.

Formaldehyde is another indoor pollutant that has been reduced by government regulations. It was a larger problem in the 1970s, when many houses were insulated with urea-formaldehyde foam; this practice has been discontinued, but smaller amounts of formaldehyde may emanate from plywood, fiberboard, carpet backing, and glues.

Furnaces, kerosene space heaters, fireplaces and wood, gas, and coal stoves can pollute indoor air, releasing carbon monoxide, nitrogen oxides, particulates, and other products of combustion. Carbon monoxide is the most dangerous of these pollutants, causing 1,500 deaths in the United States each year. To protect your health, be sure that your heaters and stoves are in top working order and that they are well ventilated.

Household cleaning products can release volatile substances such as ammonia or chlorine. *Never* mix ammonia and chlorine-containing products; they can react together to produce ammonium chloride, a toxic gas. Exercise care, too, with the use of household aerosols, especially pesticides, cleansers, paint, and varnish. Ventilation is the key to keeping your air clean as you clean your home.

Some of the steps you may now be taking in an attempt to improve your home's air quality may be having the opposite effect. Humidifiers and air conditioners can harbor molds and bacteria that live in water; their spores may be aerosolized into the air you breathe. Most of these microbes are in and of themselves harmless; but if you develop an allergy to the spores, you'll develop symptoms of asthma or pneumonia. To prevent these problems, keep your air conditioner clean, changing the filter at least once a year. Change your humidifier's water daily, and disinfect it at weekly intervals using a solution of one ounce of household chlorine bleach diluted with a pint of water; rinse thoroughly before resuming normal use.

Should you go beyond a no smoking sign, a radon check, and an open window to protect your indoor air? A new industry is capitalizing on concern about indoor pollution by marketing a variety of air-cleaning devices. Some do a good job at removing particulates, but others do not; none will remove polluting gases. Air cleaners are often expensive, and they have not been proven to prevent illness. At the present time I'd advise you to save your money. Or buy house plants. Scientists at NASA report that plants can remove carbon monoxide, benzene, and other contaminants from indoor air. The validity and health benefits of this claim have yet to be confirmed, but plants are much cheaper and prettier than commercial air cleaners. As in so many areas, use the common sense, low-tech approach to prevention before resorting to fancy devices.

The "Sick Building" Syndrome

Headaches at work are nothing new, but about 15 years ago office workers began to notice an unusually high incidence of headaches, lethargy, and irritation of the eyes, nose, and throat. These complaints have been linked to sealed, air-conditioned buildings; although the precise cause of the "sick building" syndrome has not yet been identified, indoor air pollution is the likely culprit.

Although the symptoms of the syndrome can be uncomfortable, they are rarely serious. Still, up to 1 million commercial buildings in the United States may be involved, causing distress to as many as 30 million to 70 million office workers.

Improved indoor air quality will solve the sick building syndrome, but progress must await research into the exact causes of the problem. Until then, fresh air is the most reasonable remedy: get out for a brisk walk during lunch time.

On a historical level, the sick building syndrome is an object lesson in well-intentioned technology gone awry. Sealed, air-conditioned buildings were developed to conserve energy. They are energy-efficient, but the economic benefits of reduced operating costs may be offset by decreased worker productivity. To save energy without sacrificing health we need even better technology — and we need to apply it carefully, evaluating both its benefits and its pitfalls.

■ Global Warming

Hotly debated and slow to progress, global warming is not a health hazard at present. But the only way to be sure that this will still be true in 50 or 100 years is to take preventive action now.

What Is Global Warming?

The earth's atmosphere traps heat. It allows sunlight to stream in, warming the earth. The earth in turn reflects infrared radiation back toward space. But some of this radiation is trapped by the atmosphere, retaining its heat. In this respect the earth's atmosphere functions like the glass of a greenhouse, allowing sunlight in but preventing heat from getting out.

The atmosphere regulates our planet's temperature and climate; as the atmosphere changes, so will the earth's temperature. Alterations in the amounts of five atmospheric gases suggest that the changes will be in the direction of warming. The stratospheric ozone layer normally shields the earth from the sun's ultraviolet rays, but it's being depleted. In contrast, carbon dioxide, methane, nitrogen oxides, and CFCs are trace atmospheric gases that retain the earth's heat; all four of these "greenhouse gases" are on the rise. It's a simple equation: more sunlight in (owing to ozone depletion) + less heat out (owing to greenhouse gases) = global warming.

Even though my equation is simple, the math required to predict the magnitude of global warming is very sophisticated. We know that the earth is 0.6 degrees C warmer than it was 100 years ago; computers tell us that it will be 2.5 to 5.5 degrees C warmer in another century — unless we do something to prevent it.

The Causes and Control of Global Warming

The ozone layer, 15 miles above the earth's surface, has thinned by 3 percent in just the past 20 years, and it's being destroyed at an ever faster rate. In the 10 years between 1980 and 1990, the ozone layer over the United States decreased by nearly 5 percent. The culprit: CFCs released by refrigerants, foams, and aerosols. CFCs were banned from aerosols in the United States and many other developed countries in 1978, but aerosols still account for one third of the CFCs used elsewhere in the world. An international effort to replace CFCs in coolants is being mounted, but Third World countries — and the United States! — have lagged behind, citing the economic costs of industrial reform.

CFCs do more than destroy the protective ozone layer. As they accumulate in the atmosphere, they act as greenhouse gases, reflecting heat back to earth. In all, CFCs account for about 15 percent of the greenhouse effect.

CFCs are synthetic gases that don't belong in the atmosphere. You can help get them out by avoiding CFC aerosols and by buying non-halon fire extinguishers. Because CFCs are released in the manufacture of Styrofoam, cut down on your use of foam in packaging. Avoid fabric sprays containing methyl chloroform. Be sure your refrigerators and air conditioners are in good repair so they won't leak CFCs. Above all, pressure government and industry to use alternate coolants; more expensive in the short run, they will preserve health in the long run.

Another major cause of global warming is the increase in atmospheric carbon dioxide, a greenhouse gas that retains heat in the atmosphere. Atmospheric carbon dioxide concentrations have increased 25 percent since the industrial revolution — and if they continue to increase at the present rate, they will double in the next 60 years.

There are two reasons for the increase in carbon dioxide. One is deforestation. Living plants accumulate carbon, removing carbon dioxide from the atmosphere. A forest can sequester about 5.5 tons of carbon per hectare each year. But instead of growing more trees, the peoples of the world are harvesting and burning them; the loss of forests is responsible for an extra 1 billion tons of carbon dioxide in the atmosphere each year.

The second and even more important reason for the carbon dioxide buildup is increased production. Carbon dioxide is a by-product of fossil fuel combustion. With 6 billion tons spewed into the air each year from the combustion of fossil fuels and another billion from the burning of felled forests, carbon dioxide is the world's leading waste product. And the United States is the leading producer of carbon dioxide; with only 5 percent of the world's population, we account for 23 percent of its carbon dioxide production — 18 tons annually for each American.

To reduce carbon dioxide production, we must conserve fossil fuels and develop alternative nonpolluting, renewable sources of energy. An energy policy for the nation and the world is mandatory, but you can do your part. Consider that every time you use energy you release carbon dioxide into the atmosphere. Your automobile tailpipe and home heating furnace are the obvious culprits. Remember, too, that your air conditioner adds four pounds of carbon dioxide to the atmosphere in one hour of use, your vacuum cleaner 1.75 pounds per hour, your dishwasher another 2.6 pounds per load, and your refrigerator 12.8 pounds per day. Even a 100-watt light bulb consumes enough energy to release 28 pounds of carbon dioxide in just 10 hours of use. That may not sound like much; but multiply it by all the light bulbs in the country, and you'll see that conservation really can help.

Carbon dioxide and CFCs are the major causes of global warming, but two other greenhouse gases contribute as well. Nitrogen oxides, produced by fossil fuel combustion, account for 6 percent, and methane, produced by cattle, rice fields, and landfills, accounts for another 18 percent. Atmospheric concentrations of both gases have increased substantially in the industrial age, nitrogen oxides by 19 percent and methane by 100 percent. Without corrective action the greenhouse gases will continue to rise.

Global Warming and Human Health

Are the greenhouse gases responsible for preventable illnesses? The answer is a resounding yes. Increased human exposure to ultraviolet B rays has already increased the incidence of skin cancer and cataracts. The EPA estimates that over the next 75 years ozone depletion may cause an extra — and needless — 30,000 American deaths from skin cancer and an equally preventable 3 million cases of cataracts.

Global warming will have many effects on the ecosystems that maintain human health and sustain human life. The seas will rise, the distribution of rainfall will be altered, food production will suffer, and air pollution will increase. The effects on human health are hard to foresee, but it's easy to see that they will not be good. Action is needed now — preventive medicine on a truly grand scale.

■ Climate- and Altitude-Related Illnesses

Even without another century of global warming, the world gets quite hot enough to cause illness and injury and cold enough to cause equally serious health problems. All are preventable.

Heat-Related Illnesses

These illnesses occur in three distinct patterns. *Heat cramps* are painful but temporary muscle spasms caused by dehydration and overheating during warm-weather exercise. *Heat exhaustion* is caused by similar factors but is much more serious, with profound fatigue, rapid breathing, a racing heart, light-headedness, mental fogginess, and nausea; body temperature rises to 102 degrees or more. Most serious of all is *heat stroke,* a medical emergency requiring urgent treatment to prevent death. Patients with heat stroke stop sweating. They have flushed, dry skin and body temperatures that often reach 106 degrees. Confusion, coma, and cardiovascular collapse occur in rapid sequence; abnormalities of the liver, kidneys, and blood are universal.

Heat stroke affects two very different groups of people. Young, healthy people who exercise in hot, humid weather are at risk. To prevent heat stroke, give yourself time to adjust to a warm climate before you exercise, and drink lots of water before, during, and after exercise. Most helpful of all is common sense: in warm weather you should cut back on your exercise, wear lightweight clothing, and avoid both sunshine and exertion during the midday hours; best of all, work out in an air-conditioned gym or simply call a halt to your exercise until it cools off.

People who are elderly or ill, however, are at risk for heat stroke even without any exercise at all. Heat stroke is responsible for about 1,200 excess deaths during an average American summer. To prevent these deaths we need to educate vulnerable people about the risks of extreme heat and humidity, the benefits of air conditioners, fans, hydration, and rest, and the warning symptoms of heat-induced illness.

It's been estimated that global warming would quadruple the number of heat-related deaths. But we don't have to keep the whole world cool to prevent the heat from killing. Simple, common-sense measures can protect you and your family this summer.

Cold-Related Illnesses

Cold injury results from exposure during winter months. *Frostbite* begins with whiteness and tingling of the fingers, toes, ears, and nose; numbness can disguise the fact that these tissues are at risk for permanent damage unless they are rewarmed. *Hypothermia* is even more serious; fatigue progresses to confusion, rigidity, coma, shock, and death from cardiac arrest. At particular risk are the homeless and the poor or elderly living in inadequately heated quarters. But even young, healthy people are at risk during outdoor wintertime activities. To prevent these problems, wear multiple layers of warm clothing and stay dry. Avoid extremely hostile weather, and even in moderately cold climates limit your time outdoors, stay with a companion, and know what to do in an emergency.

Altitude Sickness

Critics say that if people were intended to climb mountains, they would have been goats. It's true that altitude sickness can be prevented best by simply keeping a low profile. But heights beckon man — and travelers, tourists, trekkers, and climbers respond with their ascent. Although no rival for stratospheric gases, altitude sickness is a high-level environmental problem that can be prevented by down-to-earth measures.

The three most common types of altitude sickness are acute mountain sickness (AMS), cerebral edema (brain swelling), and pulmonary edema (fluid in the lungs). All are caused by lack of oxygen at high altitudes. All can be prevented. You don't have to stay at home to prevent altitude sickness, but you do have to plan gradual ascents when heights greater than 7,000 to 8,000 feet are involved. Avoid overexertion at altitude and remain alert for early warning symptoms. Preventive medications may also help in certain circumstances; because these are prescription drugs, you'll have to check with your doctor before your trip. And if you have medical problems, particularly heart or lung disease, you'll be wise to prevent these problems altogether by planning your high adventure at low altitude.

■ Water Pollution

Life evolved in water and continues to depend on it. Perhaps because of its abundance, however, humankind has taken its water supply for granted, overlooking its fragility and failing to protect its purity. If present trends continue, our society may someday confront the dilemma of Coleridge's ancient mariner: "Water, water everywhere / Nor any drop to drink."

The World's Water Shortage

Our supply of fresh water is at risk. Falling water tables reveal that ground water is being withdrawn from the hydrologic cycle faster than it can be replenished. Global water consumption has quadrupled since 1950, owing to the population explosion and to increased water use by industry and especially agriculture. Always among the leaders in consumption, the United States heads the list in water consumption as well, withdrawing 2,000 cubic meters per person from the water supply each year.

The Causes of Water Pollution

Air pollution causes water pollution. Particulates emitted from industry are carried by the wind and may be deposited in water. Gaseous pollutants dissolve in water and return to earth in rain and snow.

Industry causes water pollution. Heavy metals, synthetic chemicals, pesticides, and radioactive wastes are among the numberless pollutants that are discharged into lakes and rivers. Toxic chemicals in dumps leak out of soil into ground water. Oil seeps into ground water from storage tanks and refineries and spills from ships, pipelines, and drilling rigs, contaminating marine waters. Bad as they are, oil spills are at least accidental; ocean dumping of medical wastes and trash lacks even that poor excuse.

Nor are our problems confined to chemical wastes. Organic wastes from humans and animals can enter the water supply, contaminating it with a vast array of disease-producing bacteria and viruses.

Contaminants from industry, agriculture, and human waste can jeopardize our health by finding their way into drinking water. They may also cause illness indirectly by damaging marine ecosystems. Fish, one of the most naturally healthful foods, are at risk of becoming scarce, contaminated, or both.

America's Troubled Waters

According to an EPA estimate, 10 percent of America's lakes, rivers, estuaries, and coastal waters are dangerous to aquatic life because of toxic metals and chemicals. Nor are the risks confined to our underwater friends. The EPA reports that more than two thirds of the nation's 15,600 municipal water treatment plants have had some form of water quality or public health problem. According to the National Wildlife Foundation, 37 million Americans drank water that was unsafe in 1987.

Is Your Water Safe to Drink?

Americans spend more than $2 billion each year for bottled water. Should you join them? Or should you add your household to those spending more than $265 million annually for water purifiers?

The first step is to evaluate the quality of your water supply. Unfortunately, this is one area in which you cannot rely on your senses, common or otherwise. The color, odor, and taste of water do not predict its safety. Well water, for example, can be contaminated by iron and manganese; it will taste bad, look bad, and stain plumbing fixtures and clothing, but it will not harm your health. In contrast, your water may be clear and refreshing yet contain toxic concentrations of lead or radon.

You can — and should — investigate your water supply in two ways. If you use municipal water, your water company will supply a copy of its current test results; they may not like it, but the 1974 Federal Safe Water Drinking Act gives you the right to know the results. These tests will give you lots of information about the water when it left the reservoir, but that's only half the story. Your water won't get any cleaner between the reservoir and your tap, but it might become contaminated en route. As a result, it's equally important for you to test the water as it comes from your tap.

Have your water tested by an independent, state-certified lab. It's easy to do; just call your local EPA office or your municipal health department to get a list of labs and follow their directions for collecting and submitting your water specimen. Even if there is no lab in your neighborhood, you can have your water tested by mailing it to a central lab. But shop around. Testing can cost $50 to $200 depending on the information you request.

How much data do you need? You can have your water tested for hundreds of chemicals, but since most don't cause disease, the testing is wasteful. Here's what you should know about your water.

The Major Drinking Water Pollutants

Lead. We've taken the lead out of the tailpipes of American cars but not out of the water pipes of American homes. Lead does not occur naturally in water, but it can dissolve into water passing through lead pipes. Lead pipes are found most often in houses built before 1940, but they were not banned nationwide until 1986. Lead can also leak into water from lead-soldered plumbing.

Acid rain has made the lead problem worse; lead, like aluminum, cadmium, and mercury, is more soluble in acid water. In all about 25 percent of the lead absorbed by Americans comes from their drinking water.

The 1962 standards for safe water allowed up to 50 parts per billion (ppb) of lead. For perspective, consider that 55 ppb is the equivalent of 50 seconds in 32 years. But for lead in water even 50 ppb is too much. A new standard of 15 ppb was proposed in 1991; as of 1985, 42 million Americans consumed drinking water with more than that amount of lead.

If your water contains more than 15 ppb of lead, you can consider purchasing a water filter. Because water will take up extra lead if it sits in plumbing for long periods or if it runs through pipes while it's hot, you can also protect your family with some simple steps. First, let the water run for at least a minute every morning before you use it. Second, let the water run for 5 seconds before you use it later in the day. Third, use only cold water for cooking and drinking. If those simple steps don't do the job, you may have to consider a big step — replacing your home's lead-containing pipes and plumbing fixtures.

Radon. Most dangerous as a contaminant of indoor air, this radioactive gas can also dissolve in water. Because radon evaporates from water, municipal water that stands in a reservoir is safe. But well water can accumulate radon. If you depend on well water, find out if it's safe. First, test your household air (see chapter 5). If your air is safe, your water should be also. But if your air has worrisome radon levels, have your water tested. If your water radon level is high, you can lower it by installing a water aerator or carbon filter. Remember, though, to treat all the water entering your house instead of just the tap water, and don't neglect to get the radon out of your air.

Nitrates. Agriculture is the main source of nitrates, which enter the water from fertilizers and animal wastes. Rural areas using well water are at greatest risk. The EPA reports that 500,000 American households have drinking water that contains more than the recommended nitrate level of ten parts per million. Infants may develop blood disorders from nitrate exposure. Nitrates can be removed from water by distillers or reverse-osmosis filter units.

Organic chemicals. Trichloroethylene is an industrial waste that may cause neurological disorders or cancer. Trihalomethane is a possible carcinogen produced during the chlorination of surface water. The human health hazards of low concentrations are uncertain, but if your water exceeds the EPA-recommended 10 ppb, you can consider using a carbon-filter water purifier to remove organic chemicals.

Pesticides can enter the water from agricultural run-off. *PCBs, gasoline,* various *solvents,* and many other *chemicals* can enter water from industrial run-off and toxic dumps. Most water supplies are safe from these contaminants, but the few that are contaminated pose the greatest health hazards.

Bacteria, viruses, and *parasites* are the oldest contaminants of water. Originating from human and animal wastes, they are still the chief pollutants in many parts of the underdeveloped world, where they cause epidemics of diarrhea, typhoid fever, hepatitis, and other diseases; the cholera epidemic that swept through South America in 1991 is a reminder that water-borne infection can come close to home. Although water supplies in the United States are safe from the most virulent bacteria, other disease-causing microbes can spill into water from sewage and from septic tanks.

Protecting Your Water and Your Health

Water pollutants pose a formidable set of hazards. But don't panic; a simple phone call to your water company and a test of your own tap water can protect your health. The chances are good that you will not need a home water purifier; rely on objective test results rather than a salesman's pitch, however sincere, before spending your money on a filtering system. As for bottled water, if your tap water is safe, the choice is a matter of taste rather than health; in fact, bottled water is subjected to *less* stringent health and safety testing than is tap water. I drink tap water, but I'll tip my cup to whatever decision you make.

Finally, don't overlook the importance of water conservation. The long shower, the open tap while you are shaving or brushing your teeth, the half-empty washing machine, and the unnecessary car wash all waste enormous quantities of this limited resource. Drinking lots of water can help your kidneys and your health; saving lots of water can help the health of our world.

Water Additives

In our quest for purity we have come to regard all water additives as harmful. Caution and skepticism are valuable commodities when it comes to health, but they can go too far; remember that most chemicals are not toxic, especially in low doses.

Some water additives can even be beneficial. Chlorine treatment, for example, eliminates bacteria from water. It's safe in the doses used by water treatment plants, and it has prevented countless cases of diarrhea. Fluoridation of water has been controversial since its inception 50 years ago; but it has been extremely beneficial to dental health, and volumes of data prove that it's safe for humans.

I love clean water. I'll take mine chlorinated and fluoridated, thank you.

■ Acid Rain

It begins with air pollution and ends with water pollution. It has already inflicted substantial damage on forests, aquatic life, and agriculture. It even corrodes buildings and statues. If it's powerful enough to do all this, it might be powerful enough to damage human health. It is — and it does.

Acid rain begins when sulfur dioxide and nitrogen oxides are dumped from smokestacks and tailpipes into the air. Chemical reactions transform these gases into sulfuric acid and nitric acid, strong acids which dissolve in water and return to earth as acid rain, snow, fog, and dew.

Acid rain damages the environment in ways that will take their toll on human nutrition over the years. It can also damage human health right now. Fish from acidic waters may contain toxic levels of mercury, and acid drinking water may have toxic levels of lead, cadmium, aluminum, or mercury. Acoustic trauma from "heavy metal" music is one thing, but toxic damage to your internal organs from these real heavy metals is quite another.

We can apply protective coatings to statues and buildings. We can add lime to lakes and streams. We can issue air-quality pollution warnings. But the only way really to control acid rain is to reduce industrial and automotive emissions. Raise your political voice to be sure the job gets done — and do your own small but important part by conserving energy.

■ Pesticides and Fertilizers

Farmers regard pesticides and fertilizers as a boon, but to environmentalists they are a bane. Economists praise pesticides, but consumerists decry them. Nutritionists worry about them, but most doctors ignore them. As with most controversies, there is merit on both sides of the pesticide debate. And as with most controversies, the pesticide issue would benefit from more light and less heat, more information and less passion.

The Uses of Pesticides and Fertilizers

The world's grain production increased by a factor of 2.6 between 1950 and 1984. It has leveled off since, raising renewed concern about the nutritional health of the 88 million people added to the world's population each year. Human health depends on a food supply that is plentiful and economical. Improved agricultural output depends on new techniques and equipment, irrigation, new disease-resistant and climate-tolerant strains of crops, and on fertilizers and pesticides.

Pesticides do more than control plant diseases. They also combat insect-borne human diseases. Encephalitis and malaria are but two examples of grave diseases that can be contained by mosquito control.

Pesticides and fertilizers used to improve food supplies and control disease are one thing, but chemicals used simply to beautify lawns are quite another. Americans spend more than $2 billion on lawn chemicals each year, applying them to more than 25 million acres of grass, an area the size of New England. The EPA reports that it has not evaluated fully the safety of 33 of the 34 most popular lawn and garden pesticides. I'm all for green lawns, but it's clear that we need to learn if human health is endangered by the suburban passion for lush landscapes.

The Hazards of Pesticides and Fertilizers

For all the good they can do, fertilizers and pesticides can also cause harm. As nitrogen-rich compounds, fertilizers contribute to air pollution and acid rain caused by nitrogen oxides; agricultural run-off also results in ground-water pollution. Pesticides have an even greater potential for harm. They, too, can pollute water; the EPA reports that some of the drinking water in 38 states is contaminated with pesticides. Pesticides can also enter the body with food; residual amounts of agricultural chemicals are present on many fruits and vegetables. Pesticides sprayed on corn and grain used as fodder may turn up in beef, pork, and chicken. And because pesticides are applied as sprays, farmers and other residents of agricultural communities may be exposed to pesticide aerosols. Home gardeners, too, may inadvertently expose themselves to potentially toxic sprays and powders.

More than 50,000 pesticides are in use all over the world. Unfortunately, detailed data about the cancer-causing potential of many of these chemicals are lacking. For the compounds that have been studied, the risks seem low; children, however, seem to be most vulnerable. Because these chemicals are so ubiquitous, they may collectively cause up to 6,000 cases of cancer a year according to EPA estimates. The actual toll is unknown, but it is surely unacceptably high.

Controlling Pesticides and Fertilizers: The Role of Government

We can — and must — do a better job of ensuring food safety. Since it was established in 1970, the EPA has banned only 26 pesticides and fertilizers. Careful, objective evaluation of the thousands of chemicals that have been marketed without proper testing is sorely needed. The Food and Drug Administration tests less than 1 percent of fresh fruits and vegetables for pesticides, and their tests fail to detect half the pesticides in use. What's worse, food safety tests take 28 days to complete, by which time the food has long since been marketed and eaten. It is clear that we need better pesticide testing.

We also need better enforcement. Even in California, the most diligent state, fewer than 7 percent of pesticide violations result in fines, and fewer than two tenths of 1 percent are referred for possible legal action. Needed, too, are realistic disclosure laws; fruits and vegetables should be labeled with their place of origin and with the chemicals used on them while they're in the soil and after they're harvested.

No less important is the need for improved regulation of imported foods. Agricultural regulation in many parts of the world is very lax by American standards. More than 6 percent of all imported foods that are tested fail to meet our safety standards. Despite this high failure rate, fewer than 1 percent of the 1 million food shipments arriving in the United States each year are tested. But our indignation about lax standards for food imports should be tempered by the realization that the U.S. government allows American chemical manufacturers to export two pesticides (heptachlor and chlordane) that have been banned for domestic use. We can't have it both ways, selling toxins overseas and then fretting about the safety of imported foods.

Protecting Your Family from Pesticides

While working to implement regulatory reform, you can take measures to protect your family. Buy local produce when you can; because it is marketed quickly, it's less likely to have been sprayed with pesticides or treated with fungicides after harvesting. For the same reason, buying produce in season makes sense, as does favoring domestically grown foods. Carefully wash all fruits and vegetables, preferably using a brush. Peeling is even more helpful, although nutrients, taste, and texture will be sacrificed when edible peels are removed. Remember, though, that washing and peeling can remove only surface pesticides, leaving behind chemical residues that have been absorbed into the food's interior.

You can also consider switching to organically grown produce. My garden is a testimonial to the fact that growing food organically is difficult, but my neighbor's garden reminds us that it is possible. American agriculture is getting the message. Pesticide use peaked in 1982, when 880 million pounds of chemicals were sprayed on our food. Since then pesticide use has decreased but productivity has increased. The demand for pesticide-free food is slowly but surely persuading American agriculture that organic farming is good for business as well as health.

Without disputing the merits of organically grown foods, however, we should keep a few reservations in mind. Organic foods are expensive. Moreover, the term *organic* does not itself guarantee freedom from pesticides, since all carbon-containing compounds, including some synthetic petrochemical pesticides, are technically classified as "organic." "Natural" foods have no synthetic chemical additives, but even this is no guarantee that they are wholesome and safe, since they might still contain contaminants from natural sources, including bacteria, fungi, and rock minerals.

Like humans, animals can eat chemically contaminated grains; because these chemicals are often stored in body fat, it's important to remove the skin from poultry and fish and to trim all the visible fat away from meat. Be sure, too, to discard the fats and oils in pan drippings, broths, and gravies, all steps you should take to protect yourself from heart disease and cancer even if chemicals were not a concern.

Remember that pesticides and fertilizers can enter your water as well as your food; protect yourself by having your drinking water tested. You can also help by minimizing the use of chemicals on your own lawn and garden. Finally, if you do use chemicals, be sure to handle, store, and dispose of them safely.

■ Fish and Shellfish Safety

As a source of healthful protein and omega-3 polyunsaturated fats which fight heart disease, fish are an ideal food, the "vegetables of the sea." But like real vegetables, fish can become contaminated by environmental pollutants that cause human disease. It's important for you to understand seafood safety so you can balance the scales between the benefits and risks of eating fish and shellfish.

It's a sad fact that our rivers, lakes, and oceans have become the dumping grounds for industrial and agricultural chemicals. Fish process enormous volumes of water through their gills; they absorb chemicals from water and store them in their internal organs and fat. Over time, fish can build up concentrations of chemicals far higher than the original concentrations in water. These chemicals can be passed up the food chain to larger predatory fish, and ultimately to human consumers, who can also gradually accumulate chemicals in their organs. Among the many worrisome chemicals that can pass from industry to water to fish to humans are polychlorinated biphenyls (PCBs) and methylmercury, which are reproductive toxins, and PCBs, dioxins, and chlorinated hydrocarbon pesticides, which can cause cancer.

Selecting Seafood: Some Fish Are Safer Than Others

Most seafood is safe for human consumption. Although authorities reassure us that the wave of concern about seafood safety is exaggerated, we should all take steps to avoid the most dangerous fish.

Raw mollusks constitute the greatest risk to human health; one of every 1,000 people who eat raw oysters, clams, or mussels becomes ill. In this case, natural toxins are to blame. Although most shellfish poisoning is mild, serious illness can result.

Other types of raw fish rank next in the hazard list, chiefly because of microbial contamination. Thorough cooking is the only way to prevent bacterial, viral, and parasitic infection from seafood. Children, pregnant women, and patients with medical problems should never eat raw or undercooked fish. Others should understand the risks of raw fish; if they still choose to indulge, they should deal only with reputable markets and restaurants that never buy fish from contaminated waters and that handle seafood properly.

Freshwater fish pose the greatest threat of chemical contamination. Of particular concern are fish caught in waters near industrial centers. Commercial fishing is barred in the Great Lakes and other waters known to be contaminated, but sport fishermen may still catch fish in troubled waters. Bottom-dwelling species are most likely to ingest chemical contaminants, and fatty fish are most likely to accumulate toxins. Among freshwater fish, catfish, lake trout, lake whitefish, and carp are the most worrisome; perch, freshwater bass, and brook trout the least.

Ocean fish living in coastal waters are also at risk for chemical contamination. Fatty species such as herring and sardines are more likely to have high chemical concentrations than are chum salmon and pink salmon.

In general, the safest fish are the deep-water, offshore species. Because of their higher fat content, tuna, halibut, and flounder have a greater potential for contamination than leaner species such as cod, haddock, and pollock. Don't shun all oily deep-water fish, though; remember that they contain the most omega-3 fatty acids. Swordfish are a special case, since they are frequently contaminated with mercury. Even if they are caught offshore, migratory species such as striped bass and bluefish may be contaminated by PCBs.

About 25 percent of all seafood sold in the United States is canned. Because of high processing temperatures and additional inspection procedures, canned seafood appears to be the safest of all; remember, though, that canned fish can contain lots of salt. Fish raised by aquaculture techniques ("fish farms") are also safe; indeed, concerns about the safety and supply of free-living fish have revived the ancient oriental art of aquaculture, so we can expect the availability of "farmed" fish to increase in future years.

Improving Seafood Safety: Governmental Perspectives

If you think that the control of pesticides and fertilizers is lax, just wait till you hear about seafood! What's needed? Just about everything: research into the health consequences of chemical contamination, stringent standards for allowable chemical concentrations, careful inspections, and tough enforcement. Above all, of course, we need to end the wanton water pollution that got us into this sea of problems in the first place.

Another problem that needs attention is the depletion of our fish supply. Chemical contamination has taken a great toll of freshwater and coastal fish. Overfishing threatens the supply of ocean fish; at least 14 species are in serious danger of being depleted. Marine species are more resilient than land animals; still, the time has come to take steps that will ensure a safe, plentiful, and affordable supply of seafood.

Eating Seafood Safely

Despite the rising tide of concern about seafood safety, I won't flounder around with my recommendations: eat fish. All the evidence suggests that the documented health benefits of seafood, including a 50 percent reduction in the risk of heart attacks, far outweigh the potential hazards of chemical or microbial contamination. Still, you can take simple steps to ensure that your fish is safe:

- Buy your fish from reputable markets and restaurants. Even at the best markets, inspect the fish yourself before you buy it. Whole fish should have clear, bulging eyes and bright, smooth skin; the flesh should be moist and covered with a translucent sheen. Avoid fish that smells "fishy" — a strong odor is a sure sign of spoilage. Be vigilant for health alerts, particularly for shellfish. Never fish in contaminated waters.
- Handle fish properly, storing it in the coldest part of your refrigerator, at 30 to 35 degrees F. Plan to serve fish within a day or two of purchasing it.
- Cook fish thoroughly, maintaining the recommended cooking temperature for at least five minutes. Steam oysters, clams, and mussels for at least six minutes. Don't eat raw fish if you are pregnant or if you have serious medical problems. Best of all, just don't eat raw fish. Whenever possible, use a grill or rack to cook your fish, allowing fat to drip away.
- Eat a variety of species, favoring deep-water offshore fish over coastal ocean fish and freshwater fish. Pregnant women should avoid the species most likely to be contaminated with PCBs or mercury.
- Favor small, young fish, which have had less time to accumulate chemicals.
- Before you eat fish, trim away the skin and fat. Don't eat the gills or internal organs, including the green tomalley in lobster and the "mustard" in crabs.

It sounds complex, but if you eat fish as often as you should — twice a week — it will quickly become second nature. With a little care, you can enjoy healthful seafood without running aground on the perils of environmental toxins.

Final Thoughts about Food Safety

Despite its importance, chemical contamination is not the greatest threat to food safety. Bacteria, viruses, and parasites in food pose a greater risk to health. Hormones and antibiotics used in raising farm animals are also a potential concern. Most dangerous of all, however, are foods that are free of all contaminants and additives but are naturally, organically, inevitably harmful because of their fat, salt, and caloric content. Chapter 20 contains discussions of these larger considerations about food safety and good nutrition.

Should worries about chemical pollution of vegetables and fish keep you away from these foods? Certainly not! Despite valid concerns, vegetables and fish are still among the most healthful of foods. The fiber and vitamins in vegetables will reduce your risk of cancer; *not* eating vegetables poses a much greater cancer risk than does eating vegetables that may have trace amounts of pesticides. Similarly, the omega-3 fats in fish will reduce your risk of heart disease, producing a net gain in health. Still, by working to reduce the use of pesticides, to clean up our waters, and to inspect our food properly, we can make the food we eat even safer.

In a larger sense, all environmental degradations threaten the safety and supply of food. The Worldwatch Institute estimates that damage to land, water, and air is reducing global grain production by 14 million tons a year. The problem will get worse unless we all take steps to protect the environment. Our food — and our health — depend on it.

■ Wastes

"Modern living through chemistry" is not an idle boast of the advertising industry. Chemistry has contributed immeasurably to the advantages of industrialized societies. But there is a problem with chemistry: chemicals, or more specifically what do to with them. Chemical wastes, according to the U.S. Surgeon General, constitute an environmental emergency. The EPA reports that more than a ton of toxic waste is produced annually for each man, woman, and child in this country. What becomes of it? Three billion pounds are spewed into our air, 135 billion pounds are discharged into our waterways, and the rest is buried or dumped.

Chemical Wastes

Some chemicals are relatively safe, others highly toxic. The problem, though, can arise in figuring out which is which; toxicity data are just not available for 40,000 of the 50,000 chemicals registered with the EPA.

More than a dozen chemicals have been proven to cause human cancer (see table 22-2); many others cause animal tumors and are suspected causes of human cancers. We just don't know enough about the carcinogenicity of many chemical wastes; they may well contribute to the striking variations in cancer rates across the country. Toxic chemicals can also cause injury and death owing to accidents. We've been lucky in this regard compared to the citizens of Bhopal, India, where 2,000 people were killed and 200,000 injured in the 1984 industrial leak of methyl isocyanate. Still, there are about 4,000 chemical accidents in the United States each year, accounting for up to 1,000 injuries and 100 deaths.

474   STAYING WELL

In response to this ecological crisis, the government established a Superfund for toxic waste cleanup in 1980. Unfortunately, the Superfund has failed to live up to its mandate; toxic chemicals are still a major health hazard.

What should be done? Enhanced cleanup efforts are essential. But even the best cleanup is little more than locking the door on an empty barn. To avoid future contamination, industry, agriculture, and government should learn a lesson from doctors: when it comes to chemical contamination, primary prevention is best.

Remember, too, that your household may be the source of dangerous chemicals. Control your own toxic wastes, don't dump your chemicals down the drain or into the ground. In particular, solvents, petroleum products, pesticides, aerosols, oven cleaners, and batteries require safe disposal. Call your town officer or your local EPA to arrange for safe disposal of your toxins at a collection center.

Biological Wastes

Chemical wastes are a modern problem, but human wastes are an age-old issue. Even today, many parts of the world are ravaged by epidemics of typhoid, cholera, and other illnesses caused by fecal contamination of drinking water and food. We have a much better record in the United States, but contamination does occur, and many sewage-treatment facilities are becoming obsolete. We can't afford to be smug. Sewage treatment is a problem nobody likes to talk about, but it will only get worse without collective action.

Solid Wastes

When you think about air pollution, you may blame power plants and look to engineers for the solutions. When it comes to toxic dumps and chemical pollution, you may blame industry and depend on the Superfund for answers. When you consider sewage, you may think the problem starts and stops with your municipal government. In each case, of course, you'll be overlooking your own role as a consumer who creates the conditions that promote pollution. Similarly, when it comes to solid wastes, you can run but you can't hide; garbage is everybody's doing.

Americans live in an age of affluence — and effluence — in a monumentally disposable society. On average, each of us generates five pounds of trash every day. Unless you're the one carrying out the garbage, five pounds may not sound like much, but it adds up to a staggering 230 million tons of household refuse per year. Add the 5 billion tons produced by industry and agriculture, and you'll begin to understand the magnitude of the garbage crisis that threatens our world — and, ultimately, our health.

Landfills and incineration are solutions whose time has passed; turning trash into energy may offer some hope for the future, but it can hardly be expected to contain the crisis.

It's already too late for secondary prevention; we need primary prevention. The plan: generate less trash. The tactics: reuse what you can, and recycle what you can't.

How does this relate to health? Paper recycling saves 50 percent of the energy needed to make new paper while cutting air pollution by 75 percent and water pollution by 35 percent — without cutting down all those trees. Making steel from scrap metal reduces air pollution by 85 percent and water pollution by 76 percent — without generating mining wastes. Recycling glass saves 30 percent of the energy used to manufacture it from scratch, and recycling aluminum saves 95 percent. Substituting rechargeable batteries for the 2.7 billion household batteries that wind up in America's trash each year could eliminate 88 percent of the mercury and 52 percent of the cadmium in municipal dumps.

Only you can solve the problem. The average American household discards 13,000 pieces of paper, 1,800 pieces of plastic, 500 aluminum cans, and 500 glass bottles each year. Food packaging is a particularly severe problem: in 1986 Americans spent more on food packages than farmers earned for their crops. Do your part by shopping ecologically and using items wisely. Reuse what you can, and when something really is used up, send it for recycling.

I'm glad to say that recycling is catching on. But I'm sorry to say that some companies are exploiting the good intentions of consumers by trumping up claims for the biodegradability of their products. Be an ecologically shrewd consumer. The health of your environment depends on it, and a healthy world is indispensable for human health.

And, yes, this book is printed on recycled paper.

■ Radiation

Radiation is the ultimate ecological nightmare. The merest mention of radiation conjures up images of environmental disasters like Three Mile Island, health disasters like Chernobyl, and disguised disasters like Hanford. Unfortunately, entirely legitimate concerns about nuclear energy threaten to obscure the fact that even radioactivity can be used to benefit humankind if appropriate safeguards are employed. Moreover, there are many forms of *non*radioactive radiation that engender unwarranted fear just because they share the bad name "radiation." Like chemicals, some forms of radiation are very hazardous, but others are very safe.

What Is Radiation?

You don't have to be a physicist to understand that radiation is energy. But a little high school science can help you understand how that energy is transmitted through the air. All radiation is energy in the form of electromagnetic waves — so called because they are composed of an electric charge and a magnetic attraction.

Even though all electromagnetic waves carry energy in the same fash-

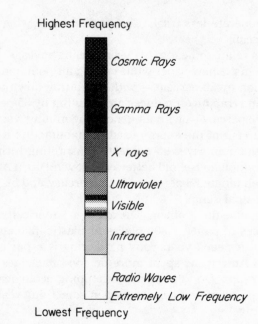

Highest Frequency

Cosmic Rays

Gamma Rays

X rays

Ultraviolet

Visible

Infrared

Figure 22-1.   Radio Waves
Radiation   Extremely Low Frequency
spectrum   Lowest Frequency

ion, they differ enormously in the amount of energy they contain. This difference is crucial for health.

The amount of energy in radiation depends on the frequency of the radiation, or the number of waves that pass through the air in a period of time. Low-frequency radiation has fewer waves, high-frequency radiation more waves. The higher the frequency, the more energy — and the greater the potential for tissue damage. Figure 22-1 displays the very different types of radiation that are part of the broad spectrum of electromagnetic energy. At the lowest end of the spectrum are the waves that carry the least energy; at the highest end are the most potent, and most dangerous, forms of radiation energy.

Although all types of electromagnetic radiation fit into this single spectrum, there is a crucial difference separating the energy into two basic types. The lower frequencies are grouped together as nonionizing radiation. More familiar, perhaps, as sunlight, microwaves, or radio transmissions, these waves do not carry enough energy to disrupt atoms. The higher frequencies are much more potent, carrying enough energy to displace electrons from their usual orbits in atoms. These powerful waves are together classified as ionizing radiation, known to most of us as radioactive energy.

Radiation can damage tissues. Its potential for causing harm depends on the intensity of its energy and the intimacy of your exposure. It will come as no surprise to you that ionizing radiation — radioactivity — is the most hazardous, with a great potential to injure or kill. Although much safer, some nonionizing radiation can still damage tissues; there is debate, however, about the potential risks of the lowest-frequency electromagnetic waves.

Low-Frequency Radiation

The lowest-frequency waves at the bottom of the energy spectrum are aptly named: extremely low frequency or ELF waves. ELF waves may be low frequency to the physicists, but they are high profile for the mass media, generating enormous controversy about their potential to cause disease.

Ordinary electric current is composed of extremely low frequency electromagnetic radiation. These ELF waves oscillate at only 60 cycles per second as the alternating current that passes through electric lines to power everything from toasters to TV sets. The current can have a shocking effect on tissues exposed directly. But the air around electric lines and appliances has always been considered safe — until the recent controversy erupted.

Sensitive measurements have detected ELF waves around electricity generators and high-voltage power lines. High-voltage electricity is, of course, very potent, but the electromagnetic fields *around* the high-voltage lines are very weak. Everyday household appliances ranging from refrigerators to electric blankets to computers also generate ELF fields, but they are even weaker, falling off to immeasurably low levels just a few inches from the appliance. In fact, the electrical fields generated by normal function of the heart and brain are three times stronger than the external ELF radiation encountered during daily life.

Damage to DNA, the genetic material in human cells, is the first step in producing cancer and birth defects. ELF waves do *not* carry enough energy to disrupt DNA. Although all scientists agree that ELF waves cannot injure DNA, some investigators report much more subtle effects on the surface membranes of animal cells. It's not known, however, if these changes really are caused by the waves, and there is no reason to suppose that these small effects would be harmful even if they are real.

Since ELF waves cannot damage DNA, why worry about them? The alarm originated with several studies which suggested that people exposed to these waves were at risk for disease. First, physicists in Denver reported a slightly higher cancer rate in people living near high-voltage transformers and power lines. Next, these same investigators reported that women using electric blankets and electrically heated waterbeds during pregnancy had a slightly increased risk of miscarriages and premature deliveries. More recently a California study reported that women working at computer screens for more than 20 hours a week during early pregnancy experienced more miscarriages than did women with less intense exposure.

These studies raise legitimate concerns. A number of individuals, however, have extended these concerns to blame ELF waves for everything from depression to cancer. Not surprisingly, the mass media have devoted extensive coverage to these alarming reports. But they fail to report that many other studies have *not* detected increased rates of cancer or leukemia in workers intensely exposed to power lines and generators or in people living nearby. Similarly, at least nine studies from around the world have found *no* link between computer use and miscarriages or birth defects.

Many of my patients have been alarmed by the warnings about ELF fields. These warnings surely are premature and exaggerated; if ELF waves are harmful at all, the risks they pose are certainly low. Media reports should not be allowed to cause fear or provoke drastic life-style changes. Even so, the warnings should not be ignored altogether. I certainly think it's prudent to stay a healthy distance from high-voltage power lines; all things being equal, it would be desirable to live one-half mile or more away from high-voltage equipment. It's reasonable, too, to put some distance between your computer screen and your body, but 12 to 24 inches should do the trick. Finally, pregnancy might be a good time to return to low-tech living, substituting a comforter for the electric blanket and a mattress for the waterbed. I can't prove that these changes are really necessary, but they do conform to a sound principle of prevention: back to basics.

Unlike higher-frequency radiation, ELF waves do not carry enough energy to generate heat, much less light. Even so, they stimulate hot debate. We need to turn down the rhetorical thermostat and wait for objective scientific studies to ferret out the facts.

Radio Wave and Microwave Radiation

It's ironic, perhaps, that some radiation containing more energy than 60-cycle ELF waves has generated less worry. The next step up on the radiation spectrum (see figure 22-1) is occupied by radio-frequency waves. AM and FM broadcasts may traumatize our ears, but this form of electromagnetic radiation is safe for tissues — so safe, in fact, that these frequencies are used to treat patients with intractable pain.

Microwaves occupy the next rung on the frequency ladder. They carry enough energy to agitate water molecules, which is how they produce heat. Microwave energy is a boon to cooking and is safe for the cook; microwave ovens are well insulated, and in any case the waves themselves can do little harm. Microwaves are so safe, in fact, that they are used medically in heat treatments for muscle spasms and other conditions. Long experience has shown that radar waves, which carry the same energy as other microwaves, are also safe.

Infrared and visible light, the next stage up in frequencies and energy, are also safe for tissues. You might want to prevent visible light from revealing more than you'd like, but you don't have to worry about preventing illness at this energy level. If anything it's the *lack* of daylight that may cause a medical problem, depression.

Ultraviolet Radiation

Ultraviolet light, at the junction of ionizing and nonionizing energy levels, is quite another story. Ultraviolet radiation *does* contain enough energy to damage DNA, and it can cause serious human diseases. But because ultraviolet radiation is responsible for an aesthetically pleasing condition, the not-so-healthy suntan, the real hazards of this form of radiation are often ignored.

Ultraviolet (UV) radiation comes in three energy levels. The highest-energy waves, UV-C, have enough energy to be very harmful, but they are screened out by the atmosphere. The lowest-frequency waves, called UV-A, are part of visible sunlight; they can penetrate window glass, but they do not carry enough energy to damage DNA. Even so, UV-A isn't entirely innocuous, since it can penetrate into the skin's elastic tissue, where it may contribute to premature skin aging.

The midfrequency UV-B waves are the main problem. Like other UV waves, they are part of sunlight. The earth is protected from UV-B waves by the stratospheric ozone layer; but as CFCs deplete the ozone layer, more UV-B waves are getting through to earth: for each 1 percent decrease in the ozone layer, human exposure to UV waves increases by 2 percent.

UV-B waves are powerful enough to disrupt DNA, injuring tissues and even causing cancer. They cannot, however, penetrate deeply into the body. As a result, the only human organs that are damaged by UV waves are the skin (sunburn, skin aging, skin cancer) and the eye (inflammation, "snow blindness," cataracts).

Clinical disease produced by ultraviolet radiation is on the increase; the dramatic rise in skin cancers, especially deadly melanomas, is particularly worrisome. To prevent these illnesses, help preserve the stratospheric ozone layer by reducing, and ultimately removing, CFCs from the atmosphere. In addition, protect yourself from sunlight. Ordinary window glass will screen out UV-B waves. Outdoor living, however, can be great for fun and great for health: you can enjoy it safely by following the simple guidelines in chapters 13 and 15.

Ionizing Radiation

Moving higher on the electromagnetic spectrum, we cross the radiation Rubicon, encountering ionizing radiation that carries enough energy to displace electrons from their normal atomic orbits — enough energy to damage DNA, enough energy to penetrate deeply into the body, and enough energy to cause human disease and death.

Cosmic Rays

Ionizing radiation is scary, but it's also part of nature. Cosmic rays are one example: produced by the sun and stars, they are largely screened out by the earth's atmosphere so they don't contribute significantly to human disease. The exception may occur in *very* frequent fliers, airline crew members who are airborne for 900 hours annually. Although the risk to crew members is very small, it may be prudent for women who are pregnant to avoid very frequent air travel. Normal travel, though, seems to be entirely safe; a flight between London and Los Angeles, for example, entails less radiation exposure than a single chest x ray.

Radon and Natural Radioactivity

The radiation risk from cosmic rays is small. But another form of natural radioactivity causes more deaths each year than any other form of radiation; it's radon. Radon is a naturally occurring radioactive gas that originates from uranium deposits in the earth's crust. It accounts for 55 percent of all the radiation received by the average American. Radon's potential role in lung cancer is often overlooked. Chapter 5 details the things you should do to keep your home safe from this radioactive gas and your lungs safe from the cancer it causes.

Uranium, thorium, radium, and other natural radioactive minerals are part of the earth's crust. Radon gas can seep up from the earth, causing a health hazard if it is retained in poorly ventilated houses. The other radioactivity in the earth's crust is harmless — unless it's stirred up. Oil drilling brings radium to the surface, exposing oil-field workers to radiation. Some oil workers are exposed to higher levels of radiation than is allowed for workers in the nuclear industry, but man-made nuclear radiation is closely monitored and regulated, whereas natural oil-field radiation is not. There ought to be a law.

Medical Radiation

Medical radiation serves as a paradigm for the entire radiation quandary: it has produced enormous health benefits, but it can also do great harm. The trick is to use it wisely. New techniques have greatly reduced the patient's radiation dose from diagnostic x rays and nuclear medicine scans. We have learned to restrict x-ray tests severely during pregnancy and to shield patients' gonadal tissues during these tests. We have also learned how to protect x-ray technicians and doctors from radiation exposure.

The final thing we need to learn is to use medical radiation judiciously. Excluding natural sources such as radon, more than 90 percent of mankind's radiation exposure results from diagnostic x rays, which now exceed 250 million examinations per year. Many are necessary to preserve health and save lives, but some are superfluous. The only *routine* x-ray tests healthy people should have are periodic mammograms and dental films. If you are sick or injured you may, of course, need diagnostic x rays; but discuss them carefully with your doctors to be sure that you get the lowest radiation dose possible.

Most doctors now understand the hazards of medical radiation, but many still order excessive testing. One particular example which merits preventive action is head and neck radiation. At one time x-ray treatments were used to treat some benign conditions such as acne, enlarged tonsils, and enlargement of the thymus gland. Unfortunately, patients who received these now abandoned treatments have an increased risk of developing thyroid cancer 5 to 30 years or more after the x-ray exposure. If you've had head and neck x-ray treatments, simply report them to your doctor, who will carefully examine your thyroid gland every year.

Nuclear Radiation

It can be difficult to balance the benefits of medical radiation against its risks: for nuclear power the balance is even trickier. As a doctor I am responsible for the first question; as a citizen I am concerned also about the second.

I don't have answers to all the complex scientific, social, environmental, and economic questions about nuclear power. But as a physician I'm very concerned about the health effects of nuclear energy. Risks may accrue to workers and to neighboring communities during normal power plant operations. Threats to health are magnified by accidents such as the partial core meltdown at Three Mile Island in 1979 and the steam-hydrogen explosion at Chernobyl in 1986. Health hazards can also persist for many years to come because of the problems intrinsic to nuclear waste disposal.

These considerations all militate against the use of nuclear power. Indeed, although 106 nuclear reactors now generate 18 percent of our nation's electricity, no new application for a nuclear plant has been filed in the United States since 1977.

Yet I am also concerned about the effects of fossil fuel combustion, effects that encompass ecology, economics, and health. The alternative to nuclear power cannot be the continued profligate consumption of fossil fuels. To forestall a return to nuclear power we must have an energy policy that stresses conservation and encourages the development of alternate, renewable, nonpolluting sources of energy. As part of such a policy, research on nuclear power plant design and waste disposal should continue so safe nuclear power will be an option for the future. Needed, too, are demanding safety standards, objective inspections, and tough penalties for violations in existing plants.

While recognizing the critical importance of national security, I must still insist that the only health impact of nuclear weapons is disaster. The deaths from radiation sickness and cancer at Hiroshima and Nagasaki are the most obvious examples. Less obvious, but no less tragic, are the leukemia and cancer deaths caused by nuclear testing. Even the production and storage of nuclear weapons pose health hazards. In the United States alone, for example, we now confront the daunting task of cleaning up no fewer than 103 contaminated laboratories, processing plants, nuclear reactors, and testing grounds that have been part of the atomic weapon industry.

Do nuclear weapons fit into the scope of preventive medicine? Yes, because they pose the greatest of all risks to human health. I am proud that 250,000 physicians in 70 countries belong to the International Physicians for the Prevention of Nuclear War, the winner of the 1985 Nobel Prize for peace. Like the other doctors in this group, I believe that nuclear weapons are too dangerous to be left in the hands of politicians. You, too, can join the effort to eliminate these weapons of mass destruction. Your efforts will help protect the health of humans and our planet.

■ Human Health and Environmental Health

All aspects of human life depend on the world around us. Human health has always depended on the natural world, but we have ignored that dependency. We have abused our bodies to create the great killers of the twentieth century, and we have abused our planet to set the stage for new killers in the twenty-first century. Both forms of abuse must stop.

We cannot take health for granted. Instead we must practice preventive medicine, largely by living as nature intended us to live. It's the only way to preserve our health.

We cannot take the environment for granted. Instead, we must practice preventive ecology to protect the planet's health. It's the only way to preserve our species.

■ 23 ■
Preventive Medical Care

Medical care is not the key to staying well.

The ancient Greeks attributed health to Aesculapius, the god of healing. But they divided his responsibilities for health between two daughters: Panacea was devoted to the use of medication while Hygeia was concerned with wise living and healthful behavior. Modern medicine, alas, has devoted much more energy to the search for pharmacological panaceas than to understanding the healthful life-style that would render many of them obsolete. To be healthy, enlist the goddess of prevention instead of the goddess of cure.

The best way to stay well is to lead the life-style recommended throughout this book. If you attend to the principles of good nutrition, balanced exercise, stress reduction, and accident prevention, you won't need much medicine, preventive or otherwise. Instead you'll be healthy, and you'll enjoy a full and varied life.

Still, you do need a doctor. Doctors should be your partners in primary prevention. Immunizations are a good example. Doctors should also strive to detect and treat problems early, before symptoms occur. Mammograms, blood pressure measurements, and cholesterol checks are examples of medical screening for secondary prevention. Most important of all, you need a doctor to treat illnesses that cannot be prevented.

An old-time runner coming to see me for his first checkup in 35 years defended his avoidance of medical care by explaining that he had "two fine doctors, my right leg and my left." I was, of course, very sympathetic to the goals of independence, self-reliance, and personal responsibility. It's your body, and it's up to you to care for it properly. Indeed, your health is too important to be left to your doctor alone. But your doctor can help. In addition to performing the crucial but rather technical roles of prevention, diagnosis, and treatment, your doctor should be a teacher, a listener, a counselor, a partner in preventive health care, and a friend.

■ Health Care in America

Health care in this country is in a period of transition. Although we often speak of "the health care system," in truth there is no system. Instead, there are many systems. Medical practice began with the model of an individual physician caring for patients and being paid directly by them. As medicine has become more complex, care has shifted from solo practitioners to groups and specialists, and from private offices to clinics and hospitals. As care has become more expensive, payment has shifted from patients themselves to private insurance companies and government agencies.

Changes notwithstanding, the key to your care is still your primary physician. Primary care practitioners include pediatricians, who provide comprehensive care for children; internists, who do the same for adults; and family practitioners, who provide basic care for both age groups. In addition, healthy young women often turn to gynecologists for primary care, an excellent arrangement as long as both patient and doctor understand what's involved.

A primary care practitioner should be your fundamental health resource. Patients often think of their primary care doctors as quarterbacks, coordinating care among various specialists. For complex situations this perception is correct. But in most cases, primary care should be more than a starting point, providing instead care that is truly comprehensive.

Primary care physicians are essential, but they are just one part of your health care team. After years of being undervalued, nurses are finally getting the recognition they deserve. Nurses can do much more than simply "follow doctor's orders." They are crucial for health screening, performing procedures such as measuring height and weight, monitoring blood pressure, and performing breast exams and Pap smears. Nurses are often excellent listeners and teachers, generally giving more time to these crucial jobs than physicians do and getting better results. Nurse practitioners and physicians' assistants have received additional training and certification; in many states, they are qualified to order diagnostic tests and formulate treatment plans, but they cannot prescribe medications and they should work in partnership with a physician. Most doctors know that their greatest assets are their nurses; many patients still don't understand that these skilled providers can also be their best medical friends.

Many other health care workers can provide valuable medical services. It's a big preventive care team with many players. How can you use the ones you need without generating confusion or conflict? Let your primary care physician be the manager of your health team. Better still, do your job as owner, not of the team but of your body; if you take good care of yourself, you'll need very few professional health services.

■ Your Doctor

You need a doctor who is skilled in diagnosing and treating disease, but your doctor should also serve as your partner in prevention. How do doctors stack up?

Two 1991 surveys of 2,610 internists belonging to the American College of Physicians give us some answers. The doctors did quite well with the problem of smoking, inquiring about this habit in 98 percent of their patients and providing information on smoking cessation to 90 percent of their patients who smoked. They did almost as well with alcohol, taking an appropriate history 94 percent of the time and providing counseling to 76 percent of their patients who drank to excess. But only 66 percent of these internists inquired about diet, and only 40 percent asked about sexual activity. Important preventive life-style advice was also hard to come by: exercise was encouraged by only 48 percent and seat belt use by 35 percent. Even when advice was provided, it was at best terse, occupying less than three minutes in most cases. These well-qualified physicians also failed to offer recommended preventive services to all their patients; they provided stool blood testing to only 76 percent, Pap smears to 71 percent, mammograms to 59 percent, and immunizations to 42 percent.

Doctors, like all people, are fallible, but some are more fallible than others. No doctor is perfect, but you can take steps to be sure you get the preventive services you need. The trick is to find the right doctor and to be a well-informed health care consumer.

Selecting a Physician

Here are some things to consider when you select a physician:

Specialty. Look for a primary care practitioner.

Education, including postgraduate training and medical board certification. Early in my practice, when I realized how few patients asked about these important qualifications, I had my diplomas and certificates framed so a glance at my office wall would answer unframed questions. If your doctor's wall is blank (or if you can't decipher Latin), feel free to ask. We've all paid plenty of tuition, and we should be proud of our training. But if asking feels awkward, a simple call to your local medical society will provide the information you need.

Age. This can be a tough call. It brings to mind the conversation between a young intern and a sage professor of medicine:

- Intern: How did you cure this patient?
- Professor: It was simple: good judgment.
- Intern: How did you develop good judgment?
- Professor: It was simple: experience.
- Intern: How did you get experience?
- Professor: It was simple: bad judgment.

Young doctors are more likely to be on top of the latest medical discoveries and to be aggressive about diagnosis and treatment. Older doctors are more likely to have seasoned clinical judgment that does, indeed, depend on experience. Choose the age that seems most comfortable to you, but if you choose an older practitioner, consider the questions of retirement and continuity.

Coverage. Your doctor should have high-quality backup coverage available at *all* times. (How does a 45-year-old doctor with 35- and 60-year-old partners sound?)

Hospital affiliations. Pick a doctor who is associated with a good hospital that has a broad network of medical and surgical specialists.

Accessibility. The best doctors in the world won't do you any good if you can't get help when you need it. Your doctor should be available to answer telephone questions and to see you in the office on short notice.

Payment plans. An ounce of prevention is worth a pound of cure — if it's covered by your health insurance. Be sure your doctor and your health coverage are compatible.

Personal health habits. Preaching is not enough. Doctors who practice prevention for themselves are the most likely to practice it for you.

Personality and style. I've confessed more than once that doctors are human. Pick a doctor with the human traits that are important to you. Warmth, frankness, and communication skills are high on the list when I pick doctors for myself and recommend them for my family. A sense of humor doesn't hurt, either. Look for doctors who are eager to answer questions, willing to admit that they don't know all the answers, and happy to seek answers and arrange consultations for second opinions.

Time. It's the most fleeting of things, and the most valuable thing a doctor can give you.

Finding the right doctor can be worrisome. When you have to find a new physician, ask for referrals from your other doctors, your county medical society, your community hospital or medical center, or from a medical school. Referrals from your relatives and friends can be even more useful, providing personal information that you can never find on sheepskins. Give it some time and thought, and give it another try if things don't work out the first time.

Relating to Your Doctor

Call it confidence, respect, or friendship. Call it trust, but never call it awe. By any name, your personal relationship with your doctor is a basic element in your health care.

Tell your doctor what you want and what you expect. Are you there for a consultation, for a one-time checkup, or to initiate long-term care? What have your previous medical experiences been like? Do you want your family to be involved in your care? Do you want to relate primarily to the doctor or the nurse? Do you want "all the facts" or just the essentials? Do you want your doctor to make the decisions, or do you want to make them yourself?

Be honest with yourself and your doctor. Too often patients are reluctant to express their real fears and concerns. Practicing medicine is hard enough without adding mind reading to its many challenges. Ask yourself if you have questions about issues that are often hard to discuss: sexuality, risks of tests and treatments, side effects of medications, costs.

Keep lists. Jot down your concerns and requests before your visit so that your doctor can deal with them completely and efficiently.

Ask questions. Doctors can examine, test, and treat, but your understanding is crucial for successful care. Don't be afraid to ask a "dumb" question; the only really dumb question is the one that remains unasked.

Take notes and ask for written information. Even doctors who are skilled communicators may not be able to explain everything in a single visit. Written information will allow you to ponder and digest all the facts and to come up with new questions for your next visit, or for a phone call or letter.

Be assertive. Doctors do not belong on pedestals; they are working for you. Don't be afraid to disagree with a physician. But remember that your doctor's advice is (I hope) based on scientific data, and understand that medical perspectives may differ from the personal testaments of your friends and relatives. If there is a conflict, the choice will be yours; but if your doctors have the data to support their views, I'd vote for medical advice over your cousin's opinion every time.

Ask for your results and keep them on file. Your medical records belong to you; a written request should allow you to obtain them at any time. Still, if you keep your own notes of your immunizations, illnesses, tests, and treatments, it will be much easier for you to fill out health forms and to consult new health care providers. Be particularly careful to note any allergies or adverse reactions that you have experienced. If you see several doctors, bring relevant information along when you see any of them. Your doctors should communicate with one another, but you're the best defense against our epistolary failures.

Be an active, informed health care consumer, not a passive patient. It's your body, and the ultimate responsibility for its health is yours. Learn as much as you can about the human body, including its marvelous strengths and its frailties. Keep up with new developments in prevention and health care (see chapter 24) so you can be sure your doctor is offering you "the latest" — if, in fact, new is really better. Knowledge *is* power, and it's also fascinating in its own right.

Don't be afraid to disappoint your doctors by letting them know that a treatment is not working out as hoped. And don't be reluctant to thank your physician if you're pleased with results; doctors always seem to find time for happy phone calls.

What to Expect from Your Doctor

No two doctors are exactly alike. For all their differences in style, however, all primary care doctors should offer you similarities in substance.

At your *initial visit* you should be asked to provide a detailed account of major illnesses in your family and of your own medical history, including illnesses, operations, immunizations, medications, and allergic reactions. Often omitted but of equal importance are questions about your life-style; your doctor should ask about your occupation, your travel, your family, your stresses and releases, your use of tobacco, alcohol, and other drugs, your use of seat belts, your understanding of safe sexual practices, your exercise schedule, and your diet.

You should be asked about your concerns and symptoms, both in general terms and with specific questions designed to elicit information about each of your body's major organ systems.

You should have a thorough physical examination that evaluates your skin, head and neck, chest, heart, abdomen, and limbs; rectal and pelvic exams are not always necessary but should be performed at certain ages even if you feel entirely well.

At your initial visit you should expect medical tests. Specific tests will depend on your medical status, but even if you're perfectly healthy, certain screening tests are beneficial while others are wasteful or even harmful.

Follow-up visits fall into two categories. *Routine checkups* should repeat the comprehensive evaluation of your initial visit. Since you've been through it once, however, these checkups will be much simpler and faster. The timing of these preventive exams and tests depends on your age, sex, and health. *Focused follow-ups* depend on your condition; healthy people don't need them at all, but sick patients will be asked to return early and often. But you don't have to be desperately ill to deserve a focused follow-up appointment. You should be given an appointment to reevaluate unexplained symptoms or other ongoing problems. A follow-up should be scheduled every time you start on a long-term medication, such as blood pressure pills. Be grateful, too, if you are asked to return to your doctor's office "just" to monitor your progress in improving your health practices (smoking, drinking, diet, exercise).

Finally, you should expect your doctor to explain how you can obtain *unanticipated health care.* You should understand how to get immediate care for emergencies and how to arrange office visits for less urgent problems. You should also learn how your doctor's office handles telephone queries.

Perhaps most important of all, you should expect to receive detailed advice on how to monitor and maintain your own health during the 99.9 percent of the time when you are not a patient but a person.

It's a lot to expect, but no admission officer ever promised a medical school applicant an easy life. Your doctors are well paid for meeting your expectations and are rewarded with enormous gratification when you stay well.

■ Preventive Services for Adults

The belief that doctors can prevent disease is as old as medicine. About 2,000 years ago the great Greek physician Galen observed that "since, both in importance and in time, health precedes disease, so we ought to consider first how health may be preserved, and then how we may best cure disease." Even today the preventive checkup is the single most common reason that patients see doctors, accounting for some 500 million office visits in the United States each year.

Both patients and doctors believe in preventive medical care. Contemporary attitudes stem not from the ancients but from Dr. George Gould, whose speech to the American Medical Association in 1900 articulated the concept that periodic medical care could prevent disease. Over the next 75 years this concept grew in popularity, fueled, no doubt, by America's love affair with the automobile and its commitment to preventive maintenance and the 10,000-mile checkup.

Routine "maintenance" and checkups are indeed important for humans. But although their value seems self-evident, they are not as helpful as we might hope.

The last two decades have witnessed a critical reappraisal of preventive medical services. Drs. Frame, Carlson, Breslow, and Sommers started the trend. The Canadian Task Force on the Periodic Health Exam took up the challenge in 1979. In the 1980s most major American health organizations issued their own recommendations. And in 1989 the U.S. Preventive Services Task Force produced the most comprehensive report, evaluating 169 separate preventive medical tests and treatments. Those guidelines have already been very helpful for clinical practice; still, they will be subjected to reappraisal in the years to come.

Tests, Tests, and More Tests

In our technological society most patients expect tests and treatments when they visit their doctors. In fact that's exactly what they get about 80 percent of the time, with only 20 percent of their visits being devoted principally to counseling. True, some tests can be life-saving — but many are unnecessary, some misleading, and a few harmful.

I need tests as much as any doctor, and I use them frequently. But as medicine becomes increasingly technical, tests are often ordered inappropriately. Sometimes the patient is responsible, asking for tests he or she doesn't really need. Sometimes the doctor is at fault, simply not understanding what a test can and cannot accomplish. In other cases doctors may feel obliged to order tests just to protect themselves from litigation ("defensive medicine"). Finally, some doctors may have a financial stake in testing, owning labs or x-ray equipment; the profession is just now starting to confront this difficult ethical dilemma.

When tests are needed, doctors should always start with the simplest, least dangerous, least expensive tests at their disposal, moving to more elaborate studies only if the basic ones fail. And we must never forget how to use the best of all diagnostic tools, our ears, eyes, and hands.

Why Have Tests?

When it comes to prevention, healthy people can benefit from good tests that are ordered appropriately. These benefits include:

Establishing a baseline. No two mammograms look exactly alike, nor do any two electrocardiograms. To find out what your normal one looks like, your doctor may order a cardiogram at about age 40 or a mammogram for women at about age 35. In the overwhelming majority of cases the tests will be normal, but they are not wasted if they can be filed away to serve as personal standards of comparison for repeat tests in later years.

Detecting clinically silent abnormalities. This is the most important role for preventive testing. The routine Pap smear is an excellent example of a good screening test: it's an inexpensive, safe, and reliable way to detect cancer of the cervix before any symptoms develop, when cure is easy.

Detecting trends. Humankind's only true constant is change. When repeated at appropriate intervals, tests can sometimes be used to detect unfavorable trends even before they cross the line between normal and abnormal. A "normal" cholesterol level of 195, for example, may merit extra dietary care if it has steadily risen from 145 over the years.

Providing reassurance. In my view the scientific committees that evaluate tests often fail to give enough weight to this potential benefit of testing. "Extra" cholesterol tests or electrocardiograms, for example, may be a great bargain if they can convince worried patients that they are indeed healthy. But an expensive or invasive test such as a cardiac catheterization should be used to provide reassurance *only* in the most extreme and unusual situations.

Motivating change. I'm sharing a trick of the trade with this one. Sometimes I will recommend a test even if its result is entirely predictable if I feel I can use the result to motivate a patient to make life-style changes. High cholesterol readings, for example, may help convince a patient that diet and exercise really are important.

Why Not Have Tests?

With so much to gain, why not have all the tests you can? Unfortunately, there is something to lose from having inappropriate tests. The drawbacks of testing include:

False alarms. Even the most specific tests will occasionally give abnormal results in healthy people. The result can be devastating; imagine how long it would take you to recover from being told that your AIDS test was positive, even if a repeat test the next day was entirely normal.

False reassurance. Even the most sensitive tests can sometimes miss early disease. In addition, normal results can sometimes be harmful if they are misinterpreted. A normal cholesterol level, for example, does not mean that it's safe for you to eat lots of animal fat, much less that you are immune to heart disease.

Inconvenience and discomfort. Most patients are willing to put up with quite a lot to have tests that "can help." But there is no reason to go through even a little discomfort if a test won't do any good in the first place.

Side effects. Most tests are safe, but no test is *perfectly* safe. Even a simple blood test can produce an unsightly, uncomfortable hematoma (black and blue mark) or a fainting spell. And when it comes to invasive tests, the side effects can be serious.

Expense. Insurance companies or government agencies pay for most tests. There may be no charge to you, but there is always a cost. Sooner or later we will all foot the bill by paying high insurance premiums and taxes. If a test is important, it's worth paying for, even out of your own pocket. But unnecessary tests are wastefully expensive even if they're "free."

To Test or Not to Test

That is the question. To help answer it, I'll describe the major preventive services and pass along suggestions for their use. But if your doctor recommends tests that are not on my list, you'll have to decide for yourself. Here are some questions you should ask:

- What are the goals of the test?
- Is the test sensitive (i.e., few false negative results) and specific (i.e., few false positives)?
- What's involved in the test? How long will it take? Is it uncomfortable?
- What are the side effects?
- What does it cost?
- Are there alternative tests?
- What are the risks of not having the test?
- Is the timing important? Should the test be done at once, or can it be postponed safely?
- Will the test lead to a treatment? Although knowledge is always a good thing, your tests should produce results as well as information.

A Core Program of Preventive Services

I can almost hear you asking the same question my patients raise after I've explained at great length the benefits and limitations of screening tests: "But, doctor, what tests should I have?" At the cost of oversimplification, I'll offer you a simple schedule of these core services. To use it appropriately, however, you must understand two things.

First, this is a schedule of preventive services for *healthy adults* with *average risk factors, no symptoms,* and *good health habits.* If you are fortunate enough to be in this group, you do not need additional exams, tests, or treatments, and you should not pay for them with your time, discomfort, money, or insurance premiums. But even healthy people may need additional services because of their family histories (high blood pressure, heart disease, breast cancer, colon cancer) or their behavior patterns (poor diet, lack of exercise, smoking, alcohol or substance abuse, unsafe sexual activity). And of course the presence of symptoms or abnormal results often calls for additional examination and testing.

Second, this schedule is *only a general guide.* Since the 1970s many expert panels have examined the benefits, risks, and costs of preventive medical services. Their findings have been extremely helpful, but their work is ongoing and their recommendations will evolve further. Because each recommendation represents a consensus hammered out in committee, it represents a conservative position. Even so, the recommendations of various groups differ. Table 23-1 presents the recommendations of the U.S. Preventive Services Task Force. When there are substantial disagreements, it also lists the positions of other major medical organizations.

How should you decide between conflicting recommendations? It's never easy, but these decisions should not produce great anxiety; they are, after all, choices between sound, responsible alternatives. And you can get help: you've gone to the trouble of finding a good doctor to get individualized recommendations based on clinical experience as well as statistics. Scientific data must be the basis for all medical recommendations, but there is room, too, for judgments based on what your doctor knows about you.

For this reason, I've added a final column to each recommendation, noting my own clinical practice patterns. They don't stray far from the official lists, but they do include a few additional tests that are noninvasive, low-risk, and inexpensive. They also include a few additional office visits, principally to build mutual understanding and rapport and to exchange information about symptoms, health habits, and new developments in prevention and clinical medicine. I'm no smarter than other doctors, and I certainly don't offer my own humble practices as superior to the advice of authoritative committees. Still, like most of my colleagues I've found these small departures helpful in taking care of real people.

Don't expect your doctor to practice cookbook medicine, simply following official recommendations by rote. But if your doctors' recipes for preventive care seem very different from the core program, ask for their reasons and think them over carefully before you have extra tests. I've explained the reasons for my recommendations in each chapter of this book. In addition to recommended tests, table 23-1 also lists a few of the major *non*recommended tests that some doctors order for patients over 40.

■ Your Role in Preventive Medical Care

Never be a passive recipient of health care; instead, always be an active patient, a true participant in your care. Your role is particularly important when it comes to preventive medical care; more than being simply your doctors' partner, you should be their senior partner.

As you've read in this chapter, current trends in medicine are pointing toward fewer "routine" doctor's visits and medical tests. There are good reasons behind these trends, but they leave a potential gap. Who can fill in for doctors and their lab tests? You can — and should. I'm not asking you to become your own doctor, but I am asking you to serve as your doctors' eyes and ears between office visits. Here's how.

Be Alert for Symptoms

Every recommendation for medical care — be it "see you in a year" or "see you in five" — is made with the understanding that you will listen to your

Table 23-1. Core Preventive Services for Healthy Adults: A Summary of Guidelines

	Source	*Recommendation*
Ages 20–39		
Women and men		
Clinical evaluation	U.S. Task Force	Weight, blood pressure every 1–3 years
		Counseling every 1–3 years, and as needed
	Other major groups	American Cancer Society: physical exam every 3 years
	My usual practice	Comprehensive health evaluation: (physical exam with review of medical history and health habits) every 5 years between ages 20 and 29 and every 3 years between ages 30 and 39
Immunizations	U.S. Task Force	Tetanus-diphtheria once every 10 years
		Measles, mumps and rubella, hepatitis B, influenza, and other vaccines as indicated by individual risk
	Other major groups	Similar
	My usual practice	Similar
Tuberculosis skin test	U.S. Task Force	Recommended only for people at above-average risk
	Other major groups	Variable
	My usual practice	At time of initial visit for all patients under 35, repeat every 1–3 years if risk is increased
Cholesterol	U.S. Task Force	Every 5 years
	Other major groups	Similar
	My usual practice	With each comprehensive health evaluation

▶

Table 23-1. (continued)

	Source	Recommendation
Ages 20–39		
Women and men		
Blood sugar	U.S. Task Force	Recommended only during pregnancy
	Other major groups	American Diabetes Association: every 3 years for high-risk individuals
	My usual practice	With each comprehensive health evaluation
Complete blood count	U.S. Task Force	Not recommended
	Other major groups	Similar
	My usual practice	With each comprehensive health evaluation
Urine analysis	U.S. Task Force	Not recommended
	Other major groups	Similar
	My usual practice	With every other comprehensive health evaluation
Electrocardiogram	U.S. Task Force	Not recommended
	Other major groups	American Heart Association: at age 20
	My usual practice	Not recommended
Dental prophylaxis	U.S. Task Force	Regular dental visits
	Other major groups	Not available
	My usual practice	Every 6 to 12 months
Eye examination with tonometry for glaucoma	U.S. Task Force	Not recommended
	Other major groups	American Academy of Ophthalmology: every 2–4 years
	My usual practice	Not recommended
Women		
Breast exam by clinician	U.S. Task Force	Not recommended
	Other major groups	American Cancer Society: every 3 years
	My usual practice	With each comprehensive health evaluation
Mammogram	U.S. Task Force	Not recommended unless high risk

Table 23-1. (continued)

	Source	*Recommendation*
Ages 20–39		
Women		
Mammogram	Other major groups	American Cancer Society: baseline exam between ages 35 and 40
	My usual practice	Baseline exam between ages 35 and 40
Pap smear	U.S. Task Force	Every 1–3 years
	Other major groups	Similar
	My usual practice	With every comprehensive health evaluation
Men		
Testicular exam by clinician	U.S. Task Force	Not recommended
	Other major groups	American Cancer Society: every 3 years
	My usual practice	With every comprehensive health evaluation
Ages 40 and above		
Women and men		
Clinical evaluation	U.S. Task Force	Every 1–3 years
	Other major groups	Variable
	My usual practice	Comprehensive health evaluation every 1–2 years between ages 40 and 49; every year above age 50
Immunizations	U.S. Task Force	Tetanus-diphtheria once every 10 years
		Influenza vaccine annually beginning at age 65; pneumococcal vaccine at age 65
	Other major groups	Similar
	My usual practice	Similar, plus annual influenza vaccine at patient request beyond age 40

▶

Table 23-1. (continued)

	Source	Recommendation
Ages 40 and above		
Women and men		
Cholesterol	U.S. Task Force	Every 5 years
	Other major groups	Similar
	My usual practice	With each comprehensive health evaluation
Blood sugar	U.S. Task Force	Not recommended
	Other major groups	American Diabetes Association: every 1–3 years for high-risk individuals
	My usual practice	With each comprehensive health examination
Complete blood count	U.S. Task Force	Not recommended
	Other major groups	Similar
	My usual practice	With each comprehensive health evaluation
Urine analysis	U.S. Task Force	Not recommended (optional for women over 60)
	Other major groups	Similar
	My usual practice	With every comprehensive health evaluation
Electrocardiogram	U.S. Task Force	Not recommended
	Other major groups	American College of Cardiology: every 5 years and at physician discretion
	My usual practice	Variable
Stress test	U.S. Task Force	Not recommended
	Other major groups	Similar
	My usual practice	Similar
Chest x ray	U.S. Task Force	Not recommended
	Other major groups	Similar
	My usual practice	Similar
Dental prophylaxis	U.S. Task Force	Regular dental visits
	Other major groups	Not available
	My usual practice	Every 6 to 12 months

Table 23-1. (continued)

	Source	Recommendation
Ages 40 and above		
Women and men		
Eye examination with tonometry for glaucoma	U.S. Task Force	Not recommended (vision tests every year over age 65)
	Other major groups	American Academy of Ophthalmology: every year
	My usual practice	Ages 40–49 every 2–3 years; over age 50 every 1–2 years
Hearing tests	U.S. Task Force	May be appropriate beyond age 65
	Other major groups	Variable
	My usual practice	Not recommended unless symptoms are present
Stool blood testing	U.S. Task Force	Not recommended
	Other major groups	American Cancer Society: every year beginning at age 50
	My usual practice	With every comprehensive health evaluation
Sigmoidoscopy	U.S. Task Force	Not recommended
	Other major groups	American Cancer Society: every 3–5 years beginning at age 50
	My usual practice	Evolving with new data; currently every 10 years, beginning at age 50
Women		
Breast exam by clinician	U.S. Task Force	Every year
	Other major groups	Similar
	My usual practice	Similar
Mammogram	U.S. Task Force	Every year
	Other major groups	Similar
	My usual practice	Similar
Pap smear	U.S. Task Force	Every 1–3 years until age 65
	Other major groups	American Cancer Society: every 1–3 years

▶

Table 23-1. (continued)

	Source	Recommendation
Ages 40 and above		
Women		
Pap smear	My usual practice	With every comprehensive health evaluation until age 65; variable thereafter
Bone density for osteoporosis	U.S. Task Force	Not recommended
	Other major groups	Similar
	My usual practice	Similar
Men		
Rectal exam to check prostate	U.S. Task Force	No recommendation for or against
	Other major groups	American Cancer Society: every year
	My usual practice	With every comprehensive health evaluation

body between office visits. Be alert for symptoms, and if they seem important, call them to your doctor's attention promptly instead of waiting for your next routine checkup.

The trick, of course, is to know what symptoms are really important. We all have aches and pains from time to time, but it won't do you much good to run to your doctor for every minor problem. In general, though, changes in your bodily functions that are unusual, unexpected, severe, or persistent *should* be evaluated — and not by your mother or cousin but by your doctor or nurse. Often a simple phone call will do the trick. Unlike tests and treatments, there are never any side effects from questions; when in doubt about a symptom, check it out.

Because this is a book about preventing illnesses rather than diagnosing and treating them, I have not tried to provide a comprehensive guide to symptoms. Still, you'll find many signs of major diseases discussed in chapters 1–18. At the risk of repetition, and at the cost of oversimplification, let me remind you of some major symptoms to watch for; remember, though that this is but a *partial, general* list:

> Heart disease — Pressure or pain in the chest, particularly following exertion, especially if pain radiates to the neck, jaw, or arms
> Undue shortness of breath, especially when lying down or with mild exertion
> Ankle swelling

	Rapid or erratic heartbeat or pulse Excessive fatigue or exhaustion Unexplained fainting
Cancer	Changes in bowel habits, particularly bleeding or pain on defecation, narrow stools, or unexplained constipation Changes in urinary function, particularly bleeding Changes in the menstrual function, particularly unexpected, excessive, or erratic bleeding Changes in the skin or mouth, particularly a sore that does not heal or one that enlarges or bleeds A swelling, thickening, or lump in the breasts, lymph glands, or other tissues Persistent unexplained cough or hoarseness Difficulty swallowing or early sensation of fullness Loss of appetite Unexplained weight loss Pallor or abnormal bleeding, especially from the gums Excessive fatigue
Vascular disease	Unexpected pain, cramps, or fatigue in a leg, particularly when walking Cold, pale, or swollen feet or legs
Neurological diseases	Weakness or impaired sensation in an arm or leg Sudden visual loss Impaired coordination or persistent tremors Impaired speech or understanding Major memory loss or personality changes Unexplained fainting Seizures
Lung diseases	Unexplained or persistent cough, especially with bleeding Excessive shortness of breath Sharp chest pain, especially when breathing deeply Wheezing
Gastrointestinal diseases	Changes in bowel habits or swallowing (see *Cancer*) Persistent or recurrent diarrhea, especially with blood, mucus, cramps, or fever

Gastrointestinal diseases (*continued*)	Persistent or recurrent nausea or vomiting, especially with bleeding or after eating
	Persistent or severe heartburn or pain in the abdomen
Liver and gall bladder diseases	Yellow discoloration of the skin or eyes
	Swollen abdomen or feet
	Pain in the upper-right abdomen, especially after eating or if accompanied by vomiting
	Abnormal bleeding
	Excessive fatigue
	Unexplained weight loss, fatigue, or confusion
Musculoskeletal diseases	Pain, swelling, or deformity of joints, bones, muscles, or back
Breast diseases	A persistent swelling, thickening, or lump
	Inward retraction of the nipple or skin
	Bleeding or discharge from the nipple
Female reproductive diseases	Abnormal vaginal bleeding
	Abnormal vaginal discharge
	Abnormal urine or bowel function
	Lower abdominal pain or swelling
Male reproductive diseases	Painful or blood ejaculation
	Changes in sex drive or potency
	Changes in urination
Urinary tract disorders	Cloudy, bloody, or malodorous urine
	Urinary frequency
	Pain on urination
	Difficulty in passing urine
Blood disorders	Pallor
	Abnormal bleeding
	Excessive fatigue or shortness of breath
Immune system disorders	Frequent, severe, or unusual infections
Diabetes	Excessive thirst, urination, or hunger
	Blurred vision
	Excessive fatigue
	Unexplained weight loss
Eye disorders	Eye pain or redness
	Impaired vision
	Abnormal tearing
Ear disorders	Impaired hearing
	Pain
	Discharge or bleeding
	Buzzing or ringing
	Loss of balance, dizziness

Teeth and mouth, throat	A sore that enlarges or does not heal Pain Swollen or discolored gums Foul breath Persistent hoarseness
Skin diseases	A sore that does not heal, particularly if it enlarges or bleeds Rash, redness, scaling Unexplained itching
Infections	Fever Chills Night sweats Loss of appetite; unexplained weight loss Cough; sputum production; cloudy, bloody, or painful urine; many other symptoms of specific organ infection
Psychological disorders	Anxiety Depression Sleep disorders Substance abuse Personality changes Family, social, or occupational conflicts Violence

It's a long list; even so, it's very incomplete. You should note, too, that most symptoms have several causes, some serious but others trivial. Don't attempt to use this list to diagnose yourself; instead, use it as a general reminder of the sorts of things you should report to your doctor.

Examine Yourself

You don't need a degree in medicine or nursing to keep an eye on yourself, nor do you need to paw over your body every day. But a few simple observations can be invaluable.

Weight	Record your weight every six to twelve months, or more often if it changes unexpectedly.
Skin	Examine your skin systematically at regular intervals.
Breast self-exam	Women should examine themselves monthly.
Testicular self-exam	Men should examine themselves about once a month, at least until age 35.
Oral self-exam	This is a bit difficult, and it's not widely recommended. Still, it's a reasonable self-exam for smokers to learn; even better, stop smoking.

Don't panic if your self-exam reveals a possible abnormality. Most often the problem is mild and its treatment effective. But don't go to the other extreme by ignoring your findings or attempting to explain them away with a homemade diagnosis. Your job is not to *interpret* your symptoms but to *report* them to your doctor.

Use Medications Properly

Use only medications that are necessary, and use them carefully. If you take nonprescription medications, be sure to read the labels carefully and to follow their directions precisely. If you are given a prescription medication, be sure you know why it's been recommended and what side effects to watch for; you can also ask for the package insert to get detailed information. Be alert for side effects, and keep a record of all medications that have affected you adversely. Before you start any new medication, be sure that your physician and pharmacist know about your other medicines.

Take Care of Yourself

The best medical care is no medical care — if you're healthy. Even as we near the end of this book, I can't resist another opportunity to remind you that preventing illness is primarily up to you. If you follow the precepts discussed in chapters 1–22, you'll need far fewer of the medical services discussed here in chapter 23.

Preventive self-care may seem complex, and there is a lot to know. But the basics remain very simple: avoid the Seven Deadly Sins. It's an old idea, and the modern seven remain startlingly close to the biblical originals. *Gluttony* and *sloth*, in fact, head both lists, while lust can be updated slightly to *unsafe sexual practices.* If we consolidate pride, covetousness, anger, and envy to their contemporary equivalent, *excessive stress,* we have room on the list for three twentieth-century health sins: *smoking, alcohol and substance abuse,* and *accident-prone behavior.* And even if you're a health sinner, don't despair. Just repent, confess to your doctor so you can get appropriate medical tests, and, above all, reform: you still have time to save yourself from needless suffering and illness.

■ 24 ■

Keeping Up with New Developments in Prevention

In *Staying Well* I've written many words about prevention — but not the last word. One of the most exciting things about medicine is that things change: new discoveries are reported every week, if not every day.

How can you keep up with new developments? The short answer is to ask your doctor. But your health is too important to be left to your doctor. You really should keep up with new developments on your own. You should also learn how to evaluate new information, looking it over carefully before you leap into the latest trend.

Staying abreast of medical developments is difficult for doctors, and it may not be easy for you. But it can be done. Here's how.

■ Medicine and the Mass Media

The fastest way to disseminate new information in our society is through the mass media, and medical information is no exception. Television and radio are often the first to publicize new advances, but they rarely provide the details you need to understand the significance of their reports.

Newspapers and magazines give you the medical headline, but they should give you the relevant details as well. Nearly every day one of my patients unfolds a crumpled newspaper to ask what I think of the latest information or advice. Often I confess that it's news to me, too, since newspapers can make it to my desk faster than medical journals. In any case I read the story carefully with my patient, trying to evaluate its message. You can learn to use the same criteria that I do.

First, ascertain the source of the information. Journalists can get medical information from many places. The least reliable source is a news conference or press release. Unfortunately, hype and hoopla have invaded science just as they've affected all human endeavors. Medical information can have enormous commercial implications; think twice about "breakthrough" stories that originate from drug manufacturers.

Journalists can also get medical information by attending lectures delivered by physicians. Many lectures are thoughtful and comprehensive, but others may be biased by the personal enthusiasm and beliefs of the speaker. The best media reports will be accompanied by interviews that elicit opinions from several authorities in the field.

Reporters can also get their scoops just the way doctors do, by attending medical meetings and reading medical journals.

Many medical advances are reported first at meetings and symposia. It's a very useful system, but it has pitfalls. Speakers are limited to 10 or 15 minutes, and the talks are scheduled on the basis of brief abstracts, so the quality of the research has not been scrutinized in detail before it's presented. Much of the work is excellent, but a lot is preliminary, and some is flawed. Unfortunately, new developments presented at meetings can sound more authoritative than they are. A little healthy skepticism on your part is good; the fact that a study is presented at a meeting of the American Heart Association does not necessarily mean that it has been scrutinized by cardiologists, much less endorsed by the association.

■ How Medical Journals Work

The best way to convey new medical information is through the medical journals. Published papers set forth methods and findings in detail so an informed reader can evaluate the quality of the work and the validity of its interpretation. Needless to say, the quality of medical journals varies substantially. The best, however, are very selective about what they print. The prestigious *New England Journal of Medicine,* for instance, evaluates more than 3,500 manuscripts each year but accepts fewer than 15 percent of them for publication. Medical journals decide which articles to print by subjecting each submission to the process of peer review, which means that each article is studied objectively by independent experts in the field before it is accepted for publication. Authors are often asked to provide clarifications requested by the reviewers. Articles that are surprising, controversial, or just plain important are often accompanied by editorials that provide perspectives on the subject.

Despite its advantages, peer review has some drawbacks, since reviewers are human and they too can make mistakes. Also, the process is slow; advocacy groups justifiably complain that it can delay the dissemination of information that may be life-saving. Medical editors are now grappling with new ways to balance the demands of quality assurance against the advantages of speed. Until they succeed, I'll do my tiny part by putting articles for review on the top of my "in" pile.

Hundreds of articles are published in peer-reviewed medical journals each month. No doctor can subscribe to all the good journals, and no science writer can read them all. Instead, we play our favorites, learning to trust a few journals that publish articles which are scientifically accurate and relevant to our clinical or research needs. Good medical writers will always identify the journals they are quoting, and you will soon identify the names of the top journals. Here are some of the publications I've found most helpful in assembling data on preventive medicine for this book:

New England Journal of Medicine
Annals of Internal Medicine
American Journal of Medicine
Archives of Internal Medicine
Journal of the American Medical Association
The Lancet
British Medical Journal
American Journal of Epidemiology
American Journal of Public Health
Preventive Medicine

It's an abbreviated list, so don't disdain information published in other excellent journals; there are dozens of them. Remember, too, that many of these journals publish letters that are *not* peer reviewed and should not be accepted as authoritative.

■ Medical Articles and Press Stories

To be published in a good medical journal, an article must survive considerable scrutiny. But that does not necessarily mean it's relevant to you. To be an intelligent information consumer, you need to think things through for yourself.

First, remember that you are reading not a medical report but a journalist's story based on that article. Victor Cohn, the former science editor of the *Washington Post*, once said that there are only two types of medical stories, "New Hope" and "No Hope." He was exaggerating, of course, but there is more than a little truth in his quip. Journalists have a natural tendency to dramatize and simplify, to omit the "ifs" and gloss over the "buts" to find a punchy moral in a complex story.

Writers and editors can also be guilty of underreporting medical information. The most dramatic example in the field of preventive medicine is the coverage — or lack of coverage — devoted to the health impacts of tobacco and alcohol. I'm sorry to say that the enormous economic clout of these giant industries has produced self-censoring by the media. Advertising revenues have been preserved, but health has suffered.

What's a reader to do? You learn to pick good medical practitioners whose work you can trust; do the same with medical journalists. But don't blindly accept the advice of your favorite writers (or, for that matter, your favorite doctors). Instead, think for yourself.

■ Major Types of Medical Research

Three types of scientific research produce information about prevention.

Laboratory experiments are apt to focus on basic mechanisms of disease. This research is essential to the progress of medicine, but it's usually years away from practical significance. Read articles about basic science to share the wonder of discovery, but don't rush to change your life-style because of test-tube triumphs, however spectacular.

Animal studies often bridge the gap between basic research and clinical observations. Only those animal studies which are really essential should be performed, and they must always be conducted in a manner that is humane and ethical. Animal studies that fulfill these criteria are essential to advance human health. When it comes to prevention, these are studies you should begin to note seriously. But once again, restraint is the watchword; if you acted on the results of every animal study, your decisions might begin to resemble those of a rat in a maze.

Clinical observations of human health and human disease are, of course, the most relevant to you. They may be observations of a single patient's illness — fascinating and instructive to your doctors, but rarely pertinent to you until many more cases have been evaluated. But clinical studies can also encompass groups of people, both healthy and ill. These studies are the most likely to produce information that should motivate you to make changes, if that information is, in fact, both scientifically accurate and personally pertinent.

■ Medical Studies: Understanding the Questions

Most medical studies that apply to prevention pose one of two questions: Does an intervention or therapy prevent a disease? And does an aspect of modern life pose a hazard to human health?

The best way to answer the first question is with a controlled clinical trial. To find out if a treatment is effective, it must be compared directly with an established treatment or with no treatment at all. Valid results depend on *randomly* assigning prospective subjects to one of the study groups.

In the best studies both the researchers and the subjects are "blinded" to the knowledge of which treatment they are receiving, thus eliminating wishful thinking and bias in interpreting results. Such "double-blinded" studies are usually done by giving the experimental group a real drug while the control group receives a placebo, or "dummy pill," which looks and tastes just like the real thing but is inert.

An excellent example of a randomized, double-blinded trial is the Physicians' Health Study discussed in chapter 2. It involves more than 22,000 volunteer subjects, all male physicians, who were randomly assigned to take either aspirin or an inert placebo. It's still in progress after more than seven years and it has cost millions of dollars. But it has found that taking one aspirin tablet every other day can cut the risk of heart attacks by 44 percent in men over 50. Now we need a similar trial for women!

Randomized clinical trials, however useful, are not always feasible — or ethical. To study the effects of smoking on health, for example, researchers might expose animals to smoke, but they could hardly randomize humans into a smoking group. Consequently, studies of health hazards rely on different techniques, utilizing epidemiological research methods. But like clinical trials, epidemiological studies require controlled observations to be valid. Many crucial insights about disease prevention have come from epidemiological studies; the links between smoking and lung cancer, cholesterol and heart disease, and high blood pressure and stroke are but a few examples.

Epidemiological studies first establish associations and test them for validity using the statistical science of probability. Next, the results must be interpreted according to strict criteria to learn if an association actually reflects causality. Finally, the importance of the link must be evaluated by determining its magnitude or relative risk.

For example, studies may show that exposure to toxin A can increase your risk of developing cancer by 10 percent. Put another way, your relative risk would be 1.1 in comparison with that of someone who has never encountered toxin A. A 10 percent increase may sound worrisome, but in fact a relative risk of 1.1 is not very substantial; even the best of studies can overlook confounding variables that could produce such small differences. Don't ignore modest relative risks, but don't get alarmed about relative risks lower than 1.5, which represents a 50 percent increase. Returning to my favorite example, cigarette smoking poses a relative risk of 2.5 for developing heart disease (a 250 percent increase) and of more than 10 (a 1,000 percent increase) for lung cancer. That's real risk!

■ Medical Studies: Understanding Their Meaning and Relevance

After reading *Staying Well*, you should understand that many of the best research studies in preventive medicine have in a sense done little more than reinvent the wheel. In most cases sophisticated, time-consuming, expensive studies have demonstrated that the best way to prevent disease is not to strike out in radical new directions but to return to the basics, to the life-style that is best matched to human genetics. Even though many studies in prevention seem to confirm the obvious, they have been necessary precisely because the norms of contemporary industrial society have drifted so far away from the basics.

You should keep up with new developments in prevention. But you should also know how to put new findings in perspective, and how to determine if *you* should follow new advice. Here are some simple criteria.

1. Understand the source of the advice. Because health is important to everybody, everybody has a theory about health. You can learn a lot from your friends and relatives as well as from nontraditional sources. Don't automatically turn up your nose at folk wisdom. Still, you should be a very cautious consumer before you buy advice based on testimonials or anecdotes. When "they say" something, ask who "they" are, as well as why they say it. Remember that advice based on scientific studies is greatly preferable to anecdotal experiences, whether they come from your doctor or your neighbor.

2. Adopt a "show me" attitude, even with recommendations based on

medical studies. Be skeptical of advice based vaguely on "impressions," "clinical experience," or "judgment." Ask for the facts. The burden of proof should rest with anyone who suggests that you undergo a new test, take a new treatment, or adopt a new life-style.

3. Be extra cautious about advice that runs counter to common sense, and your own experience. Be skeptical, too, of recommendations that would guide you away from the basics of prevention by departing from the fundamental principles of the healthful life-style. If it's not broken, don't fix it. Refer to the simple Ten Commandments of Prevention in chapter 1 to review the basics of prevention.

4. Understand that even the best medical studies require confirmation. Keep an eye out for additional evidence that may confirm, modify, or even refute earlier findings. Learn how to collect reports of new advances in prevention, and keep a file so you can compare results, opinions, and advice from several sources.

5. When evaluating new studies, ask if you fit into the population group being investigated. Findings that are based entirely on investigations of narrowly selected groups (for example, single ethnic groups, narrow age groups, selected employment categories, or single gender studies) may not apply to you and your family. Look for confirmation in studies of people more like you.

6. When evaluating the importance of newly described health risks or benefits, ask three questions:

First, what is the magnitude of risk (or benefit)? Stronger associations clearly deserve more attention.

Second, how common is the problem being studied? Small changes in the risk of contracting common diseases are more important than major changes in the risk of contracting very rare diseases.

Third, are you at risk for the condition being studied? If you are at high risk, you should pay heed to preventive strategies with even modest benefits (for example, women with a strong family history of breast cancer should be more concerned about the possible effects of alcohol use than women with no risk factors for breast cancer).

7. When considering new ways to prevent disease, ask about their costs as well as their benefits. There are always trade-offs. Ask about the side effects of anything new. Consider the costs, whether measured in money, time, or convenience. Consider, too, your personal pleasures and preferences; for example, if starting your day by eating eggs for breakfast is *extremely* important to you, you *may* decide to maintain this habit despite my advice (but please check your cholesterol, and give bran cereal an *honest* try).

8. Remember that uncertainties abound, even in the age of science. When data are incomplete, well-informed, well-intentioned authorities may give you conflicting advice (screening for colon cancer and postmenopausal hormone replacement are but two examples). Draw up your own balance sheet of pros and cons. And when the pluses and minuses seem equal,

don't be afraid to trust your doctor's personal recommendation — or your own gut instincts.

■ Sources for Additional Information about Prevention

The media and the popular press will give you the most rapid updates of new developments in prevention; in exchange for speed, however, these sources are at best sketchy, at worst misleading. Your doctor can give you more authoritative advice; the individual attention is an asset, but information based on practice norms may be excessively conservative. Don't ignore either of these resources. If you understand their advantages and limitations, they can be very useful. Consider, too, that other sources of new information are at your disposal.

Medical Newsletters

During the past 15 years medical newsletters have assumed an increasingly important role in keeping the public informed about new developments in medicine. Although they do not focus specifically on prevention, most devote extensive coverage of tactics readers can use to help themselves. Published monthly, newsletters are slower than newspapers but are still able to get information to you while it is fresh. They also have time to present a balanced view that encompasses both new developments and established facts. Typically written by teams of physicians and science writers, most are authoritative without being dull.

I'm not the only one who likes newsletters. As the public demand for them has grown, more publications have entered the field. I have worked with one of the oldest, the Harvard Health Letter, and one of the newest, the Harvard Heart Letter, and I endorse both enthusiastically. But many other medical newsletters are also excellent. Here is a partial listing.

Harvard Health Letter
Harvard Heart Letter
Harvard Mental Health Letter
164 Longwood Avenue
Boston, MA 02115

Consumer Reports Health Letter
P.O. Box 52148
Boulder, CO 80322

Mayo Clinic Health Letter
200 First Street, NW
Rochester, MN 55905

Tufts University Diet and
    Nutrition Letter
80 Boylston Street
Boston, MA 02116

University of California, Berkeley,
    Wellness Letter
P.O. Box 420148
Palm Coast, FL 32142

The Johns Hopkins Medical Letter
Health After 50
550 North Broadway, Suite 1100
Baltimore, MD 21205

U.S. Government Agencies and Private Associations

If you want detailed information about specific health topics, you can turn to specialized medical groups, both public and private. Most will send you booklets and reference materials free of charge; some will answer individual questions.

At the risk of omitting many worthy groups, I'll provide a partial list of helpful organizations; your phone book can provide others.

American Heart Association
7320 Greenville Avenue
Dallas, TX 75231
(214) 750-5300

American Cancer Society
90 Park Avenue
New York, NY 10016
(212) 599-3600

National Mental Health
  Association
1021 Prince Street
Alexandria, VA 22314
(703) 684-7722

National Osteoporosis Foundation
1625 Eye Street, NW
Washington, DC 20006
(202) 223-2226

National AIDS Information
  Clearinghouse
P.O. Box 6003
Rockville, MD 20850
(301) 762-5111

National Clearinghouse for
  Alcohol and Drug Information
P.O. Box 2345
Rockville, MD 20852
(301) 468-2600

National Arthritis and Musculo-
  skeletal and Skin Diseases
  Information Clearinghouse
P.O. Box AMS
Bethesda, MD 20892
(301) 468-3235

Food and Drug Administration
Office of Consumer Affairs
5600 Fishers Lane
HFE-88
Rockville, MD 20857
(301) 443-3170

American Diabetes Association
1660 Duke Street
Alexandria, VA 22314
(703) 549-1500

American Lung Association
1740 Broadway
New York, NY 10010
(212) 315-8700

American Medical Association
535 North Dearborn Street
Chicago, IL 60610
(312) 464-5000

Centers for Disease Control
U.S. Public Health Service
1600 Clifton Road, NE
Atlanta, GA 30333
(404) 639-3311

National Diabetes Information
  Clearinghouse
Box NDIC
Bethesda, MD 20892
(301) 468-2162

National Digestive Diseases
  Information Clearinghouse
P.O. Box NDDIC
Bethesda, MD 20892
(301) 468-6344

Environmental Protection Agency
Public Information Center
401 M Street, SW
Washington, DC 20466
(202) 382-2080

Cancer Information Service
National Center Institute
Blair Building, Room 414
9000 Rockville Pike
Bethesda, MD 20892
(800) 422-6237
(800) 4-CANCER

National Cholesterol Education
Program Information Center
4733 Bethesda Avenue, Room 530
Bethesda, MD 20814
(301) 951-3260

Dental Disease Prevention
Centers for Disease Control
1600 Clifton Road, NE
Atlanta, GA 30333
(404) 329-1830

National Highway Traffic Safety
Administration
NES-11 HL
U.S. Department of
Transportation
400 7th Street, SW
Washington, DC 20590
(202) 366-9294
Auto Hotline: (800) 424-9393

National Kidney and Urologic
Diseases Information
Clearinghouse
Box NKUDIC
Bethesda, MD 20892
(301) 468-6345

National Center for Education in
Maternal and Child Health
38th and R Streets, NW
Washington, DC 20057
(202) 625-8400

Clearinghouse for Occupational
Safety and Health Information
Technical Information Branch
4676 Columbia Parkway
Cincinnati, OH 45226
(800) 356-4674
(800) 35-NIOSH

Office on Smoking and Health
Technical Information Center
Park Building, Room 1-16
5600 Fishers Lane
Rockville, MD 20857
(301) 443-1690

Food and Nutrition Information
Center
National Agricultural Library
Room 304
Beltsville, MD 20705
(301) 344-3719

National High Blood Pressure
Education Program
Information Center
4733 Bethesda Avenue
Room 530
Bethesda, MD 20814
(301) 951-3260

Consumer Product Safety
Commission
Washington, DC 20207
(800) 638-2772

National Injury Information
Clearinghouse
5401 Westbard Avenue, Room 625
Washington, DC 20207

Consumer Information Center
Pueblo, CO 81009
Distributes consumer publications
on topics such as education,
food and nutrition, health, exercise, and weight control. The
Consumer Information Catalog
is available free from the center
at this address.

National Institute of Mental
Health
Public Inquiries Branch
Parklawn Building
Room 15C-05
5600 Fishers Lane
Rockville, MD 20857
(301) 443-4513

President's Council on Physical
Fitness and Sports
450 5th Street, NW, Suite 7103
Washington, DC 20001
(202) 272-3430

Hotlines

Additional information on prevention is just a toll-free phone call away; here are some numbers you may find handy.

National AIDS Hotline
(800) 342-AIDS

National Association for Hearing
and Speech Action Line
(800) 638-8255

Cancer Response Line
(800) ACS-2345

AIDS Clinical Trials Information
Service
(800) TRIALS-A

Organ Donor Hotline
(800) 24-DONOR

National Pesticide Telecommuni-
cations Network
(800) 858-7378

National Council on Alcoholism
(800) NCA-CALL

National Safety Council
(800) 621-7619

National Center for Sight
(800) 221-3004

Meat and Poultry Hotline
(800) 535-4555

Consumer Product Safety
Commission
(800) 638-CPSC

Cancer Information Services
(800) 4-CANCER

National AIDS Information
Clearinghouse
(800) 458-5231

Birth Control Information Line
(800) 468-3637

Chemical Referral Center
(800) CMA-8200

Alcoholism and Drug Addiction
Treatment Center
(800) 382-4357

National Highway Traffic Safety
Administration
Auto Safety Hotline
(800) 424-9393

American Diabetes Association
(800) ADA-DISC

Arthritis Foundation Information
Line
(800) 283-7800

Asthma and Allergy Foundation
of America
(800) 7-ASTHMA

Venereal Diseases Hotline
(Operation Venus)
(800) 227-8922

National Institute of Occupational
Safety and Health
(800) 356-4674

Environmental Protection Agency
Consumer Products Hotline
(800) 638-2772
Asbestos Hotline
(800) 334-8571
Safe Water Hotline
(800) 426-4791
Superfund Hotline
(800) 424-9346
Solid Waste Hotline
(800) 424-9346

■ The Last Word in Prevention

Like all areas of medicine, prevention changes as new data accumulate and old ideas fall by the wayside. Throughout this book I've tried to give you the latest information available, tempered, of course, by traditional wisdom that remains valid today. I hope you will consider seriously my recommendations. Remember, though, that some advice will change. That's why the book is printed on paper instead of being engraved in stone; buy your oat bran by the box, not the boxcar.

Remember, too, that my recommendations (and your decisions) depend on more than cold statistics and hot scientific data. *Health* derives from a word root in Old English meaning "whole." When it comes to enhancing health and preventing disease, we must look beyond the numbers to evaluate the whole picture. Clinical experience, judgment, and even personal experience can all be very important. Of course, the farther you get from hard facts, the more likely you are to face subtle biases based on personal beliefs and opinions, on hunches and hopes. Still, until we have *all* the scientific answers, judgments must sometimes suffice; each of us must decide how to live now, before the last word (or last judgment) is in.

Throughout these pages I've offered recommendations, admonitions, and even pleas. I've tried to base my advice on scientific data whenever possible, but I've called on clinical and personal experiences when necessary. I hope I've been clear about the basis for my recommendations so you can make your own informed decisions. The ultimate responsibility is, after all, yours. Doctors can advise, but it's up to you to consent or not. And that's how it should be. Your good common sense, personal experience, and thoughtful evaluation of the data are invaluable. Your health is too important to be left to a doctor — even to one who writes books!

The decisions are yours, and so is the responsibility for acting on those decisions. It's your body and your health. Understand how your body works and what can go wrong. Learn how to prevent illness whenever you can, and how best to cope with the problems you can't prevent.

It's been my privilege to try to help by providing information, motivation, and tactical tips for successful implementation. We can all look forward to learning even more about the art and science of prevention in the months and years to come. I leave you, then, to pursue the latest words in prevention with my last words:

Stay well.

Index

Accidents, 84, 298–99; airplane, 301; and alcohol abuse, 299, 301, 327; and children, 307–8; controllable factors in, 17; falls, 302–3, 327; fires, 303–5, 327; from household hazards, 305–7; motor vehicle, 299–301; occupational, 309; recreational, 301–2

ACE inhibitors, 66–67, 216

Acetaminophen: and kidney dysfunction, 188; and liver disease, 138

Acid rain, 465, 467, 468

Acne, 269

Acoustic trauma, 240–43

Addiction: to alcohol, 325, 327, 328; to drugs, 332; to tobacco, 319, 322

Additives: in food, 408; in water, 467

Adolescents, and suicide, 348

Advertising, and prevention neglect, 5

Aerobic exercise, 42, 80, 150, 212, 231, 423, 425–31; bicycling, 427, 428, 429, 434, 438–39, 445–46; and choice of sports, 436; cross-country skiing, 428, 429, 435, 436, 438; dance, 434, 438–39; and inner ear, 243; jogging and running, 428, 429, 432–33, 436, 438–39, 445–46; psychological benefits from, 352; rowing, 435, 438; skating, 428, 434–35, 436, 438; swimming and water exercises, 301, 433–34, 436, 438–39; walking, 431–32, 438–39 (*see also* Walking)

Age: and arterial disease, 68; and breast cancer, 159; and coronary artery disease, 30; and high blood pressure, 58; and kidney function, 184, 185; and obesity, 219; and osteoporosis, 144, 146; and skin, 271–72. *See also* Older persons

Agricultural diet, 8

AIDS, 285–89, 291; and blood transfusions, 200, 287; and brain, 85; from dental care, 255; and drug abuse (intravenous), 287, 289, 333, 334; and hepatitis B vaccine, 136; as immunological abnormality, 201; and leukemia or lymphoma, 199; multiple transmission routes for, 181; novelty of, 274, 279; progress against, 275; secondary prevention of, 289–91; testing for and dementia, 89; and tuberculosis, 110

AIDS-related complex (ARC), 286

Air bags (automobile), 16, 300

Air conditioners, and lung disease, 104–5

Airplane accidents, 301

Air pollution, 105–6, 454–57; asthma from, 102; and fertilizers, 468; indoor, 457–60; and water pollution, 464

Alcohol and alcohol abuse, 324–30, 361, 362; accidents from, 299, 301, 327; in balanced diet, 413; and blood disorders, 199, 327; caloric content of, 364; and cancer(s), 131, 161, 258, 259, 260, 326, 361; and cholesterol, 39; and cirrhosis, 139, 326; as controllable factor, 17; as crucial to health, 16; and dental care, 252; as escape, 351; and fire fatalities, 304; and gallstones, 140; and gout, 155; and heart disease, 52, 325, 326; and high blood pressure, 64, 326; and mental abilities, 89; morbidity from, 14; in mouthwash (and oral cancer), 251; neurological dysfunction from, 85; and osteoporosis, 144, 147, 326; and pneumonia, 109; prevalence of

(U.S.), 341; and sexual dysfunction, 178; and society, 331; and strokes, 81, 326, 361; test on, 329; as twentieth-century health sin, 502; and ulcers, 132, 326

Alcoholic liver disease, 138–39, 326

Alcoholics Anonymous (AA), 330, 355

Allergies: asthma from, 102–3; to natural vs. added chemicals, 409; to psyllium powder, 380; skin, 269–70; and toxics susceptibility, 451; and traveler's medical summary, 280

Altitude sickness, 463

Alzheimer's disease, 88, 89, 410

Amantadine, 108

Amblyopia, 237–38

Amenorrhea, secondary, 165

American Association of Retired Persons, driving course by, 300

Ammonia, danger of with chlorine, 458

Anemia, 194–98; and alcohol abuse, 327; and diet, 195–96, 362; from diverticulosis, 122; as occupational disorder, 311; pernicious, 86; runner's, 404

Aneurysms, 68–69; and strokes, 78; and tobacco abuse, 318; treatment of, 69

Angina, 27, 28; and alcohol abuse, 326; and EKG, 47; and vitamin C, 390, 392

Angiograms, 69, 82

Animal studies, 506

Anniversary reactions, 348

Antacids, and diarrhea, 128

Anxiety, 343, 344–45; and exercise, 419

Anxiety disorders, 341, 343–44

Aorta, 54; aneurysms in, 68–69

Apneas, 106

Artery(ies), 54, 67–68; carotid, 81–82, 83; diseases of, 67–70

Arthritis, 153–55; conditions misdiagnosed as, 155; and obesity, 217; rheumatoid, 155

Asbestos, 97, 311, 312, 452, 453, 458

Aspartame, 187, 211, 375–76

Aspirin, 188; and arterial disease, 69; asthma from, 102–3; and children, 138; and colon cancer, 118; and heart disease, 44–46, 48; iron loss from, 194–95; and liver disease, 138; and migraines, 87; and multiinfarct dementia, 89; and rheumatic fever, 50; and sports injuries, 442; and stool testing, 120; and strokes, 44–45, 83; and thrombophlebitis, 72

Asthma, 94, 101–4; and air pollution, 105; and diet, 361; as occupational disorder, 312; as psychosomatic, 340; and tobacco abuse, 318

Atherosclerosis, 25, 28–29; and arterial disease, 68, 70; and cerebral thrombosis, 78; in childhood, 33; controllable factors in, 18; in diabetics, 215–16; and embolic strokes, 78; and kidneys, 186; psychological factors in, 337; and smoking, 80; and strokes, 80, 81, 83

Athletes: and arthritis, 154; bone density of, 150; and exercise warnings, 420; women as, 150

Athlete's foot, 268–69

Atrial fibrillation, 78, 83

Automobile driving, 16, 299–301

Autonomic nervous system, 76

Back pain, low, 156–57

Bacteria, 275, 296; and nervous system infections, 84–85; in water, 466

Bacterial endocarditis, 52

Beta blockers, 66, 87

Beta carotene, 44, 46, 98, 361, 362, 389–90, 392, 394

Bhopal disaster, 473

Bicycling, 427, 428, 429, 434, 438–39, 445–46

Bicycling accidents, 301–2

Bikes, stationary, 437

Biological wastes, 474

Biotin, 396

Birth control pills: and cancers, 160, 168, 169; and heart attacks, 31; and migraine, 79, 87; and strokes, 79; and thrombophlebitis, 72

Blacks: and colon cancer, 115; high blood pressure in, 58, 63; life expectancy of, 15; and sickle cell anemia, 197

Bladder, 182, 183; cancer of, 186–87, 318, 362, 389, 453; infection of, 190; and menopause, 172; and occupational disorders, 311

Blindness, from diabetes, 208, 216

Blood and blood disorders, 193–94; and alcohol abuse, 199, 327; and anemia, 194–98; and exercise, 418; and leukemia, 198, 199–200, 311; and lymphoma, 199–200; recommendations on testing of, 494, 496; symptoms of disorders of, 500; and tobacco abuse, 199, 318

Blood clots (thrombosis), 28, 29, 77;
and diet, 361; and exercise, 418; in
pulmonary embolism, 71, 72
Blood pressure, 55–56; and cerebral
artery disease, 83–84; and circulation, 54–55; diastolic, 55–56, 66;
measurement of, 56–57; among
primitive peoples, 8; systolic, 55–56,
66; variations in, 57. See also High
blood pressure
Blood transfusion, 200; and AIDS, 200,
287
Blood vessels, and exercise, 417. See
also Artery; Veins
Boating accidents, 301
Bone(s), 143; alveolar, 246; and fluoridated water, 249; fractures of, 152;
and occupational disorders, 311;
osteoporosis in, 144–52
Bone marrow, 194, 198
Botulism, 295
Bowel movements: and colon cancer
detection, 119; and stool testing,
120, 497
Brain, 74–75; and alcohol abuse, 326;
cancer of, 320; two hemispheres of,
75–76. See also Nervous system
Breast(s), 158; lumpy, 158–59; symptoms of diseases of, 500
Breast cancer, 159–63; and alcohol
abuse, 161, 326; and diet, 359, 362,
385, 389, 390; and estrogen replacement, 173–74; and exercise, 419;
and obesity, 217; secondary prevention of, 21, 162–63
Breast exam: mammograms, 4, 21,
162–63, 176, 480, 494–95, 497; recommendations on, 494, 497; self-
examination, 162, 163, 501
Breathing patterns, impaired, 106
Bronchitis, 94, 100, 318. See also
Chronic obstructive lung disease
Burnout, 344
Bursas, 155

Calcitonin, 151–52
Calcium, 143, 360, 361, 362, 402–3,
404; and blood pressure, 62; and
osteoporosis, 146, 148–49, 362
Calcium channel blockers, 66–67, 87
Caloric intake: and balanced diet, 413;
and colon cancer, 117–18, 361; and
diseases, 361, 362; of fats vs. other
foods, 364; and gallstones, 140; and
osteoporosis, 146; from selected
foods (tables), 370–73, 381–83,

386–87, 391; in weight control,
225–26. See also Obesity
Cancer: and alcohol abuse, 131, 161,
258, 259, 260, 326, 361; controllable
factors in, 17; and dental care, 252;
and diet, 98, 115–18, 119, 160–61,
187, 359, 361, 362, 364–65, 385, 389,
390, 393; as disease of abuse or disuse, 10, 12, 201; emotional factors
in, 337; environmental factors in,
451–52, 453; and exercise, 118, 419;
and fluoride, 249; and obesity,
117–18, 169, 217; in safe food requirements, 408; and smoking, 95,
130, 131, 168, 180, 186, 187, 258, 259,
260, 453, 507; symptoms of, 499; and
vitamins, 116, 259, 389–90, 393; as
work-related, 308
Cancer, types of: bladder, 186–87, 318,
362, 389, 453; brain, 320; breast,
159–63 (see also Breast cancer);
cervical, 168–69, 217, 318, 359, 390;
of colon and rectum, 114–22 (see
also Colon cancer); endometrial,
169–70, 173; of esophagus, 131, 318,
319, 326, 361, 389, 390, 453; kidney,
186, 318, 319, 327, 362, 453; of larynx, 260, 318, 319, 327, 362, 453;
liver, 137–38; lung, 94–99, 318, 319,
320, 361, 453, 480; of mouth (oral),
258–59 (see also Oral cancer);
ovarian, 170, 217; pancreatic, 130,
318, 319, 361, 453; prostate, 180–81,
217, 318, 362, 364, 385, 389; skin, 264,
266–67, 479; stomach, 131, 318, 319,
326, 361, 389, 390; testicular, 178–79;
thyroid, 480; of tongue, 318; of uterus,
362, 364, 385, 389; vaginal, 170–71
Capillaries, 54
Carbohydrates, 374–77; for athletes,
445; in balanced diet, 413; caloric
content of, 364; for diabetes,
209–10, 211; and intestinal gas, 129;
and obesity, 222, 227
Carbon dioxide, 105, 449, 452, 454–55,
460, 461
Carbon monoxide, 105–6, 306, 317,
455, 458
Cardiac catheterization, 48, 51
Cardiovascular disease, 25; as cause of
death, 18; death toll from, 15; and
drug abuse, 333; morbidity from, 14;
and vitamins, 390, 392, 393; as
work-related, 308. See also Coronary artery disease; Heart disease;
High blood pressure; Strokes

Cardiovascular fitness, 417
Carotene. *See* Beta carotene
Carotid artery, 81–82, 83
Carpal tunnel syndrome, 313, 314
Cartilage, 153, 154
Cataracts, 236, 237, 362; and vitamins, 237, 392, 393
Centers for Disease Control, 284
Central nervous system, 76. *See also* Brain; Nervous system
Cerebral thrombosis, 77–78
Cerebrovascular accident, 76. *See also* Strokes
Cervical cancer, 168–69, 217, 318, 359, 390
CFCs (chlorinated fluorocarbons), 455, 460–61, 479
Charcoal broiling, 389
Chemical pollutants or wastes, 464, 473–74; as crucial to health, 16; and heart muscle disease, 52. *See also* Toxins and toxic chemicals
Chicken pox, 275
Children: and AIDS, 287; and artificial sweeteners, 376; and aspirin, 138; and atherosclerosis, 33; immunization of, 276–77, 278; and undescended testicle, 179; and urine analyses, 192
Child restraints (airplane), 301
Child restraints (auto), 300
Child safety, 307–8
Chlamydia, 181, 292–93
Chlorine, 407
Chlorine-containing products, danger of with ammonia, 458
Cholera vaccine, 281
Cholesterol, 36, 361, 363–64, 410; checking on, 33; as controllable factor, 17, 18; and coronary artery disease, 32–36, 42, 361; as crucial to health, 16; and diabetes, 210; and diet, 36–38, 49–50, 63, 363–64, 378–79, 380; gallstones from, 140; goals for, 35–36; HDL (good), 33, 34, 35 (*see also* HDL cholesterol); improving ratio of, 36–40; in Japanese vs. Japanese-Americans, 13; LDL (bad), 33, 34, 35 (*see also* LDL cholesterol); as natural toxins, 409; among primitive peoples, 8; recommendations on testing for, 493, 496; sources of (table), 370–73; and strokes, 80; understanding measurements of, 34–35
Chromium, 406, 452

Chronic obstructive lung disease, 94, 99–101; and air pollution, 105; and controllable factors, 17; death toll from, 15; as disease of abuse or disuse, 10; and smoking, 94, 100–101, 318, 319, 321
Cigarettes. *See* Smoking
Circulation: and alcohol abuse, 326; and exercise, 417; normal, 54–55; and tobacco abuse, 318
Cirrhosis, 139, 326; and diet, 362
Cleaners, household, 458–59
Climate-related illnesses, 462–63
Clinical evaluation, recommendations on, 493, 495
Clinical observations, 506
Cocaine, and heart muscle disease, 52
Cold, common, 107
Cold-related illnesses, 463
Colon, 113
Colon cancer, 114–22; and diet, 115–18, 119, 361, 364–65, 385, 389, 390; and exercise, 118, 419; and obesity, 117–18, 217
Colonoscopy, 119, 121
Computer screen (video display terminal), 86, 313, 314, 477
Condoms, 288–89
Congestive heart failure, 28
Conservation: and carbon dioxide, 461; of water, 466–67
Constipation, 125–26, 361
Consumer Product Safety Commission Hotline, 97
Contraception: and cystitis, 190, 191. *See also* Birth control pills
Cooking, 410–11; and chemical contaminants, 470; of fish, 472
Copper, 406
Coronary arteries, 27
Coronary artery (heart) disease, 25, 27–29; and alcohol, 325; and diabetes, 43, 212; and diet (cholesterol), 32–36, 42, 361; and exercise deaths, 420; and high blood pressure, 40–41, 42, 58; medications for, 44–46; psychological elements in, 339; reversing of, 49–50; risk factors in, 29–44; secondary prevention of, 46–48, 81; as stroke predictor, 80; symptoms of, 27, 48, 420, 446, 498; tertiary prevention of, 48–49; and tobacco abuse, 318. *See also* Heart disease
Cosmetics, 270
Cosmic rays, 479

Counseling, 355
Cramps, muscle, from arterial disease, 68
Cross-country skiing, 428, 429, 435, 436, 438
Cross-country ski machines, 439
Cyclamates, 187, 376, 408
Cycling (bicycling), 427, 428, 429, 434, 438–39, 445–46
Cystitis, 190–91

Dance, aerobic, 434, 438–39
"Death styles," xiii
DeCasse, Jerome, 119
Deep-breathing techniques, 354–55
Degenerative arthritis, 154
Degenerative diseases, 12–13
Dementia, 88–89; and alcohol abuse, 326
Dental care or dental work: and endocarditis, 52; guarding safety of, 255; and pneumonia, 109; preventive, 252, 480; recommendations on, 494, 496
Dental diseases, 247; and diet, 252–53, 362; periodontal disease, 254–55; symptoms of, 501; and tobacco abuse, 318; tooth decay, 247–54, 375
Depression, 346–49; and alcohol abuse, 327; and exercise, 419; and lack of daylight, 348, 478; mental slowness from, 89; and tobacco abuse, 319
Dermatitis, contact, 270
DES (diethylstilbesterol), 171; and breast cancer, 160
Diabetes, 207–13; and arterial disease, 68, 69; and controllable factors, 17; diagnosis of, 213–15; and diet, 209–11, 362, 385; as disease of abuse or disuse, 10; and exercise, 212–13, 419; forms of, 207–8; and heart disease, 43, 210, 212; and osteoporosis, 147; preventing complications of, 212, 215–16; among primitive peoples, 8; and protein consumption, 210–11, 384; secondary prevention of, 213–15; and strokes, 80, 208, 215, 216; symptoms of, 208, 500; and urinary tract infections, 190
Diabetic retinopathy, 239–40
Dialysis by artificial kidneys, 184, 208
Diarrhea, 126–28; deaths from, 15, 274; as symptom, 446; traveler's, 282–83, 295
Diet (nutrition), 360–63; American,

222, 227, 358, 359, 364, 376, 396; and anemia, 195–96, 362; and arterial disease, 69; balance in, 411–12; and cancer(s), 98, 115–18, 119, 160–61, 187, 359, 361, 362, 364–65, 385, 389, 390, 393; and cataracts, 237, 392, 393; as controllable factor, 17; as crucial to health, 16; cultural perspectives on, 358–60; and dental health, 252–53, 362; for diabetes, 209–11, 362, 385; and esophagitis, 130; for exercise, 445; and food safety, 407–11; and heart disease, 364, 385; and high blood pressure, 60–63, 80, 361, 385, 397–98; historical and genetic perspectives on, 357–58; and immune system, 201; and intestinal gas, 129; and migraine, 87; and obesity, 221–22, 362, 385; and obesity (control of), 225–30; Dr. Ornish's, 50; and osteoporosis, 144, 146, 147, 148–49, 362; of today vs. Stone Age, 10
Diet, elements of: carbohydrates, 374–77 (see also Carbohydrates); cholesterol, 36–38, 49–50, 63, 363–64, 378–79, 380 (see also Cholesterol); fats, 36–37, 222, 364–74 (see also Fat in diet); fiber, 115–17, 377–83 (see also Fiber, dietary); minerals, 396–407; protein, 185, 383–87 (see also Protein); vitamins, 116, 237, 388–96 (see also specific vitamins); water, 407 (see also Water)
Dietary supplements, 37, 394. See also Vitamins
Dieting, yo-yo, 43
Digestive system, 112–14. See also Gastrointestinal disorders
Disease (illness): causes of, 6; disparities in distribution of, 14–16; origins of (historical perspectives), 6–16; preventable, 13–14
Disease, symptoms of. See Symptoms
Disease prevention. See Preventive medical care
Diseases of abuse and disuse, 9–11, 12, 201
Diseases of contagion, 8–9, 201
Diseases of deprivation, 7–8
Diseases of environmental contamination. See Environmental diseases
Diseases of poverty, 15
Diuretics, 66
Diverticulosis, 122–23, 361, 380

Driving: accidents from, 299; healthful practices in, 16, 299–301; in tropical areas, 282

Drugs, medicinal. *See* Medication

Drugs and drug abuse, 331–34; and AIDS, 287, 289, 333, 334; categories of, 332; control of, 17, 334; as crucial to health, 16; as escape, 351; and hepatitis B, 136; and pneumonia, 109; prevalence of (U.S.), 341

Dry mouth, 256–57

Ear, 240, 244

Ear disorders, 240; acoustic trauma, 240–43; and hearing tests, 245; infections, 243–45; physical trauma, 243; symptoms of, 500

Echocardiogram, 51, 420

Edema, 71, 463

Electrical hazards, 305

Electric power lines, 477

Electrocardiogram (EKG), 47, 494, 496

ELF (extremely low frequency) radiation), 477–78

Embolic stroke, 78,

Embolism, pulmonary, 71, 72

Emotions: and coronary artery disease, 43–44. *See also* Psychological factors

Emphysema, 99–100, 318. *See also* Chronic obstructive lung disease

Encephalitis, 312

Endocarditis, 52

Endometrial cancer, 169–70; and estrogen replacement, 173

Endometriosis, 170

Endorphins, 338, 352, 418

Endothelium, 68

Energy conservation, 461

Energy policy, 481

Environment, 448–50, 482; and acid rain, 465, 467, 468; and food supply, 473; and global warming, 460–62; pesticides and fertilizers in, 467–70; radiation in, 475–81 (*see also* Radiation); and wastes, 473–75 (*see also* Wastes)

Environmental diseases, 11–12, 449–50; and air pollution, 454–60; from seafood, 470–72; and toxins, 450–54 (*see also* Toxins and toxic chemicals); and water pollution, 463

Environmental exposure, as controllable factor, 17

Environmental hazards, 6, 16

Environmental Protection Agency (EPA): address and hotline of, 510, 513; and asbestos, 97; on carbon dioxide concentration, 106; and lead poisoning, 85; and noise abatement, 241, 242; on passive smoking, 320; and radon, 96

Enzymes, digestive, 113

Epidemiology, 451, 506–7; and toxic shock syndrome, 167, 168

Esophagus, 113

Esophagus, diseases of, 130–31; and alcohol abuse, 131, 326, 361; cancer, 131, 318, 319, 326, 361, 389, 390, 453

Estrogen, 165; and body fat, 217; and menopause, 146, 165

Estrogen replacement, 30–31, 172–76; benefits and side effects of, 151; and endometrial cancer, 169; and gallstones, 140; and hot flashes, 171; and osteoporosis, 31, 146, 150–51, 172–73; and skin, 272

Etidronate, 152

Examinations. *See* Screening tests

Exercise, 416–19; aerobic-based program of, 425–36 (*see also* Aerobic exercise); and amenorrhea, 165; asthma from, 103; balanced program of, 443–47; best amount of, 424–25, 426; best form of, 423–24; best intensity of, 426–31; cardiac complications from, 27, 419–21; case study on, 19, 415–16; and cholesterol, 39, 80; and colon cancer, 118, 419; and constipation, 125; as controllable factor, 17, 18; and coronary artery disease, 41–43; as crucial to health, 16; as diabetes prevention, 212–13, 419; and endometrial cancer, 170; for flexibility, 439–40; and heat stroke, 462; and high blood pressure, 63–64, 80, 418–19; on home exercise machines, 436–39; and immunity, 202–3; injuries from, 442–43; intensity of (selected forms), 427–29; and life cycle, 421–23; and low back pain, 157; and mental fitness, 90; and myocarditis, 52–53; and obesity, 220, 230–31, 419; and osteoarthritis, 154–55; and osteoporosis, 144, 147, 150, 154, 419; and psychological factors, 351–52, 418; safety of, 42–43; for speed, 441–43; for strength, 440–41

Exercise stress tests, 47–48, 444, 496

Eye, 233–34

Eye disorders: amblyopia, 237–38; cataracts, 236, 237, 362, 392, 393; and diabetes, 213, 216; diabetic retinopathy, 239–40; glaucoma, 238–39, 494, 497; symptoms of, 500; trauma, 234–35; from ultraviolet radiation, 235–37

Failure to thrive, 245
Faith healing, 202
Falls (accidents), 302–3; and alcohol abuse, 327
Family history: and breast cancer, 159; and coronary artery disease, 30; and strokes, 80
Fat (bodily), 205–6, 217–18
Fat(s) in diet, 222, 359, 360, 361, 362, 364–74; absorption of, 205; in America, 222; animal, 364–65, 367, 368; in balanced diet, 413; and blood pressure, 62; and breast cancer, 161; in Chinese vs. Americans, 230; and colon cancer, 117; as crucial to health, 16; and diabetes, 210; and kidneys, 185; and prostate cancer, 180; saturated, 36–37, 365, 368, 370–73 (see also Saturated fat); sources of (table), 370–73; unsaturated, 36, 37, 365–67, 368; in weight control, 226–27
Fatigue: as controllable factor, 17; and diabetes, 208; and high blood pressure, 58; and memory loss, 89; (See also Sleep
Fertilizers, 409–10, 467–70
Fetal alcohol syndrome, 326
Fiber, dietary, 37, 115–16, 360, 361, 362, 375, 377–83; in balanced diet, 413; for breakfast, 228; and colon cancer, 115, 119; and constipation, 125, 126; as crucial to health, 16; for diabetes, 211; and diverticulosis, 123; and fast food, 358; and gallstones, 141; and hemorrhoids, 124; and hernias, 124; and irritable bowel syndrome, 126; sources of (table), 381–83; and ulcers, 132; and varicose veins, 70; in weight control, 227
Fibrinogen, 72
Fires, 303–5, 327
Fish (in diet), 361, 367; in balanced diet, 413; and colon cancer, 117; and heart disease, 38, 393; safety of, 470–72; and water pollution, 464
Fish oils, 36, 37–38, 62, 360, 367, 393

Flatulence, 129, 380
Flossing, dental, 251
Flu. See Influenza
Fluoride, 152, 248–50, 452, 467
Fluorine, 406
Folic acid, 197, 362, 388, 395
Food. See Diet
Food additives, 408–9
Food poisoning, 128, 295–96, 408
Food safety, 407–11, 468–73
Formaldehyde, 458
Fractures, 152; and fluoridated water, 249; hip, 144, 419; and osteoporosis, 144, 419 (see also Osteoporosis); and tobacco abuse, 318
Framingham Heart Study, 35, 61, 217
Frostbite, 463
Fruits, as crucial to health, 16
Fungal infections, 268–69
Fungi, 275

Gallbladder, 113, 133, 134, 139
Gallbladder disease (gallstones), 139–42, 217, 362, 500
Gamma globulin, 135, 137, 194, 203, 281
Garbage, 474–75
Gas, intestinal, 129, 380
Gastritis, 131–32; and aspirin, 45; and diet, 362; and tobacco abuse, 318
Gastrointestinal disorders, 112; and alcohol abuse, 326; cancer of colon and rectum, 114–22 (see also Colon cancer); constipation, 125–26, 361; diarrhea, 126–28 (see also Diarrhea); diverticulosis, 122–23, 361, 380; of esophagus, 130–31 (see also Esophagus, diseases of); gas, 129, 380; hemorrhoids, 123–24, 326, 361; hernias, 124–25, 361; irritable bowel syndrome, 126, 361; of pancreas, 129–30, 318, 319, 361, 453; of stomach and small intestine, 131–32, 326 (see also Stomach cancer); symptoms of, 499; and tobacco abuse, 318
Gastrointestinal tract, 112–14
Gender: and body fat location, 218; and coronary artery disease, 30–31; and gallstones, 140; and obesity, 219; and strokes, 80. See also Women
Genetics, and health, 6
Genetic theories of obesity, 220
Genital herpes, 181, 275, 293
Glaucoma, 238–39; recommendations on testing for, 494, 497

Global warming, 460–62
Gonorrhea, 181, 292
Gout, 155
Government agencies, for health care information, 509–12
Greenhouse gases, 460–61
Grief, 347. *See also* Depression

Hardening of the arteries, 88
Hawaii, universal health insurance in, 15
HDL (good) cholesterol, 33, 34, 35, 363; and arterial disease, 69; and exercise, 41; and menopause, 172; and smoking, 31, 318, 320
Headaches, 86–87; and high blood pressure, 58; and strokes, 78; as symptom, 87, 107, 446
Health: disparities in, 14–16; factors in, 5–6
Health (medical) care: in America, 483–84; cost of, 3, 14; and prevention, 6 (*see also* Preventive medical care)
Health crisis, 12–16
Health gap, international, 13
Health insurance, 4–5, 15, 486
Hearing loss. *See* Ear disorders
Hearing tests, 245, 497
Heart: and exercise, 417; healthy functioning of, 26–27
Heart attacks, 27–28; cost of, 25; from diabetes, 208, 215, 216; frequency of, 25; and high blood pressure, 58, 59; improved mortality rates from, 26; and menopause, 172
Heartburn, 130, 446
Heart disease, 25–26, 27; and air pollution, 105; and alcohol abuse, 52, 325, 326; as cause of death, 18; causes of, xiv; congenital, 420; controllable factors in, 17; coronary artery disease, 25, 27–44 (*see also* Coronary artery disease); cost of, 25; and diabetes, 43, 210, 212; and diet, 364, 385 (*see also* Cholesterol; Fat in diet); as disease of abuse or disuse, 10, 12, 201; and exercise, 41–43, 418; in muscle, 52–53; psychological factors in, 337; recent prevalence of, xiv, 13, 26; rheumatic, 50–51; and smoking (tobacco abuse), 31–32, 42, 318, 319, 321, 507; symptoms of, 27, 48, 420, 446, 498; valve infections, 51–52. *See also* Cardiovascular disease

Heat-related illnesses, 462–63, 467
Heavy metals, 452
Height and weight tables, 223
Heimlich maneuver, 260, 307
Hemorrhoids, 123–24; and alcohol abuse, 326; and diet, 361
Hepatitis: deaths from, 15, 274; from dental care, 255; as occupational disorder, 311, 313
Hepatitis, alcoholic, 138, 326
Hepatitis, viral, 134–35; hepatitis A, 135, 281, 296; hepatitis B, 135–37, 181, 200, 275, 278; hepatitis C, 137, 200
Hernias, 124–25, 361
Herpes, genital, 181, 275, 293
High blood pressure (hypertension), 55; and alcohol, 64, 326; as controllable factor, 17, 18; and coronary artery disease, 40–41, 42, 58; criteria for, 57, 65–66; damage from, 58–59; and diet, 60–63, 80, 361, 385, 397–98; as disease of abuse or disuse, 10; drug treatment for, 59–60, 65–67; exercise as reducing, 63–64, 80, 418–19; and kidneys, 59, 185–86; morbidity from, 14; need to check for, 57–58; from noise pollution, 243; and obesity, 63, 217; and salt, 60, 360, 361, 397–98; secondary prevention of, 65–67, 81; and smoking, 65; and stress, 57, 64, 80; and stroke, 18, 40, 59, 78, 80; testing for causes of, 59
Hip fractures, 144
HIV (Human Immunodeficiency Virus), 285, 286. *See also* AIDS
Hoarseness, and laryngeal cancer, 260
Home exercise machines, 436–39
Homeless persons, and hypothermia, 463
Homeostasis, 203
Hormones: in female reproductive system, 164–65; and liver cancer (male), 137–38; metabolic, 206; and osteoporosis, 147. *See also* Estrogen replacement
Horseback riding, 302
Hospital care, and thrombophlebitis, 71–72
Hotlines, 512–13
Household cleaning products, 458–59
Household hazards, 305–7
Human Immunodeficiency Virus (HIV), 285, 286. *See also* AIDS
Humidifier, household, 104–5, 459
Huntington's disease, 86

Hypertension. *See* High blood pressure
Hyperthermia, 463

Ibuprofen, 188, 442
Illness. *See* Disease
Imaging, 202
Immune system, 114; and alcohol abuse, 327; and blood cells, 194; and diabetes (Type I), 209; and diet, 201; disorders of, 200–201; and exercise, 202–3; and mental attitude, 202; psychosomatic influences in, 340; and stress, 201–2; symptoms of disorders of, 500
Immunizations, 276–79; childhood, 276–77, 278; as controllable factor, 17; as crucial to health, 16; for influenza, 108, 279; for Lyme disease (dogs), 294; for neurological diseases, 84, 85; for pneumonia, 109; recommendations on, 493, 495; for travelers, 278, 279, 280, 281; for tuberculosis, 110
Impotence, 178; and alcohol abuse, 326; from arterial disease, 68; and tobacco abuse, 318
Industrial chemicals, as toxic, 199
Industrial revolution, 9–10
Infectious diseases, 273–75; and agricultural age, 9; and alcohol abuse, 327; body defenses against, 275–76; control of, 296–97; and diarrhea, 128; of ear, 243–45; food poisoning, 128, 295–96, 408; immunization against, 276–79; Lyme disease, 274, 293–94, 297; and nervous system, 84–85; as occupational disorder, 311; of respiratory tract, 106–11, 294–95 (*see also* Influenza; Pneumonia; Tuberculosis); of skin, 268–69; symptoms of, 501; and tobacco abuse, 318; and travel, 279–84 (*see also* Travelers' health); of urinary tract, 190–91; and vitamins, 392. *See also* Sexually transmitted diseases; *specific diseases*
Infectious hepatitis (hepatitis A), 135, 281, 296
Infertility, male, 313
Influenza (flu), 94, 107–8, 294–95; controllable factors in, 17; immunization for, 108, 279; progress against, 275
Information on health care, associations for, 509–12

Infrared radiation, 478
Inherited diseases, 86
Injury. *See* Trauma
Insect bites, guarding against, 282
Insomnia, 352–53
Insulin, 205, 206, 207, 210, 211, 212, 229, 375
Insurance, health, 4–5, 15, 486
Interleukin-1 (IL-1), 338
International health gap, 13
Intestinal tract, 113–14, 418. *See also* Gastrointestinal disorders
Iodine, 407
Ionizing radiation, 311, 453, 476, 479–81
Iron, 194–96, 362, 403–5; and stool testing, 120
Iron-deficiency anemia, 194–96
Irritable bowel syndrome, 126, 361
Ischemia, 77; transient ischemic attacks (TIAs), 77, 78, 79, 82
Isometric workouts, 63–64

Japanese: and air-quality techniques, 456; and cancers, 115, 131, 160, 170, 180; and heart disease, 13, 30
Japan-Hawaii cancer study, 116
Jaundice, 133, 134, 138, 139
Jock itch, 268
Jogging, 428, 432–33. *See also* Running
Joints, 153; and arthritis, 153–55
Journals, medical, 504–5
Junk or fast foods, 61, 229, 358, 399

Kidney(s), 182–85; and medications, 187–89, 192; and vascular disease, 185–86
Kidney damage or disease: and alcohol abuse, 327; cancer, 186, 318, 319, 327, 362, 453; from diabetes, 208, 216; and diet, 362; from hypertension, 59, 185–86; infections, 191; as occupational disease, 311, 313; and potassium intake, 62; and protein consumption, 384
Kidney stones, 189–90

Laboratory experiments, 505–6
Lactation (nursing), 146, 147, 160
Lactose intolerance, 127–28
Larynx, disorders of, 259–60; cancer, 260, 318, 319, 327, 362, 453
Lasers, for narrowed arteries, 69
"Lazy eye" (amblyopia), 237–38
LDL (bad) cholesterol, 33, 34, 35, 363;

and arterial disease, 68, 69; and diuretics, 66; and exercise, 41; and
free radicals, 390
Lead poisoning, 198–99, 307, 452, 455;
and acid rain, 467; and drinking water, 465; and food safety, 411;
gradual effect of, 451; neurological
disorders from, 85; occupational
disorders from, 312, 313
Legionnaires' disease, 274, 297
Leg swelling and discoloration, 71
Leukemia, 198, 199–200, 311, 320
Life expectancy: and alcoholism, 328;
of black vs. white Americans, 15;
and healthy habits, 16; and history
of illness, 9, 10; prolongation of, 6;
in 20th century, 12
Life-style changes, 18–20; and atherosclerosis, 49–50; case study on, 19,
415–16; and high blood pressure,
55, 60–65, 67; and low back pain,
157; need for, 10; and physician advice, 485; preference for, 176; prevention possible from, 14; for stress
reduction, 350. *See also* Alcohol and
alcohol abuse; Diet; Drug abuse;
Exercise; Psychological factors;
Smoking
Ligaments, 153, 155
Lipoproteins, high-density. *See* HDL
cholesterol
Lipoproteins, low-density. *See* LDL
cholesterol
Liquid protein diets, 229–30
Lithotripsy, gallstone, 142
Liver, 113, 133–34, 205; and cholesterol, 36, 363
Liver diseases, 134; alcoholic, 138–39,
326; cancer, 137–38; controllable
factors in, 17; symptoms of, 500;
toxic, 138; viral hepatitis, 134–37
(*see also* Hepatitis, viral)
Low back pain, 156–57
Low-calorie diets, 229–30
Lung and respiratory tract disease, 94;
and air pollution, 102, 105–6;
asthma, 101–4 (*see also* Asthma);
cancer, 94–99, 318, 319, 320, 361,
453, 480; chronic obstructive, 94,
99–101 (*see also* Chronic obstructive lung disease); impaired breathing patterns, 106; infections,
106–11, 294–95 (*see also* Influenza;
Pneumonia; Tuberculosis); occupational, 104–5, 308, 311, 312; and
smoking (tobacco abuse), 94,

100–101, 318, 319, 321; symptoms
of, 499
Lungs, 92–93; and exercise, 104,
417–18
Lyme disease, 274, 293–94, 297
Lymphocytes, 194, 202–3, 286
Lymphoma, 199–200, 320

Magnesium, 406
Magnetic resonance imaging (MRI),
and aneurysms, 69
Malaria, 15, 274, 283–84
Mammograms, 21, 162–63; and insur-
ance, 4; recommendations on, 176,
480, 494–95, 497
Manganese, 406
Manic-depressive illness, 348
Margarine, 360, 365–66
Mass media, 503–4, 505
Measles, 277; adult immunization for,
277–78; deaths from, 15, 274; intro-
duction of to Europe, 9; and vitamin
A, 392
Meat, 117, 195, 364, 386, 408–9, 413.
See also Protein
Media, 5, 503–4, 505
Medical care. *See* Health care
Medical journals, 504–5
Medical kit, for travelers, 281
Medical newsletters, 509
Medical research, 4, 505–9
Medical training programs, 4
Medicare, and prevention, 4–5
Medication: for acne, 269; for asthma,
102; for bacterial diarrhea, 128; caution needed with, 188; and child
safety, 307; cholesterol-lowering,
38; diarrhea from, 127; dry mouth
from, 257; and esophagitis, 130–
31; for gallstones, 142; for heart
disease, 44–46; for high blood
pressure, 59, 65–67; and kidneys, 187–89, 192; for malaria,
284; and memory loss, 89; and older
persons, 302–3; and osteoporosis,
147, 151; proper use of, 502; for psychological problems, 356; and
sexual dysfunction, 178; and sports
injuries, 442; and tobacco abuse,
318; for travel, 280, 281, 282, 283;
for tuberculosis, 110. *See also*
Aspirin
Medicine, practice of: individualized
approach in, 66; standard of proof
for, 20–21, 41
Meditation, 353–54; for insomnia, 353

Melanoma, 264, 266–67, 479
Memory loss, 87–88; major, 88–89; mild, 89–90
Meningitis, 84
Meningococcal vaccine, 279
Menopause, 171–72; and coronary heart disease, 30–31; and estrogen replacement, 172–76
Menstrual cycle, 164–65
Menstrual history, and breast cancer, 160
Mental health. *See* Psychological factors
Mercury toxicity, 253, 312, 313, 452; and acid rain, 467; and Roman miners, 450
Meta-analysis, 40, 173
Metabolic fitness, 417, 418
Metabolic theories of obesity, 220
Metabolism, 204–7; and alcohol abuse, 327; and diseases of abuse or disuse, 10; and tobacco abuse, 318
Methane, 449, 455, 460, 461
Microwave cooking, 410
Microwaves, 478
Migraine headaches, 86–87; and strokes, 79
Mind-body relationship, 338
Minerals, 396; trace, 405–7. *See also specific minerals*
Molybdenum, 406
Monocytes, 194
Monounsaturated fats, 37, 62–63, 365, 366–67, 368
Morbidity, 14
Motorcycle riding, 301
Motor vehicle accidents, 299–301
Mouth, dry, 256–57
Mouth disorders: cancer, 258–59 (*see also* Oral cancer); symptoms of, 501
Mouthwash, 251
MSG, 60, 61
Multi-infarct dementia, 88–89
Mumps vaccinations, 278
Murmurs (heart), 51; and need for antibiotics, 52
Muscle relaxation techniques, 354–55; for insomnia, 353
Muscles, 155, 384
Muscular dystrophy, 86
Musculoskeletal disorders: arthritis, 153–55, 217; low back pain, 156–67; osteoporosis, 144–52 (*see also* Osteoporosis); and repetitive use, 310; symptoms of, 500. *See also* Bone
Musculoskeletal fitness, 417, 418

Myocardial infarction, 27–28
Myocarditis, 52–53, 420

Nasal disorders, occupational, 311
National Institute for Occupational Safety and Health, 310, 512
National Safety Council, driving course by, 300
Nerve damage: from diabetes, 216; as occupational disorder, 312
Nervous system, 75–76; and alcohol abuse, 326; occupational disorders of, 308, 312; and tobacco abuse, 318
Neurological diseases: infections, 84–85; nutritional deficiencies, 86; prevention of, 91; symptoms of, 499; toxic and metabolic disorders, 85–86; trauma, 84
Newsletters, medical, 509
Newspapers, 503–4, 505
Niacin (vitamin B3), 38–39, 388, 394, 395
Nicotine, 31, 316, 317. *See also* Smoking; Tobacco abuse
Nitrates, 361, 452, 466
Nitrites, 408–9
Nitrogen oxides, 312, 452, 454, 456, 460, 461, 468
Noise-induced hearing loss, 308
Noise pollution, 242–43
Nosebleeds, and high blood pressure, 58
Nuclear radiation, 481
Nurses, 484
Nursing (lactation), 146, 147, 160
Nutrition. *See* Diet
Nutritional deficiencies, 86

Oat bran, 37, 360, 378–79, 380
Obesity, 216–22; and arterial disease, 69; biological theories of, 220–21; and cancer, 117–18, 169, 217; control of, 225–30; as controllable factor, 17; and coronary artery disease, 43; and diabetes, 209, 217; and diet, 221–22, 225–30, 362, 385; and evaluation of body weight or fat, 222–25; and exercise, 220, 230–31, 419; and gallstones, 140; and hemorrhoids, 124; and high blood pressure, 63, 217; and osteoporosis, 147; among primitive peoples, 8; psychological theory of, 219–20; and strokes, 80; and thrombophlebitis, 72; and tobacco abuse, 318; and varicose veins, 70. *See also* Caloric intake

Occupational disorders, 308–9, 311–13; accidents, 309; bladder cancer as, 187; and computer screens, 313, 314, 477; eye injuries, 234–35; hearing loss, 241; illnesses, 309–10; lung disease, 104–5, 308, 311, 312; repetitive motion disorders, 310, 313–14

Older persons: and dementia, 88–89; and driving, 300; and failure to thrive, 245; in falls, 302; flu vaccination for, 108; and heat stroke, 462; and hypothermia, 463; and mild memory loss, 89–90. See also Age

Omega-3 polyunsaturated fats, 37, 62–63, 367, 470, 471, 473

Oral (mouth) cancer, 258, 259; and alcohol abuse, 327, 362; and alcohol in mouthwash, 251; and tobacco abuse, 318, 319, 453

Oral contraceptive pills. See Birth control pills

Oral hygiene, 250–52, 255; and dry mouth, 257; self-exam, 501

Organic chemicals and wastes, 452, 464, 466

Organizations for health care information, 509–12

Osteoarthritis, 153–54, 310

Osteoporosis, 144–52; and alcohol abuse, 144, 147, 326; in American vs. Chinese women, 359; and body fat, 217; and diet, 144, 146, 147, 148–49, 362; and estrogen replacement, 31, 146, 150–51, 172–73; and exercise, 144, 147, 150, 154, 419; and fluoridated water, 249; and smoking, 144, 147, 318; and testing recommendations, 498

Ovarian cancers, 170, 217

Overweight. See Obesity

Ozone, 105, 236, 264, 452, 455, 460, 479

Pancreas, diseases of, 129–30; cancer, 130, 318, 319, 361, 453

Panic attacks, 344

Pantothenic acid, 396

Pap test, 4, 168–69, 490, 495, 497, 498

Parasites, 275; and intestinal infections, 295; and malaria, 283, 284; in water, 466

Parkinson's disease, 312

Particulates, 105, 452, 455

Peer review process, 504

Periodontal disease, 251, 254–55, 318; and diabetes, 208

Peripheral nervous system, 76; and alcohol abuse, 326

Peripheral vascular disease, diabetic, 215, 216

Pernicious anemia, 86

Personal behaviors, 6. See also Lifestyle changes

Personality. See Psychological factors

Pesticides, 408, 409–10, 452, 466, 467–70; and fish, 408, 470

Phobias, 344

Phosphorus, 407

Physicians, 484; and prevention, xiii–xiv, 484–88; selecting of, 485–86

Physicians' Health Study, 45

Plaque, dental, 248, 251, 375

Plaques (artery), 28–29, 68, 78

Plasma, 193

Platelets, 193; and exercise, 80; and smoking, 31, 320; and thrombophlebitis, 72

Pneumonia, 94, 100, 108–9, 294–95; controllable factors in, 17; deaths from, 15, 274

Pneumococcal pneumonia, immunization for, 279

Poisonings: child, 307; lead, 198–99, 307, 455 (see also Lead poisoning)

Polio immunizations, 279

Pollution: air, 102, 105–6, 454–60, 464, 468; noise, 242–43; water, 463–67

Polyps, in colon, 115, 119

Polyps, vocal cord, 260

Polys, 194, 202

Polyunsaturated fats, 37, 365–67, 368; omega-3, 37, 62–63, 367, 470, 471, 473

Post-traumatic stress disorder, 344

Potassium, 361, 399, 402, 403; and blood pressure, 61–62

Poverty, diseases of, 15

Pregnancy: and AIDS, 287, 290–91; and alcohol, 325; and artificial sweeteners, 376; and breast cancer, 160; and cosmic rays, 479; diabetes of, 207–8, 209, 214, 215; drug abuse during, 333; and ELF radiation, 478; and fish, 472; and gallstones, 140; and hemorrhoids, 124; and hepatitis B testing, 137; and immunizations, 278; and osteoporosis, 146, 147; and reproductive toxicity, 452; and smoking, 318, 320, 321; and thrombophlebitis, 72; unintended, 165–66; and urine analysis, 192; and varicose veins, 70

Preventable illnesses, 13–14
Preventive medical care, 483–84, 513; complexity of, 6; core program of, 491–92, 493–98; and environment, 449–50, 482 (*see also* Environment); implementing of, 18–19; information sources on, 509–13; life-style changes in, 18–20 (*see also* Lifestyle changes); and mass media, 5, 503–4, 505; and medical journals, 504–5; and medical research, 505–9; neglect of, 3–5; patient's role in, xiii–xiv, 21–22, 492, 498–502, 513; physician in, xiii–xiv, 484–88; prevalence of, 488–89; profit lacking in, 4; scope of, 20–21; self-examination in, 501–2; and socioeconomic conditions, 110; strategies for, 16–18; and tests, 489–91; three stages of, 21
Primary prevention, 21, 22, 46, 450; of coronary artery disease, 29–47; and environment, 450
Private associations for health care information, 509–12
Products, hazardous, 306–7
Prostate gland, disorders of, 179–81; cancer, 180–81, 217, 318, 362, 364, 385, 389; recommendations on checking for, 498
Prostate-specific antigen (PSA) test, 181
Protein, 185, 362, 383–87; in balanced diet, 413; in blood, 193; caloric content of, 364; and cancers, 117, 361, 389; and diabetes, 210–11, 384; in energy storage, 205; and kidney disorders, 184–85, 189; sources of (table), 386–87
Protozoa, 283
Psychological disorders: prevalence of in U.S., 341; symptoms of, 501; work-related, 308
Psychological factors, 337; anxiety, 343–45; and coping strategies, 350–56; and coronary artery disease, 43–44; depression, 346–49; and exercise, 351–52, 418; and mind-body relationship, 338; stress, 341–43, 344–45 (*see also* Stress, psychological)
Psychological fitness, 417, 418
Psychosomatic illnesses, 339–40
Publications on health care, 509–12
Pulmonary embolism, 71, 72
Pulse, taking of, 430

Race: and gallstones, 140; and life expectancy, 15. *See also* Blacks
Radiation, 475–77; as controllable factor, 17; as crucial to health, 16; infrared and visible, 478; ionizing (radioactivity), 311, 453, 476, 479–81; low-frequency, 477–78; medical, 480; natural, 480; nuclear, 481; radio wave and microwave, 478; ultraviolet, 16, 235–37, 263–64, 271, 452, 453, 478–79
Radon, 452, 458, 465–66, 480; and lung cancer, 95–97, 453, 480; and occupational disorders, 311
Recklessness, as controllable, 17
Records, medical, 487
Recreational accidents, 301–2
Recycling, 475
Relaxation techniques, 64; deep breathing, 355; for headache, 86; and high blood pressure, 64; meditation, 353–54; progressive muscle relation, 354–55
Repetitive motion disorders, 310, 313–14
Reproductive system, female, 163–65
Reproductive system, male, 176–77
Reproductive system disorders, female: and alcohol abuse, 326; breast cancer, 159–63, 173–74 (*see also* Breast cancer); cervical cancer, 168–69, 217, 318, 359, 390; endometrial cancer, 169–70, 173; endometriosis, 170; exams recommended for, 494–95, 497–98; lumpy breasts, 158–59; and menopause, 171–76; ovarian cancer, 170, 217; psychosomatic influences in, 340; and reproductive cycle, 165; symptoms of, 500; and tobacco abuse, 318; toxic shock syndrome, 167–68; uterine cancer, 362, 364, 385, 389; vaginal cancer, 170–71; as work-related, 308
Reproductive system disorders, male, 176; and alcohol abuse, 326; prostate gland disorders, 179–81, 217, 318, 362, 364, 385, 389; psychosomatic influences in, 340; recommended services for, 495, 498; sexual dysfunction (impotence), 68, 178, 318, 326; symptoms of, 500; testicular cancer, 178–79; and tobacco abuse, 318
Reproductive toxicity, 452
Research, medical, 4, 505–9

Respiratory tract, 92–93
Respiratory tract diseases. *See* Lung and respiratory tract disease
Retin-A, 271–72
Retinopathy, diabetic, 239–40
Reye's syndrome, 138
Rheumatic heart disease, 50–51
Rheumatoid arthritis, 155
Ringworm, 268
Rowing, 435, 438
Rowing machines, 439
Rubella (German measles) immunizations, 278
Running, 429, 432–33, 436, 438–39; and safety, 445–46

Saccharine, 376
Saliva, 256–57
Salmonella, 128
Salt, 60–61, 360, 361, 396–99; and arterial disease, 69; as crucial to health, 16; and high blood pressure, 60, 360, 361, 397–98; and kidneys, 183, 185; reducing consumption of, 61
Sanitation, against food poisoning, 296
Saturated fat, 361, 365, 367, 368; and blood pressure, 62–63; and cholesterol, 36–37, 363; and colon cancer, 117; as natural toxins, 409; and prostate cancer, 180; sources of (table), 370–73
Scalding, 305–6
Screening tests: for AIDS, 290; for alcohol abuse, 329; for breast cancer/mammogram, 4, 21, 162–63, 176, 480, 494–95, 497; for cervical cancer/Pap test, 4, 168–69, 490, 495, 497, 498; for cholesterol, 33–35; for colon cancer/stool testing, 120–22, 497; as crucial to health, 16; dental x rays, 252; for diabetes, 213–15; for glaucoma, 239; and hearing, 245; for heart disease/electrocardiogram or stress test, 47–48, 444, 494, 496; for kidney and urinary disorder, 191–92; for lung cancer/chest x rays, 98–99, 496; neglect of guidelines for, 4; for osteoporosis, 152; for prostate cancer, 181; for sickle cell anemia and thalassemia, 197, 198; for testicular cancer, 178–79; for tuberculosis, 110
Seafood. *See* Fish; Shellfish
Sealants (for teeth), 250

Seasonal affective disorder (SAD), 348
Seat belts, 16, 17, 300
Secondary prevention, 21, 47, 81; of AIDS, 289–91; of breast cancer, 21, 162–63; of cervical cancer, 168; of colon cancer, 118–22; of coronary artery disease, 46–48, 81; of cystitis, 191; of diabetes, 213–15; of gallbladder disease, 141–42; of glaucoma, 239; of high blood pressure, 65–67, 81; of lung cancer, 98–99; of oral cancer, 259; of osteoporosis, 152; of prostate cancer, 180–81; of strokes, 81–82; of tuberculosis, 110. *See also* Screening tests
Selenium, 406
Self-examination, 501–2; breast, 162, 163, 501; for skin cancer, 267, 501; testicular, 178–79, 501
Self-expression, 350
Senility, 88
Serum hepatitis, 136
Set-point theories of obesity, 220–21, 231
Seven Countries Study, 359
Seven Deadly Sins, 502
Sewage: and hepatitis A, 135; treatment of, 474
Sexual dysfunction. *See* Impotence
Sexually transmitted diseases, 181, 291; AIDS, 285–91 (*see also* AIDS); AIDS transmission aided by other, 287; cervical cancer as, 168; chlamydia, 181, 292–93; as crucial to health, 16; genital herpes, 181, 275, 293; gonorrhea, 181, 292; hepatitis B as, 136, 181; syphilis, 9, 181, 292; and tropical travel, 282
Shellfish, 360, 409; and hepatitis A, 135, 296; safety of, 470
Shock, 57
Sick building syndrome, 459–60
Sickle cell anemia, 6, 109, 197–98
Sigmoidoscopy, 120–21, 497
Silent ischemia, 27
Sinuses, infection of, 111
Skating, 428, 434–35, 436, 438
Skiing, cross-country, 428, 429, 435, 436, 438
Skin, 261–63; acne on, 269; aging of, 271–72, 319; and alcohol abuse, 327; allergies of, 269–70; cancer of, 264, 266–67, 479; dry, 267–68; infections of, 268–69; psychosomatic influences in, 340; self-examination of, 501; and smoking, 271, 319; and

Skin (*continued*)
sunburn, 263–66; symptoms of diseases of, 501; and toxic chemicals, 270–71, 310, 313; and work-related disorders, 308
Sleep, 352; and depression, 347
Sleep-apnea syndrome, 106
Smallpox: elimination of, 15, 274, 275, 277; introduction of to Europe, 9
Smog, 105, 454
Smoke detectors, 304
Smoking and tobacco use or abuse, 316–21; and arterial disease, 68, 69; and blood disorders, 199, 318; and cancer(s), 95, 130, 131, 168, 180, 186, 187, 258, 259, 260, 453, 507; cessation from, 320–23; and cholesterol, 39; as controllable factor, 17, 18; cost of, 14; as crucial to health, 16; and dental care, 252; different forms of, 319; as escape, 351; and fires, 299, 304; and heart disease, 31–32, 42, 318, 319, 321, 507; and high blood pressure, 65; and lung disease, 94, 100–101, 318, 319, 321; morbidity from, 14; neurological damage from, 85–86; and osteoporosis, 144, 147, 318; passive, 32, 85–86, 95, 168, 319–20, 458; and routine urine analysis, 192; and skin aging, 271, 319; and society, 320, 323–24; and strokes, 79, 80, 318, 319, 321; and toxic particles, 104; as twentieth-century health sin, 502; and ulcers, 132, 318, 321. *See also* Tobacco
Social isolation, as risk factor, 44, 337
Sodium, 398–99, 400–402, 409, 410; and diabetes, 211; and high blood pressure, 60, 64; and kidney function, 183. *See also* Salt
Solid wastes, 474–75
Somatic nervous system, 76
Spinal cord, 75
Sports, competitive, 436, 438
Sports injuries, 235, 256, 442
Stair climbers, 437–38
Starches, 211, 374–75, 376–77
Stomach: and alcohol abuse, 326; and aspirin, 45; gastritis and ulcers in, 131–32
Stomach cancer, 131; and alcohol abuse, 326; and diet, 361, 389, 390; and tobacco abuse, 318, 319
Stone Age, health and diet in, 7–8
Stool testing, 120, 121–22, 497

Strep throat, 50, 51
Stress, psychological, 341–43, 344–45; and amenorrhea, 165; asthma from, 103; as controllable factor, 17; and coronary artery disease, 43–44; as crucial to health, 16; and eating, 219, 228; and exercise, 416; and gastrointestinal illnesses, 127, 132, 340; and headaches, 86; and high blood pressure, 57, 64, 80; identifying sources of, 350; and immunity, 201–2; origins of, 8; thyroid overactivity from, 340
Stress test, 47–48, 444, 496
Strokes, 76–81; and alcohol abuse, 81, 326, 361; aspirin for, 44–45, 83; controllable factors in, 17; decreased mortality from, 18; from diabetes, 80, 208, 215, 216; and diet (cholesterol), 80, 361; as disease of abuse or disuse, 10, 12; and estrogen replacement, 172; and exercise, 419; functions remaining intact in, 75; and high blood pressure, 18, 40, 59, 78, 80; and multi-infarct dementia, 88; psychological factors in, 337; secondary prevention of, 81–82; and smoking, 79, 80, 318, 319, 321; tertiary prevention of, 82–84; and TIAs, 77, 78, 79, 82
Substance abuse, 315, 351, 502. *See also* Alcohol and alcohol abuse; Drugs and drug abuse; Smoking
Sugars, 211, 222, 253, 362, 375, 409, 413
Suicide, 17, 348
Sulfites, 103, 409
Sulfur dioxide, 312, 452, 454, 456
Sunburn, 263–66
Sunscreens, 264–66
Sweeteners, artificial, 375–76; and bladder cancer, 187; and diabetes, 211
Swimmer's ear, 244
Swimming, 433–34, 436, 438–39; safety in, 301; while traveling, 282
Symptoms, 498–501; of AIDS and AIDS-related complex, 286; of bladder cancer, 186; of cancer, 499; of colon cancer, 119; of cystitis, 190; of diabetes, 208, 500; of diverticulosis, 122; of endometrial cancer, 169; of food poisoning, 295; headaches as, 87, 446; of heart disease, 27, 48, 420, 446, 498; hoarseness as, 260; of influenza, 107; of lung disease, 100; of Lyme disease, 294; of malaria, 283;

patient's alertness to, 492, 498; of
pneumonia, 108; of problem drinking, 328; of sexually transmitted diseases, 292, 293; of skin cancer, 267;
and testicular cancer, 179
Syphilis, 9, 181, 292

Tartrazine sensitivity, 103
Teeth, 246–47; trauma against, 256.
See also Dental diseases
Teflon, 411
Telephone hotlines, 512–13
Temperomandibular joint syndrome,
257–58
Ten Commandments of Prevention,
16–17, 19, 508
Tendons, 155
Tension, mental. *See* Stress
Tertiary prevention, 21, 82; of asthma,
102; of coronary artery disease,
48–49; of diabetes, 215–16; of lung
cancer, 98, 99; of strokes, 82–84
Testicular cancer, 178–79
Testicular exam or self-exam, 495, 501
Testosterone, 146, 177, 178, 269
Tests (medical), 489–91
Tests, screening. *See* Screening tests
Tetanus-diphtheria immunization, 277
Thalassemia, 198
Third World population explosion, 166
Throat disorders, 259–60, 501
Thrombophlebitis, 71–73
Thrombosis. *See* Blood clots
Thrombotic strokes, 77–78
Thyroid cancer, 480
Thyroid gland, 206–7
TIAs (transient ischemic attacks), 77,
78, 79, 82
Ticks, 294
Tobacco: commercial power of,
323–24. *See also* Smoking
Toxic liver disease, 138
Toxic shock syndrome, 167–68, 274,
297
Toxins and toxic chemicals, 85,
270–71, 450–54, 473–75; in acid
rain, 467; and blood disorders,
198–99; as controllable factor, 17; in
fish, 470, 471; food poisoning from,
295; and heart muscle disease, 52;
and kidneys, 186, 187; liver cancer
from, 137; and lung disease, 104;
mercury as, 253 (*see also* Mercury
toxicity); as occupational hazard,
309–10, 311–13; as wastes, 473–74;
in water, 464, 465, 466

Trachea, 92, 93
Tranquilizers, 342
Trans-fatty acids, 360, 366, 368
Transient ischemic attacks (TIAs), 77,
78, 79, 82
Trauma: and alcohol abuse, 326, 327;
and arthritis, 155; on ears (acoustic), 240–43; on ears (physical), 243;
on eye, 234–35; need to prevent,
152; neurological, 84; sports injuries, 235, 256, 442; on teeth, 256; and
tobacco abuse, 319; as work-related,
308
Travelers' health, 279–84; and altitude
sickness, 463; and cosmic rays, 479;
immunization for, 135, 278, 279, 281;
and middle-ear infection, 244; and
sinus infection, 111; traveler's diarrhea, 282–83, 295
Treadmills, 438–39
Tretinoin, 271–72
Triglycerides, 34, 217, 218
Tropical oils, 36, 365
Tuberculosis, 109–11, 294–95; deaths
from, 274; as occupational disorder,
311; skin test for, 493
TV viewing, and obesity, 230
Type A personality, 43–44, 339–40
Typhoid vaccinations, 281

Ulcers, 131–32; and alcohol abuse,
132, 326; and aspirin, 45; and diet,
362; and tobacco abuse, 132, 318,
321
Ultrasound, and aneurysms, 69
Ultraviolet radiation, 263–64, 271, 452,
453, 478–79; as crucial to health, 16;
eye disorders from, 235–37
United States: accidents in, 298–99;
diet in, 222, 227, 358, 359, 364, 376,
396; health care in, 483–84; health
crisis in, 12–16; health disparities
in, 14–16; medicine vs. health in, 3;
obesity in, 218–19; preventive medicine training in, 4; psychological
disorders in, 341; water pollution in,
464
Unsaturated fats, 36, 365–67, 368; polyunsaturates vs. monounsaturates,
37, 365
Upper respiratory tract infection, 111
Urinary tract, 182–83; infections of,
190–91; symptoms of disorders of,
500
Urine analysis, 191–92; for diabetes,
213; recommendations on, 494, 496

U.S. government agencies, for health
  care information, 509–12
Uterine cancer, 362, 364, 385, 389

Vaccination. *See* Immunizations
Vaginal cancer, 170–71
Varicose veins, 70–71, 361
Vascular disease: and kidneys,
  185–86; symptoms of, 499; (*See also*
  Arteries; Atherosclerosis; High
  blood pressure; Veins
Vasodilators, 66
Vegetable oils, 36, 365–66, 368
Veins, 54; diseases of, 55, 70–73
Video display terminal (computer
  screen), 86, 313, 314, 477
Violence, 303. *See also* Trauma
Viruses, 274–75; and nervous system
  infections, 85; in water, 466
Vitamin A, 46, 364, 388, 389–90, 391,
  392, 394, 413; and acoustic trauma,
  243; and bladder cancer, 187; and
  breast cancer, 161; and colon cancer, 117
Vitamin B$_1$ (thiamine), 86, 388, 395
Vitamin B$_2$ (riboflavin), 395
Vitamin B$_3$ (niacin), 38–39, 388, 394, 395
Vitamin B$_6$ (pyridoxine), 388, 394, 395
Vitamin B$_{12}$, 86, 89, 196–97, 362, 388,
  393, 395
Vitamin C (ascorbic acid), 46, 361, 388,
  389, 390, 391, 392, 394, 395, 413; and
  blood pressure, 63; and colon cancer, 117; iron absorption helped by,
  195; and stool testing, 120
Vitamin D, 361, 364, 388, 390, 394, 395;
  and bones, 143; and breast cancer,
  161; and colon cancer, 116, 117; and
  osteoporosis, 146, 149; and ultraviolet radiation, 263–64
Vitamin E, 46, 361, 364, 388, 389, 390,
  394, 396
Vitamin K, 364, 388, 396; and osteoporosis, 146, 149
Vitamin-deficiency anemias, 196–97
Vitamins, 388–94; and cancers, 116,
  259, 389–90, 393; as cataract prevention, 237, 392, 393; glossary of,
  394–96; and heart disease, 46; high
  doses of as toxic, 394

Walking, 427, 428, 431–32, 433, 436,
  438–39, 443; and arterial disease,

69; vs. running, 432; and safety,
  445–46; as warm-up, 426
Warfarin therapy, 83
Wastes, 473; biological, 474; chemical,
  16, 52, 464, 473–74; organic, 464,
  466; solid, 474–75; (*see also* Toxins
  and toxic chemicals
Water, 407; additives in, 467; and bladder cancer prevention, 187; as cystitis prevention, 191; and fiber in diet,
  116, 126, 383; for kidney stone prevention, 189; safety of, 464–66, 470,
  474; in tropics, 281
Water exercises, 433. *See also*
  Swimming
Water pollution, 463–67
Weight: evaluation of, 222–25; self-examination of, 501; and smoking,
  321. *See also* Obesity
Weight control or loss, 217; and cholesterol, 39; and diabetes, 209; and
  gallstones, 140–41
Wernicke-Korsakoff syndrome, 86
Wine bottles, and lead, 411
Women: and anemia, 195, 196; and aspirin for heart disease, 45; and athletic amenorrhea, 150; and calcium,
  149, 402–3 (*see also* Calcium); and
  cystitis, 190–91; exams recommended for, 494–95, 497–98; and
  high blood pressure, 58; and iron,
  404–5; and osteoporosis, 144, 146,
  172–73, 359 (*see also* Osteoporosis);
  and Sjogren's syndrome, 257. *See
  also* Gender; Reproductive system,
  female
Work, and leg veins, 71
Work disorders. *See* Occupational
  disorders
World Health Organization, international travel booklet of, 284

X rays: chest, 98–99, 496; dental, 252,
  480; mammograms, 4, 21, 162–63,
  176, 480, 494–95, 497; and safety,
  480

Yellow Dye Number Five, 103
Yellow fever immunization, 281

Zinc, 406